OPHTHALMOLOGY CLINICS-I
for Postgraduates

OPHTHALMOLOGY CLINICS-I
for Postgraduates
SECOND EDITION

Editors

Prafulla Kumar Maharana MD DNB
Additional Professor
Department of Ophthalmology
Dr Rajendra Prasad Centre for Ophthalmic Sciences
All India Institute of Medical Sciences
New Delhi, India

Namrata Sharma MD
Professor
Department of Ophthalmology
Dr Rajendra Prasad Centre for Ophthalmic Sciences
All India Institute of Medical Sciences
New Delhi, India

Atul Kumar MD FAMS FRCS (Ed)
Medical Director
Department of Ophthalmology
AK Institute of Ophthalmology
New Delhi, India

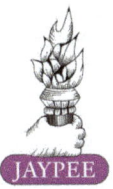

JAYPEE BROTHERS MEDICAL PUBLISHERS
The Health Sciences Publisher
New Delhi | London

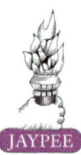 **Jaypee Brothers Medical Publishers (P) Ltd.**

Headquarters
Jaypee Brothers Medical Publishers (P) Ltd
EMCA House, 23/23-B
Ansari Road, Daryaganj
New Delhi 110 002, India
Landline: +91-11-23272143, +91-11-23272703
+91-11-23282021, +91-11-23245672
Email: jaypee@jaypeebrothers.com

Corporate Office
Jaypee Brothers Medical Publishers (P) Ltd
4838/24, Ansari Road, Daryaganj
New Delhi 110 002, India
Phone: +91-11-43574357
Fax: +91-11-43574314
Email: jaypee@jaypeebrothers.com

Overseas Office
JP Medical Ltd.
83, Victoria Street, London
SW1H 0HW (UK)
Phone: +44 20 3170 8910
Fax: +44 (0)20 3008 6180
Email: info@jpmedpub.com

Website: www.jaypeebrothers.com
Website: www.jaypeedigital.com

© 2024, Jaypee Brothers Medical Publishers

The views and opinions expressed in this book are solely those of the original contributor(s)/author(s) and do not necessarily represent those of editor(s) or publisher of the book.

All rights reserved. No part of this publication may be reproduced, stored or transmitted in any form or by any means, electronic, mechanical, photocopying, recording or otherwise, without the prior permission in writing of the publishers.

All brand names and product names used in this book are trade names, service marks, trademarks or registered trademarks of their respective owners. The publisher is not associated with any product or vendor mentioned in this book.

Medical knowledge and practice change constantly. This book is designed to provide accurate, authoritative information about the subject matter in question. However, readers are advised to check the most current information available on procedures included and check information from the manufacturer of each product to be administered, to verify the recommended dose, formula, method and duration of administration, adverse effects and contra indications. It is the responsibility of the practitioner to take all appropriate safety precautions. Neither the publisher nor the author(s)/editor(s) assume any liability for any injury and/or damage to persons or property arising from or related to use of material in this book.

This book is sold on the understanding that the publisher is not engaged in providing professional medical services. If such advice or services are required, the services of a competent medical professional should be sought.

Every effort has been made where necessary to contact holders of copyright to obtain permission to reproduce copyright material. If any have been inadvertently overlooked, the publisher will be pleased to make the necessary arrangements at the first opportunity.

Inquiries for bulk sales may be solicited at: jaypee@jaypeebrothers.com

Ophthalmology Clinics-I for Postgraduates

First Edition: 2017
Second Edition: **2024**

ISBN: 978-93-5696-877-6

Dedicated to

My parents, Mr Devendra Maharana and Mrs Binadini Maharana

– **Prafulla Kumar Maharana**

My parents, Dr Ramesh C Sharma and Mrs Maitreyi Pushpa
My husband, Dr Subhash Chandra; and Daughter, Vasavdatta

– **Namrata Sharma**

My late parents, Mr Sanat Kumar and Mrs Swarna Kumar
My wife, Mrs Parul Kumar; and, Children, Aman and Arshi

– **Atul Kumar**

Contributors

Aafreen Bari MD
Senior Resident
Dr Rajendra Prasad Centre for Ophthalmic Sciences
All India Institute of Medical Sciences
New Delhi, India

Adarsh Shashni MD

Aditi Dubey MBBS MS (Ophthalmology)
Associate Professor
Department of Ophthalmology
Gandhi Medical College
Bhopal, Madhya Pradesh, India

Amar Pujari MD
Senior Resident
Dr Rajendra Prasad Centre for Ophthalmic Sciences
All India Institute of Medical Sciences
New Delhi, India

Ananya PR MD
Senior Resident
Cornea, Cataract, Refractive and Ocular Oncology Services
Dr RP Centre for Ophthalmic Sciences
All India Institute of Medical Sciences
New Delhi, India

Anasua Ganguly Kapoor
MD DNB FICO
Consultant, Head of Campus
Department of Ophthalmic Plastic Surgery and Ocular Oncology
LV Prasad Eye Institute, Kode Venkatadri Chowdary Campus
Vijayawada, Andhra Pradesh, India

Anu Malik MS
Assistant Professor
Dr RP Centre for Ophthalmic Sciences
All India Institute of Medical Sciences
New Delhi, India

Ashi Gupta MBBS
Junior Resident
Dr RP Centre for Ophthalmic Sciences
All India Institute of Medical Sciences
New Delhi, India

Ashish Markan
MD (AIIMS, Delhi) MCh (Vitreoretina, PGI, Chandigarh) FRCS (Glasgow) DNB FICO (UK) FICO (Vitreoretina) FAICO (VR) FAICO (Uvea)
Consultant
Department of Vitreoretina
Eye7 Hospitals
New Delhi, India

Ashutosh Kumar Gupta MS
Graded Specialist
Department of Ophthalmology
Military Hospital
Agra, Uttar Pradesh, India

Aswini Kumar Behera MD
Founder and Director
NAITRIKA Super Specialty Eye Care
Berhampur, Odisha, India

Atul Kumar MD FAMS FRCS (Ed)
Medical Director
Department of Ophthalmology
AK Institute of Ophthalmology
New Delhi, India

Bijnya Birajita Panda
MS FICO (UK) FAICO (Oculoplasty Surgery) FRCS (Glasgow Part 2)
Assistant Professor
Department of Ophthalmology
All India Institute of Medical Sciences
Bhubaneswar, Odisha, India

Brijesh Takkar MD FICO
Associate Ophthalmologist
Anant Bajaj Retina Institute
LV Prasad Eye Institute
Hyderabad, Telangana, India

D Satyasudha MBBS

Deepali Singhal
MD DNB FICO FICO Cornea Fellowship Refractive Surgery
Medical Director and Chief Consultant
Department of Cataract, Cornea and Refractive Surgery
Anil Eye Hospital
Thane, Maharashtra, India

Devesh Kumawat MD (Ophthalmology)
Assistant Professor
Dr Rajendra Prasad Centre for Ophthalmic Sciences
All India Institute of Medical Sciences
New Delhi, India

Devika S Joshi MS
Fellow
Narayana Nethralaya
Bengaluru, Karnataka, India

Dewang Angmo MD FICO FRCS
Additional Professor
Dr Rajendra Prasad Centre for Ophthalmic Sciences
All India Institute of Medical Sciences
New Delhi, India

Dhaval Patel MD
Consultant
Centre for Sight
Vadodara, Gujarat, India

Dheepak Sundar MD

Divya Agarwal
MD DNB MNAMS FICO FAICO (Retina)
Vitreoretina, Uvea and ROP Consultant
Department of Ophthalmology
Vikalp Eye and Retina Centre
Bareilly, Uttar Pradesh, India

Esha Agarwal MD (Ophthalmology) FAICO DNB
Consultant
Department of Cataract and Refractive Surgery
The Sight Avenue
New Delhi, India

Gunjan Saluja
MD (AIIMS, Delhi) DNB FRCS (Glasgow) FICO FAICO (Pediatric Ophthalmology and Strabimsus)
Consultant
Strabismus, Oculoplasty and Neuro-ophthalmology Services
Bhatia Netralaya
Bhilai, Chhattisgarh, India

Harathy Selvan MBBS

Harika Regani MD
Consultant
Department of Oculoplasty, Ocular Oncology and Facial Aesthetics
iFOCUS Superspeciality Eye Hospital
Vijayawada, Andhra Pradesh, India

Jeewan S Titiyal MD
Chief and Dean (Research)
Dr Rajendra Prasad Centre for Ophthalmic Sciences
All India Institute of Medical Sciences
New Delhi, India

Jennil Shetty MBBS DNB

Jyotiranjan Mallick MS (Ophthalmology)
Senior Resident
Department of Ophthalmology
All India Institute of Medical Sciences
Bhubaneswar, Odisha, India

Karthikeya R MBBS MD DNB FICO MRCSEd
Consultant
Department of Vitreoretina
Sharp Sight Eye Hospitals
New Delhi, India

Manasi Tripathi MD
Senior Resident
Department of Ophthalmology
Dr Rajendra Prasad Centre for Ophthalmic Sciences
All India Institute of Medical Sciences
New Delhi, India

Mandeep S Bajaj MD
Professor
Dr Rajendra Prasad Centre for
Ophthalmic Sciences
All India Institute of Medical Sciences
New Delhi, India

Manpreet Kaur MD
Associate Professor
Department of Cornea, Cataract and Refractive Surgery
Dr Rajendra Prasad Centre for Ophthalmic Sciences
All India Institute of Medical Sciences
New Delhi, India

Namrata Sharma MD
Professor
Department of Ophthalmology
Dr Rajendra Prasad Centre for
Ophthalmic Sciences
All India Institute of Medical Sciences
New Delhi, India

Neelima Aron MD DNB FICO

Nitika Beri
MS (Ophthalmology) DNB (Ophthalmology) FAICO (Glaucoma)
Senior Research Associate
Glaucoma Unit
Dr Rajendra Prasad Centre for Ophthalmic Sciences
All India Institute of Medical Sciences
New Delhi, India

Patil Mukesh Prakash MBBS MD FICO

Prafulla Kumar Maharana MD DNB
Additional Professor
Department of Ophthalmology
Dr Rajendra Prasad Centre for
Ophthalmic Sciences
All India Institute of Medical Sciences
New Delhi, India

Prakhar Goyal
MBBS DNB FICO (UK) FVRS
Retina, Uvea and ROP Specialist
Goyal Netra Chikitsalaya
Narnaul, Haryana, India

Pranayee Behera MS FICO
Consultant Ophthalmology
Burnpur Hospital, SAIL-ISP
Asansol, West Bengal, India

Pranita Sahay
MD (AIIMS) FRCOphth FRCS (Glasgow) FICO (Cornea) FAICO (Ref Sx) DNB
Assistant Professor
Guru Nanak Eye Centre
Maulana Azad Medical College
New Delhi, India

Prateek Kakkar
MD (Ophthalmology, AIIMS, New Delhi) DNB FICO FAICO (Vitreoretina)
Medical Director
Reticure Eye Centre
New Delhi, India

Priyanka Ramesh MBBS

Pulak Agarwal MD FICO
Director
JRM Multispecialty Hospital
Bikaner, Rajasthan, India

Raghav Ravani
MBBS MD FICO FAICO (Vitreoretina)
Medical Director
ASG Eye Hospital
Surat, Gujarat, India

Rajesh Pattebahadur
MD (Ophthalmology)
Associate Professor
Department of Ophthalmology
All India Institute of Medical Sciences
Nagpur, Maharashtra, India

Contributors

Ritika Mukhija MBBS MD FRCOphth
Consultant
Department of Ophthalmology
Sussex Eye Hospital
Brighton, UK

Ritu Nagpal MD
Consultant
Cornea, Cataract and Refractive Surgery Services
Goyal Eye Group of Eye Hospitals
New Delhi, India

Ruchir Tewari MD FICO
Senior Consultant
Vitreous Retina, Uvea and ROP Services
Tewari Eye Center
Ghaziabad and Noida, Uttar Pradesh, India

Ruchita Falera
MBBS MD (Ophthalmology) FICO (UK)
Consultant Ophthalmologist
Department of Cornea and Refractive Surgery
Dr Agarwal Eye Hospital
Bengaluru, Karnataka, India

Sagnik Sen MBBS

Sandeep Gupta MS DNB MNAMS
Associate Professor
Department of Ophthalmology
Armed Forces Medical College
Pune, Maharashtra, India

Sanjana M DNB
Fellow
Department of Ophthalmic Plastic Surgery and Ocular Oncology
LV Prasad Eye Institute, Kode Venkatadri Chowdary Campus
Vijayawada, Andhra Pradesh, India

Sapna Raghuwanshi MS (Ophthalmology)
Associate Professor
Department of Ophthalmology
Atal Bihari Vajpayee Government Medical College
Vidisha, Madhya Pradesh, India

Saranya Devi K MD DNB FICO

Shipra Singhi MD
Consultant
ASG Eye Hospital
Jodhpur, Rajasthan, India

Shorya Vardhan Azad MS
Additional Professor
Dr Rajendra Prasad Centre for Ophthalmic Sciences
All India Institute of Medical Sciences
New Delhi, India

Shreyas Temkar MD DNB FICO FAICO

Swati Phuljhale MD
Additional Professor
Dr Rajendra Prasad Centre for Ophthalmic Sciences
All India Institute of Medical Sciences
New Delhi, India

Talvir Sidhu MD DNB
Assistant Professor
Department of Ophthalmology
Government Medical College
Patiala, Punjab, India

Tushar Agarwal MD
Professor
Dr Rajendra Prasad Centre for Ophthalmic Sciences
All India Institute of Medical Sciences
New Delhi, India

Vaishali Ghanshyam Rai MBBS DNB

Varsha Varshney MBBS MS

Yamini Attiku MBBS MD

Preface to the Second Edition

A Big Thank You to Everyone!

Dear readers, we are overwhelmed by the response to our book received from you all. A lot of hard work was involved while bringing out the first edition of this book. The best satisfaction is "when hard work pays off."

The revised edition of the book has several additions. We have included several new chapters. Besides, classification systems of all the disorders have been updated as per the current literature. Similarly, treatment approaches have been revised to include the updated protocols. In the instruments section, several new instruments including images have been included. We have added as many flowcharts and tables as possible to help the readers.

There were several errors in our earlier edition. I would like to thank the readers across India who communicated with us about these errors. We have tried our best to correct all the errors in the previous edition and to avoid any errors in the current edition.

The goal of the book is to help the Diploma/DNB/MS/MD (Ophthalmology) students appearing in various examinations across the world. I hope this edition of the book will be helpful to the readers and it will receive the same appreciation as our previous edition.

Lastly, in spite of all the efforts, there may still be some errors, I request the readers to communicate with me so that we can make the necessary corrections.

All the Best!

Prafulla Kumar Maharana

Preface to the First Edition

"The whole art of medicine is in observation."
– **Sir William Osler**

Postgraduate examination is one of the most difficult and stressful milestones in the medical profession. It entails a tremendous amount of stress on the candidates who appear for the examination. The never-ending knowledge of ophthalmology makes it quite difficult to revise all the cases from the standard textbooks before the examinations. Further, the presentation of cases—long case or short case—is completely in a different format from what is given in the standard textbooks. Most of the time, the candidate fails to present the case properly in spite of good theoretical knowledge. The primary reason for this is that the format in which a topic is discussed in textbooks is completely different from that required for a practical examination.

This book attempts to present the important topics in a format that is exactly same as required in the practical examinations. The primary focus is on history taking and proper clinical examination of the cases. Every effort has been made to describe the procedures of clinical examinations in such a way that the candidate can perform these examination techniques accurately in front of the examiner. Special emphasis has been given to the differential diagnosis of the cases, which is often a favorite question amongst the examiners. Clinical photographs of the cases as well as the important signs and investigation findings have been provided that will help the students for better understanding of the cases. The cases are being selected after discussing with experts in this field as well as candidates who have recently appeared in various postgraduate examinations. Each chapter ends with a section on viva-voce questions that will help the candidates to mentally prepare for the viva before the final examination. In addition, a chapter on instruments has been included which is invariably a part of all postgraduate practical examinations. The editors and all the contributors have made sincere efforts to make things simple and concise and to facilitate quick and thorough revision. However, it must be remembered that this is not a substitute for standard textbooks. The readers are encouraged to read standard textbooks before going through this book. This will make their understanding and application of this book more rewarding.

The editors wish the best of luck to the students for their examinations!

Prafulla Kumar Maharana
Namrata Sharma
Atul Kumar

Contents

1. OCULOPLASTY 1

LONG CASES

- **Proptosis** *1*
  Varsha Varshney, Sanjana M, Anasua Ganguly Kapoor, Mandeep S Bajaj

- **Lid Tumors** *9*
  Sapna Raghuwanshi, Anasua Ganguly Kapoor, Mandeep S Bajaj

- **Ptosis** *15*
  Aditi Dubey, Sanjana M

- **Contracted Socket** *24*
  Varsha Vashney, Aditi Dubey, Amar Pujari

- **Blowout Fracture of Orbit** *30*
  Aditi Dubey, Sanjana M

- **Thyroid-associated Ophthalmopathy** *35*
  Aditi Dubey, Prafulla Kumar Maharana

- **Lacrimal Gland Tumors** *43*
  Varsha Vashney, Amar Pujari

SHORT CASES

- **Congenital Ptosis** *51*
  Aditi Dubey, Amar Pujari

- **Ectropion** *55*
  Aditi Dubey, Bijnya Birajita Panda, Sanjana M

- **Entropion** *59*
  Aditi Dubey, Ritu Nagpal

- **Blepharophimosis, Ptosis, Epicanthus Inversus Syndrome** *63*
  Amar Pujari, Aditi Dubey

- **Sebaceous Gland Carcinoma** *67*
  Amar Pujari, Sapna Raghuwanshi

- **Pyogenic Granuloma** *70*
  Sapna Raghuwanshi, Bijnya Birajita Panda

- **Lagophthalmos** *71*
  Varsha Varshney, Ritu Nagpal

- **Dermoid Cyst** *77*
  Shipra Singhi, Deepali Singhal

- **Orbital Hemangioma** *82*
  Aditi Dubey, Sanjana M, Rajesh Pattebahadur
- **Coloboma of Eyelid** *85*
  Shipra Singhi, Anasua Ganguly Kapoor

2. CORNEA AND CONJUNCTIVA 90

LONG CASES

- **Corneal Ulcer** *90*
  Prafulla Kumar Maharana, Shipra Singhi, Ritu Nagpal, Tushar Agarwal, Namrata Sharma
- **Keratoconus** *109*
  Prafulla Kumar Maharana, Sapna Raghuwanshi, Manasi Tripathi,
  Ritu Nagpal, Namrata Sharma
- **Corneal Stromal Dystrophy** *121*
  Shipra Singhi, Divya Agarwal, Prafulla Kumar Maharana
- **Fuchs' Endothelial Corneal Dystrophy** *133*
  Prafulla Kumar Maharana, Sapna Raghuwanshi, Manasi Tripathi, Ritu Nagpal,
  Namrata Sharma
- **Acute Graft Rejection** *140*
  Ritu Nagpal, Vaishali Ghanshyam Rai, Prafulla Kumar Maharana

SHORT CASES

- **Pterygium** *147*
  Aafreen Bari, Ritu Nagpal
- **Keratoglobus** *151*
  Prafulla Kumar Maharana, Sapna Raghuwanshi, Aafreen Bari
- **Pellucid Marginal Degeneration** *155*
  Aafreen Bari, Sapna Raghuwanshi, Namrata Sharma
- **Band-shaped Keratopathy** *158*
  Manpreet Kaur, Sapna Raghuwanshi, Ritu Nagpal
- **Spheroidal Degeneration** *161*
  Sapna Raghuwanshi, Aafreen Bari, Ritu Nagpal
- **Congenital Hereditary Endothelial Dystrophy** *164*
  Prafulla Kumar Maharana, Vaishali Ghanshyam Rai
- **Iridocorneal Endothelial Syndrome** *167*
  Vaishali Ghanshyam Rai, Neelima Aron, Prafulla Kumar Maharana
- **Peters' Anomaly** *170*
  Shipra Singhi, Neelima Aron, Manpreet Kaur
- **Limbal Dermoid** *174*
  Prafulla Kumar Maharana, Deepali Singhal, Aafreen Bari

3. GLAUCOMA 182

LONG CASES

- **Primary Angle Closure Glaucoma** *182*
  Vaishali Ghanshyam Rai, Talvir Sidhu, Dewang Angmo

SHORT CASES

- **Sturge-Weber Syndrome** *190*
  Vaishali Ghanshyam Rai, Aditi Dubey, Ritika Mukhija, Dewang Angmo
- **Buphthalmos** *193*
  Vaishali Ghanshyam Rai, Aditi Dubey, Nitika Beri
- **Neovascular Glaucoma** *197*
  Jennil Shetty, Talvir Sidhu, Anu Malik
- **Angle Recession Glaucoma** *203*
  Prakhar Goyal, Nitika Beri, Divya Agarwal, Talvir Sidhu
- **Steroid-induced Glaucoma** *206*
  Vaishali Ghanshyam Rai, Talvir Sidhu, Nitika Beri
- **Pseudoexfoliation Glaucoma** *209*
  Ashi Gupta, Vaishali Ghanshyam Rai, Dewang Angmo

4. RETINA 214

LONG CASES

- **Vitreous Hemorrhage** *214*
  Ritu Nagpal, Ashi Gupta, Shipra Singhi, Brijesh Takkar
- **Central Retinal Vein Occlusion** *222*
  Ashish Markan, Esha Agarwal, Brijesh Takkar
- **Branch Retinal Vein Occlusion** *229*
  Pulak Agarwal, Shorya Vardhan Azad
- **Proliferative Diabetic Retinopathy** *236*
  Brijesh Takkar, Dhaval Patel, Rajesh Pattebahadur
- **Nonproliferative Diabetic Retinopathy** *242*
  Dhaval Patel, Brijesh Takkar, Rajesh Pattebahadur
- **Retinitis Pigmentosa** *251*
  Jyotiranjan Mallick, Prafulla Kumar Maharana
- **Macular Hole** *258*
  Vaishali Ghanshyam Rai, Brijesh Takkar
- **Retinal Detachment** *267*
  Pranayee Behera, Rajesh Pattebahadur, Raghav Ravani
- **Age-related Macular Degeneration** *280*
  Ritu Nagpal, Shipra Singhi, Raghav Ravani

- **Intermediate Uveitis** *293*
  Raghav Ravani, Karthikeya R, Harathy Selvan, Atul Kumar
- **Choroidal Melanoma** *299*
  Karthikeya R, Raghav Ravani, Prateek Kakkar, Atul Kumar

SHORT CASES

- **Cherry-red Spot** *309*
  Rajesh Pattebahadur, Brijesh Takkar
- **Central Serous Chorioretinopathy** *312*
  Vaishali Ghanshyam Rai, Ashish Markan, Raghav Ravani
- **Diabetic Macular Edema** *317*
  Brijesh Takkar, Dhaval Patel, Ashish Markan
- **Epiretinal Membrane** *323*
  Dhaval Patel, Brijesh Takkar
- **Fundal Coloboma** *327*
  D Satyasudha, Ruchir Tewari, Atul Kumar
- **Giant Retinal Tear** *335*
  Ashish Markan, Brijesh Takkar
- **Posterior Segment Cysticercosis** *339*
  Harika Regani, Karthikeya R, Yamini Attiku, Atul Kumar
- **Cataract in Silicone Oil-filled Eyes** *343*
  Sagnik Sen, Esha Agarwal, Raghav Ravani, Atul Kumar
- **Silicone Oil-induced Secondary Glaucoma** *347*
  Ashish Markan, Esha Agarwal, Raghav Ravani, Atul Kumar
- **Posterior Dislocated Lens** *351*
  Shipra Singhi, Brijesh Takkar
- **Stargardt Disease** *356*
  Aswini Kumar Behera, Ruchir Tewari
- **Traumatic Retinal Detachment** *361*
  Priyanka Ramesh, Shreyas Temkar, Dheepak Sundar, Atul Kumar

5. NEURO-OPHTHALMOLOGY AND STRABISMUS 367

LONG CASES

- **Third Cranial Nerve Palsy** *367*
  Adarsh Shashni, Shipra Singhi
- **Sixth Cranial Nerve Palsy** *375*
  Shipra Singhi, Swati Phuljhale
- **Fourth Cranial Nerve Palsy** *381*
  Gunjan Saluja, Shipra Singhi, Patil Mukesh Prakash

- **Optic Neuritis** 387
  Ritu Nagpal, Adarsh Shashni
- **Esodeviation** 394
  Ritika Mukhija, Adarsh Shashni
- **Exodeviation** 405
  Shipra Singhi, Adarsh Shashni

SHORT CASES

- **Duane Retraction Syndrome** 411
  Shipra Singhi, Saranya Devi K
- **Ocular Myasthenia Gravis** 414
  Shipra Singhi, Adarsh Shashni
- **Monocular Elevation Deficit** 418
  Gunjan Saluja, Anu Malik
- **Dissociated Vertical Deviation** 420
  Gunjan Saluja
- **Optic Disc Edema** 422
  Gunjan Saluja, Anu Malik
- **Optic Atrophy** 425
  Gunjan Saluja, Anu Malik

6. LENS 428

LONG CASES

- **Zonular Cataract** 428
  Manpreet Kaur, Ashutosh Kumar Gupta, Jeewan S Titiyal
- **Ectopia Lentis** 434
  Prafulla Kumar Maharana, Ananya PR, Ruchita Falera, Manpreet Kaur

SHORT CASES

- **Lenticonus** 442
  Manpreet Kaur, Prafulla Kumar Maharana, Jeewan S Titiyal
- **Posterior Polar Cataract** 445
  Manpreet Kaur, Ananya PR, Jeewan S Titiyal, Sandeep Gupta
- **Microspherophakia** 449
  Manpreet Kaur, Devika S Joshi, Prafulla Kumar Maharana
- **Posterior Capsular Opacification** 453
  Prafulla Kumar Maharana, Manpreet Kaur
- **Traumatic Cataract** 457
  Deepali Singhal, Ruchita Falera, Manpreet Kaur

7. INSTRUMENTS 462

- **Ophthalmic Instruments** 462
  Pranita Sahay, Devesh Kumawat

8. SUPPLEMENTARY CHAPTER OF GLAUCOMA 487

- **Primary Open Angle Glaucoma** 487
  Dewang Angmo, Vaishali Ghanshyam Rai, Ritika Mukhija

Index 497

CHAPTER 1

Oculoplasty

LONG CASES

PROPTOSIS

Varsha Varshney, Sanjana M, Anasua Ganguly Kapoor, Mandeep S Bajaj

■ INTRODUCTION

Proptosis is defined as an abnormal forward protrusion of one or both eyeballs with respect to the orbit. Among adults, the usual distance from the lateral orbital rim to the corneal apex is approximately 16–21 mm.[1,2] Proptosis is said to be present when the following criteria are present:
- Protrusion >22 mm beyond the orbital rim
- An asymmetry of >2 mm between the eyes

Proptosis is one of the common topics given as a long case in examinations.

■ HISTORY

Chief Complaints

A case of proptosis usually presents with following complaints:
- Protrusion of one or both the eyes
- *Loss of vision:* It indicates *optic nerve compression*/involvement (by *intrinsic lesions* of optic nerve such as meningiomas or optic nerve gliomas or *external compression*, e.g., tumors located in the orbital apex, such as a hemangioma and Graves' disease) or *induced astigmatism* due to globe compression or *exposure keratopathy*.
- Rare presentation includes diplopia, restricted ocular motility, and redness/pain/discharge due to associated exposure keratopathy.

History of Present Illness

Following points must be noted while examining a case of proptosis:
- *Age of onset:* Age of onset can point toward the probable diagnosis as shown in **Table 1**.
- *Nature of onset:*
  - *Sudden (hours to days):* It suggests inflammatory and infective process, trauma (orbital emphysema, fracture of the medial orbital wall, orbital hemorrhage), or rupture of ethmoidal mucocele.
  - *Gradual (over many months to years):* It suggests tumors and lymphoma—proliferative disorders
- *Progression:*
  - *Slow continuous:* It suggests tumor, however, gradual progression with sudden increase in proptosis can harbor malignant transformation.
  - *Rapid progression:* It indicates infection/inflammation/hemorrhage/malignant transformation

Table 1: Causes of proptosis based on the age of onset.

Newborn	Children	Young adults	Middle age	Senile
• Orbital cellulitis • Orbital neoplasm	• Rhabdomyosarcoma • Hemangioma • Dermoid cyst • Orbital cellulitis • Optic nerve glioma • Craniosynostosis lymphomas	• Thyroid ophthalmopathy • Pseudotumor • Orbital cellulitis • Osteomas • Infiltrative tumors	• Pseudotumor • Endocrine • Malignant lymphomas/leukemias • Optic nerve sheath meningiomas • Mucocele	• Malignant and metastatic tumor of orbit • Pseudotumor • Leukemia • Lymphomas • Sarcomas

– *Intermittent:* Intermittent proptosis can be due to following causes:
  ♦ Periodic orbital edema
  ♦ Recurrent orbital hemorrhage/chocolate cyst and highly vascular tumors
  ♦ Increases during attacks of common cold/upper respiratory infections—lymphangioma
  ♦ Postural (associated with bending forward) or with Valsalva suggests orbital varices
  ♦ Increases on crying capillary hemangiomas in young children
• *Pain:* Depending upon presence of pain, proptosis can be as follows:
  – *Painful:* Infective, acute inflammations, chocolate cyst, orbital hemorrhages
  – *Painless:* Tumor, endocrinopathy (pain can be there in some malignant tumors that show perineural spread, such as adenoid cystic carcinoma of the lacrimal gland)
• *Laterality:*
  – *Unilateral:* Unilateral proptosis is seen in tumors, cysts, and vascular anomalies.
  – *Bilateral:* The different causes of bilateral proptosis are summarized in **Table 2**.
• *Special characteristics:* Rarely, patient can give a history of feeling the *pulsation* within the orbit or periorbital area. An example of such cases include arteriovenous (AV) malformation, caroticocavernous fistula, and saccular aneurysm of ophthalmic artery or due to *transmitted cerebral pulsations* in conditions associated with deficient orbital roof such as congenital meningocele or meningoencephalocele and traumatic or operative hiatus.

Table 2: Common causes of bilateral proptosis.

Pathology	Etiologies
Inflammations	• Thyroid orbitopathy • Wegener granulomatosis • Idiopathic inflammatory pseudotumor • Myositis • Sarcoidosis • Sjögren syndrome
Neoplasia	• Lymphoma • Leukemia • Metastatic carcinoma • Optic nerve glioma
Vascular lesions	• Arteriovenous shunts • Varix

History of Past Illness

A careful past history can point toward the provisional diagnosis. Following points must be asked in history of past illness:
• Systemic inflammatory disease such as thyroid disorder and sarcoidosis
• Malignancy—lungs, breasts, and prostate
• Trauma
• Periocular tumors

Past Surgical History

Prior periorbital surgery or history of surgery for intraocular malignancy such as malignant melanoma might point to the possibility of orbital extension or metastasis.

EXAMINATION

General Examination/Specific Systemic Examination

Look for signs of Graves' disease/sarcoidosis/any malignancy/any infective foci.

Ocular Examination

The points that must be noted in an ocular examination are described below.

Visual Acuity

In general, visual acuity is not affected with orbital diseases except in cases with optic nerve compression, refractive changes due to pressure on back of the eyeball or exposure keratopathy.

Eyeball

A case of proptosis should be examined under following headings:

Inspection:
- Head posture, facial asymmetry, and shape of the skull
- Differentiate between pseudoproptosis
- Signs of trauma
- Periocular ecchymosis—trauma and neuroblastoma
- *Protrusion of the eye:* In unilateral cases, there will be obvious disparity between the two eyes. In bilateral cases, some difficulty may be there in early cases of proptosis. Following two methods are useful in detection of proptosis:
    1. *Naffziger method:* Relative protrusion can be observed by simply standing behind a seated patient and gazing downward (tangentially) toward the chin from the forehead to assess protrusion of the eye beyond the orbital rim.
    2. *Worm eye view:* It is similar to Naffziger method but the difference is that the examiner examines up from below with the patient's head tilted back.
- *The direction of proptosis:* The direction of proptosis can indicate the probable etiology. The direction can be following:
    - *Axial:* Thyroid-related ophthalmopathy, glioma of optic nerve **(Fig. 1)**, optic nerve sheath, meningioma, and cavernous hemangioma
    - *Nonaxial/Eccentric:*
        - *Down and out:* Dermoid, dermolipoma, frontal and ethmoidal mucocele, and meningocele
        - *Down and in:* Lacrimal gland tumor and dermoid
        - *Upward:* Carcinoma of maxillary sinus, lacrimal sac tumors, lymphoma, maxillary sinus tumor, and metastatic tumors
        - *Outward:* Lesion of anterior ethmoidal sinus, nasopharyngeal tumor, lymphangioma **(Fig. 2)**, lethal midline granuloma, metastatic tumors, and secondary tumor

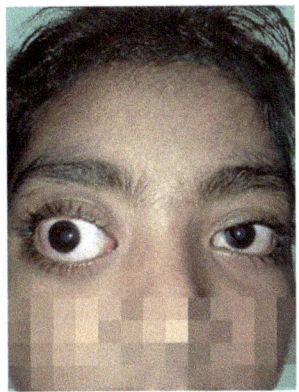

Fig. 1: Axial proptosis due to optic nerve glioma.

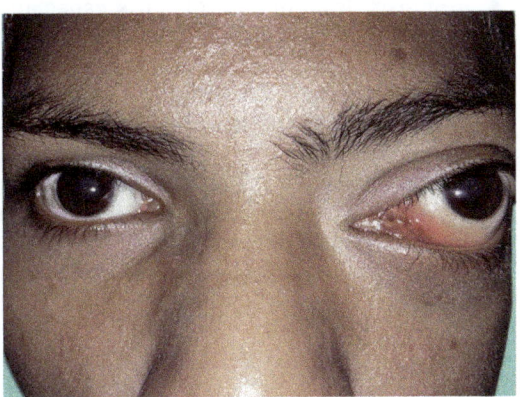

Fig. 2: Abaxial proptosis due to medial orbital lymphangioma.

- *Medial displacement:* Dermoid cyst, lacrimal fossa tumors and cysts, and sphenoid wing meningioma
- *Laterality:* Unilateral or bilateral
- *Ocular motility:* Ocular motility disturbance can be due to the following reasons:
  - Involvement of the rectus or oblique muscles directly
  - Affecting nerve supply of rectus or oblique muscles
  - From restriction of the orbital fascial connective tissue septae
- *Eyelids:* Lids can be affected by direct involvement of the levator muscle or the 3rd cranial nerve (CN), or because of associated proptosis. Examination of lid is especially important in thyroid-associated eye disease. The various lid signs and their terminology have been described in **Table 3**.
- *Periorbital inflammation:* Look for inflammatory signs (erythema, edema, chemosis, and dilated vessels) of the periorbital structures that can be associated with infections and acute inflammatory diseases.
- *Nose/roof of mouth* (sinus disease or when intranasal source is suspected) and neck (for goiter)
- *Valsalva:* Orbital varix or highly vascular lesions such as capillary hemangiomas will enlarge with increase in arterial pressure. This can be elicited with the Valsalva maneuver or by asking the patient to bend forward.
- Lagophthalmos, Bell's phenomena, and exposure keratopathy

Palpation: It should be carried out to confirm the findings of inspection and also for following reasons:
- *Retropulsion:* In a retropulsion test, thumb/two fingers/palm is used to gently push on the globe through the upper eyelid to know compressibility/resistance of the tumor. While hemangioma, lymphangioma, orbital varices give a soft consistency, optic nerve glioma may give a firm consistency. Resistance to retropulsion suggests retrobulbar tumor or thyroid ophthalmopathy.
- *Orbital thrill/Pulsation:* Place your index and middle finger over the orbit (with closed lids) and observe the following:
  - *True pulsation:* Finger will raise and separated
  - *Transmitted pulsation:* Finger will raise only
- *Swelling/mass around the eyeball:* If present, its size, site, shape, consistency, fixity (skin/bone/muscle), signs of inflammation (*Rubor*—redness; *color*—raised temperature, check with your back surface of hand; *dolor*—pain/tenderness; *tumor*—swelling; *functionless*—loss of function), and overlying skin changes must be noted carefully.
- *Regional lymph nodes:* Palpate the submandibular and preauricular lymph nodes.
  - Medial and central lower lid (along the facial vein), medial upper lid, central upper lid, and medial canthus drain into the submandibular lymph nodes.
  - Lateral upper lid and lateral lower lid drain into the preauricular parotid lymph nodes.
- *Orbital rim/margin* with index finger to look for any mass, or erosion (malignancy), irregularity (previous trauma)
- *Reducibility of the mass:* Check for reducibility of the mass lesion. It can provide a clue about the probable etiology, for example, vascular tumors and schwannoma are reducible masses but lacrimal gland tumor and pseudotumor are not reducible.
- *Infraorbital/supraorbital anesthesia:* Perineural invasion by a tumor can result in pain, numbness, and paresthesia in infraorbital or supraorbital area. Adenoid cystic carcinoma (ACC) of the lacrimal glands often presents with orbital pain and paresthesia as this type of tumor is frequently associated with perineural spreading (Remember, the *lacrimal nerve* is the smallest of the three branches of the ophthalmic division of the trigeminal nerve. It passes through the lacrimal gland, then pierces the upper lid and supplies the supraorbital area. It provides sensory innervations for the lacrimal gland, conjunctiva, and the lateral upper eyelids and adjacent supraorbital area, and partly the zygomaticotemporal area just adjacent to the orbital rim. Hence, in case ACC, these areas must be checked for sensory abnormalities).

Table 3: Lid signs in proptosis.

Sign	Description
Abadie's sign	Elevator muscle of upper eyelid is spastic
Ballett's sign	Paralysis of one or more extraocular muscle (EOM)
Beck's sign	Abnormal intense pulsation of retina's arteries
Boston's sign	Jerky movements of upper lid on lower gaze
Cowen's sign	Extensive hippus of consensual pupillary reflex
Dalrymple's sign	Upper eyelid retraction
Enroth's sign	Edema especially of the upper eyelid
Gifford's sign	Difficulty in eversion of upper lid
Goldzieher's sign	Deep injection of conjunctiva, especially temporal
Griffith's sign	Lower lid lag on upward gaze
Hertoghe's sign	Loss of eyebrows laterally
Jellinek's sign	Superior eyelid folds is hyperpigmented
Joffroy's sign	Absent creases in the forehead on upward gaze
Jendrassik's sign	Abduction and rotation of eyeball is limited also
Knies' sign	Uneven pupillary dilatation in dim light
Kocher's sign	Spasmodic retraction of upper lid on fixation
Loewi's sign	Quick mydriasis after instillation of 1:1,000 adrenaline
Mann's sign	Eyes seem to be situated at different levels because of tanned skin
Means' sign	Increased scleral show on upgaze (globe lag)
Moebius's sign	Lack of convergence
Payne/Trousseau sign	Dislocation of globe
Pochin's sign	Reduced amplitude of blinking
Rieseman's sign	Bruit over the eyelid
Movement's cap phenomenon	Eyeball movements are performed difficultly, abruptly and incompletely
Rosenbach's sign	Eyelids are animated by thin tremors when closed
Saiton's sign	Frontalis contraction after cessation of levator activity
Snellen-Rieseman's sign	When placing the stethoscope's capsule over closed eyelids' a systolic murmur could be heard
Stellwag's sign	Incomplete and infrequent blinking
Suker's sign	Inability to maintain fixation on extreme lateral gaze
Tellas's sign	Inferior eyelid might be hyperpigmented
Topolanski's sign	Around insertion areas of the four rectus muscles of the eyeball a vascular band network is noticed and this network joins the four insertion points
von Graefe's sign	Upper lid lag on downgaze
Wilder's sign	Jerking of the eye on movement from abduction to adduction

Auscultation: Auscultation is done with the help of a stethoscope, over eyeball and temporal area, to look for a bruit. A bruit can be seen in cases of AV malformation.

Transillumination: It is helpful in evaluating anterior orbital lesions. It is usually performed using a penlight. Interpretation is based on the opacity of the mass relative to surrounding tissues as follows:
- *Bright:* The area lights up more than the surrounding tissues, for example, cyst filled with clear liquid, dacryops
- *Equal:* The area lights up to the same degree as surrounding tissues, for example, lipoma
- *Indeterminate:* The area seems darker than surrounding tissues to a variable degree, for example, inclusion cyst, dermoid cyst
- *Dark:* The area is clearly opaque, creating a shadow effect. Aneurysm, for example, solid tumors (lacrimal gland tumors) and osteoma
- Remember some clinicians interpret transillumination test as positive or negative; in that case first two categories can be considered positive while the last two as negative transillumination test.

Exophthalmometry: The most common type exophthalmometer used in clinical practice is Hertel's exophthalmometer. Other exophthalmometers used in clinical practice are Luedde scale, Naugle exophthalmometer, and Gormaz exophthalmometer. However, in the absence of any of these, an ordinary transparent ruler can be used to measure proptosis. The measurement, in Hertel's exophthalmometer, is done from the lateral orbital rim to the anterior corneal surface. A difference of >2 mm between an individual patient's eyes suggests proptosis. Procedure—following points must be considered while using Hertel's exophthalmometer:
- The patient and the examiner must be at the same level, eye to eye.
- Locate the orbital notch with patient's eyes closed (the deepest points on orbital rim) on the temporal side of the orbital rim near the lateral canthus.
- The prisms or the mirrors are slide across the bar to adjust the footplates to fit on the orbital rim. The exophthalmometer is opened so that the grooves are placed in the orbital notch.
- The separation of the exophthalmometer (baseline reading) is very important and must always be noted and the exophthalmometer must always be set at that separation on future or repeated readings.
- The patient is then asked to open the eyes and look straight ahead.
- Look into the exophthalmometer, the red lines should overlap to avoid the parallax. Look into the mirrors located at each end of the exophthalmometer. Now note the millimeter mark corresponding to the corneal apex position on the scale and the readings on the cross bar for baseline reading.

Limitations: There are several limitations to Hertel's exophthalmometer. The readings are unreliable in presence of poor fixation, uncooperative patients with convergence or repeated head movements. In addition, in presence of depressed/fractured lateral orbital rim, it cannot be done.

Luedde's exophthalmometer: It is a transparent plastic ruler which is thicker than the normal ruler. It has several advantages over an ordinary plastic ruler such as the reading starts from the apex and the apex fits the orbital notch accurately. It is more accurate than Hertel's exophthalmometer in presence of facial asymmetry.

Naugle exophthalmometer: It uses fixation points slightly above and below the superior and inferior orbital rims (cheekbones and forehead). Naugle exophthalmometer measures the difference in proptosis between the two eyes rather than absolute measure with the Hertel method. It is preferred in presence of an orbital fracture or after lateral orbitotomy.

Interpretation: The normal range is 12–21 mm. A difference of >2 mm between the two eyes is significant. In pediatric age group, the readings may vary depending upon the age; <4 years old (13.2 mm), 5–8 years old (14.4 mm), 9–12 years old (15.2 mm), and 13–17 years old (16.2 mm).

Conjunctiva: Examine carefully (with a slit lamp) for the following factors:
- Dilated or tortuous blood vessels, chemosis, dilated lymphatics, vascular malformation, and inflammation
- Hyperemia over the insertions of the horizontal rectus muscles—one of the earliest sign of thyroid eye disease (TED)

- Corkscrew-shaped tortuous dilated episcleral vessels high-flow AV malformations or a carotid cavernous fistula
- Subconjunctival mass—anterior extension of a deeper orbital tumor such as a lymphoma or intraocular melanoma with extraskeletal orbital extension (a dark subconjunctival mass)—salmon patch

Cornea: Look for signs of exposure keratopathy. Fluorescein staining can reveal early stage of exposure keratopathy showing multiple punctate defects. The corneal sensation must be checked in all cases of proptosis.

Sclera/Iris: Careful examination is carried out to look for signs of inflammation and any nodules.

Pupil: Examination of the pupil is extremely important as it often provides the first clue of a probable optic nerve involvement. The presence of relative afferent pathway defect (RAPD) must be ruled out in all cases. Any intraconal mass compressing optic nerve or any tumor intrinsic to optic nerve (optic nerve glioma) can lead to RAPD.

Intraocular pressure (IOP): If possible, IOP should be recorded in different gaze (ideally in all gazes and at least in primary and superior) especially in cases of suspected thyroid ophthalmopathy (in case of thyroid ophthalmopathy variable IOP in upgaze can be an early sign due to an involvement of inferior rectus muscle). The IOP may vary due to the restricted mobility of extraocular muscles—dancing mires for CCF.

Lens: Lens is usually clear except the effect of aging.

Vitreous: Usually normal except in cases of intraocular tumor.

Fundus: Carefully look for signs of globe compression such as venous engorgement, choroidal folds, and papilledema or optic atrophy.

Choroidal folds and opticociliary shunts may be seen in patients with meningiomas. In cases with cavernous sinus thrombosis retinal edema, exudates and engorged retinal veins can be seen due to increased venous pressure.

■ DIFFERENTIAL DIAGNOSIS

Based upon history and clinical examination the differential diagnosis has to be made.

The commonly seen diseases in clinical practice include the following:
- Vascular (cavernous fistula, cavernous hemangiomas)
- Endocrine (TED)
- Inflammatory (orbital cellulitis, orbital inflammatory disease, and orbital cysticercosis)
- Infections
- Neoplastic (ON glioma, ON meningiomas, lacrimal gland tumors, and frontal sinus mucocele)

■ INVESTIGATIONS

The line of investigation depends on upon the differential diagnosis arrived. Following tests must be done routinely in a case of proptosis:
- Thyroid function tests
- Complete blood count (CBC), peripheral smear (leukemia/lymphoma), erythrocyte sedimentation rate (ESR), and blood sugar

Specific Tests

Imaging Technique

Noninvasive techniques:
- *Plain X-rays:* It is often the initial radiological examination, especially when other modalities are not available. Commonly done exposures are in the Caldwell view, the Water's view, a lateral view, and the Rhese view (for optic foramina). The findings of orbital diseases in X-ray include enlargement of orbital cavity, calcification, hyperostosis, and enlargement of optic foramina.
- *Ultrasonography (USG):* It is a nonradiational noninvasive, completely safe, and extremely valuable initial scanning procedure for orbital lesions. In the diagnosis of orbital lesions, it is superior to computed tomography (CT) scanning in actual tissue diagnosis and can usually differentiate between solid, cystic, infiltrative, and spongy masses. The limitations of USG are limited ability to evaluate orbital bones, periorbital sinuses, and the orbital apex due to poor distance penetration.
- *CT scanning:* It is extremely helpful in determining the location and size of an orbital mass. A combination of axial and coronal cuts

enables a three-dimensional visualization. In addition to globe, extraocular muscles, and optic nerves visualization, it can show areas adjacent to the orbits such as orbital walls, cranial cavity, paranasal sinuses, and nasal cavity. Mass lesions in the orbit usually appear as an abnormal density within the typically low-density orbital fat. The lesion may be well defined with sharp borders (e.g., cavernous hemangioma), or infiltrative with diffuse borders (e.g., pseudotumor). CT can give information about adjacent bone erosion (suggestive of malignancy), remolding or fossa formation (encapsulated benign lacrimal gland tumor such as pleomorphic adenoma, encapsulated malignant lacrimal gland tumor, orbital dermoid), or displacement of adjacent bony orbital walls. Its main disadvantage is the inability to distinguish between pathologically soft tissue masses that are radiologically isodense. In addition, the risk of radiation exposure [in contrast to magnetic resonance imaging (MRI)] is always there.

- *MRI:* MRI is very sensitive for detecting differences between normal and abnormal tissues. Advantages of MRI over CT include:
  - Better soft tissue visualization, especially in the region of the orbital apex, optic canal, and cavernous sinus
  - Various fat suppression techniques allow the visualization of gadolinium-enhanced lesions that are often difficult to see the normally high signal-generating orbital fat
  - Better tissue differentiation
  - No radiation exposure

Invasive procedures:
- *Orbital venography:* It is useful in orbital varix. It confirms the diagnosis and also outlines the size and extent of the lesion that helps in proper surgical planning.
- *Carotid angiography:* It is useful in cases of pulsatile proptosis and in those associated with a bruit or thrill. It helps to identify the location and extent of ophthalmic artery aneurysms and AV malformations. It is also helpful in identifying the feeding vessels thus, for planning surgery in cases of vascular orbital tumors.

Histopathology

The exact diagnosis of many orbital lesions cannot be made without the help of histopathological studies, which can be accomplished by following techniques:
- *Fine-needle aspiration biopsy (FNAB):* It is quick, reliable, and relatively accurate. The biopsy aspirate is obtained under direct vision (when there is an obvious mass) or guided by CT/USG using a 23-gauge needle.
- *Incisional biopsy:* The scope of incisional biopsy in the diagnosis of orbital masses is not clearly defined. It is often contraindicated due to the risk of tumor seeding or increased risk of malignant transformation (e.g., benign lacrimal gland tumor).
- *Excisional biopsy:* It is the procedure of choice especially when the mass is well encapsulated or circumscribed. It is performed by orbitotomy.

■ CLASSIFICATION/STAGING/SCORING

It depends upon the individual disease.

■ MANAGEMENT

The management depends upon the individual diseases.

VIVA QUESTIONS

Q.1. Explain pseudoproptosis.
Ans. Pseudoproptosis is either the simulation of an abnormal prominence of the eye or a true asymmetry that is not caused by a mass, a vascular abnormality, or an inflammatory process.

Causes are multiple and include:
- *Enlarged globe:*
  - Myopia
  - Trauma
  - Glaucoma
- *Asymmetric orbital size:*
  - Congenital
  - Postradiation
  - Postsurgical
- *Asymmetric palpebral fissure:*
  - Contralateral ptosis
  - Lid retraction

- Facial nerve paralysis
- Lid scar, ectropion, entropion
- *Extraocular muscle abnormalities:*
  - Postsurgical muscle recession
  - Paralysis or paresis
- *Contralateral enophthalmos:*
  - Contralateral orbital fracture
  - Contralateral small globe
  - Contralateral cicatricial tumor

Physiological proptosis: It is proptosis in infants due to the fact that orbital cavities do not attain their full size so rapidly as the eyes.

Q.2. Most common cause of proptosis.
Ans.
- *Unilateral proptosis:* TED
- *Bilateral proptosis:* TED

Q.3. Causes of pulsatile proptosis.
Ans. *True vascular:*
- Carotid cavernous fistula
- AV fistula in the orbit between ophthalmic artery and orbital vein, in the neck—carotid artery and jugular vein
- Highly vascular orbital tumor
- Orbital varies

Transmitted:
- Congenital failure in the development of roof of the orbit, for example, encephalocele/encephalomyelocele
- Traumatic or operative hiatus in orbit roof resulting in the formation of meningocele

Q.4. What are the 6 P's of the orbital history and physical examination?
Ans. Useful in the diagnostic process:
- Pain
- Proptosis
- Progression
- Palpation
- Pulsation
- Periocular changes

Q.5. Few facts about orbit dimensions.
Ans. The facts are as follows:
- Volume—30 cc
- Horizontal entrance width—40 mm
- Height at orbital rim—35 mm
- Orbital depth (rim to the optic strut)—45–55 mm
- Orbital segment of optic nerve—25 mm

REFERENCES

1. Albert DM, Miller JW, Azar DT, Blodi BA. Albert and Jakobiec's Principles and Practice of Ophthalmology, 3rd edition. Philadelphia: Saunders/Elsevier; 2008.
2. Bowling B. Kanski's Clinical Ophthalmology: A Systematic Approach, 8th edition. Edinburgh: Elsevier; 2015.

LID TUMORS

Sapna Raghuwanshi, Anasua Ganguly Kapoor, Mandeep S Bajaj

INTRODUCTION

Lid tumors can arise from the epidermis, dermis, or adnexal structures of the eyelid. Malignant lesions are common around the eyes because many are induced by sun exposure or develop from sun-related benign lesions. Typically, most of these are small and slowly growing.

The common periocular malignancies are basal cell carcinoma (BCC), squamous cell carcinoma (SCC), sebaceous gland carcinoma (SGC), and malignant melanoma. In western literature, BCC constitutes around 85% of the cases because of fair complexion. Whereas in India, all three major variants constitute around 33% each.[1,2]

HISTORY

Demography

Commonly, present in 5th to 6th decade of life with site of involvement:
- Involvement pattern in BCC (lower eyelid, caruncle, upper eyelid, and lateral canthus) **(Fig. 1)**
- Involvement pattern in sebaceous CC (upper eyelid and lower eyelid) **(Fig. 2)**

Oculoplasty

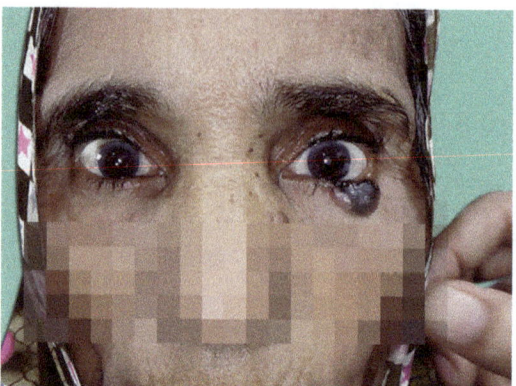

Fig. 1: Pigmented basal cell carcinoma of the left lower eyelid.

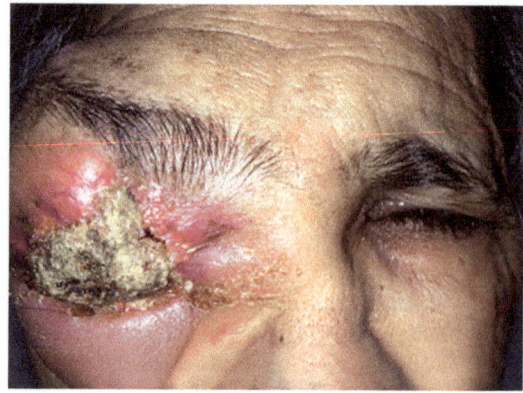

Fig. 3: Squamous cell carcinoma of the eyelid with extensive periorbital involvement.

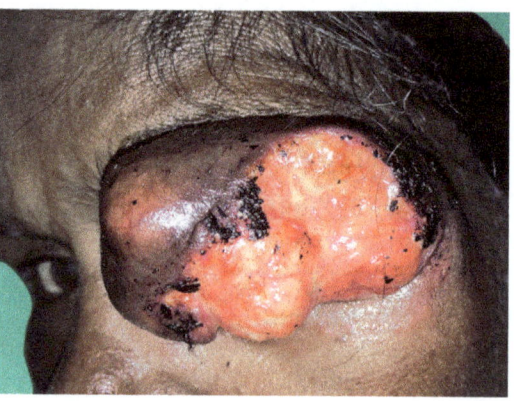

Fig. 2: Sebaceous gland carcinoma of the left upper eyelid.

- Involvement pattern in squamous CC (lower eyelid, caruncle, and upper eyelid) **(Fig. 3)**.

Chief Complaints

A case of lid tumor can present with presents with following complaints:
- Slow, generally painless growth on lid margins
- Ulceration of the lid margins
- Loss of eyelashes
- Distortion of eyelid margin
- Ectropion/retraction (secondary due to lid growth or skin contracture)
- Increasing pigmentation of eye lid margins
- Palpebral preauricular lymph nodes
- Dilated blood vessels (telangiectasias)

History of Present Illness

Following points must be noted for a lid tumor:
- *Onset:* Common lid tumors are insidious in onset
- *Progression:* Progression is usually slow
- Any deterioration of vision
- Diplopia or restriction of eye movements (frozen globe)
- Any other swelling around the head and neck region (preauricular and cervical lymph node for metastasis)
- Systemic features of metastasis

Past History

Predisposing factors: Following are the predisposing factors for lid tumors:
- Ultraviolet exposure (UV-B)
- Ionizing radiation
- Arsenic exposure
- Psoralen plus ultraviolet A (PUVA)
- Human papilloma virus
- Genetic diseases (albinism, xeroderma pigmentosum risk factor for BCC)
- Recurrent chalazion (could be sebaceous cell carcinoma)
- Previous surgery for eyelid malignancies
- Topical chemotherapy

Important Examination Findings

- *Eyelid:* Careful examination of the eyelid for signs of lid malignancy

- Eyelid should be examined carefully for depth or plane of involvement, lid margin involvement, and medial and lateral canthal involvement.
- *Bulbar and palpebral conjunctiva:* In cases of sebaceous cell carcinoma, look for "Pagetoid spread" (Intraepithelial spread of tumor cells)
- *Cornea:* Again in case of sebaceous cell carcinoma
- *Look for scleral invasion and globe integrity:* In cases where the tumor is extending beyond the orbital septum
- *Lymph nodes*

■ DIAGNOSIS

The best way to confirm the diagnosis is excision biopsy.

Histopathology

- *BCC:* The tumor cells arise from the basal layer of the epidermis. The cells proliferate downward thus exhibiting palisading at the periphery.
- *SCC:* The tumor arises from the squamous layer of epidermis, well-differentiated tumors show characteristic keratin "pearls."
- *Sebaceous cell carcinoma:* The tumor shows irregular lobules consisting of sheets of cells with varying degrees of sebaceous differentiation. The malignant cells show foamy, multivacuolated cytoplasm, secondary to intracytoplasmic lipid.

Biopsy Methods

- *Incision biopsy:* Where only a part of the tumor is removed using either blade or biopsy punch
- *Excision biopsy:* Here the entire tumor is removed
- *Impression cytology:* After drying the area to be examined, nitrocellulose filter paper is applied, and then firmly pressed with Goldmann tonometer head. Peel off paper with forceps and place in appropriate fixative solution for examination.
- *Fine needle aspiration cytology (FNAC):* In case of large tumor as a preliminary modality or in cases of lymph node involvement.

Imaging

Computed tomography is indicated in cases with postseptal extension to know the extent of orbital spread and bony involvement. Positron emission tomography (PET) and single photon emission computed tomography (SPECT) are done in cases to study the status of sentinel lymph nodes.

■ STAGING

Staging is required to plan the treatment strategy and prognosis. The most common staging system for carcinoma of the eyelid is the TNM system.

The TNM system applies for all three common eyelid carcinomas, but melanoma of the eyelid is staged in the manner as skin melanomas. TNM stands for tumor, nodes, and metastasis. This describes the size of the primary tumor, the number and location of any regional lymph nodes and metastatic foci anywhere in the body.

■ MANAGEMENT

Surgical Excision with Standard Frozen Section Control

This technique is performed by noting the clinical boundaries of the tumor edges and excising an additional 3 mm cuff of normal appearing tissue followed by histopathological assessment of the excised specimen for tumor-free margins.

Mohs' Micrographic Surgery

This technique involves removal of the gross mass of the tumor plus a small peripheral margin of normal tissue. A thin layer of tissue, approximately 2 mm thick, is further excised from the entire base and edges of the wound. The initial specimen is divided into 4-7 μm thick portions on glass slides; the edges are marked with different colored dyes to maintain orientation. Frozen sections are obtained from the under surface and skin edge of each specimen. Locations of residual tumor are marked on a map and only those areas are re-excised. Surgical resection is continued until there is a microscopically proven tumor-free plane. The defect is then reconstructed by the oculoplastic surgeon.

Cryosurgery

It is useful for small lesions, but less effective for larger and deeply invasive tumors.

Contraindications of Cryosurgery

- Involvement of the conjunctival fornix
- Fixation of tumor to periosteum
- Sensory or motor denervation
- Cold intolerance—cryoglobulinemia or cold urticaria
- Deeply pigmented skin
- Indistinct margins
- Diameter of lesion >10 mm
- Sclerosing or multicentric type

Complications

- Depigmentation
- Hyperpigmentation
- Eyelid notching
- Hypertrophic scar
- Pseudoepithelial hyperplasia
- Ectropion
- Punctal and canalicular stenosis
- Lash loss

With conjunctival involvement: The adjuvant methods followed are:
- Local application of cryotherapy
- Topical mitomycin C application or interferon

Extensive disease: Exenteration for orbital involvement and extended exenteration with radical neck dissection for metastatic disease beyond the orbit with lymph node involvement.

Radiotherapy: Indication of radiotherapy includes following:
- Inoperable disease
- Multiple medical problems
- Elderly patients unable to tolerate surgical resection
- Patients in whom surgery will result in extensive disfigurement with potential loss of useful ocular function.
  Complications of radiotherapy include:
  - Skin atrophy
  - Ectropion
  - Entropion
  - Nasolacrimal duct stenosis
  - Keratitis
  - Conjunctival keratinization
  - Cataract
  - Loss of eyelashes
  - Globe perforation
- *Chemotherapy:* Used in cases of systemic involvement
- Others such as photodynamic therapy and CO_2 laser treatment are rarely used.

■ PROGNOSIS

Following are the poor prognostic factors:
- Duration of symptoms >6 months
- Vascular and lymphatic infiltration
- Orbital extension
- Poor tumor differentiation
- Multicentric origin intraepithelial carcinomatous changes of the conjunctiva, cornea, or skin
- Location in the upper eyelid
- Tumor diameter >2 cm
- Location on central face or ears
- Long-standing presence prior to initial treatment
- Incomplete excision
- Aggressive subtype
- Perineural or perivascular involvement
- *Recurrent tumor:*
  - BCC of the eyelid rarely spreads to lymph nodes or other organs, so the prognosis for this type of tumor is usually very good.
  - SCC can be more aggressive than BCC and can spread to the orbit, lymph nodes, or other organs. However, the prognosis is good if SCC of the eyelid is detected early and can be completely removed.
  - The mortality rate (the number of people who die from the disease each year) for SGC of the eyelid is about 5–10%. However, sebaceous gland tumors are often not diagnosed early and have a high rate of recurrence and spread (metastasis).

VIVA QUESTIONS

Q.1. Key points of individual malignancies.
Ans. *Basal cell carcinoma:*
- It is the common type of eyelid tumor.
- It usually affects adult population.

- It commonly involves the lower eyelid due to exposure to sunlight.

Inherited conditions predisposing to BCC:
- Albinism
- Xeroderma pigmentosum
- Basal cell nevus syndrome or Gorlin syndrome
- Bazex syndrome
- Rombo syndrome

Sebaceous gland carcinoma (SGC) (Sebaceous gland carcinoma, Meibomian gland carcinoma) [also see short case]:

Important clinical points:
- These arise from the Meibomian glands in the eyelid.
- It is more often in elderly women than men and often present late due to less malignant course.
- These tumors commonly arise from the upper eyelid followed by the lower eyelid the caruncle and bulbar conjunctiva. The upper eyelid is more prone due to more number of Meibomian glands in the upper eyelid (20–25) as compared to that in the lower eyelid (15–20).
- SGC can be multifocal due to peculiar pattern of spread called "Pagetoid spread" where there is an intraepithelial spread of the tumor.
- The gross appearance resembles yellowish nodular mass.
- It may resemble blepharoconjunctivitis.
- It can involve the orbit and regional lymph nodes.

Q.2. Signs of lid malignancy
Ans. Following are the signs:
- Destruction of lid architecture
- Involvement of both anterior and posterior lamella
- Ulceration of the lid margins
- Loss of eyelashes
- Distortion of eyelid margin
- Ectropion/retraction (secondary due to lid growth or skin contracture)
- Increasing pigmentation of eye lid margins
- Palpebral preauricular lymph nodes
- Dilated blood vessels (telangiectasias)

Q.3. Differentiation of three lid malignancies based on clinical findings.
Ans. *See* text.

Q.4. Sentinel lymph node biopsy.
Ans. Sentinel lymph node (SLN) biopsy is used for identifying the microscopic nodal metastasis from a malignant tumor. Tumors may preferentially spread to a first draining or "sentinel" lymph node before they spread to distant sites.[3]

Preoperatively: 99mTc-Sulfur colloid ($t_{1/2}$ 6 hours) will be injected around the tumor and hybrid SPECT/CT is performed to locate sentinel lymph nodes (Preauricular, intraparotid, and submandibular).

Intraoperatively: In the first setting based on the previous SPECT/CT images, maximal radioactive counts were identified by handheld gamma probe, followed by injection of 1% isosulfan blue dye perilesionally followed by gentle massage to augment lymphatic drainage. An incision will be made over the area of highest radioactive count and lymph nodes are dissected. In the second setting, eyelid tumors are excised and reconstruction done.

Q.5. Map biopsy.
Ans. *See* text.

Q.6. Reconstruction of the eyelid defects.
Ans. Lid reconstruction:

Anterior lamella reconstruction:
- Primary closure
- Full thickness skin grafts
- Musculocutaneous flap
- Advancement flap
- Transposition flap
- Rhombic flap.

Posterior lamella reconstruction:
- Buccal mucosa (preferred)
- Hard palate mucosa
- Tarsoconjunctival graft

Full thickness lid defect—See **Table 1**.

Q.7. Different histological types of BCC.
Ans. *See* **Table 2**.

Table 1: Full thickness lid reconstruction.

Size of the lid defect	Repair
<25%	Direct closure
25–50%	Direct closure with cantholysis
33–66%	Semicircular flap (Tenzel flap) alone or along with the periosteal flap
50–75%	• Cutler Beard (Upper eyelid defect) • Hughes procedure (Lower eyelid defect)
75–100%	• Lower eyelid (Tarsoconjunctival flap with skin grafting) • Upper eyelid (Median forehead flap with mucus membrane grafting)

Table 2: Lid manifestation of basal cell carcinoma (BCC).

Nodular-ulcerative	Pigmented	Morphea or sclerosing	Superficial	Fibroepithelioma
• Most common lesion pink or pearly papule or nodule • Overlying telangiectatic vessels present • Central ulceration with rolled border "rodent ulcer"	• Similar to the noduloulcerative type in morphology • Brown or black pigmentation • More common in dark complexion persons	• Least common • Flat, indurated, yellow-pink plaque with ill-defined borders • Aggressive and may invade the dermis deeply • Invade into the paranasal sinuses and orbit • Mimic blepharoconjunctivitis	• Scaling patch with a raised pearly border • Arise on the trunk rather than the eyelid	• Pedunculated or sessile smooth, pink nodule • Arise on the trunk rather than the eyelid

Table 3: Lid manifestation of malignant melanoma.

Lentigo malignant melanoma	Superficial spreading melanoma	Nodular melanoma	Acral lentiginous melanoma
Slowly expanding pigmented, flat, nonpalpable, tan to brown macule with irregular borders	Plaque with irregular outline, variable pigmentation	• Blue-black nodule with normal surrounding skin • May be nonpigmented	Occurs on the palms, soles, and distal phalanges as well as on the mucous membranes

Q.8. Different lid manifestations of malignant melanoma.

Ans. *See* **Table 3**.

■ REFERENCES

1. Albert DM, Miller JW, Azar DT, Blodi BA. Albert and Jakobiec's Principles and Practice of Ophthalmology, 3rd edition. Philadelphia: Saunders/Elsevier; 2008.
2. Bowling B. Kanski's Clinical Ophthalmology: a Systematic Approach, 8th edition. Edinburgh: Elsevier; 2015.
3. Lokdarshi G, Vuthaluru S, Pushker N, Kumar R, Kashyap S, Mathur S. Sentinel lymph node biopsy in malignant eyelid tumor: hybrid single photon emission computed tomography/computed tomography and dual dye technique. Am J Ophthalmol. 2016;162: 199-200.

PTOSIS

Aditi Dubey, Sanjana M

■ INTRODUCTION

Drooping of the eyelid is known as ptosis or blepharoptosis. It is a common pathology seen in all age groups. It is given as both long and short case in the examination. The most important part in a case of ptosis is its examination.

■ HISTORY

Chief Complaints

A case of ptosis can present with following complaints:
- Adult patient commonly complains of drooping of the upper lid.
- In children, parents often complain of an affected eye being smaller in comparison to another eye.
- Diminution of vision is not a common complaint and amblyopia is associated only with severe ptosis due to stimulus deprivation. The prevalence of amblyopia is around 12–20% in cases with severe congenital ptosis.[1-4]

History of Present Illness

It is important to note about following points:
- The age of onset and duration (congenital or acquired)
- Progression of ptosis (chronic progressive external ophthalmoplegia)
- Any head position (e.g., chin lift)
- History of trauma
- Associated symptoms can often indicate the underlying cause.

For example:
- Associated double vision points toward 3rd CN palsy/aberrant regeneration
- Alteration in an amount of ptosis with jaw movements (jaw-winking phenomenon) can be seen in Marcus Gunn syndrome
- Difficulty in deglutition is seen in oculopharyngeal muscular dystrophy
- Limitation of ocular motility can be seen in myasthenia gravis (MG) and Kearns-Sayre syndrome
- Worsening of ptosis as the day progresses is seen in MG [Levator palpebrae superioris (LPS) weakness compensated for by Müller's muscle in myasthenia, which fatigues with progression of the day]
- Associated recurrent allergic conjunctivitis can cause mechanical ptosis

Past History

Following points must be noted in history in a ptosis case:
- Recurrent episodes of ptosis can be seen in recurrent 3rd nerve palsy, for example, ischemic neuropathy associated with diabetes or hypertension
- Contact lens wear (ill-fitting contact lens may cause blepharospasm and small palpebral aperture which may be confused with ptosis)
- Drug intake such as neostigmine can point toward the possible diagnosis
- Trauma (lid or facial trauma mat cause scarring or LPS damage) to rule out traumatic ptosis
- Medical conditions, for example, MG, myotonia, muscular dystrophies, diabetes, and hypertension
- Spectacle use or amblyopia therapy during childhood is important when there is associated vision loss.

Past Medical History

Diabetes mellitus (DM), hypertension, bleeding diathesis (important for surgery), recurrent stye/chalazion/vernal keratoconjunctivitis (mechanical ptosis), and any neurological disorder must be ruled out.

Past Surgical History

Peribulbar block for any intraocular surgery and cataract surgery can lead to ptosis. Any previous squint surgery or ptosis surgery must be recorded.

Birth History

History pertaining to pregnancy, delivery, neonatal period, and early development are important in congenital ptosis. Birth history such as instrument/forceps delivery can toward the cause of ptosis.

Family History

Positive family history can be present in blepharophimosis syndrome.

■ EXAMINATION

Visual acuity: Visual acuity and refractive error must be assessed in all cases of congenital or childhood ptosis in order to identify and treat the child with concomitant amblyopia. Amblyopia can result from anisometropia, high astigmatism, strabismus, or occlusion of a pupil. Amblyopia occurs in approximately 12–20% of patients with congenital ptosis.

Facial symmetry and orbit: Look for the following features:
- *Head posture:* Chin elevation is seen in cases of bilateral moderate to severe ptosis.
- *Frontalis overaction:* Raised eyebrows to compensate for ptosis.
- *Pseudoptosis:* Ipsilateral microphthalmos or contralateral lid retraction can lead to pseudoptosis.
- The presence of strabismus must be ruled out by Cover-Uncover test.
- Extraocular muscle function should also be assessed in primary and secondary gazes. The presence of motility abnormalities is seen in congenital conditions such as double elevator palsy (combined superior rectus and LPS muscle maldevelopment) and congenital oculomotor palsy and acquired conditions such as ocular or systemic MG, chronic progressive external ophthalmoplegia, oculopharyngeal dystrophy, and oculomotor palsy with or without aberrant regeneration.
- Signs of trauma

Eyelid: Following points must be noted:
- If ptosis is unilateral **(Figs. 1 and 2)** or bilateral
- Signs of previous trauma such as eyelid scar
- Mechanical causes of ptosis such as eyelid tumors, multiple chalazia, and giant papillae
- Lagophthalmos—important for surgical planning
- Pupillary reaction—pupillary involvement can be seen in cases of 3rd CN palsy and Horner syndrome

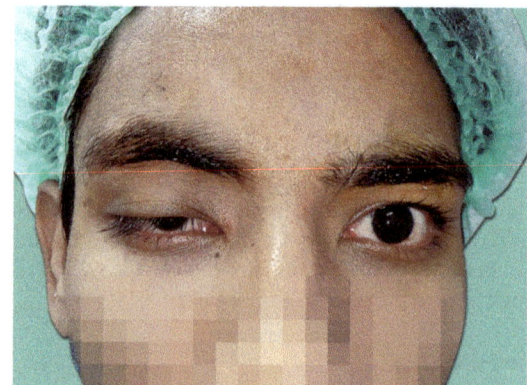

Fig. 1: Simple severe congenital ptosis before surgery.

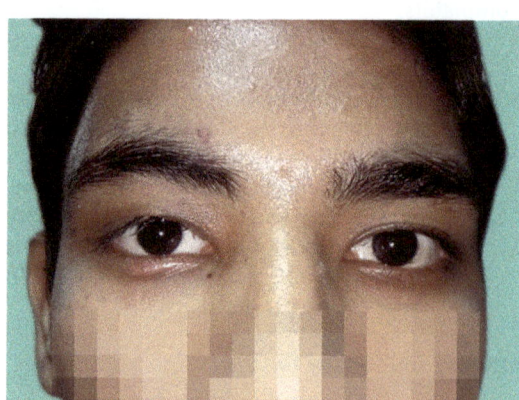

Fig. 2: Simple severe congenital ptosis after surgery.

- The position of the lids should be noted in the different position of gaze. Variability of ptosis in the different position of gaze is an indication of aberrant regeneration after the 3rd nerve palsy.
- Also note the speed of saccades: slow saccades are indicative of myopathic muscles.
- Variation in the amount of ptosis with extraocular muscle or jaw muscle movements (synkinesis) should be noted. Synkinesis may be seen in Marcus Gunn jaw-winking ptosis, aberrant regeneration of the 3rd CN, or the VII CN, and some types of Duane syndrome.

Measurement of Ptosis

- *Margin-reflex distance 1 (MRD1):* It is the distance from the upper eyelid margin to the

corneal light reflex in the primary position. It is the *single most important measurement* in describing the amount of ptosis. The MRD1 is also checked in the reading position.
- *Margin-reflex distance 2 (MRD2):* The MRD2 is the distance from the corneal light reflex to the lower eyelid margin. MRD2 is a measure of lower eyelid retraction (or scleral show).
- *Palpebral aperture:* The vertical interpalpebral fissure is measured at the widest point between the lower eyelid and the upper eyelid. This measurement is taken with the patient fixating on a distant object in primary gaze. Normally, the palpebral fissure height in males is 7–10 mm, and in females, it is 8–12 mm. *Remember the sum of the MRD1 and the MRD2 should equal the vertical interpalpebral fissure height.*
- *Margin crease distance (MCD):* It is the distance from the upper eyelid crease to the eyelid margin. The insertion of fibers from the LPS muscle into the skin contributes to the formation of the upper eyelid crease. High, duplicated, or asymmetric creases may indicate an abnormal position of the levator aponeurosis. The upper eyelid crease is 8–9 mm in males and 9–11 mm in females. The crease is usually elevated in patients with involutional ptosis and is often shallow or absent in patients with congenital ptosis. The height of the crease on the normal side should be measured and compared to the ptotic eyelid in downgaze. In patients, when more than one lid crease is present, *the most prominent* one should be considered.
- *LPS function Berke's method (lid excursion):* LPS function is estimated by measuring the upper eyelid excursion from downgaze to upgaze with frontalis muscle function negated. Fixating the brow with digital pressure minimizes contributions from accessory elevators of the eyelids such as the frontalis muscle. Failure to negate the influence of the frontalis muscle results in an overestimation of LPS function. LPS function can be graded according to Beard's classification
  – *Normal:* >15 mm
  – *Good:* 12–14 mm
  – *Fair:* 5–11 mm
  – *Poor:* <4 mm

Putterman's method: This is carried out by the measurement of the distance between the middle of upper lid margin to the 6 o'clock limbus in extreme upgaze. This is also known as the margin limbal distance (MLD). Normal is about 9.0 mm.

Assessment in children:
- Assessment of LPS function in small children is a difficult task, as the child allows no formal evaluation. Following methods may help
- The presence of lid fold and increase or decrease in its size on a movement of the eyelid gives us a clue to the LPS action.
- The presence of anomalous head posture like the child throwing his head back suggests a poor LPS action.
- *Iliff test:* This test can be performed in the first year of life to evaluate the levator function. The upper eyelid of the child is everted as the child looks down. If the levator action is good, lid reverts on its own.

Lagophthalmos: The patient should be assessed for lagophthalmos and if it is present, the degree should be noted, checking head position, chin elevation, brow position, and brow action in attempted upgaze. Lagophthalmos and poor tear film quantity or quality may predispose a patient to complications of ptosis repair such as dryness and exposure keratitis.

Bell's phenomenon: It is an upward and outward movement of the eye when an attempt is made to close the eyes. Bell's phenomenon is a normal defense reflex.
- *Demonstration:* Ask the patient to close the eye forcibly (as if the patient wants to sleep). The examiner then lifts the patient's upper eyelid manually. In a patient with a normal Bell's phenomenon, the globe will rotate upward and outward and the eyelid will cover the cornea.
- *Significance:* If a patient does not have a good Bell's phenomenon, a cautious ptosis correction should be undertaken to prevent subsequent corneal exposure, especially when planning for sling surgery.
- Bell's phenomenon is graded into three grades:
  1. *Good:* Less than one-third of the cornea visible
  2. *Fair:* One-third to one-half of the cornea visible

3. *Poor:* More than one-half of the cornea visible
- *Inverse Bell's phenomenon:* If the cornea is not in upgaze or if it moves to other position of gaze, such as downgaze on closing the eyes, then it is called inverse Bell's phenomenon.

Cornea

- The corneal sensation must be checked in all cases. A normal corneal sensation is essential for normal blink reflex and prevention of exposure keratitis the following surgery.
- Quantity and quality of the tear film must be documented in the initial examination. Schirmer test, tear break-up time (TBUT) and tear meniscus must be recorded in all cases of ptosis. Dry eye syndrome is a contraindication for ptosis surgery; especially sling surgeries as it may cause corneal damage postoperatively.

Pupil: Pupillary examination is important in the evaluation of ptosis. Pupil abnormalities are present in some acquired and congenital conditions associated with ptosis (e.g., Horner syndrome, 3rd CN palsy). Miosis that is most apparent in dim illumination is seen in Horner syndrome and mydriasis is seen in some cases of 3rd CN palsy.

Fundus: Fundus examination after mydriasis is essential for any concomitant fundus abnormality.

Rest of the findings such as iris, lens, sclera, and IOP are usually within normal limits.

To rule out myasthenia—fatigue and ice-pack test can be done.

■ DIFFERENTIAL DIAGNOSIS

A case of ptosis must be differentiated from pseudoptosis. Pseudoptosis is apparent eyelid drooping due to ocular or adnexal diseases and should be differentiated from true ptosis. On elevating the ptotic lid, the other eyelid droops slightly in true ptosis while remains at the same level in pseudoptosis. Causes of pseudoptosis includes following:
- *Unilateral:*
  - Hypertropia
  - Enophthalmos
  - Microphthalmia
  - Anophthalmia
  - Phthisis bulbi
  - Superior sulcus defect
  - Dermatochalasis
- *Contralateral:*
  - Upper eyelid retraction
  - Proptosis
  - Buphthalmos

■ INVESTIGATIONS

A case of ptosis usually does not need any special investigation other than routine tests done before surgery. Investigations such as visual field may be required in special situations as discussed under Viva questions.

■ CLASSIFICATIONS

Based on the onset:
- *Congenital ptosis:* It is present since birth. It can be further categorized into following:
  - Congenital simple ptosis
  - Complicated:
    • With oculomotor abnormalities
    • With blepharophimosis syndrome
    • Synkinetic ptosis
  - Marcus Gunn jaw-winking
  - Misdirected 3rd nerve ptosis
- *Acquired ptosis:* True acquired ptosis is the result of some disturbance of the upper lid retractors, the levator or Müller's muscle, or both, and is best classified according to its primary cause, which includes mechanical **(Fig. 3)**, myogenic, neurogenic, and aponeurotic. Differentiating points between

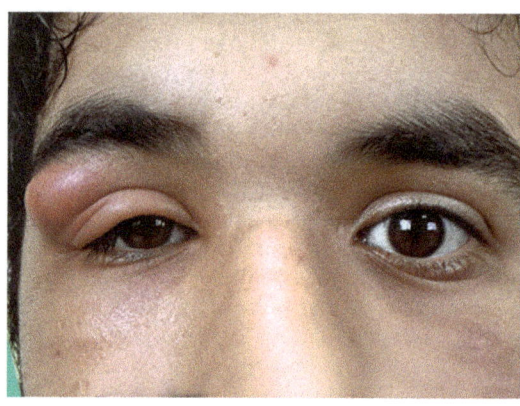

Fig. 3: Right upper eyelid mechanical ptosis.

congenital and acquired ptosis are given in **Table 1**.

Bases on pathogenesis: The classification is shown in **Table 2**.

■ STAGING/SCORING

The amount of ptosis can be determined by:
- The difference in MRD1 of the two sides in unilateral cases.
- The difference from normal in bilateral cases gives the amount of ptosis.

Grading

- *Mild ptosis:* ≤2 mm
- *Moderate ptosis:* 3 mm
- *Severe ptosis:* ≥4 mm

Table 1: Differences between congenital and acquired ptosis.

Parameters	Congenital ptosis	Acquired ptosis
MRD1	Mild-to-severe ptosis	Mild-to-severe ptosis
Upper eyelid crease	Weak or absent crease in normal position	Higher than normal crease
LPS function	Reduced	Near normal
Downgaze	Eyelid lag (lid lag sign)	Eyelid drop
Palpebral aperture	Greater in downgaze	Less in downgaze

(LPS: levator palpebrae superioris; MRD: margin-reflex distance)

Table 2: Classification of ptosis based on pathogenesis.

Type	Mechanism	Example
Myogenic	• Maldevelopment of elevators • Myopathic conditions involving the LPS or myoneural junction • Direct damage to LPS or myoneural junctions	• Congenital simple ptosis • Blepharophimosis syndrome • Double elevator palsy • Congenital ocular fibrosis syndrome • Chronic progressive external ophthalmoplegia • Oculopharyngeal dystrophy • Muscular dystrophy • Traumatic
Neurologic	• Dysfunction of the 3rd cranial nerve • Dysfunction of sympathetic innervation to Müller muscle • Aberrant regeneration after oculomotor nerve palsies	• Oculomotor nerve palsy • Horner syndrome • Myasthenia gravis • Marcus Gunn jaw-winking phenomenon
Aponeurotic	• Dehiscence in the central part of the aponeurosis • Disinsertion of the aponeurosis from the tarsus • Thinning and stretching, termed attenuation or rarefaction, of the aponeurosis attenuation or rarefaction, of the aponeurosis	• Involutional (aponeurosis dehiscence) • Post-traumatic • Postsurgical blepharochalasis • Chronic, recurrent edema • Pregnancy • Chronic ocular inflammation • Rigid contact lens wear
Mechanical	• Excessive weight	• Dermatochalasis • Eyelid mass • Giant papillae/VKC • Multiple chalazion • Orbital mass • Scarring

(LPS: levator palpebrae superioris; VKC: vernal keratoconjunctivitis)

MANAGEMENT

The aim of the surgery is to lift the ptotic lid above the pupillary aperture when the eyes are in the primary position. The height of the two lids regardless of whether the ptosis is unilateral or bilateral should be equal. There should also be adequate mobility of the lid when blinking, a normal lid fold, and no diplopia. The surgical procedures and their indications are as follows:

- *Fasanella Servat operation:*
  - Mild ptosis (≤2 mm)
  - Levator action >10 mm
  - Well-defined lid fold—no excess skin
- *Levator resection:*
  - Mild/moderate ptosis
  - Levator action ≥4 mm
- *Brow suspension ptosis repair:*
  - Severe ptosis
  - Levator action <4 mm
  - Jaw-winking ptosis or blepharophimosis syndrome

The treatment of congenital ptosis has been described in detail in chapter congenital ptosis (short case). The treatment of acquired ptosis depends upon the cause.

VIVA QUESTIONS

Q.1. What are visual problems due to ptosis?
Ans. Ptosis is a common cause of reversible peripheral visual loss. Although the superior visual field is most often involved, central vision can also be affected. Patients with ptosis complain of difficulty with reading because the ptosis worsens in downgaze. Ptosis has also been shown to decrease the overall amount of light reaching the macula and therefore can reduce visual acuity, especially at night.
- The restricted peripheral visual field is a contraindication for issuing of driving license and jobs requiring broader fields in western countries. Visual fields <10 degrees in the better eye with the best correction are considered as legal blindness.

Q.2. What is the normal position of upper lid?
Ans. The vertical interpalpebral fissure is measured at the widest point between the lower eyelid and the upper eyelid. Normally, the UL should cover 1/6th or 2 mm of the cornea and lower lid should just touch the limbus.

Q.3. Classification of ptosis.
Ans. Ptosis can be classified as following:
- *Based on onset:* Congenital or acquired
- *Based on etiopathogenesis:* Myogenic, aponeurotic, neurogenic, mechanical, and traumatic

The most common type of congenital ptosis results from a poorly developed levator muscle LPS (myogenic). The most common type of acquired ptosis is that caused by stretching or disinsertion of the levator aponeurosis (aponeurotic).

Q.4. Differentiate between congenital and acquired ptosis
Ans. *See* **Table 1**.

Q.5. What is blepharophimosis epicanthus inversus ptosis syndrome (BPES)?
Ans. Details in short cases.

Q.6. What is Bell's phenomenon and its grading?
Ans. See examination.

Q.7. Explain the importance of Hering's law in ptosis.
Ans. In cases with bilateral ptosis and with one side having marked ptosis compared to the other side, following surgical correction on the greater ptotic side, the side with minimal ptosis may droop more. This is due to the Hering's law. This is important to predict the postoperative results of ptosis surgery. Patient has to be warned that the contralateral eye may droop following correction of the greater ptotic lid to avoid any postoperative unrealistic expectation by the patient.

Q.8. What should be the sequence of surgery if ptosis and strabismus coexist?
Ans. As correction of the strabismus may relieve the ptosis, strabismus surgery should be performed before treatment of ptosis. An exception may be made for cosmetically acceptable strabismus for which only ptosis needs to be treated. If the patient has horizontal strabismus with ptosis,

surgery for both strabismus and ptosis can be performed at the same sitting because the result of one is unlikely to influence the result of the other.

Q.9. How to demonstrate and grade Marcus Gunn jaw-winking?

Ans. Synkinesis is best demonstrated by having the patient move the jaw to the opposite side of the ptotic eye, but widely opening the mouth or moving the jaw forward would also elevate the eyelid.

Grading of Marcus Gunn jaw-winking phenomenon is based on the amplitude of lid movement:
- *Mild:* ≤2 mm
- *Moderate:* 3–6 mm
- *Severe:* ≥7 mm

Q.10. What are the other ancillary tests that should be done in ptosis?

Ans.
- *Visual field testing* with the eyelids untaped (in the natural, ptotic state) and taped (artificially elevated) helps determine the patient's level of functional visual impairment. Comparison of the taped and untaped visual fields gives an estimate of the superior visual field improvement that can be anticipated following surgery.
- Pharmacologic testing may be helpful in confirming the clinical diagnosis of Horner syndrome and MG. Fluctuating ptosis that seems to worsen with fatigue or prolonged upgaze, especially when accompanied by diplopia or other clinical signs of systemic MG.
- *Phenylephrine test:* One drop of phenylephrine 2.5% is installed in the upper fornix, stimulates the alpha-receptors in Müller muscle, causing its contraction and hence lid elevation. It is possible to demonstrate the potential outcome of surgery to a patient with a positive response to phenylephrine. One can also unmask a coexisting ptosis in the so-called normal eye, which appeared normal due to increased LPS stimulation (Hering's law).

Q.11. Explain the significance of pupillary examination in ptosis.

Ans.
- A small pupil (miotic) indicates Horner syndrome.
- A large pupil might be a sign of 3rd nerve palsy.
- In aberrant 3rd nerve palsy, the size of a pupil may change in different position of gaze.

Q.12. What is MRD3?

Ans. MRD3 is the distance from the ocular light reflex to the central UL margin when the patient looks in extreme upgaze. In unilateral ptosis, the difference between normal and abnormal MRD3 multiplied by three approximately shows the amount of LPS that must be resected.

Q.13. What are the bedside tests to rule out myasthenic ptosis?

Ans.
- *Fatigability:* Ask the patient to look up and down for about 1 minute to induce fatigue or sustained upgaze for 1 minute will achieve the same result. Progressive ptosis will ensue in a myasthenic patient. MRD1 is measured before and after these fatigue tests. Note that myasthenic patients might also develop diplopia with this test.
- *Cogan twitch sign:* The patient is first asked to look down for 15 seconds. A small upshoot of the eyelid is noted as a myasthenic patient then moves back to the primary position.
- *Ice-pack test:* Apply an ice-filled glove to the affected eye for 10 minutes. In a myasthenic patient, the ptosis improves by ≥2 mm.

Tests to confirm myasthenia:
- *Edrophonium chloride test or tensilon test:* This test is done in doubtful cases where an acquired ptosis due to MG is suspected. In adults, 2 mg of edrophonium is injected slowly in 15–30 seconds. The needle is left in situ and the remaining 8 mg is injected slowly if no untoward incident is observed within 1 minute. The effect occurs in 1–5 minutes and if myasthenia

is the cause, ptosis improves after edrophonium injection.
- *Acetylcholine receptor antibody test* when positive has 100% specificity.
- *Single-fiber electromyogram* (EMG: 100% sensitivity) and muscle biopsy are other more invasive tests that are helpful in identifying the site of pathology in myopathic and myasthenic ptosis.

Q.14. Postsurgical ptosis.

Ans. The incidence of ptosis after cataract surgery has been reported to be as high as 13%.[3] Although it can be seen following any intraocular surgery, it is often seen following cataract and vitreoretinal surgery. It can be *transient/acute ptosis* that resolves after surgery or *chronic/persistent ptosis* that persists after surgery.

Etiopathogenesis: Postsurgical ptosis can be due to the following:
- Myogenic due to the process of injecting anesthetic into the muscle or myotoxic effects of the anesthesia
- *Aponeurotic:* Due to use of a bridle suture or rigid lid speculum
- *Neurogenic:* Due to the prolonged effects of anesthetic on the neuromuscular junction, causes transient neurogenic ptosis
- *Mechanical:* May be due to edema or hematoma formation in the eyelid
- *Traumatic:* Due to blunt or sharp trauma to the levator aponeurosis

Prevention: Prevention of postsurgical ptosis is an essential part of the modern ocular surgery.
- Topical anesthesia eliminates all problems with local anesthesia including hematoma and edema of the eyelid and myotoxic effects on the levator.
- Use of ocular massage and compression decreases the amount of eyelid edema and hematoma formation.
- Limit surgical time and thus eyelid complications secondary to ocular inflammation or compressive effects of prolonged use of a lid speculum.
- Disuse of bridle sutures or a rigid speculum.
- Superior approach to surgery has a greater risk compared to a temporal approach.

Treatment: After a thorough examination in which the etiology is determined, one must decide whether to intervene. In most cases, postsurgical ptosis resolves with time, and therefore observation is the most prudent form of intervention. This form of ptosis typically improves within 6 months. Ptosis that does not resolve is typically secondary to aponeurotic dehiscence; this is readily repaired surgically.

Q.15. What is traumatic ptosis?

Ans. Trauma to the levator aponeurosis or the LPS muscle may also cause ptosis through myogenic, aponeurotic, neurogenic, or mechanical defects. Eyelid lacerations exposing preaponeurotic fat indicate that the orbital septum has been transected and suggest the possibility of damage to the levator aponeurosis. Exploration of the LPS muscle or aponeurosis is indicated in these patients if LPS function is diminished or ptosis is present. Orbital and neurosurgical procedures may also lead to traumatic ptosis. The ophthalmologist normally observes the patient for 6 months before considering surgical intervention.

Q.16. What is myogenic ptosis?

Ans. *Congenital myogenic ptosis:* This type of ptosis is due to dysgenesis of the LPS muscle. Congenital ptosis caused by maldevelopment of the LPS muscle is characterized by decreased LPS function, eyelid lag, and sometimes, lagophthalmos. The upper eyelid crease is often absent or poorly formed, especially in cases of more severe ptosis. Congenital myogenic ptosis associated with a poor Bell's phenomenon or with vertical strabismus may indicate concomitant maldevelopment of the superior rectus muscle (double elevator palsy, or monocular elevation deficiency).

Acquired myogenic ptosis: It is uncommon and results from localized or diffuse muscular diseases such as muscular dystrophy, chronic progressive external ophthalmoplegia, MG, or oculopharyngeal dystrophy. Surgical correction may be difficult, requiring frontalis sling procedures.

Q.17. What is aponeurotic ptosis?

Ans. It is the most common form of acquired ptosis. It results from stretching or dehiscence of the levator aponeurosis or disinsertion from its normal position. Common causes are involutional attenuation or repetitive traction on the eyelid, which may occur with frequent eye rubbing or prolonged use of rigid contact lenses. It can also occur due to intraocular surgery or eyelid surgery. The characteristic sign is a high or an absent upper eyelid crease secondary to upward displacement or loss of the insertion of LPS fibers into the skin. Thinning of the eyelid superior to the upper tarsal plate can also be present. LPS function in aponeurotic ptosis is usually normal (12–15 mm) and worsens in downgaze.

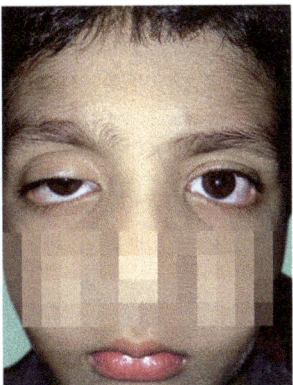

Fig. 4: Right-sided severe complicated ptosis.

Q.18. Describe neurogenic ptosis.

Ans. *Congenital neurogenic ptosis* is caused by innervational defects during embryonic development. It is rare and commonly associated with congenital 3rd CN palsy, Horner syndrome, or Marcus Gunn jaw-winking syndrome. It manifests as ptosis together with an inability to elevate, depress, or adduct the globe. The pupils may also be dilated.

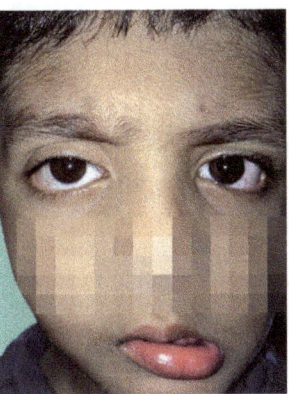

Fig. 5: Right-sided severe complicated ptosis with improvement in ptosis after chewing movement.

- *Congenital Horner syndrome* is a manifestation of an interrupted sympathetic nervous chain. It is associated with mild ptosis, miosis, anhidrosis, and decreased pigmentation of the iris on the involved side. Decreased sympathetic tone to the inferior tarsal muscle in the lower lid (the analog of the Müller muscle) results in elevation of the lower eyelid. This phenomenon is called *lower eyelid reverse ptosis*. The combined upper and lower eyelid ptosis decreases the vertical interpalpebral fissure and may confuse with enophthalmos. The pupillary miosis is most apparent in dim illumination.
- *Marcus Gunn jaw-winking syndrome* **(Figs. 4 and 5)** is the most common form of congenital synkinetic neurogenic ptosis.
- Some forms of Duane retraction syndrome also cause elevation of a ptotic eyelid with the movement of the globe.

Acquired neurogenic ptosis results from interruption of normally developed innervation and is most often secondary to an acquired 3rd nerve palsy, to an acquired Horner syndrome, or MG. Less common causes of acquired neurogenic ptosis include myotonic dystrophy, chronic progressive external ophthalmoplegia, Guillain-Barré syndrome, and oculopharyngeal dystrophy. Botulinum toxin injection in the forehead or orbital region to ameliorate benign essential blepharospasm can also lead to this form of ptosis.

Q.19. What is mechanical ptosis?

Ans. Mechanical ptosis usually refers to the condition in which an eyelid or orbital mass weighs or pulls down the upper eyelid. It can be caused by a congenital abnormality, such as a plexiform neurofibroma or hemangioma, or by an acquired neoplasm such as a large chalazion, skin carcinoma, or orbital mass. Postsurgical or post-traumatic edema can also cause temporary mechanical ptosis.

■ REFERENCES

1. Bowling B. Kanski's Clinical Ophthalmology: A Systematic Approach, 8th edition. Edinburgh: Elsevier; 2015.
2. Albert DM, Miller JW, Azar DT, Blodi BA. Albert and Jakobiec's Principles and Practice of Ophthalmology, 3rd edition. Philadelphia: Saunders/Elsevier; 2008.
3. Oral Y, Ozgur OR, Akcay L, Ozbas M, Dogan OK. Congenital ptosis, and amblyopia. J Pediatr Ophthalmol Strabismus. 2010;47:101-4.
4. Skuta GL, Cantor LB, Weiss JS. Basic and Clinical Science Course. Orbit, Eyelids, and Lacrimal System. San Francisco: American Academy of Ophthalmology; 2011-2012.

CONTRACTED SOCKET

Varsha Vashney, Aditi Dubey, Amar Pujari

■ INTRODUCTION

The contracted socket is defined as the shrinkage and shortening of all or a part of orbital tissues causing a decrease in depth of fornices and orbital volume ultimately leading to inability to retain prosthesis. It is characterized by extensive loss of conjunctival surface area, deep cicatrix formation, atrophy of the orbital fat, fornix contraction, and volume redistribution leading to postenucleation syndrome.

In examinations, it can be given as a long or short case.

■ HISTORY

Chief Complaints

Patient is usually an adult with history previous enucleation or evisceration surgery for any cause with or without prosthesis with complaints of:
- Poor cosmetic appearance
- Repeated extrusion of prosthesis
- Previously fitting prosthesis not fitting now
- The patient sometimes may be a child with a history of the underdeveloped socket.

History of Present Illness

Note about following factors:
- *Age at onset:* To differentiate between congenital and acquired anophthalmic socket
- *Preceding surgery:* Type of surgery performed and its details from the record if available
- *Progression:* Whether the implant or prosthesis was fitting earlier, and if the implant size has been changed over time.

History of Past Illness

Past history may give a clue about the probable cause, therefore following points must be noted in past history:
- Ocular insult such as chemical or radiation injury may be present
- Panophthalmitis requiring evisceration
- Severe ischemic ocular disease
- Cicatrizing conjunctival diseases may lead to progressive forniceal shortening
- Chronic inflammation and infection that might have led to the surgery
- Mutilating trauma to eye in which evisceration might have done to prevent sympathetic ophthalmia.

Surgical History

History of prior surgery such as enucleation/evisceration and multiple socket reconstruction and the details of the procedure can identify the reason for contracted socket.

History of Systemic Illness

History of hypertension, DM, vascular diseases, and any previous cerebrovascular accident must be noted carefully. Any neurological event may indicate the intracranial spread of the disease, for which the surgery have been done, such as infection or malignancy.

■ EXAMINATION

Systemic Examination

Most of the time the surgery is carried out to remove an intraocular malignancy in an advanced stage, for example, stage E retinoblastoma. Thus, a detailed systemic examination is carried out to rule out any systemic metastasis, especially the nervous system.

Ocular Examination

Ocular examination includes following:
- *Eyelids:*
  - Eyelid notches and abnormalities need to be looked out for. In long-standing cases, there may be stretching and lengthening of the lower lid, which would need to be tackled simultaneously.
  - Eyelid closure needs to be looked for too.
  - The lower eyelid should be evaluated for laxity. Lash position and lid margin position should be noted, as entropion can indicate socket contracture.
  - The superior sulcus should be checked for deepening and symmetry with the opposite side. The upper eyelid position should be noted for ptosis, and levator function should be evaluated.
- *Assessment of the socket:* The following parameters are evaluated:
  - General appearance and symmetry compared to the other normal side should be noted carefully.
  - *Area of the socket:* The area is assessed particularly the depth of the fornices. The depth of the fornices can be calculated by inserting a blunt lacrimal probe into each of the fornices and noting down the length to which it can be inserted. The inferior fornix is the most important as it has to support the prosthesis. The other fornices also need to be adequate to ensure the prosthesis fitting.
  - *Entropion*
  - *The volume of the socket:* The volume is assessed by noting the relative depth of the socket compared to the fellow eye. Another practical way of assessing the volume is to inject saline into the socket drop by drop till it overflows. The superior sulcus deformity and presence of ptosis with prosthesis and enophthalmos are also indicators of volume loss.
  - *Dry or wet socket:* Look for any discharge from the socket. There should be no active discharge from the socket. Dry fibrotic conjunctiva indicates a poorly vascularized socket.
  - *Movements:* The movements of the muscles are looked for. In a case of dermis fat grafting, suturing the muscles to the graft ensures better survival.
  - The tone of the orbicularis and tarsal sulci.
  - Cicatricial bands and degree of contracture within the socket.
  - Associated any bony contracture must be checked for.
  - Look for signs of inflammation, excessive mucus, giant papillary conjunctivitis under the upper eyelid, and pyogenic granulomas.
  - Palpation of the socket is done to for the presence or absence of an implant and the position of the implant should be noted.
  - *Prosthesis:* With the prosthetic in place, the patient should be evaluated for fit, size, and its appearance with respect to the fellow eye. The movement of the prosthetic should be evaluated compared to the other eye. The prosthetic can then be removed and evaluated for type, size, smoothness, and cleanness.

■ INVESTIGATIONS

- *Microbiological investigations* to rule out any infection
- *Radiological investigation* to look for any fracture in orbit or search of buried implant

GRADING

- *Gopal Krishna classification*:
  The soft tissue sockets were divided into five grades for the sake of convenience in the management of contracted sockets.
  1. *Grade-0:* Socket is lined with the healthy conjunctiva and has deep and well-formed fornices.
  2. *Grade-I:* Socket is characterized by the shallow lower fornix or shelving of the lower fornix. Here the lower fornix is converted into a downward sloping shelf, which pushes the lower lid down and out, preventing retention of an artificial eye. Common causes are physical injuries, endophthalmitis, and retinoblastoma.
  3. *Grade-II:* Socket is characterized by the loss of the upper and lower fornices. The common causes are physical injuries, endophthalmitis, panophthalmitis, and retinoblastomas.
  4. *Grade-III:* Socket is characterized by the loss of the upper, lower, medial, and lateral fornices. Common causes are chemical injuries and panophthalmitis.
  5. *Grade-IV:* Socket is characterized by the loss of all the fornices and reduction of a palpebral aperture in horizontal and vertical dimensions. Common causes are chemical injuries and panophthalmitis.
  6. *Grade-V:* In some cases, there is the recurrence of contraction of the socket after repeated trial of reconstruction. Common causes are thermal and chemical injuries of the eye.
- *Byron Smith classification:* Socket contraction may also be graded as follows:
  - *Mild:* Includes grade I and II where only one fornix is involved and there is a shortening of the posterior lamella of the lids.
  - *Moderate:* Includes grade III where both superior and inferior fornices are involved.
  - *Severe:* Comprises cases in which all fornices are involved along with phimosis of palpebral aperture.
  - *Malignant contracted socket:* It is the most severe variety of contracted socket *and associated bony contraction,* resulting from severe trauma or multiple surgeries.

Table 1: Morphological classification of contracted socket.

Type	Examples
Anophthalmic contracted socket	Most common seen after enucleation and evisceration surgery
Ophthalmic contracted socket	Following chemical and irradiation injury
Microphthalmic contracted socket	In association with microphthalmos and microcornea
Hypoplastic contracted socket	Congenital under development of bony socket

- *Morphological classification: Guibor* has classified clinically contracted socket into four morphological types as shown in **Table 1**.

TREATMENT

The primary aim of management is to create a socket so as to maintain a prosthesis with a good cosmetic appearance. Before commencing a definitive therapy, it is necessary to identify, classify, and eliminate any precipitating factors leading to contracture.

General considerations before socket reconstruction are as follows:
- Informed consent must be obtained.
- The prognosis and aim of surgery must be well explained.
- In cases oral mucosa grafting is planned, the patient should have mouthwashes started at least 2 weeks prior to the surgery.
- Ensure the that the socket is free of any infection.
- *Mild contracted socket:* This can usually be managed by deepening the inferior fornix with fornix formation sutures.
- *Management of moderate-to-severe contracted socket:* These cases are usually managed with a graft. Grafts that can be used for socket reconstruction include mucosa, split skin, and dermis—fat grafts. The socket needs to be healthy and vascularized for the grafts to take up. For mucous membrane grafts, mucus can be taken from buccal cavity

- (lip or cheek), rectum, or vagina. The buccal cavity is preferred as it is easy to access.
- *Management of severe contracted socket:* These cases usually require both area and volume replacement thus a composite graft is required. The commonly used graft is the dermis fat graft wherein the fat provides the volume and the dermis provides the surface area of the socket. The graft is taken from the hip. Although autogenous dermis fat orbital implantation is an effective means of orbital reconstruction, there is a 30% chance of atrophy of at least half of the graft volume when it is implanted in an avascular socket. Introducing a pedicle flap into the orbit as a vascular bed for an autogenous dermis fat graft may increase the prospect of graft survival, as well as supply additional volume to fill the socket. Temporalis muscle graft is supplied by a superficial temporal artery, a branch of an external carotid artery and it can be used as a pedicle graft.
- *Treatment of moist socket:* Partial thickness mucous membrane grafts are more susceptible to shrinkage and contracture. Full thickness mucous membrane contracts less and may be obtained with minimal postoperative complications at the donor site. However, mucosal contracture and submucosal scar formation increase with the size of the oral mucous membrane harvested and mucous membrane lacks the rigidity needed for grafting the palpebral surface. A full thickness mucous membrane graft is obtained from oral mucosa of cheeks and lips (most common), hard palate, preputial skin, and the skin of labia. The graft should be 40–50% larger than anticipated to allow for subsequent contracture with healing. It is helpful to harvest the graft at the beginning of the procedure so that it can be soaked in antibiotic solution before use.

Amniotic membrane can also be used instead of the mucosa. It has less patient morbidity, faster recovery, and better fitting of a prosthesis. No contracture is observed with an amniotic membrane as against mucous membrane. It is cheap and easily available and has no significant complications associated with it.

- *Treatment of dry socket:* The socket is lined with a split thickness skin graft in these cases. The skin graft is placed around an orbital mould with the epithelial surface toward it and perforations are made in the graft. The mould is sutured into the socket. After 1-month, the graft is split open in the area of palpebral fissure. The mould is kept for at least 4 months after which a permanent prosthesis is placed.
- *Management of recalcitrant cases:* A socket that has undergone multiple unsuccessful operations and has excessive scar tissue is unlikely to benefit from further repair. For such sockets, exenteration of the eyelid and residual socket material to create a cavity into which a prosthesis is fitted can be done. Optical methods to improve the appearance includes spectacle prosthesis or smoked lenses, plus or minus lenses to magnify a micro-ophthalmic socket to minimize buphthalmic socket, prisms to change the apparent horizontal or vertical position of malpositioned prosthesis or socket.

Management can also depend on volume or surface loss.
Volume: Implants—porous or non porous, dermis fat graft, fornix formation suture
Surface: AMG, MMG, autologous serum
Volume and surface: Dermis fat graft

VIVA QUESTIONS

Q.1. What are the causes of contracted socket?
Ans. Causes of contracted socket can be congenital or acquired **(Table 2)**.
- *Congenital:* Conditions such as microphthalmos **(Fig. 1)** or congenital anophthalmos **(Fig. 2)** usually lead to a contracted socket as the stimulus of the eyeball is essential for healthy growth of the orbit.
- *Acquired:* Acquired causes are described here:
  - *Enucleation without implant:* A poorly done enucleation, particularly without implant, can lead to a contracted socket. This is more so in children as in the absence of the stimulus of either eyeball or implant, there is a

Table 2: Mechanism of contracted socket.

Etiology	Factors
Etiology-related	Alkali burns, radiation therapy leading to severe damage to the socket and fibrosis
Surgery-related	• Fibrosis from the initial injury • *Poor surgical techniques:* Extensive dissection of the orbital tissue • *No implant or undersized implant:* In children, the absence of the stimulus of either eyeball or implant can lead to bony contraction as well • Excessive sacrifice of the conjunctiva and Tenon capsule • Traumatic dissection within the socket leading to scar tissue • Multiple socket operations
Site-related	• Poor vascular supply • Severe ischemic ocular disease in the past • Cicatrizing conjunctival diseases • Chronic inflammation and infection
Implant and prosthesis-related	• Undersized implant • Implant migration • Implant exposure • *Not wearing a conformer/prosthesis:* Confirmer keeps the fornices stretched and prevents fornicial shallowing • Ill-fitting prosthesis

bony contraction as well. The implant needs to be carefully selected, both in terms of size and material.
- *Delay in use of conformer:* In both enucleation and evisceration procedures, conformer should be fitted immediately. This keeps the fornices stretched and prevents fornicial shallowing. The conformer should be on the correct side, of adequate size, and have multiple holes to allow flushing and drainage of secretions.
- *Trauma:* Extensive lacerations of the lids and orbital tissue can lead to tissue loss and fibrosis resulting in socket contraction. Injuries with alkali/acid can also cause fibrosis.
- *Radiotherapy:* Postoperative radiotherapy for retinoblastoma can cause fibrosis and a grossly contracted socket. These sockets are usually poorly vascularized and difficult to reconstruct.
• *Infection:* Socket/implant infection can lead sloughing of the conjunctiva and shortening of the fornices.

Q.2. What precautions should be taken to prevent contracted socket?

Ans. Socket contraction should be prevented as far as possible by taking some precautions at the primary surgery.
• Proper dissection at the time of initial procedure

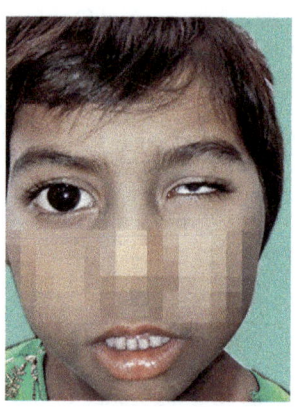

Fig. 1: Unilateral microphthalmia with contracted socket.

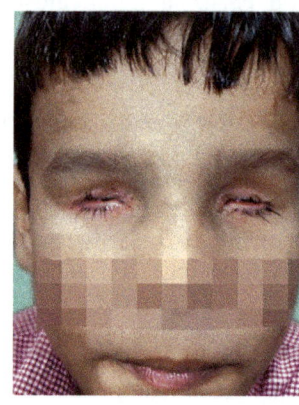

Fig. 2: Bilateral anophthalmia with contracted socket.

- Preserving as much conjunctiva and Tenon capsule as possible during enucleation
- Secure closure of all layers over the implant without tension or superior displacement of the inferior fornix
- Avoidance of ill-fitting or roughened prosthesis as it may cause a more rapid contracture, symblepharon formation, and total abandonment of prosthesis
- Elimination of any source of chronic infection that may arise from lid margin, socket, canaliculi, lacrimal sac, chemical, or thermal injury
- Identification of conjunctival cicatrizing diseases such as pemphigoid, Stevens–Johnson syndrome
- Avoidance of oversized prosthesis so as to prevent migration of the implant into the inferior fornix and thereby obliteration of inferior cul-de-sac
- *Conformer:* A conformer should always be placed at the end of the surgery. This is replaced by the prosthetic eye 4–6 weeks later. If the socket has undergone prior irradiation, chemical, or thermal injury, the conformer has to be left for a much longer time.
- Radiotherapy if required should be used with fractionation of dose.

Q.3. What are the characteristics of an ideal orbital implant?

Ans. Ideal orbital implant should be:
- Light weight
- Nonantigenic
- Inert
- Biocompatible
- Affordable
- Mimic the motility of the normal globe
- Minimum complications such as infection, extrusion, and migration

Q.4. Types of orbital implants.

Ans. Presently all implants are broadly classified as:
- *Nonintegrated implants:* Are nonporous and are not integrated and have no direct muscle attachment, for example, silicon and acrylic implants
- *Semi-integrated implants:* Allow attachment of muscle in tunnels on the anterior surface for better motility. Examples include Allens, Iowa, etc.
- *Biointegrated implants:* These allow fibrovascular ingrowth in the porous channels and result in direct biological integration with orbital contents. Examples include hydroxyapatite, porous polyethylene implants, aluminum oxide, and alpha sphere.
- *Biogenic implants:* An autograft or allograft of natural tissue with direct biological integration with orbital structures but not prosthesis. For example, dermis fat graft, mucous membrane graft.

Porous implants are presently the material of choice as vascularization leads to the integration of implants. But porous implants are significantly more expensive than acrylic and silicon implants.

Q.5. Postenucleation socket syndrome/volume deficient socket.

Ans. Typically seen following the enucleation and characterized by following:
- Enophthalmos
- An upper eyelid sulcus deformity
- Ptosis or eyelid retraction
- Laxity of the lower eyelid
- A backward tilt of the ocular prosthesis
- Unhappy with cosmetic appearance

■ **BIBLIOGRAPHY**

1. Krishna G. Contracted sockets-I (Aetiology and types). Indian J Ophthalmol. 1980;28:117-20.
2. Nesi FA, Lisman RD, Levine MR. Evaluation and current concepts in the management of anophthalmic socket. Smith's Ophthalmic Plastic and Reconstructive Surgery, 2nd edition. US: Mosby; 1998. pp. 1079-124.

BLOWOUT FRACTURE OF ORBIT

Aditi Dubey, Sanjana M

■ INTRODUCTION

Orbital injury forms an important aspect of ocular trauma. The blowout fracture is the most common type of orbital fracture. The term pure orbital blowout fracture is used to describe fracture of the orbital floor, the medial wall or both, with an intact bony margin and intact posterior ledge and orbital strut. The term impure orbital blowout fracture is used when such fractures occur in conjunction with a fracture of the orbital rim. The most common site for orbital blowout fracture is the posteromedial aspect of the orbital floor medial to the infraorbital neurovascular bundle where the maxillary bone is very thin (0.25–0.50 mm). As the lamina papyracea is also very thin, the medial orbital wall is also prone to fracture, either in isolation or in association with a fracture of the orbital floor or other facial bones. In examinations, it can be given as a long case.

■ HISTORY

Chief complaints: It depends upon the duration following trauma, after which the patient presents. When the patient presents immediately following trauma, the complaints include:
- *Eyelid ecchymosis* (**Fig. 1**)/*periorbital hematoma:* Usually present but signs may be absent as seen in the "white-eyed blowout fracture"

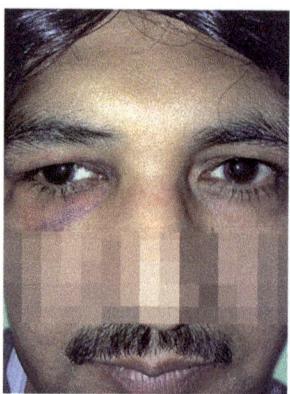

Fig. 1: Orbital floor fracture.

- *Subcutaneous emphysema:* If a blowout fracture communicates with an air-filled sinus, it may result in emphysema. Commonly seen in medial orbital wall blowout fractures. It may result in palpable crepitus. Patients should be advised not to blow their nose.
- Proptosis of variable degree can also be seen initially due to orbital edema and hemorrhage.
- Other complaints such as epistaxis, pain, and loss of vision can be there depending on the damage to adjacent structures.
- Diplopia can be there due to muscle entrapment.
- Small or inward displacement of an eyeball (enophthalmos) can be there due to soft tissue prolapse into adjacent sinuses.
- In cases, where the presentation is delayed, the complaints are usually of a small or shrunken eyeball, limitation of movements, or diplopia.
- *Oculocardiac reflex:* Bradycardia

History of Present Illness

A detailed history regarding mode of injury should be taken to assess the mechanism and extent of an injury. In cases of delayed presentation, progression must be noted carefully. The decision for surgical intervention largely depends upon the course of the symptoms over time.

Past history: Past history of poor vision in the affected eye, repeated trauma should be noted.

Systemic history: Past history of DM, hypertension, bleeding disorders, and neurological problems must be noted. This will be helpful while planning surgery, especially under general anesthesia.

■ EXAMINATION

Systemic examination: General condition of a patient and another nonocular injury should be checked. Life-threatening injuries must be taken care of first before proceeding for ocular examination.

Ocular examination: Following points must be noted in a case of orbital fracture.

Visual acuity: Visual acuity at presentation has medicolegal importance in ocular trauma cases. Uncorrected as well as best corrected visual acuity must be noted in all cases of trauma.

Orbit

- Palpate orbital rim to look for deformity and crepitus. Subcutaneous emphysema with crepitus seen in fractures communicating with air-filled sinuses. The malar eminences should be palpated and any depression should be noted. The patient should be asked to open and close his mouth to rule out pain or trismus that may be associated with a zygomatic complex fracture.
- Paresthesia or sensory loss over ipsilateral lower lid, cheek, and upper lip pathognomonic. Neurosensory loss occurs in the area supplied by the infraorbital nerve. This occurs because the fracture extends along the infraorbital groove or canal injuring the infraorbital nerve. These sensory defects tend to resolve spontaneously with time but may get aggravated by surgery in the area.
- *Ocular motility:* Full orthoptic assessment should be performed in nine positions of gaze. Limitation of ocular motility can occur due to following causes:
  - Entrapment of orbital contents such as connective tissue, septa, extraocular muscle (inferior rectus most commonly) within the fracture
  - Hematoma/edema in the orbital fat adjacent to the fracture
  - Hematoma or contusion of the extraocular muscle itself
  - Palsy of an extraocular muscle due to neuronal damage
  - Volkmann's ischemic contracture of an entrapped extraocular muscle
  - Inferior rectus muscle leads to motility restriction especially in upgaze (vertical diplopia)

Eyelid: Pseudoptosis occurs due to loss of support. Look for other signs of trauma such as laceration or scar.

Conjunctiva: Subconjunctival hemorrhage and conjunctival chamois may be there.

Cornea: Trauma can lead to corneal abrasion and corneal laceration.

Iris and anterior chamber: Trauma may be associated with iritis, miosis or mydriasis, and hyphema

Pupil: Presence of RAPD indicates optic nerve injury that needs urgent intervention in the form of pulse steroid therapy

Lens: Trauma may be associated with subluxation and dislocation of lens

Fundus: Look for effects of trauma such as dialysis, tear, retinal detachment, or vitreous hemorrhage

Special Tests

- *Hertel exophthalmometer:* Exophthalmometry is done to document enophthalmos.
- *Force duction test (FDT):* FDT is useful in determining whether dysmotility is restrictive or paralytic. In a blowout fracture with inferior rectus, entrapment FDT is "positive" indicating a mechanical cause.
- *Force generation test (FGT):* In testing force generation, the muscle insertion is grasped and the patient is asked to look into the muscle's field of action. A paretic muscle will feel weak when compared with the fellow eye.
- *Diplopia charting:* With red-green glass, diplopia charting with streak light shows diplopia worsening in upgaze.
- *Hess screen or Lee screen tests* were done document the muscle involved.

■ INVESTIGATIONS

- *Plain X-rays:* Easily available and cost-effective imaging modality. *Water's view* is the most useful projection for detecting an orbital floor fracture. X-ray shows bone discontinuity in the orbital floor with herniation of soft tissue in maxillary antrum seen as *"hanging drop" sign.*
- *CT scanning:* CT gives the detailed visualization of bony and soft tissue injury where entrapment of muscle can be appreciated **(Fig. 2)**. Coronal sections are particularly useful and can show antral soft tissue densities, such as prolapsed orbital fat, extraocular muscle, or hematoma with 3D reconstruction.

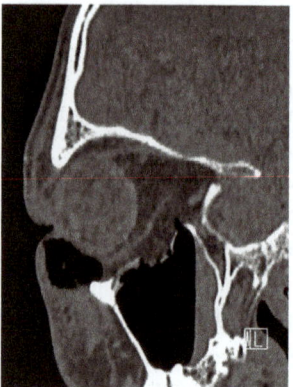

Fig. 2: Fracture of orbital floor on a computed tomography (CT) scan.

- *MRI:* It can be utilized when there is the need for greater soft tissue evaluation. MRI is insufficient in assessing the bony structures and therefore needs to be combined with CT.

MANAGEMENT

Treatment includes both medical and surgical management:
- *Medical management/observation:* It consists of oral antibiotics, analgesics, and a short course of oral prednisone. Oral steroid benefits the patient by reducing the edema of the orbit and muscle. This also may allow for a more thorough assessment of the relative contribution to enophthalmos or entrapment from the fracture versus that from edema. Medical management is indicated in following conditions:
  - No significant enophthalmos (<2 mm)
  - Lack of marked hypo-ophthalmos
  - Absence of an entrapped muscle or tissue
  - Fracture <50% of the floor
  - No diplopia
  - The patient must be advised to avoid nose blowing, to avoid creating, or worsening orbital emphysema. Nasal decongestants can be used if not contraindicated. Ice packs may be applied for initial 48 hours to reduce the pain and tissue edema.
- *Surgical treatment:* Surgical intervention is indicated in following cases:
  - *Immediate intervention:*
    • Diplopia present with CT evidence of an entrapped muscle or periorbital tissue and associated with a nonresolving oculocardiac reflex: Bradycardia, heart block, nausea, vomiting or syncope
    • "White-eyed blow-out fracture." Young patients (<18 years), history of periocular trauma, little ecchymosis or edema (white eye), marked extraocular motility vertical restriction, and CT examination revealing an orbital floor fracture with entrapped muscle or perimuscular soft tissue
    • Early enophthalmos/hypoglobus causing facial asymmetry.
- *Within 2 weeks:* Patients with diplopia are usually observed for 2 weeks. If the diplopia resolves with a small fracture evident on CT, no surgical intervention is required. It is advisable to wait for 2–3 weeks for resolution of orbital edema/hematoma. However, surgery is indicated in the following scenario:
  - Symptomatic diplopia with positive forced ductions, evidence of an entrapped muscle or perimuscular soft tissue on CT examination, and minimal clinical improvement over time.
  - Large floor fracture causing latent enophthalmos
  - Significant hypo-ophthalmos
  - Progressive infraorbital hypoesthesia

Surgical principle: The basic steps of surgery includes assessing the orbital floor, releasing the soft tissue and muscle entrapment and strengthening the floor with use of implants.

The orbital floor can be approached through following ways:

Subciliary approach: Incision given 2–3 mm below the lash line. It has the advantage of better scar camouflage. The disadvantage is postoperative ectropion and lower lid retraction.

Subtarsal approach: Incision below tarsal plate over orbital rim. The advantage is it gives direct access to the floor with good exposure. The disadvantage is it leads cosmetically unacceptable scar.

Transconjunctival approach: Incision given in lower fornix 3 mm below the tarsal plate and can be combined with a lateral canthotomy for better exposure. The advantage is it gives no visible scar.

Transantral approach: Orbital floor reached via the maxillary sinus using Caldwell-Luc incision. It is a difficult technique and it is not a favored by an ophthalmologist.

Endoscopic approach: Transmaxillary and transnasal endoscopies have been described which eliminate the need for eyelid incisions and gives improved visualization of fractures. However, it is difficult and often clumsy.

The orbital floor is reinforced with either autogenous or synthetic implant **(Table 1)**. The surgeon should size the implant to cover the defect adequately and to prevent displacement or extrusion later. While cutting the implant, it should be tapered posteriorly to fit the orbital floor configuration.

Table 1: Examples of implant materials used in orbital floor repair.

Implant material	Advantage	Disadvantage
Membranous bone	Autogenous	• Morbidity at donor site • Extended operation time • Resorption unpredictable
Cartilage	Autogenous	• Morbidity at donor site • Extended operation time • Resorption unpredictable
Titanium mesh	Biocompatible stable	• Foreign material that remains in the body • Combination with bone recommended
Porous polyethylene (Medpore) sheets	Easy to shape and handle, Biocompatible stable	Foreign material that remains in the body
Silicon sheet	Easy-to-handle and cheap	Extrusion rates higher
Silastic sheet (Teflon)	Easy-to-shape and handle	Foreign body reaction and extrusion common

VIVA QUESTIONS

Q.1. What is a pure and impure blowout fracture?

Ans. A pure orbital blowout fracture is used to describe fracture of the orbital floor, the medial wall or both, with an intact bony orbital margin. Impure orbital blowout fracture is used when such fractures occur in conjunction with a fracture of the orbital rim.

Q.2. Most common site for the blowout fracture of orbit?

Ans. The *posteromedial aspect* of the orbital floor medial to the infraorbital neurovascular bundle where the maxillary bone is very thin (0.25–0.50 mm) is the most common site.

Q.3. What is the etiopathogenesis of blowout fracture?

Ans. There are two theories to explain the possible mechanism of orbital fracture:
1. *Retropulsion theory/hydraulic theory:* It states that the backward displacement of the globe caused by a blunt nonpenetrating object raises the intraorbital pressure sufficiently to fracture the posteromedial orbital floor and/or the lamina papyracea of the ethmoid.
2. *Buckling theory/transmission theory:* A transient deformation of the orbital rim transmits the force of injury directly to the orbital wall. During the course of injury, the force that is transmitted to bony walls of the orbit may also cause concussion ocular trauma leading to angle recession, hyphema, vitreous hemorrhage, commotio retinae, etc.

Q.4. Expanded orbit syndrome.

Ans. Multiple fractures in and around the orbit may lead roomy orbit with extensive prolapse of orbital tissues. This expansion can be seen in orbital fracture along with midfacial fracture as in tripod or Le Fort type III. Clinically patient has gross enophthalmos, inferior displacement of the globe (hypoglobus), deep superior sulcus, eyelid asymmetry, and diplopia.

Q.5. What are the features of medial wall fracture?

Ans. Blowout fracture of a medial wall is much less common than a floor and usually seen along with nasoethmoid fractures rather than as an isolated entity. Horizontal diplopia is usually the primary complaint when medial orbital tissues are involved. However, a vertical or oblique component can also be found in such cases.

Q.6. What is "white-eyed" blowout fracture?

Ans. The bones of a child's orbit are more elastic than adults. Thus, injury in children causes more anteroposterior buckling creating a fracture with overlapping segments. This leads to "trapdoor-type" fracture where prolapsed orbital tissue is caught in the fracture site leading to severe motility restriction and diplopia in absence of marked congestion or ecchymosis. The condition is also called the "white-eyed" blowout fracture. It is seen in orbital blowout fracture in children.

Q.7. Boundaries of the orbital floor and contents.

Ans.
- The adult orbital floor is formed by the maxillary, zygomatic bones anteriorly, and palatine bones posteriorly.
- Orbital floor measures about 35–40 mm anteroposteriorly and it is the shortest of all the walls. It forms the roof of the maxillary sinus.
- The floor of the orbit contains infra-orbital groove that forms infraorbital foramen. Infraorbital nerve, a branch of the maxillary division of trigeminal nerve passes through the groove, providing sensory innervations to the ipsilateral orbital floor, mid face, and posterior upper gingival area. The infraorbital artery, a branch of the maxillary artery, and the infraorbital vein also are found within the infraorbital groove.

Q.8. What are common complications of floor repair surgery?

Ans.
- Intraoperative bleeding
- Residual or new-onset diplopia
- Extraocular muscle dysfunction
- Postoperative neuralgia
- Residual enophthalmos
- Implant extrusion
- Possible loss of vision.

Q.9. How to treat persistent diplopia?

Ans. Some patients may have persistent diplopia even after adequate surgical repair of floor fracture. Diplopias in primary gaze and in downgaze (functional gaze) are more troublesome. Such cases will require muscle surgery. To correct diplopia in down gaze, "Reverse Knapp procedure" is performed placing medial and lateral recti behind the inferior rectus muscle. Fresnel prisms can be employed in selective cases.

Q.10. How to treat postoperatively cosmetically unacceptable enophthalmos?

Ans. A repeat surgery with adequate size orbital implant, if the downward sinking of an eye along with enophthalmos is unacceptable to patient, may have to be done. The pseudo-ptosis can be corrected with Müllerectomy, which will increase palpebral height.

BIBLIOGRAPHY

1. Burnstine MA. Clinical recommendations for repair of isolated orbital floor fractures: An evidence-based analysis. Ophthalmology. 2002;109(7):1207-10.
2. Principles and Practice of Ophthalmology: Albert and Jakobeic, Vol. 6, 2nd edition, Pgs. 5303-9.
3. Smith B, Regan WF. Blowout fracture of the orbit (mechanism and correction of internal orbital fracture). Am J Ophthalmol. 1957;44:733-9.
4. Yadav P, Pushker N, Bajaj M, Chandra M, Shrey D, Lohiya P. Orbital blow out fracture. DOS Times. 2008;8(14):2.

THYROID-ASSOCIATED OPHTHALMOPATHY

Aditi Dubey, Prafulla Kumar Maharana

INTRODUCTION

Thyroid-associated ophthalmopathy (TAO) is the most common cause of proptosis in adults. TAO is a self-limiting autoimmune disease associated mainly with hyperthyroidism, but also with hypothyroid and euthyroid states. Although it can affect any age, it most commonly presents during the fourth and fifth decades of life. It is one of the most important long case given in practical examinations. In TED, it is important to record a proper history and elicit the signs associated with it.

HISTORY

Demography

It can affect any age group. Patients with TAO are more likely to be female by a 2:1 ratio, following the usual predominance of autoimmunity in women. However, male Graves' disease are at the same, if not higher, risk of TAO development, which is usually of a more severe form and occurs at a more advanced age than in their female counterparts. Asians are having a lower likelihood of developing the disease than Europeans.[1,2]

Chief Complaints

A case of TAO can present with following complaints:
- Excessive lacrimation, a gritty sensation, discomfort, and photophobia are often present in early course of the disease.
- Bilateral upper lid retraction is the most common presenting feature of the thyroid eye disease.
- Bilateral proptosis can also be the presenting feature.
- At times, it may be detected accidentally or referred by the endocrinologist.
- Decrease in visual acuity can be a presenting feature when it is associated with optic nerve compression, exposure keratopathy, or induced astigmatism due to globe compression.
- Patients may also complain of general symptoms such as weight loss, sweating, heat intolerance, weakness, fatigue, and palpitation along with ophthalmic complains.

Approximately 5–10% of Graves' orbitopathy patients are euthyroid at presentation and some of them may not have a history of thyroid dysfunction. In approximately 40% of patients with TAO, the signs of the eye disease occur simultaneously with the first symptoms of hyperthyroidism.

History of Present Illness

The history of present illness must include all the points described in the chapter of proptosis.
- The patient of TED presents with the bilateral upper lid retraction and or exophthalmos. A careful history can reveal history of irritation, foreign body sensation, watering, and recurrent lid edema in past that is often ignored by the patient. As the disease progresses, the full blown picture of TED develops.
- Cigarette smoking has been considered the strongest risk factor for developing TED. Hence, a detailed history of smoking must be asked.
- Females are having more predominance in TED (2:1). However, males presents with more severe disease and usually at a later age.
- Patient may be in hyperthyroid or hypothyroid state, but 5–10% cases are euthyroid at the time of presentation.

Past History

- History of DM, hypertension, asthma, and thyroid abnormality should be noted.
- In a case of diagnosed TAO, past history of steroid, radiotherapy, orbital decompression, or any thyroidectomy must be recorded.

Personal History

Personal history of alcohol intake, smoking, tobacco chewing or any other if present should be noted, because smoking is considered as important risk factor for the TED.

EXAMINATION

Examination of a case of TAO is similar to that of a case of proptosis. Salient features of TAO are described here.

Systemic Examination

General examination may show the signs of hyperthyroidism such as tachycardia, fine hand tremor, warm and sweaty skin, pretibial myxedema, finger clubbing, alopecia, and vitiligo. A detailed examination of cardiovascular system, respiratory system, gastrointestinal system, and central nervous system has to be done as these systems get affected by Graves' disease. Check for neck swelling.

Ophthalmic Examination

The ocular examination is similar to a case of proptosis. Important points to note are as follows:
- Proptosis is usually axial.
- Globes are mostly aligned.
- The most characteristic signs are eyelid erythema and swelling, caruncular, and conjunctival injection and edema **(Fig. 1)**.
- Some patients may have restriction of the eye movements leading to squint. The most commonly affected muscle is inferior rectus followed by medial, superior, levator, and lateral rectus **(Fig. 2)**. The muscles affected result in ocular misalignment and diplopia. Strabismus is also common, and it often presents as hypotropia or esotropia.
- *Eyelid:* Various lid signs can be seen in thyroid ophthalmopathy **(Table 1)**. All signs may not be present in a single patient. Lid retraction, also known as Dalrymple sign, occurs most commonly as lid sign, in about 37–92% of patients **(Fig. 3)**.
- Eyelashes are usually normal.
- Conjunctiva may show mild congestion due to the dry eye caused by the excessive evaporation of the tears due to the lid retraction.
- Inflammation along recti muscle (tendonitis) can be an early sign of the disease.
  - Cornea may have exposure keratopathy. Causes of exposure keratopathy include:
    ◆ Inadequate eyelid closure leading to excessive moisture loss as a consequence of proptosis and eyelid dysfunction
    ◆ Diminished tear production resulting from lacrimal gland infiltration
    ◆ Lagophthalmos from proptosis
    ◆ Loss of Bell's phenomenon from inferior rectus infiltration
- Pupillary reaction may or may not be normal. Presence of RAPD or APD suggests optic nerve compression.
- Variable IOP can be there in different gazes due to restrictive myopathy. An IOP rise >8 mm Hg on upgaze is significant and warrant treatment. Glaucoma can also result from decreased episcleral venous outflow.
- Lens do not show any specific changes.
- Fundus examination may show signs of globe compression—disc edema and macular folds.

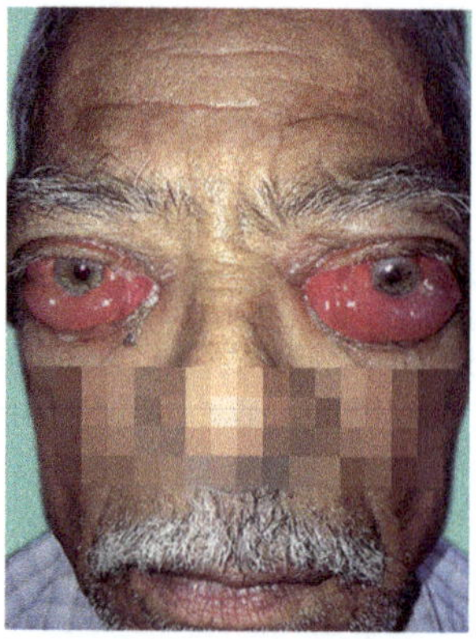

Fig. 1: Severe bilateral proptosis due to thyroid eye disease.

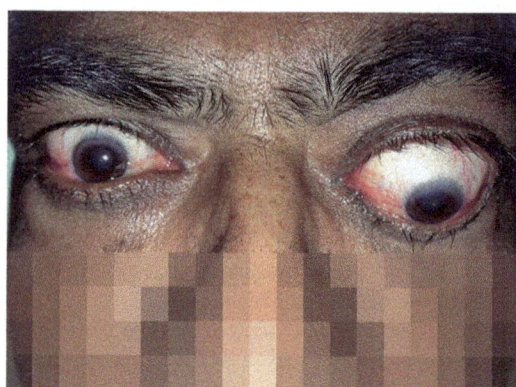

Fig. 2: Thyroid eye disease with disproportionate proptosis and inferior dystopia in the left eye.

Table 1: Lid signs in proptosis.

Sign	Description
Abadie's sign	Elevator muscle of upper eyelid is spastic
Ballett's sign	Paralysis of one or more extraocular muscle (EOM)
Beck's sign	Abnormal intense pulsation of retina's arteries
Boston's sign	Jerky movements of upper lid on lower gaze
Cowen's sign	Extensive hippus of consensual pupillary reflex
Dalrymple's sign	Upper eyelid retraction
Enroth's sign	Edema especially of the upper eyelid
Gifford's sign	Difficulty in eversion of upper lid
Goldzieher's sign	Deep injection of conjunctiva, especially temporal
Griffith's sign	Lower lid lag on upward gaze
Hertoghe's sign	Loss of eyebrows laterally
Jellinek's sign	Superior eyelid folds is hyperpigmented
Joffroy's sign	Absent creases in the forehead on upward gaze
Jendrassik's sign	Abduction and rotation of eyeball is limited also
Knies' sign	Uneven pupillary dilatation in dim light
Kocher's sign	Spasmodic retraction of upper lid on fixation
Loewi's sign	Quick mydriasis after instillation of 1:1,000 adrenaline
Mann's sign	Eyes seem to be situated at different levels because of tanned skin
Means' sign	Increased scleral show on upgaze (globe lag)
Moebius's sign	Lack of convergence
Payne/Trousseau sign	Dislocation of globe
Pochin's sign	Reduced amplitude of blinking
Rieseman's sign	Bruit over the eyelid
Movement's cap phenomenon	Eyeball movements are performed difficultly, abruptly and incompletely
Rosenbach's sign	Eyelids are animated by thin tremors when closed
Saiton's sign	Frontalis contraction after cessation of levator activity
Snellen-Rieseman's sign	When placing the stethoscope's capsule over closed eyelids a systolic murmur could be heard
Stellwag's sign	Incomplete and infrequent blinking
Suker's sign	Inability to maintain fixation on extreme lateral gaze
Tellas's sign	Inferior eyelid might be hyperpigmented
Topolanski's sign	Around insertion areas of the four rectus muscles of the eyeball a vascular band network is noticed and this network joins the four insertion points.
von Graefe's sign	Upper lid lag on downgaze
Wilder's sign	Jerking of the eye on movement from abduction to adduction

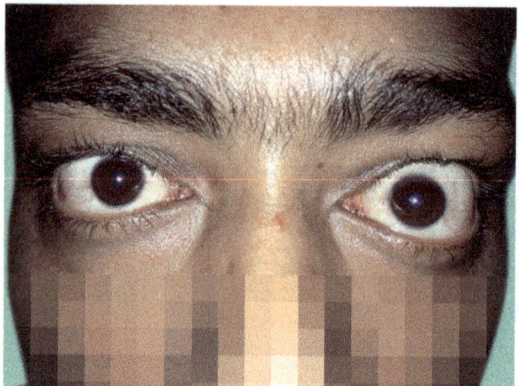

Fig. 3: Thyroid eye disease with lid retraction.

Compressive optic neuropathy occurs in <5% of patients with thyroid ophthalmopathy resulting in slowly progressive visual loss. It occurs due to compression from the oversized recti and orbital fat causing compartment syndrome at the apex of orbit. It is characterized by decrease in vision, color vision, contrast sensitivity, and relative afferent papillary defect. Visual loss may progress undetected due to insidious onset and subtlety of neuropathy. Risk factors for optic neuropathy include:
- Older age
- Smoking
- Male gender
- Significant strabismus with mild proptosis.
- *Visual field:* Central and inferior arcuate scotoma and generalized constriction may be seen in advanced cases ophthalmopathy.

■ DIFFERENTIAL DIAGNOSIS

The diagnosis is often straightforward. The characteristic signs and systemic signs are difficult to miss. However, in early course of the disease, following diseases may mimic TAO:
- Orbital myositis
- Nonspecific orbital inflammatory disease (NSOID)
- MG
- Chronic progressive external ophthalmoplegia
- Carotid-cavernous fistula
- Specific inflammatory orbitopathy
- Orbital tumors

- Lid retraction, characteristic of TAO can also be seen in number of other diseases as given here.

Upper Lid Retraction
- Congenital
- *Neurologic disorders:* Midbrain disease, hydrocephalus
- *Postsurgery:* Ptosis surgery, lid reconstruction
- Marcus Gunn phenomenon, faulty regeneration of CN III
- Parinaud syndrome
- Sympathomimetic drugs
- Cirrhosis

Lower Lid Retraction
- Idiopathic senile flaccidity of lower lid
- Post-traumatic impairment
- Congenital abnormality
- Postsurgical lesion—recession of the inferior rectus muscle and repair of a blowout fracture
- Facial nerve lesion

■ INVESTIGATIONS

Following investigations are carried out in a case of TAO:
- CBC, thyroid function test [Tri-iodothyronine (T3), free thyroxin (T4), serum thyroid-stimulating hormone (TSH), thyrotropin receptor antibodies (TRAb), ESR]
- *USG:* On cross-section, there is an increase in thickness of the extraocular muscles. USG of the globe and the orbit can help in visualization of the tendinous intersections. This also helps to differentiate between active and inactive disease. By comparing the muscle thickness, ultrasound may help in confirming the diagnosis in unilateral cases. It also helps in differentiating associated diseases presenting with similar clinical features.
- *CT scan:* Typical radiological features seen on CT are muscle belly enlargement that is classically described as "tendon sparing," an increase in orbital fat volume, and crowding of the optic nerve at the orbital apex in severe cases. It helps in assessing the relationship between the optic nerve and muscles at the apex that helps in planning for the surgical

intervention, if needed. CT is more sensitive than MRI in identifying enlarged extraocular muscles. As a standard, 2 mm cuts should be requested for, along with coronal and axial slices. Orbital fat is imaged in CT as a black, low-density area that contrasts with the higher density image of extraocular muscles and the optic nerve. CT scans allow for better delineation of the bony orbit and therefore are invaluable in planning orbital decompression.

- *MRI:* Demonstrates fusiform rectus enlargement and orbital fat expansion. It assesses water content in the muscles that correlates with the active inflammation. In the active phase, the extraocular muscles appear isointense in T1-weighted images and hyperintense in T2-weighted images, whereas in the chronic phase, they appear hypointense on T2-weighted images.
- Visual field testing is important for detecting early damage to the optic nerve due to apical crowding around the optic nerve. The changes on visual fields are reversible if the crowding is relieved early, either surgically or medically. Usually, the patterns of visual field loss vary, the most common being central, paracentral, and/or inferior.

CLASSIFICATION

Different classification systems have been proposed, however there is no consensus on the best way to classify TAO:
- *NO-SPECS classification:*
    - Proposed by Werner et al. and adopted by the American Thyroid Association **(Table 2)**
    - Based upon clinical presentation
    - *Limitation:* Relies on subjective evaluation, does not take into account the severity of manifestations, patient may fall into >1 particular class, may not progress in an orderly fashion from class 1 to class 6, and is relatively insensitive to subtle changes, hence less preferred.
- *RELIEF classification* of soft tissue signs and symptoms:
    R—Resistance to retropulsion
    E—Edema of conjunctiva and caruncle
    L—Lacrimal gland enlargement
    I—Injection over the horizontal rectus muscle insertions

Table 2: NO-SPECS classification of thyroid-associated ophthalmopathy.

Class	Grade	Clinical features
0		N—No signs symptoms
1		O—Only signs
2		S—Soft tissue involvement
	O	Absent
	A	Minimal
	B	Moderate
	C	Marked
3		P—Proptosis
	O	<23 mm
	A	23–24 mm
	B	25–27 mm
	C	≥28 mm
4		E—Extraocular muscle involvement
	O	Absent
	A	Limitation of motion in extremes of gaze
	B	Evident restriction of movement
	C	Fixed eyeball
5		C—Corneal involvement
	O	Absent
	A	Stippling of cornea
	B	Ulceration
	C	Clouding
6		S—Sight loss
	O	Absent
	A	20/20–20/60
	B	20/70–20/200
	C	<20/200

E—Edema of the eyelids
F—Fullness of the eyelids

Staging/Scoring

- *Clinical activity score (CAS):*
    - It is one of the widely utilized grading system described by Mourits and colleagues.
    - It attempts to identify patients with active disease who are likely to respond to medical therapy.
    - *The CAS is generated by the addition of 1 point for the presence of each the following features:* Chemosis, eyelid swelling, eyelid erythema, conjunctival erythema, caruncular swelling, pain in primary gaze, and pain with ocular movement.

In addition, if the patient has been examined within the 3 months prior, additional points may be given for decreased visual acuity, worsened diplopia, and increased proptosis compared with that visit.
- TAO is considered active in patients with a CAS of ≥3 out of 7 (if no previous assessment is available), or 4 out of 10 on the complete scale.
- This scale has a specificity of 86%, sensitivity of 55%, positive predictive value of 80%, and negative predicative value of 64% for predicting the activity of the disease.

Limitation: It is subjective (depends on both patient and practitioner) and it fails to account for active improvement or worsening of the disease.

- *European Group on Graves' orbitopathy (EUGOGO):* It is one of the commonly used scoring systems. It recommends the following classification of patients with thyroid ophthalmopathy.[3]

Mild GO: They usually present with ≥1 of the following signs:
- Minor lid retraction (<2 mm)
- Mild soft tissue involvement
- Exophthalmos <3 mm (above the normal range for the race and gender)
- Transient or no diplopia

Corneal exposure responsive to lubricants *moderate-to-severe GO:* These patients usually have any ≥1 of the following:
- Lid retraction >2 mm
- Moderate or severe soft tissue involvement
- Exophthalmos >3 mm above normal for race and gender
- Inconstant or constant diplopia

Sight-threatening GO:
- Patients with dysthyroid optic neuropathy and/or corneal breakdown
- Other infrequent conditions are ocular globe subluxation, severe forms of frozen eye, choroidal folds, and postural visual darkening
- This category warrants immediate intervention
- As a rule of thumb, it is considered that all patients who do not have a mild or a sight-threatening ophthalmopathy present a moderate-to-severe disease

- *VISA scoring:*
  - Developed by Dolman and Rootman and adopted with modifications by the International Thyroid Eye Disease Society (ITEDS)
  - It is based on symptoms (subjective) and signs (objective) inputs
  - *Four severity parameters are analyzed:* V (vision), I (inflammation/congestion), S (strabismus/motility restriction), and A (appearance/exposure)
  - Each feature is considered and graded independently
    * *Vision:* 1 point
    * *Inflammation/congestion:* 10 points
    * *Strabismus:* 6 points (diplopia: 3 points plus restriction: 3 points)
    * *Appearance/exposure:* 3 points
    * A global severity grade, with maximum score is 20 points, is the sum of each of the involved systems graded independently.
- *Vision (V):* Evaluates the visual problems, especially due to associated dysthyroid optic neuropathy. It is assessed through visual acuity, pupillary reflexes, color vision, visual fields, optic nerve examination, and visual evoked potentials.
- Soft tissue *inflammation/congestion (I)* evaluation is graded according to the worst score for the eye or the eyelid with the Inflammatory Index as shown in **Table 3**. Patients with moderate inflammatory index (less than 4 of 10) are managed conservatively. Patients with high scores (above 5 of 10) or with evidence of progression (as documented on subsequent visits) in the inflammation are offered a more aggressive therapy.
- *Strabismus/motility restriction (S)* is documented by three aspects:
  1. Diplopia that is graded from 0 to 3 (0 = no diplopia, 1 = diplopia with horizontal or vertical gaze, 2 = intermittent diplopia in straight gaze, and 3 = constant diplopia in straight gaze)
  2. Ocular ductions are measured to the nearest 5° in four directions using the corneal light reflex technique. Any change of ≥12° in any direction can be considered progression

Table 3: VISA inflammatory index.	
Sign or symptom	**Score**
Caruncular edema	0: Absent 1: Present
Chemosis	0: Absent 1: Conjunctiva lies behind the gray line of the lid 2: Conjunctiva extends anterior to the gray line of the lid
Conjunctival redness	0: Absent 1: Present
Lid redness	0: Absent 1: Present
Lid edema	0: Absent 1: Present but without redundant tissues 2: Present and causing bulging in the palpebral skin, including lower lid festoon
Retrobulbar ache: • At rest • With Gaze	 0: Absent; 1: Present 0: Absent; 1: Present
Diurnal variation	0: Absent; 1: Present

3. Ocular restriction can be graded from 0 to 3 based on the range of ductions (0 = duction > 45°, 1 = 30–45°, 2 = 15–30°, and 3 <15°) quantified by prism cover testing.

- *Appearance/exposure (A):*
  - Symptoms include appearance concerns (such as bulging eyes, eyelid retraction, and fat pockets) and those derived from ocular exposure (such as gritting sensation, photophobia, dryness, and secondary tearing)
  - Signs include measurements of eyelid retraction (millimeters from the pupillary light reflex to the lid margin); scleral show (millimeters from the limbus to the lid margin); levator palpebrae superioris function; lagophthalmos (incomplete eyelid closure); and proptosis with the Hertel exophthalmometer. Signs of corneal exposure are best assessed with the slit-lamp microscope and may include punctate epithelial erosions, ulcerations, and, in severe cases, corneal thinning and risk of perforation.

The VISA and CAS were designed to determine the clinical *activity*. In comparison, the NO SPECS and EUGOGO classification assess the clinical *severity*. Both VISA (particularly in US) and EUGOGO (European countries) are currently used for deciding upon treatment and also monitoring response to treatment.[3-5]

■ MANAGEMENT

Treatment of Thyroid Gland Dysfunction

It is the most important aspect of treatment of thyroid ophthalmopathy. Frequent monitoring of thyroid status (every 4–6 weeks) is imperative in the initial phases of treatment when changes in thyroid status are expected.

Treatment of Ophthalmopathy

Treatment should follow the sequence of (V-I-S-A), that is, first take care of visual disturbance then ISA (of VISA scoring).

Treatment Options

- *Supportive measures:*
  - *Artificial tears:* Lubricant eye drops during the day and lubricant ointments at night time
  - *Sunglasses:* To avoid photophobia
  - *Patients with symptomatic diplopia:* Fresnel prisms or occlusion therapy
  - *Botulinum toxin injection may be considered for upper lid retraction*
  - *Topical adrenergic blocking agents such as 5% guanethidine sulfate drops transiently improve mild eyelid retraction but not of much use*
  - *Cool compresses*
  - *Head elevation*: To reduce periorbital edema
  - *Stop smoking and selenium supplements*
- *Medical management:*
  - *Corticosteroids:* Systemic steroids are indicated in patients with severe inflammation or compressive optic neuropathy. Intravenous glucocorticoids

are required for patients with advanced thyroid-associated orbitopathy. Intravenous glucocorticoids seem to be associated with higher success rate and better tolerability as compared to oral glucocorticoids.
  – *Steroid-sparing immunosuppressive drugs:* Cyclosporine and methotrexate, intravenous administration of immunoglobulin, tumor necrosis factor-α blockers, and anti-CD20 monoclonal antibodies (rituximab) have been found useful. However, these are inferior to steroids as monotherapy and considered only when steroid is contraindicated.
- *Radiation therapy:* Acts by a nonspecific anti-inflammatory effect. RT is effective in patients who have active eye disease with recent progression and ineffective in inactive stages of the disease. The lymphocytes infiltrating the orbit have high radio sensitivity. Usually a dose of 20 Gy is given per eye fractionated over a 2-week period. However, RT can be associated with transient exacerbations of inflammation, hence simultaneous glucocorticoids must be started. Although the evidence regarding the efficacy of radiation therapy in the management of TAO is limited, it is still one of the widely used treatment modality.
- Surgical management
  – *Orbital decompression:* It is indicated in cases with compressive optic neuropathy not improving with medical treatment. It enlarges the existing space of the orbit by partial removal of bony walls and periosteum. The most commonly done decompression involves the posteromedial wall followed by floor and lateral wall.

Treatment

It depends upon the stage and severity:
- *Mild TED:* Only supportive therapy is required. Progression from mild-to-moderate-to-severe TED occurs in about 15%. The side effects of immunosuppressive treatment or radiation do not weigh against the expected beneficial effects.
- *Moderate-to-severe TED:* Moderate-to-severe TED is defined as no threat to vision but sufficient impact on daily life to justify the risks of immunosuppression. Corticosteroids are the treatment of choice with a response rates up to 80%. Intravenous prednisolone treatment is recommended because it has better results compared with high-dose oral therapy and it is associated with less side effects such as diabetes or weight gain. Prior to starting high-dose steroid possible contraindications for high-dose prednisone treatment, such as gastrointestinal ulcer disease, severe osteoporosis, latent tuberculosis or hepatitis B or C positivity, uncontrolled diabetes/hypertension must be ruled out. The cumulative dose of prednisolone should not exceed 8 g in one course of therapy. However, the exact dose of prednisolone that yields satisfactory therapeutic effect without adverse events is not exactly known.
- *Very severe TED:* Very severe TED should be treated with 1 g methylprednisolone IV daily for 3 consecutive days, repeated after 1 week, followed by an oral tapering dose. When there is clinical deterioration, urgent orbital decompression should be considered. Indications for surgical decompression include the following:
  – Patients with active disease who have refractory or progressing corneal ulcer
  – A stretched optic nerve
  – Prevention of further corneal damage
  – Cosmetic in acceptability.

In orbital decompression, part of the bony walls is removed to provide more room for the extraocular muscles and orbital fat. Associated diplopia usually requires surgery of the extraocular muscles. But after the orbital decompression surgery, diplopia surgery should be postponed till effect of the previous is established. Eyelid surgery such as lengthening (in case of upper eye lid retraction) may be a final step in the rehabilitation of the patient with TED.

VIVA QUESTIONS

Q.1. What are the risk factors for TAO?
Ans. *Genetics:* The TED is considered be an autoimmune disease because of its clinical

association with Graves' disease, an associated condition known to be caused by TRAb.

Tobacco smoking: Smoking is the risk factor most consistently linked to either development or deterioration of TAO. Overall, more than 40% of smokers either developed or worsened TAO, which was almost double the rate of nonsmokers. Cigarette smoke extract increases production by orbital fibroblasts of glycosaminoglycans, hydrophilic macromolecules that accumulate in TAO orbital tissues.

Therapy for TED with radioactive iodine (RAI): TAO has 15 and 39% risk for development or progression after RAI therapy for hyperthyroidism. The majority of patients developing TED after RAI treatment had mild and transient disease requiring no treatment.

Thyroid dysfunction: Both hyper- and hypothyroidism have been shown in multiple reports to be associated with increased risk for development or deterioration of TAO.

Thyroxine and tri-iodothyronine levels: Some studies have suggested that circulating tri-iodothyronine (T3) or thyroxine (T4) may also be associated with TAO.

Q.2. What is Rundle's curve/natural course of TAO?

Ans. Rundle conceptualized two distinct phases for TED, which is graphically represented in his famous "Rundle's curve." Rundle's curve represents the natural course of TED. It helps in understanding and managing TED. It has two stages:

1. An initial *active inflammatory phase* that is associated with by periorbital erythema and edema, conjunctival chemosis, orbital inflammation and congestion, associated with upper lid retraction, proptosis, and occasionally diplopia. The inflammatory phase typically lasts for a period between 6 and 24 months
2. This is followed by a quiet, minimally inflammatory chronic fibrotic phase, which is associated with orbital fibrosis, glycosaminoglycan deposition, and enlarged extraocular muscles. There are usually no active inflammatory episodes in this phase.

REFERENCES

1. Stan MN, Bahn RS. Risk factors for development or deterioration of Graves' ophthalmopathy. Thyroid. 2010;20:7.
2. Bhatt R, Nelson CC, Douglas RS. Thyroid-associated orbitopathy: Current insights into the pathophysiology, immunology and management. Saudi J Ophthalmol. 2011;25(1): 15-20.
3. Barrio-Barrio J, Sabater AL, Bonet-Farriol E, Velázquez-Villoria Á, Galofré JC. Graves' Ophthalmopathy: VISA versus EUGOGO Classification, Assessment, and Management. J Ophthalmol. 2015;2015:249125.
4. Bahn RS. Graves' ophthalmopathy. N Engl J Med. 2010;362(8):726-38.
5. Dolman PJ. Evaluating Graves' orbitopathy. Best Pract Res Clin Endocrinol Metab. 2012;26(3):229-48.

LACRIMAL GLAND TUMORS

Varsha Vashney, Amar Pujari

INTRODUCTION

The lacrimal gland is situated in the superotemporal orbit and it consists of two lobes, the orbital lobe and the much smaller palpebral lobe. The palpebral lobe can be visualized in the superior fornix on lid eversion but not the orbital lobe. Thus, any pathology that affects the orbital lobes only may be missed for a long period. Lacrimal gland tumors account for about 10–15% of all orbital tumors.[1] The clinician should consider the axiom: *"Half and a half; then half again."* Approximately half of all lacrimal fossa masses are inflammatory, and the other half is neoplastic. Out of the neoplastic group, half are the aggressive adenoid cystic carcinoma (ADCC) variety.[1,2]

In examinations, it can be given as a long case.

■ HISTORY

Demography

Lacrimal gland tumors are seen more frequently in the third to fourth decade of life (may present from childhood to old age), and the second bimodal peak is in the teenage years.

Chief Complaints

The presentation varies from patients who are asymptomatic but have a slight fullness in the temporal upper lid to those who present with frank proptosis, diplopia, and an encroaching mass lesion.

History of Present Illness

All points as described in section proptosis must be recorded carefully while taking history. In addition, following points must be noted:
- History of a long-standing (>1–2 years), noninfiltrating lacrimal gland lesion suggests a benign tumor, such as a pleomorphic adenoma.
- A shorter history suggests either an inflammatory or a malignant process.
- Pain most commonly is seen with inflammatory lesions of the lacrimal gland, but adenoid cystic carcinomas and other malignancies also can present with pain secondary to perineural or bony involvement.
- Malignant lesions characteristically present with a subacute course of proptosis and temporal sensory loss in the distribution of the lacrimal nerve in one-third of the patients.
- Limitation of eye movement, diplopia, and diminished visual acuity can be seen with large tumors due to distortion of the globe by the firm tumor mass.
- Benign lesions commonly present with painless inferonasal globe displacement and fullness of the superotemporal lid and orbit. Old photographs may be helpful in establishing the duration of displacement.
- Acute onset of a painful, erythematous, and indurated eyelid suggests inflammation.
- Other symptoms that may present include facial asymmetry noted by friends, epiphora, exposure symptoms.

History of Past Illness

Past ocular history may uncover an episode of trauma, prior periorbital surgery, or periocular tumors that could relate to the present illness. A history of intraocular malignancy such as malignant melanoma might point to the possibility of orbital extension or metastasis.

Surgical History

History of surgical removal of similar mass may be there (recurrence is found in pleomorphic adenoma). Incomplete excision of pleomorphic adenoma can lead to relentless recurrences and malignant transformation **(Fig. 1)**. Thus the previous history of biopsy (such as incisional or needle) is important in such cases.

History of Systemic Illness

The past general medical history may elicit important diagnostic information. For example, a history of breast cancer might suggest metastasis. A history of systemic inflammatory disease such as sarcoidosis should raise concern for a related orbital inflammatory process.

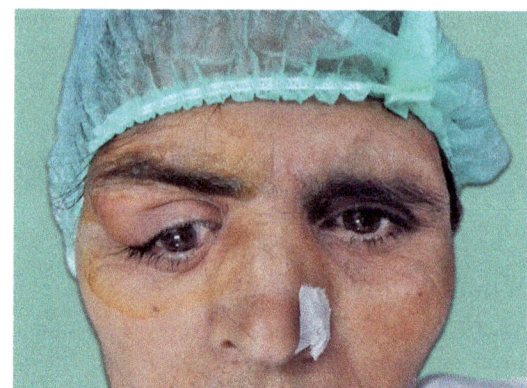

Fig. 1: Adenoid cystic carcinoma of lacrimal gland.

EXAMINATION

Systemic Examination

A detailed general examination is carried out to rule out any systemic metastasis. Preauricular lymphadenopathy from regional metastasis in malignant lesions must be ruled out. Signs of primary elsewhere in the body must be looked for.

Ocular Examination

Following points must be noted in ocular examination:
- *Visual acuity:* Diminished visual acuity can be seen with rapidly progressive lesions. Patients with induced hyperopia from an orbital mass may show a significant asymmetric refractive error.
- *Eyeball:* Displacement of the globe with or without proptosis can occur. The displacement is characteristically nonaxial with *inferomedial globe displacement.*
- *Ocular balance and ductions:* Binocular patients should be examined for latent or manifest ocular deviations and the approximate extent of uniocular ductions in the four cardinal positions estimated. A forced duction (traction) test under topical anesthesia will assist differentiation of neurological from mechanical causes of restricted eye movements. Likewise, retraction of the globe during an active duction suggests fibrosis of the ipsilateral antagonist muscle, this being a common sign with chronic orbital myositis.
- *Lids:* An S-shaped contour to the upper lid (the lateral half of the eyelid lies lower than the medial half) is characteristic for lacrimal gland lesions, but it is relatively nonspecific to the type of tumor. A firm, rubbery, nontender mass can be seen with either benign or lymphoproliferative lesions.
- Complete examination of mass should be done (as discussed in chapter proptosis), which includes size, shape, site, margins, edges, consistency, mobility, adherence to overlying skin and underlying bone, color of skin, temperature of skin, reducibility and compressibility, increase in size with Valsalva maneuver, pulsations, and transillumination.
- *Conjunctiva, cornea:* Signs of inflammation such as congestion and chemosis may be present with dacryoadenitis, tumors, or infiltration of the lacrimal gland. A *"salmon patch"* subconjunctival lesion may be present and is characteristic of lymphoma. Signs of exposure keratopathy (punctate defects or epithelial defect with infiltrates) may be present. A reduced Schirmer test may indicate toward an inflammatory lesion (e.g., Sjögren syndrome).
- *Pupils:* Usually the pupillary reaction is normal. RAPD may be present if the mass is compressing or infiltrating the optic nerve.
- *Anterior segment:* Usually normal. Raised IOP may be present due to globe compression.
- *Posterior segment:* (Slit-lamp biomicroscopic examination using a 90D/78D lens and indirect ophthalmoscopy)
  - *Vitreous, optic disc, and macula:* Are usually normal
  - Choroidal folds may be present, resulting from globe indentation by an orbital mass.

INVESTIGATIONS

The investigating modalities used in a suspected case of lacrimal gland tumor are described below.

High-resolution Computed Tomography

- *Benign tumors:* Pleomorphic adenomas appear as well-defined, sometimes nodular and nonhomogeneous lesions that show moderate enhancement with intravenous contrast. Palpebral lobe tumors lie anterior to the orbital rim, whereas expansion of the lacrimal fossa with preservation of intact cortical bone is seen in most cases of orbital lobe adenoma. Molding of the lacrimal gland fossa on CT scan is a *hallmark* of benign growth. Discrete calcification may also be present in a minority of cases, and indentation of the globe is common with larger tumors.
- *Malignant tumors:* These are poorly defined margins, with infiltration into surrounding tissues, and bone. Calcification occurs in about one-third of carcinomas, but is diffuse compared to pleomorphic adenomas. In contrast to the hard pleomorphic adenomas

that flatten the globe, rapidly growing and softer lesions (such as carcinoma and lymphoma) tend to mold to its surface.

Histologic Findings

Histologic examination of pleomorphic adenomas reveals evidence of both epithelial and mesenchymal differentiation. The proliferation of benign epithelial cells usually is arranged in a double layer to form lumens. Stromal differentiation can be seen in the formation of bone and cartilage.

ADCC are derived from duct cells, and they form spaces into which basement membrane-like material is deposited. This confers a *cribriform or "Swiss cheese" appearance to the tissue*, which is characteristic of ADCC.

Immunohistochemistry

This may be helpful in distinguishing between inflammatory, benign, and malignant lymphoproliferative lesions. Immunohistochemistry is a laboratory modality that uses special markers to demonstrate the presence of specific antigens in target tissues. Benign inflammatory lesions (pseudotumor) have a polyclonal morphology, whereas the lymphoid lesions tend to be monoclonal.

■ DIFFERENTIAL DIAGNOSIS

- The differential diagnosis of a lacrimal gland mass has been described in **Table 1**.
- *Key features* are described in **Table 2**.

Benign Tumors

- *Pleomorphic adenoma:* It has following important features:
- Most common intrinsic lacrimal gland lesion
- Painless, progressive, slow growing
- Well-circumscribed mass with absence of bony destruction
- Remove with pseudocapsule intact to decrease risk of recurrence or malignant transformation
- *Histopathologically, comprised of two cell components:* Benign epithelial cells arranged in double layer forming ducts stellate spindle cells contained in loose stroma

Table 1: Differential diagnosis of lacrimal gland mass.

Non-neoplastic	Neoplastic
• Dacryops/ dacryoadenitis • Dermoid cysts • Hemangioma • Amyloid	*Lymphoproliferative diseases*: • Benign lymphoid hyperplasia • Atypical lymphoid hyperplasia • Malignant lymphoma *Benign tumors:* • Pleomorphic adenoma (benign mixed tumor) • Benign fibrous histiocytoma • Oncocytoma • Myoepithelioma • Cystadenoma *Malignant tumors:* • Adenoid cystic carcinoma • Malignant mixed tumor (carcinoma expleomorphic adenoma) • Adenocarcinoma • Mucoepidermoid carcinoma • Squamous cell carcinoma • Acinic cell carcinoma • Malignant oncocytoma • Lung and breast metastases

Myoepithelioma

- Rare tumor with biological behavior similar to that of a pleomorphic adenoma
- *Five subtypes:* Spindle, plasmacytoid, epithelial, clear, and mixed

Oncocytoma

- Rare tumor secondary to metaplasia of ductular cells (epithelial origin)
- Large, eosinophilic cells rich in mitochondria "Warthin tumor" (cystadenolymphoma)
- Commonly presents as an epithelial neoplasm of the salivary glands (lacrimal gland is an unusual location)
- Epithelial columnar cells arranged in solid nests or lining cystic spaces

Malignant Tumors

Adenoid Cystic Carcinoma

- Bimodal distribution with peak incidences in second and fourth decades of life

Table 2: Summary of major lacrimal gland tumors.

Types of lesions	Clinical features	Imaging features	Histopathologic features	Treatment
• Pleomorphic adenoma (benign mixed tumor) • Most common epithelial tumor	• Painless, progressive, slow-growing mass on superotemporal area of upper eyelid • Nontender, firm, well-contoured mass • Variable proptosis, diplopia loss of vision rare	• CT—round to oval well circumscribed mass in the lacrimal fossa, with bony expansion and excavation, no bony destruction • USG—round to oval mass with medium to high reflectivity and regular internal structure	• Two morphologic cell components: Benign epithelial cells arranged in a double forming ducts and stellate spindle cells contained in a loose stroma • Epithelial cells in the stroma can undergo metaplasia with cartilaginous, fibrous, or myxoid characteristics	Modified lateral orbitotomy and excision using an extraperiosteal approach for the lateral portion for an anteriorly situated palpebral lobe tumor, isolated dacryoadenectomy via a transcutaneous or transconjunctival approach
Oncocytoma	Rare affects elderly females; caruncle most common site		Large, eosinophilic cells rich in mitochondria	Complete surgical excision
Cystadenoma (Warthin tumor)	• Rare • Clinical characteristic is similar to pleomorphic adenoma	Similar to those of a pleomorphic adenoma	• Epithelial columnar cells arranged in solid nests or lining cystic spaces • Often contains an exudative fluid component and a lymphoid infiltrate with focal follicular organization	Complete excision of the globular cystic mass with preservation of the thin capsule
Adenoid cystic carcinoma	• Periocular pain, mild ptosis, proptosis, brow numbness, and diplopia • Rapid progression symptoms are typically present for 6 months, and almost always <1 year	• Globular lacrimal gland mass with irregular borders, bony erosion, bone destruction, and soft tissue calcification • Contiguous tumor extension to adjacent area	Sheets of epithelial cells arranged in either solid or cribriform patterns with spaces into which basement membrane like material is deposited (Swiss-Cheese)	• *En bloc*, excision of the orbit and its contents, including the orbital roof, the lateral wall, the lids, and the anterior portion of the temporalis muscle where the zygomatico-frontal and zygomatico-temporal nerves extend • Adjunctive postoperative radiotherapy

Contd...

Contd...

Types of lesions	Clinical features	Imaging features	Histopathologic features	Treatment
Malignant mixed tumor	The average age at diagnosis is 50 years. This tumor may arise *de novo* because of malignant transformation following an incomplete excision of a benign adenoma, or as malignant transformation years after diagnosis of a presumed benign adenoma	Similar to adenoid cystic carcinoma, may show a bilobed appearance	Histopathologically, the malignant component may be attached to and arise from the benign mixed aspect of the tumor, yielding a bilobed appearance	• Complete surgical resection • Mortality is high
Mucoepidermoid carcinoma	• Rare • Locally aggressive • Average age at presentation of 49 years • Male:Female 2:3	Similar to adenoid cystic carcinoma	• Epidermoid and mucus-secreting cells arranged in a pattern of cords and islands • The mucus-secreting cells and cystoid spaces within the specimen stain positively with mucicarmine, alcian blue stain, and Periodic acid-Schiff reaction	• Excision with or without adjuvant radiotherapy • Advanced stage has a worse prognosis, requires exenteration and radiotherapy
Carcinosarcoma	Carcinosarcoma may arise from a pleomorphic adenoma		Considered in the differential diagnosis of a lacrimal gland mass, if sarcomatous components are encountered on histologic examination	Management requires complete excision of the lesion

(CT: computed tomography; USG: ultrasonography)

- Periocular pain (severe pain due to perineural spread), mild ptosis, proptosis, downward and inward displacement of the globe
- Bony erosion, bone destruction, and soft tissue calcification on CT
- High mortality rate (intra-arterial cytoreductive chemotherapy may improve survival)
- Sheets of epithelial cells arranged in solid or cribriform pattern resembling a glandular structure is characteristic

Primary Adenocarcinoma

- Rare tumor with clinical findings similar to adenoid cystic carcinoma

- Pleomorphic, mitotically active cells arranged in sheets and cords

Pleomorphic Adenocarcinoma (Malignant Mixed Tumor)

- May arise de novo as consequence of malignant transformation following incomplete excision of benign adenoma or as malignant transformation of a presumed benign adenoma
- Well circumscribed, pseudocapsulated **(Table 3)**

■ TREATMENT[3-5]

Pleomorphic Adenoma

It should be excised intact with a cuff of normal tissue. Palpebral lobe tumors can be resected through an upper lid skin crease incision Stallard-Wright incision (anterior orbitotomy). Orbital lobe tumors can be approached through a lateral orbitotomy approach. It is important to avoid any intraoperative spillage during surgery. Thus, a buffer of normal tissue should always be maintained around the tumor mass. If intraoperative spillage of cells occurs through cautery and lavage of the operative field has to be done. If the periosteum is already destroyed, the breach should be treated by strict surgical isolation and cyanoacrylate glue may be applied to minor capsular breaches during surgery. Excision of the orbital lobe alone with preservation of palpebral lobe reduces the incidence of dry eye and secondary corneal disease.

Biopsy (other than excision) *should not be attempted* in any suspected case of pleomorphic adenoma. If it has been inadvertently biopsied, the biopsy tract and the tumor should be meticulously excised as recurrent pleomorphic adenoma is typically infiltrative and may need extensive tissue resection or exenteration.

Adenoid Cystic Carcinoma

It depends upon the extent of the tumor. For tumors that are localized to the orbit, excision of the tumor and adjacent tissues should be done. Advanced tumors require surgical resection followed by external beam radiation therapy (EBRT). ADCC is often extensive and requires orbital exenteration or midfacial resection. EBRT delays the growth or recurrence of the tumor. Brachytherapy (locally implanted radioactive plaques seeds) may also give results similar to EBRT. Chemotherapy does

Table 3: Difference between pleomorphic adenoma and adenoid cystic carcinoma.

Features	Pleomorphic adenoma	Adenoid cystic carcinoma
Pain	Painless	Periocular pain often sever
Course	Slow-growing mass	Fast growing
Proptosis	Variable	Proptosis with downward and inward displacement of the globe
Associated features	Decreased vision and diplopia rare	Brow numbness is characteristic, diplopia, mild ptosis
Palpation	Nontender, firm, well contoured mass	Firm irregular bordered mass
Histological features	Benign epithelial cells arranged in a double layer forming ducts and stellate spindle cells contained in a loose stroma	Sheets of epithelial cells arranged in either solid or cribriform patterns (Swiss-Cheese pattern) that mimic glandular structure
Radiological features	• Round to oval well-circumscribed mass in the lacrimal fossa • Bony expansion and excavation but no bony destruction • The posterior edge of the lesion typically exhibits a curved contour that molds to the adjacent orbital bone	• Globular lacrimal gland mass with borders that are irregular • Associated with bony erosion, bone destruction, and soft tissue calcification • Tumor extension toward the medial orbit, apex, and the temporalis fossa

not have a recognized role in the treatment of adenoid cystic carcinoma.

The malignant mixed tumor is treated with local excision followed by irradiation.

Metastatic tumor carries a poor prognosis. The target is to provide palliative therapy through orbital irradiation or chemotherapy.

VIVA QUESTIONS

Q.1. Most common lacrimal gland tumors.

Ans.
- Pleomorphic adenomas account for almost all benign tumors of the lacrimal gland.
- Adenoid cystic carcinoma is the most common (76%) malignant epithelial tumor.
- Carcinoma arising in pre-existing pleomorphic adenoma (malignant mixed tumor) is the second most common malignancy of the lacrimal gland.
- Lymphoma accounts for about 10–14% of all lacrimal gland masses and may be part of a systemic disease.

Q.2. Where do you find a "salmon patch lesion"?

Ans. A salmon patch subconjunctival lesion is a characteristic nontender firm reddish fleshy mass of conjunctival lymphoma. It may be an extension of orbital or intraocular lymphoma. Only 25% patients of orbital/adnexal lymphoma have conjunctival involvement. Most commonly, it is confused with chronic follicular conjunctivitis. Histologically, these are non-Hodgkin lymphoma of low-grade B-cell variety.

Q.3. Differential diagnosis of a lacrimal fossa mass.

Ans. Refer to differential diagnosis.

Q.4. How do you differentiate pleomorphic adenoma from adenoid cystic carcinoma?

Ans. *See* Table 3.

Q.5. What is "Swiss cheese" pattern of ADCC?

Ans. It refers to the microscopic picture of ADCC. Closely packed, small, densely stained cells aggregate around large ovoid spaces containing hyaline or mucin. This resembles the Swiss cheese pattern and hence the description.

Q.6. Prognosis of ADCC.

Ans. The prognosis is poor in cases of ADCC. The overall 5-year survival rate of all adenoid cystic carcinomas was 47%. This number reduces to 20% after 13 years and 22% after 15 years. Most cases recur within 2 years of treatment. Intracranial spread can occur due to the propensity of perineural invasion that results in the death of the majority of patients.

REFERENCES

1. Albert DM, Miller JW, Azar DT, Blodi BA. Albert and Jakobiec's Principles and Practice of Ophthalmology, 3rd edition. Philadelphia: Saunders/Elsevier; 2008.
2. Bowling B. Kanski's Clinical Ophthalmology: A systematic approach, 8th edition. Edinburgh: Elsevier; 2015.
3. von Holstein SL, Coupland SE, Briscoe D, Le Tourneau C, Heegaard S. Epithelial tumors of the lacrimal gland: a clinical, histopathological, surgical and oncological survey. Acta Ophthalmol. 2013;91(3):195-206.
4. Bernardini FP, Devoto MH, Croxatto JO. Epithelial tumors of the lacrimal gland: an update. Curr Opin Ophthalmol. 2008;19(5):409-13.
5. Alkatan HM, Al-Harkan DH, Al-Mutlaq M, Maktabi A, Elkhamary SM. Epithelial lacrimal gland tumors: A comprehensive clinicopathologic review of 26 lesions with radiologic correlation. Saudi J Ophthalmol. 2014;28(1):49-57.

SHORT CASES

CONGENITAL PTOSIS

Aditi Dubey, Amar Pujari

■ INTRODUCTION

Drooping of the eyelids is known as ptosis. It may be present at birth, or it may develop later in life. If a droopy eyelid is present at birth or within the first year of life, the condition is called congenital ptosis. In most cases of congenital ptosis, the problem is isolated and does not affect the vision.[1-3]

Congenital ptosis can be given as a short case in examinations.

■ HISTORY

All pediatric patients presenting with either unilateral droopy eyelid or bilateral droopy eyelids need a thorough history and examination (kindly see the section of ptosis, long case).

Chief Complaint

Parents usually bring the child with the history of drooping of the eyelid **(Fig. 1)** or narrow palpebral fissure since birth.

History of Present Illness

The onset, progression, and other associated abnormalities such as deviation of eyes, nystagmus, face turn, and any relation to the amount of ptosis to jaw movement.

Medical History

A careful medical history regarding malignancy should be obtained. Metastatic or primary orbital tumors can result in malpositioning of the eyelid.

Family History

A patient with a strong family history of congenital ptosis may not need an extensive work-up. Family photographs can help determine onset or variability of the ptosis.

History of Drug or Allergic Reactions

A history of drug or allergic reactions may be helpful. Allergic reactions can result in eyelid edema and droopy eyelid.

History of Trauma

Orbital wall fractures (pseudoptosis with enophthalmos) or cranial nerve III palsy from trauma may result in ptosis.

■ EXAMINATION

A case of congenital ptosis must be evaluated in detail as described in the chapter of long case ptosis. In cases of congenital ptosis, following should be taken care of:
- *Visual acuity:* Risk of amblyopia is there in case of severe ptosis. The amblyopia can occur due to occlusion amblyopia or rarely due to astigmatism induced by the compression of the droopy eyelid.
- Refractive error and cycloplegic refraction should be recorded in all cases.
- In infants, make sure that the baby can fixate and follow objects with each eye individually.

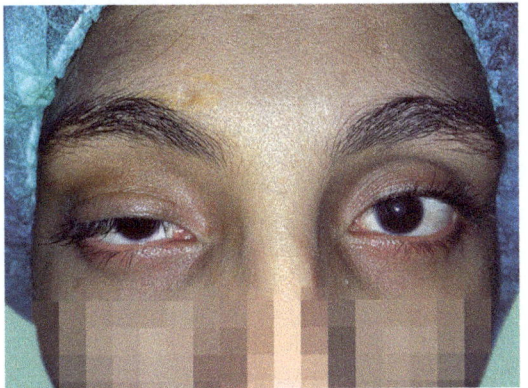

Fig. 1: Simple severe congenital ptosis.

- The patient should be evaluated for strabismus (misalignment).
- Serial external photographs of the eyes and the face may be included in the patient's record for documentation.
- Tear function should be evaluated.
- Corneal sensitivity should be tested (if possible); may be a difficult test in young pediatric patients.
- The pupillary size and the iris color differences between the eyes should be examined for Horner syndrome.
- Palpebral fissure distance.
- Lid position in downgaze (the ptotic lid appears higher in downgaze)
- Bells and Lid crease height.

Levator Function

Measurement of the levator function in small children is a difficult task, as the child allows no formal evaluation. The presence of lid fold and increase or decrease its size on the movement of the eyelid gives us a clue to the levator action. The presence of anomalous head posture like the child throwing his head back suggests a poor levator action.

Iliff Test

This test can be performed in the first year of life to evaluate the levator function. The upper eyelid of the child is everted as the child looks down. If the levator action is good, lid reverts on its own.

■ INVESTIGATION

A routine case does not require any specific investigations except those required for general anesthesia if surgery planned (hemoglobin, urea, creatinine, bleeding, and clotting time). Neuroimaging [magnetic resonance imaging (MRI) or computed tomography (CT)] is indicated in following conditions:
- If history not consistent and onset not clear
- Other neurologic findings along with ptosis are present
- Orbital wall fracture suspected with history of trauma
- Visible or palpable lid mass
- Suspected orbital tumors (e.g., lymphoma, leukemia, and rhabdomyosarcoma)
- New onset of Horner syndrome with or without other neurologic findings
- New onset of third cranial nerve palsy with or without other neurologic findings
- Globe displacement with either enophthalmos or proptosis

Differential diagnosis/classification/management has been covered in detail in the long case, ptosis part.

■ MANAGEMENT

The points considered while performing the surgery are discussed here.

Timing of Surgery

It is advisable to wait till *4–5 years of age* for surgical correction when the tissues are mature enough to withstand the surgical trauma and a better assessment and postoperative care is possible due to improved patient cooperation.[2,3] *Urgent surgery* is indicated in children with severe ptosis developing amblyopia. In such cases, sling surgery is done.

Surgical Approach

It is based on whether the:
- Ptosis is unilateral or bilateral
- Severity of ptosis
- Levator action
- Presence or absence of abnormal ocular motility, jaw-winking phenomenon, or blepharophimosis syndrome.

Aim of Surgery

Target is to lift the ptotic lid above the papillary aperture when the eyes are in the primary position. The height of the two lids regardless of whether the ptosis is unilateral or bilateral should be equal. There should also be adequate mobility of the lid when blinking, a normal lid fold, and no diplopia.

Surgical Procedure

The choice of surgery is given below:
- *Fasanella-Servat operation:*
    - Mild ptosis (≤2 mm)

Table 1: Berke's criteria for levator resection.			
Degree of ptosis	Levator function	Amount of levator resection	Ideal preoperative correction
1.5–2 mm (mild)	• Good (≥8) • Good (≥8)—usual	• Small (10–13) • Moderate (14–17)	Under correct by 1–3 mm
3 mm (moderate)	• Fair (5–7) • Poor (rare, ≤4)	• Large (18–22) • Maximal (≥23)	Match the level of normal lid and correct ptosis fully
≥4 (severe)	• Fair (Sometimes, 5–7) • Poor (usual, ≤4)	• Super maximal (≥27) • Frontalis sling	Over correct by 1–2 mm

- Levator action >10 mm
- Well-defined lid fold—no excess skin
- *Levator resection:*
  - Mild/moderate/severe ptosis
  - Levator action ≥4 mm
- *Brow suspension ptosis repair/Frontalis flap or supramaxial resection:*
  - Severe ptosis
  - Levator action <4 mm
  - Jaw-winking ptosis [along with levator palpebrae superioris (LPS) excision] or blepharophimosis syndrome.

In cases with bilateral congenital ptosis, simultaneous bilateral intervention in the two eyes is needed. However, in cases where gross asymmetry exists between the two eyes, the eye with a greater ptosis is operated first and the other eye is operated after 6–8 weeks when the final correction of the operated eye can be assessed.

Levator resection is the most commonly performed procedure, there are different criteria to determine the amount of levator resection required. The two important and widely used guidelines are Berke's **(Table 1)** and Putterman's **(Table 2)** method.

Contraindications to Surgery

Ptosis surgery is relatively contraindicated in presence of following:
- Poor orbicularis muscle function (lagophthalmos and corneal exposure)
- Loss of blink reflex
- Loss of corneal sensitivity
- Significant dry eye
- Poor Bell's phenomena.

Table 2: Putterman's criteria for amount of levator resection.	
Levator action	Recommended lid placement
2–4 mm	1 mm above the limbus
5–7 mm	1 mm below the limbus
≥8 mm	2 mm below the limbus

VIVA QUESTIONS

Q.1. What are the causes of congenital ptosis?
Ans. Following are important causes of congenital ptosis:
- Idiopathic
- *Blepharophimosis syndrome [blepharophimosis, ptosis, and epicanthus inversus syndrome (BPES)]:* Short palpebral fissures, congenital ptosis, epicanthus inverses, and telecanthus
- Third cranial nerve palsy
- *Horner syndrome: Ipsilateral* findings of mild ptosis, miosis, and anhidrosis characterize this syndrome
- *Marcus Gunn jaw-winking syndrome:* The motor nerve to the *external pterygoid muscle* is misdirected to the *ipsilateral levator muscle.* Lid elevation occurs with mastication or with the movement of the jaw to the opposite side.
- Birth trauma
- *Periorbital tumor:* Neuroblastoma, plexiform neuromas, lymphomas, leukemias, rhabdomyosarcomas,

neuromas, neurofibromas, or other deep orbital tumors may produce ptosis and proptosis.
- *Kearns–Sayre syndrome:* Progressive external ophthalmoplegia, heart block, retinitis pigmentosa, and central nervous system manifestations. This condition begins in childhood but is rarely present at birth.
- Myotonic dystrophy
- *Blepharochalasis:* Infiltrative processes that thicken the lids and produce ptosis
- *Myasthenia gravis:* A defect at the neuromuscular junction
- *Pseudotumor of the orbit:* Ptosis due to inflammation and edema of the eyelid
- *Pseudoptosis:* Less tissue in the orbit (e.g., unilateral smaller eye, fat atrophy, blowout fracture) produces the appearance of ptosis secondary to the decreased volume of orbital contents.

Q.2. Describe the pathology in congenital ptosis.

Ans. Histologically, the levator muscles of patients with congenital ptosis are dystrophic. The levator muscle and aponeurosis tissues appear to be infiltrated or replaced by fat and fibrous tissue. In severe cases, little or no striated muscle can be identified at the time of surgery. This suggests that congenital ptosis is secondary to local developmental defects in muscle structure. Congenital ptosis may occur through autosomal dominant inheritance. Common familial occurrences suggest that genetic or chromosomal defects are likely.

Q.3. Complications of the sling surgery.

Ans. Complications associated with the frontalis suspension procedure for congenital ptosis repair include the following:
- Granuloma
- Lid asymmetry
- Overcorrection with exposure keratopathy
- Undercorrection
- Infection.

Q.4. What is the prognosis after surgery?

Ans. The repair of congenital ptosis can produce excellent functional and cosmetic results. With careful observation and treatment, amblyopia ptosis can be treated successfully. Patients who require surgical intervention, ≥50% may require repeat surgery in 8–10 years following the initial surgery.

Q.5. Management of complicated ptosis.

Ans. The management of simple congenital ptosis associated with other anomalies is as follows:
- *Ptosis with oculomotor abnormalities:* In cases with superior rectus involvement (usually associated with severe ptosis), an inferior rectus recession at times combined with superior rectus resection is carried out on the affected side as the first procedure. To correct the ptosis levator resection with bilateral brow suspension is done later. *Knapp's procedure* may be done for ptosis associated with double elevator palsy where lateral and medial rectus tendons are transplanted to the area of superior rectus insertion. This does not cause significant limitation of adduction or abduction. Ptosis is corrected *3 months later.*
- *Blepharophimosis syndrome:* The following sequence is followed:
  - Y-V plasty mustard's double "Z" plasty with transnasal wiring is done as a primary procedure. This gives a good surgical result both in terms of correction of telecanthus as well as deep placement of the medial canthus. The results are long-lasting.
  - Brow suspension is carried out *6 months after* the first procedure for correction of ptosis.
- *Marcus Gunn ptosis:* Mild cases of jaw-winking where the jaw-winking is minimal can be treated satisfactorily by Fasanella-Servat operation while severe cases or cases where jaw-winking is prominent require bilateral resection of levator aponeurosis and terminal levator with fascia lata brow suspension.

- *Misdirected third nerve ptosis:* In cases of misdirected third nerve ptosis where treatment is imperative levator resection with bilateral fascia lata, sling is the procedure of choice. Ptosis associated with third nerve palsy is difficult to manage because of poor Bell's phenomenon. A crutch glass may be prescribed or a conservative sling surgery may be performed.

REFERENCES

1. Bernardini FP, Devoto MH, Priolo E. Treatment of unilateral congenital ptosis. Ophthalmology. 2007;114(3):622-3.
2. Shields M, Putterman A. Blepharoptosis correction. Curr Opin Otolaryngol Head Neck Surg. 2003;11(4):261-6.
3. Yilmaz N, Hosal BM, Zilelioglu G. Congenital ptosis and associated congenital malformations. J AAPOS. 2004;8(3):293-5.

ECTROPION

Aditi Dubey, Bijnya Birajita Panda, Sanjana M

INTRODUCTION

Ectropion is characterized by an eversion or outward turning of the eyelid margin away from the globe. It is a commonly encountered eyelid malposition. It is characterized by rotation of lid margin outward resulting in its fall away from the globe.[1] To make things worse, the constant wiping and rubbing of the eyes irritated by the epiphora further aggravates the condition. The underlying factor may vary in each case and an appropriate identification of the type of ectropion and the factor responsible for its occurrence are important in choosing the correct surgical intervention.[2,3]

In examinations, it is usually given as a short case or spot case.

HISTORY

Chief Complaints

Watering, irritation, grittiness, foreign body sensation, or chronic red eye are the chief complaints. Symptoms are caused by ocular exposure and inadequate lubrication.

Past History

Facial palsy, lid trauma, ocular allergy, previous lid surgery, and chemical injury should be taken.

EXAMINATION

The routine examination is carried out and the conjunctiva, cornea, and anterior chamber are examined for any signs of inflammation.

Eyelid: There is outward turning of the lid margin. There may be signs of chronic blepharitis.

Conjunctiva: Keratinization and hypertrophy.

Cornea: Changes secondary to exposure may be present.

Lagophthlamos

Schirmer's test: To rule out dry eye.

Syringing and Jones test I and II (to rule out lacrimal passage obstruction).

Tests for Ectropion

Pinch Test

To determine the amount of lid laxity. If the lid can be pulled >6 mm away from the globe, the lid is lax. If the medial and lateral canthal tendons are lax as well, the lid can be pulled away up to 20–25 mm.

Snap-back Test

Downward traction is applied to the lower lid and then released; the lid should revert to its normal position without the aid of a blink in a normal person. However, when laxity is present, the lid is not opposed to the globe.

Grading of lid laxity according to the snap-back test is as follows:
- *Normal:* The lid returns to its position immediately on release
- *Grade 1:* Approximately 2–3 s
- *Grade 2:* 4–5 s
- *Grade 3:* >5 s but returns to position on blinking
- *Grade 4:* Continues to hang down.

Inferior Lid Retractor Laxity

Retractor weakness can be demonstrated by observing the lower lid as the patient looks down. Reduction in inferior movement on down gaze and a deep inferior fornix occurs due to laxity or loss of retractor attachment in this area.

Medial Canthal Tendon Laxity

The lateral excursion of the inferior punctum is measured by pulling the lid laterally. The punctum lies lateral to the caruncle at rest and should not be displaced more than 1–2 mm with lateral lid traction. If pulling on the medial canthus allows the punctum to be stretched, it suggests medial canthal tendon (MCT) is lax. Laxity is graded as following:
- *Mild:* Up to the limbus
- *Moderate:* Up to the pupil
- *Severe:* Beyond the temporal pupillary border.

Lateral Canthal Tendon Laxity

The lateral canthal angle should be evaluated with the lid at rest. The lateral canthus should have an acute angular contour and should lie 1–2 mm medial to the lateral orbital rim. A rounded appearance of the canthus indicates laxity. The lateral part of the lid if pulled medially should not result in >1–2 mm movement of the lateral canthal angle in absence of laxity.

Position of the Lacrimal Puncta

Punctum alone can be everted or the whole lid may be everted. In a normal lid, the inferior punctum is directed posteriorly against the globe and should not be visible without pulling the lid downward. Direction of the punctum away from the globe is the earliest sign of medial lid ectropion and can be graded as follows:
- *Mild:* Puncta are not opposed to the globe on looking up
- *Moderate:* Puncta are not opposed to the globe even in primary gaze
- *Severe:* Palpebral conjunctiva and fornix are exposed.

Cicatricial Skin Changes

Vertical shortening of the anterior lamella—like signs of repair of lid laceration or scar of excision of the tumor should be looked for.

Lid margin examination: Keratinization or trichiasis or distichiasis

Orbicularis Muscle Weakness

The facial nerve must be examined to rule out ectropion due to paralysis of the seventh nerve. Lagophthalmos and reduced force of contraction on forced eyelid closure demonstrate orbicularis muscle weakness. Other signs of facial palsy such as brow ptosis, loss of forehead wrinkles, absent nasolabial fold, and drooping of the angle of the mouth should also be looked for.

■ CLASSIFICATION

Ectropion can be classified as following:
- *Congenital ectropion:* Rare, associated with congenital epiblepharon
- *Acquired ectropion:* Can be further classified as following on the basis of pathogenesis:
  - *Involutional ectropion:* It is the most common variety. Multiple factors are responsible for its development, for example, horizontal lid laxity, medial canthal tendon laxity, etc., which are all normal aging changes of the lid (**Fig. 1**).
  - *Cicatricial ectropion:* Lid margin is pulled away from the globe due to the shortage of skin, for example, congenital shortage (**Fig. 2**), trauma, burns, cicatrizing skin tumors, allergies, etc.; it may be unilateral or bilateral/localized or generalized depending on the cause.
  - *Mechanical ectropion:* Tumor or cyst near the lid margin mechanically pulling down the lid
  - *Paralytic ectropion:* VII nerve palsy resulting in sagging and downward displacement of paralyzed orbicularis muscle.

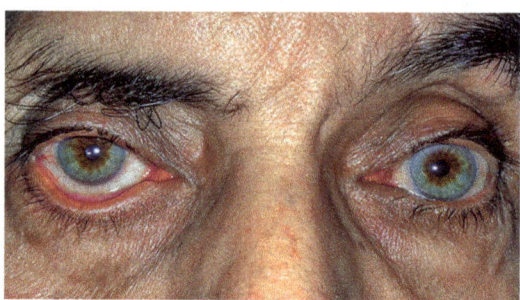

Fig. 1: Senile ectropion.

Oculoplasty

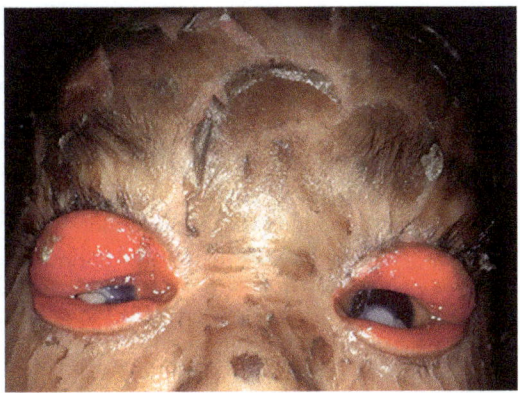

Fig. 2: Paralytic ectropion due to tight skin in a collodion baby.

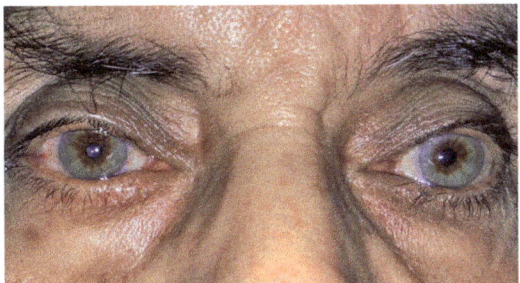

Fig. 3: Cicatricial ectropion (Fig. 1) after surgery (lateral tarsal strip procedure).

GRADING

Grade of Orbito-lid Apposition

- *Grade 0:* With normal lid-globe apposition
- *Grade 1:* With punctal eversion
- *Grade 2:* With partial lid eversion and scleral show
- *Grade 3:* With conjunctival hyperemia and thickening
- *Grade 4:* As for grade 3 with exposure keratitis.

Grades of Ectropion

- *Grade 1:* Punctal eversion
- *Grade 2:* Eversion of sharp posterior lid margin
- *Grade 3:* Palpebral conjunctival exposure
- *Grade 4:* Exposure of the fornix.

TREATMENT

Factors considered for selection of surgery for ectropion:
- *Basic cause* of ectropion
- Secondary mechanisms coexisting with the basic pathology
- Grade of ectropion
- *Identify* the defects in various components of lid lower
- Excess lid skin
- Laxity of lateral canthal tendon (LCT)/MCT and its severity
- Shortening of posterior lamella comprising of tarsoconjunctiva
- Any mass lesion in lid causing ectropion
- Any scarring whether localized or generalized
- Systemic disease causing scarring of tarsoconjunctiva.

Surgical Management of Ectropion

Involutional Ectropion

- *Mild-to-moderate ectropion mainly affecting lateral lid:* Full thickness pentagonal wedge resection of the lid
- *Mild ectropion with an excess of skin:* Modified Kuhnt-Szymanowski procedure—blepharoplasty with a base up lateral triangle and excision of full thickness wedge of lid beneath the blepharoplasty flap
- *Moderate ectropion—generalized or affecting lateral lid:*
  - *Lateral tarsal strip:* In this, a horizontal incision is made and inferior crus of LCT is cut, triangular portion of the temporal lid is resected sparing tarsus and the tarsal strip is sutured with a mattress suture in a superotemporal direction to the periosteum. Smith and Lisman propose an alternative method where after excising the anterior lamella of the lid on temporal aspect the periosteum is exposed in a superotemporal direction and the tarsal strip is sutured to it **(Fig. 3)**.
- *Marked ectropion:* Double wedge resection with lateral tarsal strip
- *Extreme ectropion:* Temporalis muscle transfer involutional ectropion affecting only the medial aspect
- *Only punctal eversion present and no lid laxity:* Medial conjunctivoplasty

- *Horizontal lid laxity is present but MCT is not lax: Lazy-T* (Excision of tarsoconjunctiva combined with full thickness wedge excision of lid)
- *Horizontal lid laxity which is due to MCT laxity:* MCT plication or resection depending on severity of laxity
- *Lateral canthal resuspension.*

Management of Cicatricial Ectropion

Correction of a cicatricial ectropion requires lengthening of the cutaneous surface and correction of any associated factors—resection of subcutaneous cicatrix or horizontal lid lengthening. Following surgeries have been described:
- *Localized: Z-plasty* (Elschnig's operation)
- *V-Y operation*
- *Severe or generalized cicatricial ectropion:* Releasing the scar and full thickness skin grafting or a monopedicle flap.

Management of Paralytic Ectropion

Management involves giving support to the lower lid or strengthening of the lower lid. Support can be given medially, laterally, or to the lower lid as a whole. In long-standing cases associated with cheek ptosis, a cheek lift/mid-face lift may be necessary. Following surgeries have been described:
- *Only medial ectropion:* Medial canthoplasty
- *Generalized lid laxity:* MCT plication + lateral canthal sling
- *Medial with MCT laxity:* MCT resection.

Management of Mechanical Ectropion

Masses near the lid margin causing the ectropion should be excised. Excision should be as vertical as possible and it is important to avoid scar formation/skin shortening.

VIVA QUESTIONS

Q.1. Pathogenesis of involutional ectropion.

Ans. Ectropion involves the lower lid more commonly than the upper lid. There is decreased resilience and increased laxity of periocular tissues due to age-related microinfarction and secondary atrophy. This inadequate support and effect of gravity cause more pronounced stretching of the lower lid increasing the burden on suspensory canthal tendons and resulting in ectropion. Primary abnormality is laxity of the lateral canthal tendon. Other contributory factors include the following:
- Horizontal lid laxity
- Medial canthal tendon laxity
- Punctal malposition
- Vertical tightness of the skin
- Lower lid retractors disinsertion or laxity.

Q.2. Congenital ectropion.

Ans. Congenital ectropion is a rare entity. It is more often associated with blepharophimosis syndrome (BPES type 2), Down syndrome, or ichthyosis. In rare cases, congenital ectropion occurs as an isolated finding. It is caused by a vertical insufficiency of the anterior lamella of the eyelid. Complications include chronic epiphora and exposure keratitis. Management is as follows:
- Mild congenital ectropion—no treatment
- Severe and symptomatic—horizontal tightening of the lateral canthal tendon and vertical lengthening of the anterior lamella by means of a full-thickness skin graft.

A complete eversion of the upper eyelids occasionally occurs in premature infants transiently due to orbicularis slippage/lamellar slippage, inclusion conjunctivitis, anterior lamellar inflammation or shortage, or Down syndrome. Treatment includes topical lubrication, short-term patching of eyes, full-thickness sutures, or a temporary tarsorrhaphy.

Q.3. What are the disadvantages of lid resection procedures?

Ans.
- Does not correct the underlying physiological abnormality
- Causes lid notching
- Causes lid shortening
- Causes loss of meibomian glands.

REFERENCES

1. Bosniak SL, Zilkha MC. Ectropion. In: Nesi FA, Lisman RD, Levine MR (Eds). Smith's Ophthalmic Plastic and Reconstructive Surgery, 2nd edition. St Louis: Mosby; 1998. pp. 290-307.
2. Bergin DJ. Anatomy of the eyelids, lacrimal system, and orbit. In: McCord CD, Tanenbaum, Nunery WR (Eds). Oculoplastic Surgery, 3rd edition. New York: Raven Press; 1995. pp. 51-84.
3. Robinson FO, Collin RO. Ectropion. In: Yanoff M, Duker JS (Eds). Ophthalmology, 2nd edition. India: Mosby. 2006. pp. 676-83.

ENTROPION

Aditi Dubey, Ritu Nagpal

INTRODUCTION

Entropion is a condition in which eyelid turns inward. This causes the eyelashes or the eyelid margin to rub against the eyeball and results in irritation, watering, redness, keratitis, and even corneal perforation. It may occur at any age but occurs primarily because of advancing age. It can be missed easily and thus one should specifically look at the eyelid to diagnose it.[1-3]

In examination, it can be given as a short case.

HISTORY

Chief Complaints

Patients with entropion commonly complain of the following:
- Foreign body sensation
- Frequent eye infections
- Red eyes
- Watering.

Past History

History of onset is important to rule out congenital component.
- *Age of patient:* In children, congenital entropion is rare and should be definitely differentiated from epiblepharon
- History of ocular trauma, facial burn, Stevens–Johnson syndrome is important for cicatricial entropion
- History of ocular surface irregularity or any other painful ocular pathology (acute spastic entropion).

EXAMINATION

- Lid margin is found in-turned (**Fig. 1**). Depending upon the degree of in turning it can be divided into the following three grades:
  - *Grade I:* Only the posterior lid border is in rolled
  - *Grade II:* Entropion includes in turning up to the intermarginal strip
  - *Grade III:* The whole lid margin including the anterior border is in turned.
- *Lid laxity:*
  - *The pinch test:* To determine the amount of lid laxity. If the lid can be pulled >6 mm away from the globe, the lid is lax. If the medial and lateral canthal tendons are lax as well, the lid can be pulled away up to 20–25 mm.
  - There may a hump on lower eyelid due to overriding of preseptal orbicularis over the pretarsal part.
  - It is often associated with an absence of the downward excursion of the eyelid in

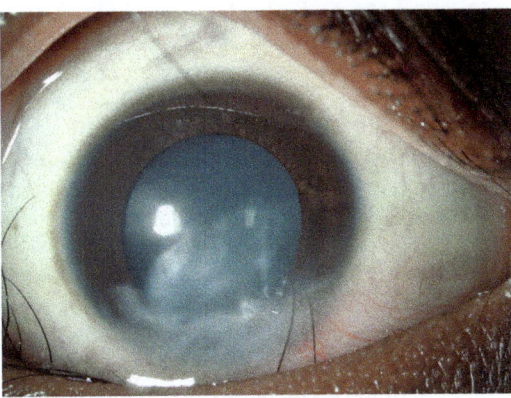

Fig. 1: Entropion.

down gaze due to the weakness of the lower lid retractors. Excursion of the lower lid in down gaze usually 3–4 mm—loss of movement indicates retractor weakness/disinsertion.
- *Snap-back test:* Perform this test by pulling the lower lid away and down from the globe for several seconds. If the lid resumes position, note the time required for the lid to return to its original position without the patient blinking. The snap-back test provides a good idea of relative lower lid laxity. Lids with normal laxity immediately spring back to original position; the longer this takes, the more laxity is present.
  - Grades:
    - *Normal:* Lid returns immediately on release
    - *Grade 1:* Approximately 2–3 s
    - *Grade 2:* 4–5 s
    - *Grade 3:* >5 s but returns to position on blinking
    - *Grade 4:* Continues to hang down
- *Medial canthal laxity test:* Perform this test by pulling the lower lid laterally from the medial canthus. Measure displacement of the medial punctum. Greater distance equates to more laxity. Normal displacement ranges from only 0–1 mm.
  - Grades:
    - Mild—up to the limbus
    - Moderate—up to the pupil
    - Severe—beyond the temporal pupillary border.
- *Lateral canthal laxity test:* Perform this test by pulling the lower lid medially from the lateral canthus. Measure displacement of the lateral canthal corner. Greater distance equates to more laxity. Normal displacement ranges from only 0–2 mm. Assign grades on a scale from 0–4 (0 = normal laxity, 4 = severe laxity).
- *Bell phenomenon:* Instruct the patient to attempt eye closure while the examiner holds lids open. If eyes move up, the test indicates a positive result for Bell phenomenon.
- *Orbicularis muscular tone:* Ask the patient to squeeze eyes shut. Note how much worse the entropion is immediately after opening.
  - Grades of orbicularis muscle tone:
    - Grade 0 = no paralysis
    - 1 = weak
    - 2 = normal
    - 3 = overactive
    - 4 = spastic
- *The digital eversion test can be done to distinguish cicatricial component:* Observe directly by everting the lids. It can also be ascertained by pulling the lid superiorly if it does not reach 2 mm above lower limbus; lid is vertically deficient.
- *Slit-lamp examination:* To look for corneal status and other evidence of dryness, punctuate keratopathy due to blepharitis, meibomitis, trichiasis, foreign bodies, corneal scarring **(Fig. 2)**, and dry eyes.
- *Fluorescein staining:* This test is essential when looking for signs of corneal damage. It can detect damage from lashes or lid skin rubbing on the cornea.
- *Schirmer test:* To rule out other causes of dryness
- *Lid margin examination:* Keratinization or trichiasis or distichiasis
- *Lacrimal system patency assessment:* Done by syringing, dye disappearance test, and Jones Dye Test I and II.

CLASSIFICATION

Entropion can be classified into congenital, involutional, cicatricial, and acute spastic.[1-3]
- *Congenital entropion:* Occurs due to hypertrophy of the anterior lamella. Mostly mild and resolves with time.

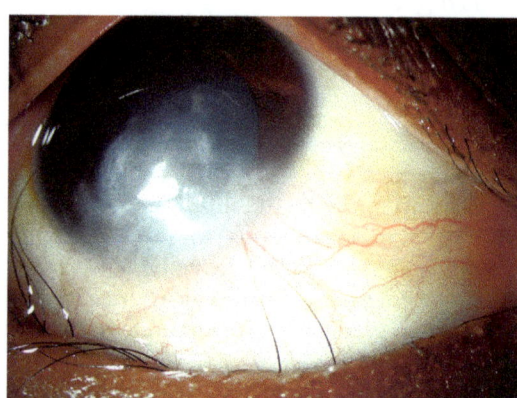

Fig. 2: Entropion with eyelash rubbing cornea causing keratopathy.

- *Involutional entropion:* An age-related condition caused by the laxity of tarsus, its medial and lateral canthal tendons, lower lid retractors, along with the over-riding of the orbicularis oculi muscle.
- *Cicatricial entropion:* Occurs due to scarring and shortening of the posterior lamella due to chemical injury, infection, or Stevens–Johnson syndrome.
- *Acute spastic entropion:* Follows ocular irritation or inflammation.

Most Common Types of Entropion
- Lower lid—involutional entropion
- Upper lid—cicatricial entropion.

■ MANAGEMENT
Nonsurgical Management
In cases before proceeding to the definitive surgery, the following medical management plans can be followed:
- Eyelid taping to the malar eminence
- Injecting Botox into the orbicularis muscle.

Surgical Management
Senile Entropion
- Rotational sutures or everting sutures
- Lateral tarsal strip—if there is horizontal laxity
- Lower eyelid retractor reinsertion.

Spastic Entropion
First, treat the underlying condition that might cause infection or irritation of ocular surface. Followed by either rotational sutures can be passed or Botox can be injected.

Cicatricial Entropion
- Tarsal fracture
- Transverse blepharotomy with marginal rotation
- For severe cases, posterior lamellar lengthening using mucous membrane grafting
- Anterior lamellar recession with or without mucus membrane graft.

Surgery Names
- Weiss procedure (transverse blepharotomy with everting sutures)
- Quickert everting sutures
- Jones retractor plication.

VIVA QUESTIONS

Q.1. Congenital entropion.
Ans.
- Extremely rare
- Inversion of entire tarsus and lid margin
- Epiblepharon and horizontal tarsal kink are to be differentiated
- *Surgery (Hotz procedure):* Minimal ellipse of skin and orbicular is excised from the medial two-thirds of the lower lid. Skin is fixed to the lower edge of the tarsus.

Q.2. Differentiate between congenital entropion and epiblepharon?
Ans. *See* Table 1.

Q.3. Involutional entropion.
Ans.
- Often seen in elderly patients, particularly women.
- Causes great discomfort as well as problems with clear vision due to constant watering.
- The appropriate procedure depends on the degree of entropion, keratinization, and distortion of the lid margin and eyelashes and analysis of posterior lamellar shortening and scarring.
- For cases with mild-to-moderate degree of cicatrization—tarsal wedge resection or the tarsal fracture procedure.
- *In severe or recurrent cases:* Posterior lamellar grafting procedure to lengthen the posterior lamella.

Q.4. Causes of cicatricial entropion.
Ans.
- Trachoma
- Acid and alkali burn
- Ocular pemphigus
- Leprosy
- Severe membranous conjunctivitis
- Stevens–Johnson syndrome.

Table 1: Differences between congenital entropion and epiblepharon.

Features	Epiblepharon	Congenital entropion
Extrafold of skin	Fold of skin overlapping the lid margin is present medially	Absent
Occurrence	Common	Rare
Lid affected	Lower lid	Both
Lid margin	Not turned inward	Entire lid margin turned inward
Direction of eye lashes	Straight up and lie flat against the cornea	Turned inward
On pulling down the skin	Lashes turn out but the margin of the lid remains in apposition to the globe	Lid margin also pulls away from the globe
Treatment	Spontaneous resolution	May require surgical correction

Q.5. Causes of spastic entropion.

Ans.
- Senile
- Ocular surface disorder, for example, dry eye
- Enophthalmos
- Loss of orbital fat
- Tight bandage
- Enucleation socket

Management of acute spastic entropion:
- Treatment of the underlying cause—break the irritation-entropion cycle.
- Taping of the inturned eyelid to evert the margin, various suture techniques afford temporary relief for most patients.
- Additional definitive surgical repair to correct the underlying involutional changes.
- In selected cases, botulinum toxin injection can be used to paralyze the overriding preseptal orbicularis muscle.

Q.6. Role of botulinum toxin in management of entropion.

Ans.
- Works very well in correcting spastic entropion.
  - Also, in selected cases of involutional entropion with significant preseptal muscle override when the patient is not willing for surgery or is bedridden and not fit for surgery.
- *Dose and procedure:* 2.5 units of botulinum toxin are injected at two or three places below the lower lid margin. Injected directly into the muscle by pinching it taking care not to go deep to avoid trauma to extraocular muscles (especially medially as it may cause inferior oblique muscle paresis and lead to diplopia).
- *Disadvantage:* May take around 4–7 days for its effect to appear. Short-term; not a permanent solution.

Q.7. The material of choice for the spacer graft for entropion correction.

Ans.
- Hard palate mucosal graft
- Donor sclera
- Buccal mucous membrane
- Amniotic membrane.

REFERENCES

1. Tenzel RR. Orbit and Oculoplastics. Textbook of Ophthalmology. London: Gower Medical Publishing; 1993.
2. Beyer-Machule CK, Von Noorden GK. Atlas of Ophthalmalmic Surgery. New York: Thieme; 1985.
3. Albert DM, Jakobiec FA (Eds). Principles and Practice of Ophthalmology. US: WB Saunders; 2000.

BLEPHAROPHIMOSIS, PTOSIS, EPICANTHUS INVERSUS SYNDROME

Amar Pujari, Aditi Dubey

■ INTRODUCTION

First described by Komoto in 1921, BPES is a dominantly inherited disorder characterized by the presence of above features (i.e., blepharophimosis, ptosis, and epicanthus) at birth. The main findings of this disorder are eyelids that are abnormally narrow horizontally (blepharophimosis), a vertical fold of skin from the lower eyelid up either side of the nose (epicanthus inversus), and drooping of the upper eyelids (ptosis). It can be given as a short case in the examination.

■ HISTORY

Chief Complaints

The parents bring the child with anyone or a combination of the following complaints:
- Drooping of eyelid
- Abnormal head posture (chin up due to ptosis)
- Small size of eyeball
- Abnormal eyelid
- *Diminution of vision:* Blurring of vision is related to refractive error, astigmatism
- Absence of eyeball
- Bluish colored swelling (in case of cryptophthalmos)
- Epiphora (due to displaced tear ducts).

Past History

A careful past history should be taken for any:
- Perinatal and pregnancy history
- Family history of congenital eyelid colobomas or other congenital anomalies, especially facial (e.g., cleft lip/palate)
- History of other birth defects
- Pediatric review of systems
- Facial asymmetry
- Hearing loss
- Recurrent infection
- Menstrual history (in case of late presentation).

Past Surgical History

The previous history of ocular surgery (attempts to correct any of the lid deformity or squint) may or may not be present.

■ EXAMINATION

Systemic Examination

Features frequently observed in both BPES type I and type II are a broad nasal bridge, low-set ears, and a short philtrum.

This condition is sometimes associated with ovarian failure although breast development is often normal. Secondary sexual characteristics are usually normal in both BPES type I and type II. In BPES type I, menarche is usually normal, followed by oligomenorrhea and secondary amenorrhea.

Other malformations that can be seen includes (also known as BPES plus):
- Contractures
- Low nose bridge, micrognathia, and microcephaly
- *Ear abnormalities:* Incomplete ear development/cupped ears, posteriorly rotated ears
- Infertility in females, premature menopause, and primary gonadal failure
- Reduced muscle tone—only early in life
- Mental defects, severe psychomotor retardation, and growth retardation
- Genitourinary malformations, cryptorchidism, and syndactyly.

Ocular Examination

Visual acuity: It is variably impaired depending on the severity of ptosis, astigmatism. Cycloplegic refraction is a must in all such cases as the significant refractive error may be seen in almost one-third of these cases and if untreated can lead to amblyopia. Amblyopia can also occur due to stimulus deprivation (in a case of severe ptosis) but rare.

Head posture: To compensate for the ptosis, affected person assumes a characteristic posture with the head tilted backward, the brow furrowed, and the chin arched upward. Frontalis overaction may be there (eyebrows are increased in their vertical height and they are drawn up into a pronounced convex arch).

Eyeball: The eyeball may show microphthalmos, anophthalmos, and cryptophthalmos. The palpebral fissure is reduced in both horizontal and vertical dimensions. The normal horizontal fissure length in adults is 25–30 mm whereas in this syndrome it is usually 20–22 mm. Telecanthus is seen in the majority of patients. This refers to a lateral displacement of the inner canthi leading to a widening of the intercanthal distance. The interpupillary distance (IPD) is usually normal. The patient may have esotropia, divergent strabismus, or nystagmus.

Eyelids: Eyelids are often covered by the smooth skin without eyelid folds and deficient amounts of skin in both eyelids may be found **(Fig. 1)**. Frequently, the upper and lower lacrimal puncta are displaced laterally or duplication of puncta can be seen.

Blepharoptosis literally means a falling of the lids. The palpebral fissure is abnormally small in the vertical dimension. It is caused by the absence or impairment of the function of the levator palpebrae superioris muscle and is usually bilateral and symmetrical [Kindly see the examination part of ptosis in chapter ptosis for a detailed examination of ptosis].

Dysplastic eyelids: Eyelids are often covered by the smooth skin without eyelid folds and deficient amounts of skin in both eyelids may be found. The upper eyelid margin may show "S"-shaped curve. The lower lid margin usually has an abnormal concavity downwards, particularly laterally where an ectropion might occur. Trichiasis can also occur in BPES.

Epicanthus inversus: A small skin fold that arises from the lower lid and runs inward and upward characterizes it. Associated with this are an increased length of the medial canthal ligament and a lack of the normal depression seen at the internal canthus.

Conjunctiva: It is usually normal.

Cornea: It may show micro cornea occasionally. Corneal sensation should be checked.

Lens/Sclera/Iris/Fundus: Usually normal.

■ INVESTIGATIONS

Diagnosis of the disease is straightforward based on the clinical signs. Molecular genetic testing and specific laboratory studies are indicated in cases of associated syndromes. A pelvic ultrasound examination and measurement of bone mineral density are indicated if at ovarian insufficiency is suspected.

■ CLASSIFICATION

Two types of BPES have been described:
1. *BPES type I:* It is the more common type in which males transmit the syndrome only and affected females are infertile. It is associated with an early loss of ovarian function (primary ovarian insufficiency) in women, which causes their menstrual periods to become less frequent and eventually stop before age 40 years. Primary ovarian insufficiency can lead to difficulty conceiving a child (subfertility) or a complete inability to conceive (infertility).
2. *BPES type II:* Both affected females and males transmit this variant. It is not associated with female infertility.

Both types are inherited as an autosomal dominant trait. There is complete penetrance (100%) in type I and slightly reduced (96.5%) penetrance in type II. Both types I and II include the eyelid malformations and other facial features.[1-3]

■ DIFFERENTIAL DIAGNOSIS

Differential diagnosis includes those conditions in which ptosis or blepharophimosis are a major

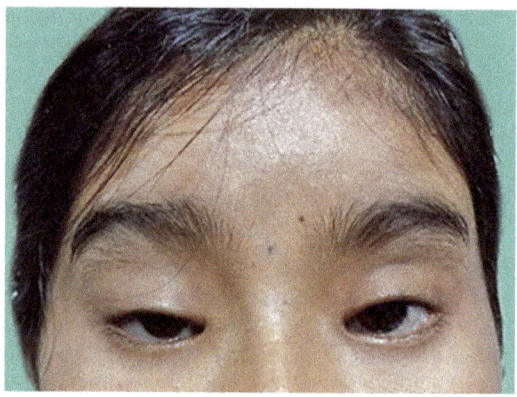

Fig. 1: Blepharophimosis epicanthus inversus syndrome.

feature (**Table 1** describes the features of these syndromes):
- Congenital simple ptosis
- Ptosis with external ophthalmoplegia
- Noonan syndrome
- Marden–Walker syndrome
- Schwartz–Jampel syndrome
- Dubowitz syndrome
- Smith–Lemli–Opitz syndrome.

The characteristic combination of signs usually clinches the diagnosis.

■ MANAGEMENT

Management requires the input of specialists including a clinical geneticist, pediatric ophthalmologist, oculoplastic surgeon, (pediatric or adult) endocrinologist, reproductive endocrinologist, and gynecologist.

Management of BPES is primarily surgical if indicated. However, any refractive error must be corrected to avoid amblyopia. The indication of surgery is moderate to severe ptosis, amblyopia, and trichiasis, which may cause the corneal lesion, cosmesis, and strabismus. Care should be given to treat associated amblyopia.

The timing of eyelid surgery is controversial; it involves weighing the balance of early surgery to prevent deprivation amblyopia and late surgery to allow for more reliable ptosis measurements, the latter of which provides a better surgical outcome. Furthermore, ptosis surgery is hampered by the dysplastic structure of the eyelids. The surgical management is traditionally performed in two stages and involves a medial canthoplasty for correction of the blepharophimosis, epicanthus inversus, and telecanthus at about the age of

Table 1: Syndromes associated with BPES.

Association	Inheritance	Features
Hereditary congenital ptosis 1 (PTOS1)	AD	Ptosis
Hereditary congenital ptosis 2 (PTOS2)	XL	Ptosis
Ohdo blepharophimosis syndrome	AD	Blepharophimosis, ptosis, mental retardation, congenital heart defects, teeth abnormality (hypoplastic teeth)
3MC syndrome 1 (Michels syndrome)	AD	Blepharophimosis, ptosis, epicanthus inversus, corneal abnormality, cleft lip/palate, skeletal abnormalities
Ptosis with external ophthalmoplegia	AR	Ptosis, ophthalmoplegia, miosis. Decreased accommodation
Noonan syndrome	AD	Ptosis, short stature, heart defects, clotting abnormalities
Marden–Walker syndrome	AR	Ptosis, blepharophimosis, growth retardation, mental retardation
Schwartz–Jampel syndrome	AR	Intermittent ptosis, blepharophimosis, telecanthus, cataract, short stature, skeletal anomalies, muscle hypertrophy
Dubowitz syndrome	AR	Ptosis, blepharophimosis, lateral telecanthus, short stature, intellectual disability, immunodeficiencies
Smith–Lemli–Opitz syndrome	AR	Ptosis, epicanthus, cataract, growth retardation, intellectual disability, genitourinary, cardiac, gastrointestinal anomalies
KANSL1-related intellectual disability syndrome	AR	Developmental delay, intellectual disability, long face, high forehead, ptosis, blepharophimosis, large low-set ears, bulbous nasal tip, pear-shaped nose, cardiac septal defects, seizures, cryptorchidism

(AD: autosomal dominant; AR: autosomal recessive; BPES: blepharophimosis, ptosis, epicanthus inversus syndrome; XL: X-linked)

4–5 years and correction of the ptosis about 9–12 months later. Early surgery may be necessary for amblyopia.

Epicanthus fold and telecanthus: The various procedures for correction of epicanthus fold and telecanthus include double Z or Y-Z plasties (**Fig. 2**) and transnasal wiring of the medial canthal tendons. If the epicanthal folds are small, a Y-V canthoplasty is traditionally used; if the epicanthal folds are severe, a double Z-plasty is used. An alternate technique for medial canthoplasty has been described recently using the skin redraping method, which has a simple flap design, less scarring, and the effective repair of epicanthus inversus and telecanthus.[3]

Ptosis: Generally, it is corrected with brow suspension procedure. Supermaximal resection and frontalis suspension is the preferred method as it leads to a good cosmetic outcome as well as to an improved muscle function.

Although traditional management of blepharophimosis syndrome includes medial canthoplasty between the ages of 3 and 5 years, followed by ptosis correction about 6 months later, patients with severe ptosis may need early surgery to prevent amblyopia. Traditional multiple surgeries may delay the amblyopia management and influence the visual outcome. Thus, many surgeons suggest correction of ptosis first, even at a very early age, to prevent amblyopia. Soft tissue medial canthal and lateral canthal surgery can wait until the face is grown.[3] Treatment of associated abnormalities: it includes management of ovarian failure, hormone replacement therapy, and embryo cryopreservation. Management of amblyopia (i.e., with/without spectacle wear/contact lens) must be continued after surgical intervention to obtain optimal results.

Patient education: Genetic consultation is highly recommended, especially for patients with associated syndromes.

VIVA QUESTIONS

Q.1. What is the sequence of surgeries for ptosis and epicanthus in BPES?
Ans. *See* management part.

Q.2. When should the BPES be repaired?
Ans. *See* management part.

Q.3. What are the syndromes associated with ptosis?
Ans. *See* **Table 1**.

Q.4. Classify BPES.
Ans. Already given in classification.

Q.5. Genetics of BPES.
Ans. Both types are caused by mutations in the *FOXL2* gene. The *FOXL2* gene provides instructions for making a protein that is active in the eyelids and ovaries. The *FOXL2* protein is likely involved in the development of muscles in the eyelids.

REFERENCES

1. Alao MJ, Lalèyè A, Lalya F, Hans Ch, Abramovicz M, Morice-Picard F, Arveiler B, Lacombe D, Rooryck C. Blepharophimosis, ptosis, epicanthus inversus syndrome with translocation and deletion at chromosome 3q23 in a black African female. Eur J Med Genet. 2012;55(11):630-4.
2. Batista F, Vaiman D, Dausset J, Fellous M, Veitia RA. Potential targets of FOXL2, a transcription factor involved in craniofacial and follicular development, identified by transcriptomics. Proc Natl Acad Sci USA. 2007;104(9):3330-5.
3. Beckingsale PS, Sullivan TJ, Wong VA, Oley C. Blepharophimosis: a recommendation for early surgery in patients with severe ptosis. Clin Experiment Ophthalmol. 2003;31(2):138-42.

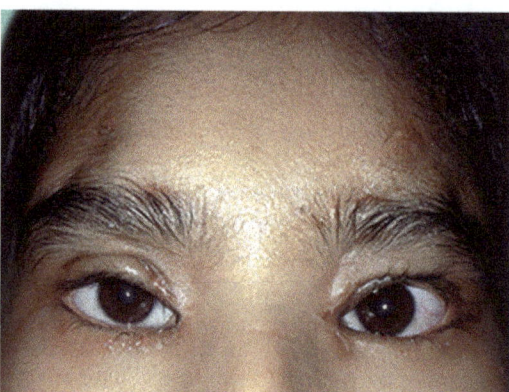

Fig. 2: Blepharophimosis, ptosis, epicanthus inversus syndrome (**Fig. 1** patient) after bilateral Y-V plasty and bilateral sling surgery.

SEBACEOUS GLAND CARCINOMA

Amar Pujari, Sapna Raghuwanshi

INTRODUCTION

Sebaceous gland carcinoma (SGC) is third most common eyelid malignancy of the eyelids. Most sebaceous carcinomas arise from the meibomian glands, Zeiss gland, and Moll gland of the eyelid; usually occur between fifth and ninth decades of life; and women are more affected than man.[1-3] It mostly involves the upper lid **(Fig. 1)**.

In examination, it can be given as a long case or short case.

HISTORY

Kindly see the section of lid tumors also.

Chief Complaint

Patients may present with the following complaints:
- Slowly enlarging, firm, and painless mass or nodule at the lid margins (most common presentation)
- Yellowish nodule at eyelid margin or caruncle
- As chronic blepharoconjunctivitis (irritation, redness, or foreign body sensation)
- Recurrent chalazion
- Chronic blepharitis with loss of cilia
- Skin or conjunctival ulcer
- Advanced cases may present as eyelid mass with a destruction of marginal cilia and lid architecture

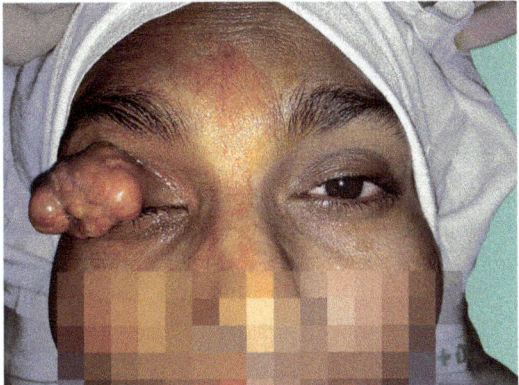

Fig. 1: Sebaceous gland carcinoma.

- Proptosis due to local invasion (anterior orbital mass or lacrimal gland tumor).

Past History

A careful history about the onset, progression, and association with pain must be recorded (similar to that described under long case section for lid tumors).

The risk factors of sebaceous cell carcinoma must be ruled out in history such as the following:
- Recurrent chalazion
- Previous radiotherapy
- Chronic blepharoconjunctivitis
- Immunosuppression
- Asian race
- Prolonged use of thiazide diuretics
- Older age (5th to 9th decade, average age 60–69 years)
- Female sex (55–57% cases are females)

EXAMINATION

Ocular Examination

Eyelids: Eyelid may have a nodule with following features:[1]
- Slowly enlarging, firm, and painless mass affecting the tarsal plate or the eyelid margin (as the meibomian gland is buried deep in the tarsus, initially the tumor will form a firm mass, and may be misdiagnosed as a chalazion. As the tumor invades more superficially, a yellowish cast may be visualized through the skin); involves both anterior and posterior lamella
- *Location:*
  - *Upper lid:* 60–70%, most common site, involved two to three times more frequently than the lower lid **(Fig. 1)**. This is due to the presence of a greater number of meibomian glands in the upper lid (50 glands in upper eyelids, 25 in lower approximately).
  - *Caruncle:* 5–11%
  - *Eyebrow:* 2%
  - *Simultaneous involvement of both lids:* 6–8%

- Lesions may also exhibit varying degrees of yellow coloration/yellowish cast due to the presence of lipid within the mass.
- Lesions originating from the Zeis glands appear as small, yellowish nodules located at the eyelid margin anterior to the gray line. At times, it may form a papilloma or cutaneous horn.
- Tumors arising from sebaceous glands of the caruncle usually appear as a subconjunctival, multilobulated, yellow mass.
- Eyelids are diffusely thickened.
- Skin appears indurated, usually skin is movable on the mass until late stages.
- Small telangiectasias over the mass.
- Loss of eyelashes (Disruption of eyelid architecture and lash loss can occur as the tumor destroys lash bulbs).
- Rarely can present as anterior orbital mass or lacrimal gland tumor.

Enlarged lymph nodes: Submandibular, submental, preauricular, and cervical.

Conjunctiva: Conjunctival inflammation and superior limbic keratoconjunctivitis can be seen.

Cornea: Superficial keratitis may be present if tumor cells invade corneal epithelium.

Other findings are usually within normal limits.

■ DIFFERENTIAL DIAGNOSIS

The following diseases must be differentiated from the sebaceous cell carcinoma:
- Blepharoconjunctivitis
- Blepharitis
- Chalazion
- Superior limbic keratoconjunctivitis
- Basal cell carcinoma
- Squamous cell carcinoma.

The characteristic features of sebaceous cell carcinoma that help in differentiating from these lesions are yellowish discoloration and telangiectatic blood vessels on the surface. At times, it is often difficult to differentiate, especially in early cases and excisional biopsy is the best way to arrive at a conclusion.

■ INVESTIGATION

A case of SGC needs following investigations.

Routine tests: Including complete blood count and renal and liver function tests.

Metastatic work-up: X-ray chest/ultrasonogram (USG) abdomen.

Positron emission tomography (PET)-CT: Brain and orbit.

CT orbit: When there is proptosis or posterior extent not seen.

Fine needle aspiration cytology (FNAC): Lymph node (lipid stains).

Conjunctival impression biopsy (for pagetoid spread).

Map biopsy: SGC must be confirmed by a full-thickness wedge biopsy of the affected eyelid. Because of multicentric spread, multiple biopsy specimens should be taken from the adjacent bulbar and palpebral conjunctiva and the other ipsilateral eyelid to form a map of the extent of tumor spread across an ocular surface. After histologic confirmation of sebaceous carcinoma, the surgeon must consider the extent of possible pagetoid involvement of the bulbar conjunctiva. Map conjunctival biopsies were taken in all four quadrants.[1-3]

■ MANAGEMENT

- *Nodular sebaceous carcinoma without pagetoid involvement:* Lesion can be removed by following techniques:
    - Full thickness eyelid resection with 4 mm clear margin with frozen section control of margins with cryotherapy
    - Mohs' micrographic technique: Excision of the visible tumor with a 5 mm margin of clinically normal tissue on either side
- Nodular sebaceous carcinoma of one eyelid with evidence of pagetoid spread:
    - Excision of the nodular lesion with conjunctive and superficial keratectomy/cryotherapy of the lesion.
    - Mitomycin C (MMC) can be tried to control conjunctival tumor. MMC 0.4% four times per day for a week and then were

medication free for 1 week; this cycle was repeated until resolution of malignancy.
- *If bulbar conjunctiva is involved extensively by tumor and reconstruction is not possible:* Exenteration is recommended.
- *If both upper and lower eyelids are involved by tumor without an involvement of the conjunctiva:* Remove both eyelids and reconstruct the defect.
- *Concomitant involvement of eyelids and conjunctiva:* It requires exenteration.
- *Orbital disease with no metastasis:* Orbital exenteration.
- *Ocular disease with lymphatic metastasis:* Neoadjuvant chemotherapy, mass resection/exenteration, radical neck dissection, and postoperative radiation.
- Systemic chemotherapy may is required in the management of metastatic disease; however, there is little in the literature on the efficacy of postsurgical chemotherapy for metastatic disease.

■ PROGNOSIS

- Poor compared to basal cell carcinoma (BCC)
- *Five-year mortality:*
   - Early disease: 15% (6–30%)[1-3]
   - Metastatic disease: 50–67%[1-3]
- *Five-year recurrence rate:* 9–36%[1-3]

VIVA QUESTIONS

Q.1. Histopathology.

Ans. Dysplasia and anaplasia of the sebaceous lobules in the meibomian glands are seen in SGC, associated with the destruction of tarsal and adnexal tissues. As the neoplastic nodule enlarges, it may erupt toward the eyelid skin to initiate the intraepidermal growth phase, wherein the sebaceous cells spread diffusely throughout the epidermis. This "pagetoid" epidermal invasion is a distinctive feature of sebaceous carcinomas.

Specific characteristics on histopathology are as follows:
- Stains with oil red O and Sudan IV
- Cytoplasm is frothy and vacuolated
- Cells are larger vesicular and have prominent nucleoli.

Histopathologic subtypes: Lobular (lobules of sebaceous architecture), comedocarcinoma (characterized by a central necrotic core), papillary (papillary projections and areas of sebaceous differentiation), and mixed (features of any subtype). It can also be described as well differentiated, moderately differentiated, and poorly differentiated.

Q.2. Metastasis.

Ans. An invasive, potentially lethal tumor, SGC may cause an extensive local destruction of eyelid tissues. It carries a risk of metastasis to preauricular and submandibular lymph nodes or may spread hematogenous to distant sites. It may invade locally into the globe, the orbit, the sinuses, or the brain. The frequencies of the spreads are:[1-3]
- *Direct extension:* Orbit, lacrimal glands—6–17%
- *Lymphatic:* Regional nodes—17–28%
- *Hematogenous:* Rare, <1%, lungs, liver, skull, and brain

Pagetoid spread: Intraepithelial or intraepidermal spread of malignant cells similar to that observed in Paget's disease of the nipple or extramammary Paget's disease. Spread along skin or conjunctiva, producing individual cell clusters are characteristic. It is seen in almost 47% of the cases.

Risk factors for subclinical spread include:
- Duration of symptoms >6 months
- Vascular and lymphatic infiltration
- Orbital extension
- Poor tumor differentiation
- Multicentric origin intraepithelial carcinomatous changes of the conjunctiva, cornea, or skin
- Location in the upper eyelid.

Q.3. Prognostic factors.

Ans.
- Site:
   - Lower lid tumor (better) > Upper lid tumor > Both upper and lower lids (worst)
   - *Conjunctival tumor:* Metastatic disease

- *Tumor size:* Increased size, worse prognosis >10 mm
- *Delay in diagnosis:* Delay >6 months, bad prognosis
- *Histology:*
  - Vascular invasion
  - Lymphatic invasion
  - Highly infiltrative pattern
  - Poor differentiation
  - Pagetoid spread
  - Multicentric origin
  - Orbital invasion.

Q.4. What is Muir–Torre syndrome?

Ans.
- It is an autosomal dominant condition in which there are sebaceous (oil gland) skin tumors in association with internal cancer.
- The most common organ involved is the gastrointestinal tract, with almost one-half of the patients having colorectal cancer. The second most common site is cancer of the genitourinary tract.
- Following skin lesions are associated with this syndrome:
  - Sebaceous adenomas
  - Sebaceous epitheliomas
  - Sebaceous carcinoma
  - Keratoacanthoma
  - Squamous cell carcinoma
  - Multiple follicular cysts
- It is now thought to be a hereditary nonpolyposis colorectal cancer syndrome due to mutations in the DNA mismatch repair genes *MSH2* or *MLH1*.

Q.5. Sebaceous carcinoma in systemic disease.

Ans. Sebaceous gland carcinoma is seen in association with following:
- Familial retinoblastoma after radiotherapy
- Immunosuppression in HIV disease
- Muir–Torre syndrome.

■ REFERENCES

1. Wali UK, Al-Mujaini A. Sebaceous gland carcinoma of the eyelid. Oman J Ophthalmol. 2010;3(3):117-21.
2. Mulay K, Aggarwal E, White VA. Periocular sebaceous gland carcinoma: A comprehensive review. Saudi J Ophthalmol. 2013;27(3):159-65.
3. Albert DM, Miller JW, Azar DT. Albert & Jakobiec's Principles and Practice of Ophthalmology, 3rd edition. Philadelphia: Saunders/Elsevier; 2008.

PYOGENIC GRANULOMA

Sapna Raghuwanshi, Bijnya Birajita Panda

■ INTRODUCTION

Pyogenic granuloma is an inflammatory vascular response of the tissue that usually occurs after a previous insult, typically either inflammatory or trauma. It is the most common acquired vascular lesion to involve the eyelids. It also involves the conjunctiva. The name is a misnomer because this lesion is neither pyogenic nor granulomatous.[1,2]

In examination, it can be given as a short case.

■ HISTORY

Chief Complaints

The patient may present with the following complaints:

- Rapidly growing mass over eyelids and conjunctiva
- Lesion readily bleeds with minor contact
- Pain (associated with superficial ulceration).

Past History

Following points must be noted in history:
- Minor trauma
- Surgery (Limbal surgery for pterygium, squamous cell carcinoma, phthisis, and squint surgery)
- Chalazion
- Microbial infection
- Pterygium
- Chemical burns.

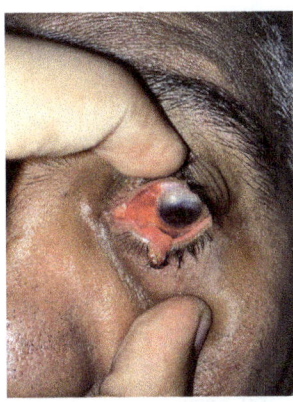

Fig. 1: Pyogenic granuloma.

■ EXAMINATION

Eyelids: Raised, red, and smooth surfaced lesions with a narrow base **(Fig. 1)**.

Conjunctiva: If conjunctiva is involved, conjunctival inflammation may be present **(Fig. 1)**.

Other findings are usually within normal limits.

■ DIFFERENTIAL DIAGNOSIS

- Kaposi sarcoma—slow growing, in immunocompromised patient in contrast to fast growing pyogenic granuloma and associated risk factors
- Intravascular papillary endothelial hyperplasia
- Squamous papilloma
- Conjunctival lymphoma
- Ocular lymphangiectasia.

■ HISTOPATHOLOGY

Lesion consists of a mass of granulation tissue, prominent capillaries, and acute and chronic inflammatory cells.

■ MANAGEMENT

- Surgical excision
- *Topical or intralesional corticosteroids:* It is better to give a short course of steroid therapy before proceeding with surgery.

■ REFERENCES

1. Bowling B. Kanski's Clinical Ophthalmology: A systematic approach, 8th edition. Edinburgh: Elsevier; 2015.
2. Albert DM, Miller JW, Azar DT. Albert & Jakobiec's Principles and Practice of Ophthalmology, 3rd edition. Philadelphia: Saunders/Elsevier; 2008.

LAGOPHTHALMOS

Varsha Varshney, Ritu Nagpal

■ INTRODUCTION

Lagophthalmos is a condition in which the eyelids do not close to cover the eye completely. The term lagophthalmos actually comes from the Greek word for hare (lagoos) and derives from a myth that hares sleep with their eyes open.[1,2] In examinations, it can be given as a short or spot case. A normal, healthy eye is covered by a film of tears that protects the surface and washes away dust and particles. Dry eyes that result from lagophthalmos are not only uncomfortable but are also subject to injury or infection from foreign objects landing in and abrading the eye surface. Left untreated, lagophthalmos can lead to permanent loss of vision.

■ HISTORY

Chief Complaints

Lagophthalmos patients commonly complain of inability to close lids completely **(Figs. 1 and 2)**. Associated features are as follows:
- Foreign body sensation
- Increased tearing
- Photophobia
- Pain may be worse in the morning due to increased corneal exposure and dryness during sleep
- Blurry vision, which results from unstable tear film
- In cases of advanced keratopathy and corneal ulceration, the symptoms and presentation may be severe.

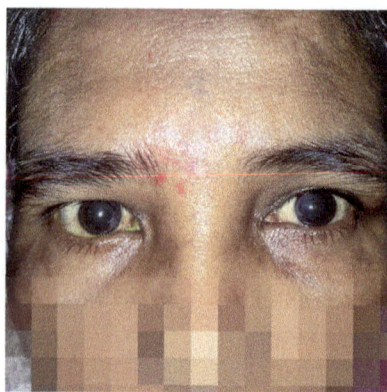

Fig. 1: Normal lid opening.

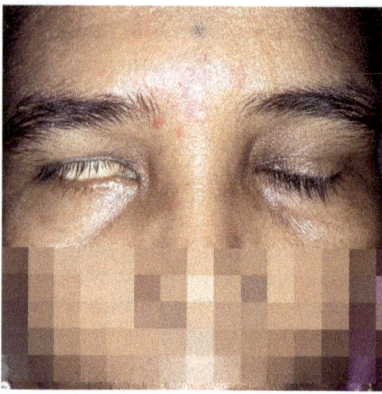

Fig. 2: Lagophthalmos on lid closure in a case (**Fig. 1**).

History of Past Illness

- The recent history of trauma or surgery involving the head, face, or eyelids should be documented with special attention to fractures to the skull base (a petrous portion of the temporal bone) or mandible that could affect facial nerve.
- Past infections should be reviewed, with particular attention to any history of herpes zoster infection.
- It is also important to document any past symptoms suggestive of thyroid disease or obstructive sleep apnea (*Floppy eyelid syndrome*).

History of Systemic Illness

History of systemic diseases such as diabetes (diabetic neuropathy), any neurological disorder (polio, Guillain-Barré syndrome, and leprosy), and cerebrovascular accidents.

■ EXAMINATION

Systemic Examination

Complete neurological examination should be performed.

Ocular Examination

Visual acuity: Usually, normal. The blurring of vision may be present due to tearing or dryness.

Eyeball: Usually, normal.

Lids: Ask the patient to look down and gently close both eyes. Lagophthalmos is present when space remains between the upper and lower eyelid margins in extreme downgaze. Document the degree of lagophthalmos by measuring this space, in millimeters, with a ruler. In addition, following points must be recorded carefully:
- Record the blink rate as well as the completeness of the blink.
- Carefully test ocular motility and the strength of the orbicularis oculi muscle. The latter can be assessed by evaluating the force generated on attempted eyelid closure.
- Bell's phenomenon.
- Scar marks of previous trauma or surgery or infections may be present.

Conjunctiva: Diffuse or ciliary congestion may be there in presence of dry eye and exposure keratopathy.

Cornea: Following points must be recorded:
- Corneal sensitivity by applying a wisp soft cotton to the unanesthetized cornea and comparing the blink reaction with that of the fellow eye.
- Fluorescein staining with cobalt blue filter to find out the presence of punctate epithelial erosions or abrasions. Pay particular attention to the inferior cornea where lid excursion ends.
- Tear breakup time.
- Any epithelial defects or corneal ulcers should be carefully documented.
- *Schirmer test:* The Schirmer test is used to assess tearing function. The degree of tearing can be compared between the paralyzed and normal sides.

Pupils: Pupillary reflexes are usually normal unless other cranial nerves are involved.

Anterior segment: Normal chamber depth and contents.

Posterior segment: Slit-lamp biomicroscopic examination using a 90D/78D lens and indirect ophthalmoscopy—usually normal.

■ INVESTIGATIONS

Blood Investigations

To rule out any systemic disease or infection following tests can be performed:
- CBC, blood sugar
- Thyroid function test
- Human immunodeficiency virus (HIV) enzyme-linked immunosorbent assay (ELISA)/western blot
- Venereal disease research laboratory (VDRL)/RPR.
  The tests advised must be based on the history and clinical findings.

Radiological Investigations

Preferably gadolinium-enhanced MRI: To rule out any neurological causes such as fracture damaging the nerve, mass compressing the nerve, and ischemic areas involving facial nerve origin (geniculate ganglion).

Conduction Testing and Electromyography

The tests are most useful when performed 3–10 days after the onset of paralysis. Comparison to the contralateral side helps to demonstrate the extent of nerve injury and has prognostic implications. Nerve conduction responses are abnormal if a difference of 50% in amplitude between the paralyzed and normal side is detected; a difference of 90% between the 2 sides suggests a poorer prognosis.

Electroneurography

It is a physiologic test that objectively measures the difference between potentials generated by the facial musculature on both sides of the face in response to a supramaximal electrical stimulation of the facial nerve.

Electrodiagnostic Testing

Measures the facial nerve degeneration indirectly. If a patient does not reach 90% degeneration within the first 3 weeks of the onset of paralysis, some studies suggest that the prognosis is excellent, with over 80–100% of the patients recovering with excellent function.

Brainstem Auditory Evoked Response

It may be obtained in patients with peripheral facial nerve lesions and other neurologic involvement. This test measures the transmission of response through the brainstem and is effective in detecting, notably, retrocochlear lesions.

Blepharokymographic Analysis

A high-speed eyelid motion-analysis system has been used to evaluate movement of the eyelids. The computer-based analysis may prove helpful in diagnosing Bell palsy, predicting prognosis, and evaluating response to therapeutic measures such as placement of a gold weight in the affected upper eyelid (used in cases in which spontaneous recovery has been limited).

All these investigations must be conducted in consultation with a neurologist.

■ DIFFERENTIAL DIAGNOSIS

Lagophthalmos can be due to a variety of causes, careful history and neuroimaging often help in arriving at a diagnosis. Following points must be kept in mind:
- Most common cause is Bell's palsy.
- If another cranial nerve, motor, or sensory symptoms are present, then other neurologic diseases should be considered (e.g., stroke, Guillain–Barré syndrome, basilar meningitis, and cerebellar pontine angle tumor).
- Symptoms associated with seventh nerve neoplasm include slowly progressive paralysis, facial hyperkinesis, severe pain, recurrent palsy, and other cranial nerve involvement.
- Cerebellopontine tumors may affect the seventh, eighth, and fifth cranial nerves simultaneously.
- Patients with a progressive paralysis of the facial nerve lasting longer than 3 weeks should be evaluated for neoplasm.

- Recurrent ipsilateral facial paralysis must raise the suspicion of a tumor of the facial nerve or parotid gland. Tumors in the temporal bone, such as facial nerve neuromas, meningiomas, hemangiomas, and malignant primary and metastatic lesions, should be considered as well.
- If a patient reports the sudden onset of hearing loss and severe pain with the onset of facial paralysis, Ramsay Hunt syndrome must be considered. Typically, these patients will also have an erythematous vesicular rash involving the ear canal, auricle, and/or oropharynx.

Bilateral cases: Bilateral simultaneous Bell palsy is a rare (<1% of that of unilateral facial nerve palsy) condition. Examples include Guillain–Barré syndrome, sarcoidosis, Lyme disease, meningitis (neoplastic or infectious), or bilateral neurofibromas (in patients with neurofibromatosis type 2).

TREATMENT

Medical Treatment and Supportive Care for Corneal Exposure

Nonpreserved artificial tears should be administered frequently (at least four times per day) in order to supplement the patient's tear film. Ointments can be applied to the cornea once at bedtime or throughout the day in cases of severe corneal exposure. Prophylactic antibiotics (preferably nonepitheliotoxic such as chloramphenicol 0.3%) can be added to the regimen. In addition, following measures can be used:
- Moisture goggles also may be used.
- Punctal plugs may be helpful if dryness of the cornea is a persistent problem.
- Infectious corneal ulcers should be treated with appropriate antibiotic therapy.
- Patching the eye in the night time with simple micropore or a Frost suture for temporary protection of the cornea can also be helpful.
- Botulinum toxin can be injected transcutaneously or subconjunctivally at the upper border of the tarsus to paralyze the levator muscle to produce complete ptosis and to protect the cornea.

Tarsorrhaphy

A *temporary tarsorrhaphy* is performed if recovery of the eyelid closure is expected within a few weeks. In most cases, the cornea can be protected adequately by suturing the lateral one-third of the eyelids together. Ideally, a small opening remains so that the patient can retain useful vision, the health of the cornea may be assessed and lubrication or antibiotic therapy can be applied to the eye.

A *permanent tarsorrhaphy* is performed if a protracted clinical course is expected. If the patient regains useful function of the orbicularis oculi muscle, the adhesions can be lysed. The limitation of tarsorrhaphy is poor cosmetic appearance.

Gold Weight Implantation

Gold weights can be implanted into the upper eyelid to treat paralytic lagophthalmos. It enhances eyelid closure in a gravity-dependent fashion. Gold is considered an ideal substance because it is inert and it is not visible through the thin skin of the eyelid. Gold weights range from 0.6 to 1.6 g (in 0.2-g increments). The appropriate weight is chosen preoperatively by taping weights of varying sizes onto the external lid above the tarsus and observing the closing and opening of the lids. Properly chosen, the ideal weight will allow full closing and the opening of the lids while avoiding ptosis in primary gaze. Gold weight implantation is usually well-tolerated. However, astigmatic shift, as well as migration and/or extrusion of the gold weight, are its limitations. In cases of allergy to gold, platinum may be used.

Upper Eyelid Retraction and Levator Recession

The recession of the upper eyelid retractors (levator and Müller muscles) is a useful procedure in patients with lagophthalmos related to upper eyelid retraction from thyroid ophthalmopathy. Also, a combination of full-thickness skin grafts, advancement flaps, tarsal-sharing procedures, and release of scar bands can be performed on patients with lagophthalmos from cicatricial or postsurgical lid shortening.

Lower Eyelid Tightening and Elevation

Laxity of the lower eyelid may occur in conditions such as facial nerve palsy and floppy eyelid syndrome. A tightening procedure such as a lateral tarsal strip will improve apposition of the lower eyelid to the globe and decrease tearing. This is also helpful in cases where upper eyelid restructuring procedures fail.

Other Surgical Procedures

In cases of severe lagophthalmos, various other procedures have been described such as elevation of the midface using a variety of materials such as autogenous fascia slings, temporalis muscle transposition/transfer, nerve grafts and anastomoses, palpebral springs, soft tissue repositioning, and suborbicularis oculi fat lifts.

VIVA QUESTIONS

Q.1. What are the ocular symptoms and signs of Bell's palsy?

Ans. Bell's palsy is the most common cause of unilateral facial paralysis. Ocular manifestations have been described in **Table 1**. Two-thirds of the patients complain about epiphora, which is due to punctal eversion and the reduced function of the orbicularis oculi in transporting the tears (fewer tears arrive at the lacrimal sac, and overflow occurs).

Q.2. Discuss etiology of lagophthalmos.

Ans. Lagophthalmos can occur due to a pathology in the facial nerve or in the lid. The different causes are summarized in **Table 2**.

Q.3. Relevant anatomy of facial nerve and eyelid.

Ans. *Facial nerve:* The facial nerve (seventh cranial nerve) innervates both the frontalis

Table 1: Ocular manifestations of Bell's palsy.

Early	Late
• Lagophthalmos • Paralytic ectropion of the lower lid • Tear overflow • Brow ptosis • Upper eyelid retraction • Dry eye—poor tear distribution • Corneal exposure, erosion, infection, and ulceration (rare)	• Narrow palpebral fissure—generalized mass contracture of the facial muscles (after several months) • Aberrant regeneration of the facial nerve with motor synkinesis • Reversed jaw-winking—twitching of the corner of the mouth or dimpling of the chin occurring simultaneously with each blink • Crocodile tears—tearing with chewing

Table 2: Causes of lagophthalmos.

Pathology	Etiology	Factors/mechanism
Facial nerve	Trauma	• Fractures to the skull base (petrous portion of the temporal bone) or mandible • Neurosurgical procedures
	Bell's palsy	Acute viral infection or reactivation of herpes simplex virus
	Tumors	• Acoustic neuromas in the cerebellopontine angle • Metastatic lesions
	Cerebrovascular accidents	Blockage of anterior inferior cerebellar artery
	Infectious, immune-mediated causes	Lyme disease, chickenpox, mumps, polio, Guillain–Barré syndrome, leprosy, diphtheria, and botulism
	Mobius syndrome	Characterized by cranial nerve palsies (sixth and seventh cranial nerve), motility disturbances, limb anomalies, and orofacial defects

Contd...

Contd...

Pathology	Etiology	Factors/mechanism
Eyelids	Cicatrices	Chemical or thermal burns, ocular cicatricial pemphigoid, Stevens–Johnson syndrome, mechanical trauma
	Eyelid surgery	• Excessive removal of eyelid skin or muscle; blepharoplasty, tumor excision • Overcorrection in ptosis repair
	Proptosis	Exophthalmos of one or both globes may inhibit eyelid closure
	Enophthalmos	• Posterior displacement of the eye may affect eyelid apposition and closure • Causes include orbital blowout fractures; orbital fat atrophy (trauma, infection, inflammation, aging, scleroderma, HIV-AIDS); phthisical eye; scirrhous carcinomas
	Floppy eyelid syndrome	Severe laxity and flexibility of the superior and inferior tarsal plates

(AIDS: acquired immunodeficiency syndrome; HIV: human immunodeficiency virus)

muscle, which raises the eyebrow, and the orbicularis oculi muscle, which closes the eyelids. In addition, the 7th nerve innervates the muscles of the facial expression such zygomaticus muscles, which elevate the cheeks as well as the corrugator supercilii and procerus muscles, which depress the eyebrow.

Eyelids: The upper and lower eyelids contain seven structural layers. Beginning anteriorly, these comprise (1) skin and subcutaneous tissue, (2) orbicularis oculi muscle, (3) orbital septum, (4) orbital fat, (5) muscles of retraction, (6) tarsus, and (7) conjunctiva. Damage to or degeneration of any of these tissues may inhibit good eyelid closure.

Q.4. Discuss treatment options for Bell's palsy.

Ans. Treatment options for Bell's palsy includes following:

Pharmacologic therapy: The most widely accepted treatment for Bell's palsy is corticosteroid therapy. However, the use of steroids is still controversial because most patients recover without treatment. The recommended dose of prednisone for the treatment of Bell's palsy is 1 mg/kg or 60 mg/day for 6 days, followed by a taper, for a total of 10 days.

Antiviral agents: Such as acyclovir (Zovirax) and valacyclovir (Valtrex) have shown limited benefit.

Surgical options: Surgical options for Bell's palsy include the following: Facial nerve decompression, subocularis oculi fat (SOOF) lift, implantable devices (e.g., gold weights) placed into the eyelid, tarsorrhaphy, transposition of the temporalis muscle, facial nerve grafting, and direct brow lift.

■ REFERENCES

1. Pereira MV, Glória AL. Lagophthalmos. Semin Ophthalmol. 2010;25(3):72-8.
2. Vásquez LM, Medel R. Lagophthalmos after facial palsy: current therapeutic options. Ophthalmic Res. 2014;52(4):165-9.

DERMOID CYST

Shipra Singhi, Deepali Singhal

■ INTRODUCTION

A dermoid cyst (epidermal dermoid cyst) is an epithelial-lined structure with dermal appendages in its wall and keratin and hair in its lumen. It can be found in any subcutaneous location but >80% are located in the region of the head, with the majority in the eyelid and orbital area, usually superotemporally near the zygomaticofrontal suture.

It can be given as a short case or spot case in examination.

■ HISTORY

Chief Complaint

The presenting feature depends upon the location of dermoid. It can present in following manner:
- *Superficial dermoid:* Well-defined painless lesion and ptosis
- *Deep dermoid:* Proptosis, diplopia, or EOM restriction
- Painless fullness of upper eyelid or a mass lesion, most commonly at lateral orbital rim can be the presenting feature in an anteriorly located dermoid.
- A posteriorly located dermoid can present with painless, progressive proptosis, and diplopia.
- Rarely there can be associated ptosis and limitation of the movement.
- *Diminution of vision:* Blurring of vision is related to size and nerve compression and the presence of complications. It is usually progressive and painless.
- Sometimes patient may present with symptoms including the rapid onset of unilateral pain, redness, and watery discharge due to a ruptured cyst.
- Intermittent increase in size during chewing indicated extension to the temporalis muscle of deep dermoid. However, this mode of presentation is very rare.

In adults, dermoids may become symptomatic for the first time and grow considerably over a year. Based on this fact, some conclude that these lesions may be dormant for many years or have intermittent growth.

History of Present Illness

The onset, progression, association with pain, and any preceding events such as trauma must be noted. Dermoid cyst usually has an insidious onset, painless, and progresses slowly over a period of years. Rapid onset of unilateral pain, redness, and watery discharge suggests a ruptured cyst.

Past History

A careful past history should be taken of any mass (tumor), nerve paresis, infection, trauma, and ocular inflammatory diseases.

Past Surgical History

Previous history of any intraocular surgery should be enquired.

■ EXAMINATION

Ocular examination: Ocular examination should include following:

Visual acuity: Visual acuity is variably impaired depending on the site of involvement, size, and compression of nerve and the presence of complications.

Eyeball:
- Proptosis is usually nonaxial. Extension into intracranial fossae is possible if the frontal or sphenoid bones are involved. Temporal fossa involvement is rare but reported; this may result in intermittent proptosis associated with chewing, as positional changes of the temporalis muscle during chewing transmit pressure to the lesion and, hence, to the orbit.
- *Mass:* A mass lesion due to dermoid cysts have the following characteristics:
  – Firm in consistency
  – Margins are smooth
  – Nontender

- Mobile preseptal masses without fixity to skin or muscle
- Superotemporal quadrant is the most common site, less commonly, the superonasal quadrant is affected.
- Many of them have variable periosteal attachment near the underlying frontozygomatic or frontoethmoidal sutures.
- Occasionally, the dermoid will pass into or through defects in the neighboring bone and may communicate intracranially.
- A dermoid cyst can rupture spontaneously or with trauma, inciting an intense inflammatory response in the orbital soft tissues. This response may be limited to injection of the conjunctiva or may be severe and mimic orbital cellulitis.
- Occasionally, subconjunctival droplets of fat are seen. In some cases, a secondary fistula between the cyst and the skin may allow the contents of the cyst to drain intermittently.

• Rarely the dermoid is incompletely separated from the skin surface and presents as a chronically inflamed and discharging sinus.
• Dermoid cyst can also be associated with motility deficits and diplopia when the extent is large.

Eyelids: When dermoid is located anteriorly, it can lead to ptosis.

Anterior segment: Generally normal. Occasionally, subconjunctival droplets of fat are seen in case of rupture of cyst.

Tonometry: Intraocular pressure (IOP) is usually unaffected.

Fundus: There may be compressive neuropathy or choroidal folds especially in cases of posterior dermoid.

■ DIFFERENTIAL DIAGNOSIS

Differential diagnosis depends upon the location of the dermoid:
• *Lateral anterior dermoid:*
  – Lacrimal gland mass
  – Lipodermoid
  – Teratoma
  – Plexiform neurofibroma
• *Medial anterior dermoid:*
  – Mucocele
  – Encephalocele
• *Cyst with spontaneous rupture:*
  – Orbital cellulitis
  – Orbital pseudotumor
• *Deep dermoid with mass effect:*
  – Orbital tumors
  – Thyroid ophthalmopathy.

■ INVESTIGATION

Classic dermoid cysts located at the frontozygomatic suture whose posterior aspect can be palpated may be diagnosed clinically without imaging. Medial lesions require imaging to rule out an encephalocele or mucocele before surgical excision. Deep orbital lesions also require imaging for diagnostic purposes and to help with surgical planning.

Computed Tomography Scan

A dermoid cyst typically has a hyperdense wall and a hypodense cavity that remains nonenhancing with contrast. The central cavity may appear heterogeneous as a result of keratin and other cystic debris. CT imaging is especially useful in delineating bony changes such as *smooth pressure erosion (scalloped) near the affected suture or fossa, clefts, and full-thickness bony channels*, seen in as much as 85% of cases. A dumbbell cyst have a typical appearance with a component on either side of the bone and a bony communication between them.

Magnetic Resonance Imaging

The lesions are generally hypointense on T1-weighted imaging with respect to fat and are best visualized using fat-suppression techniques. It appears as a well-defined, round-to-ovoid structure of variable size. The lesions tend to be hyperintense on T2-weighted imaging. These lesions typically do not enhance with contrast due to lack of blood vessels in the cyst. MRI has the advantage of not exposing the patient to radiation, hence extremely useful in pediatric age group.

Ultrasonography

Ultrasound characteristics of dermoid cysts include a smooth contour and variable echogenicity.

Color Doppler Imaging

Color Doppler imaging of dermoid cysts shows no intralesional blood flow, which can help differentiate them from hemangioma and rhabdomyosarcoma.

■ MANAGEMENT

A small, asymptomatic orbital epidermal dermoid cyst requires no immediate treatment. In many cases, however, the cyst slowly enlarges or ruptures, and eventually requires treatment. The treatment of orbital dermoid cysts is surgical excision. The primary goal of excision is to remove the dermoid with the cyst wall intact without causing an iatrogenic rupture. Leakage of the cystic contents into the orbit can result in significant inflammation and recurrence, while lesions removed in their entirety rarely recur.

The surgical approach depends upon the location of the lesion. An anterior orbital epidermal dermoid cyst can be removed through anterior orbitotomy (superior eyelid crease incision). A posterior orbital epidermal dermoid cyst can be removed through lateral orbitotomy. The use of a cryoprobe can help in the delivery of the cyst intact in these cases. Deeper lesions are approached based upon their location in the orbit and relationship to adjacent structures. Intracranial extension requires a multidisciplinary surgical approach for complete excision.

Great care should be taken to remove the cyst with the capsule intact, using meticulous dissection at the site of the attachment of the cyst to the bony sutures. If the cyst is accidentally ruptured at the time of surgery, copious irrigation and attempted removal of the cyst remnants should be done.

In the rare case of dermoid cyst at the orbital apex, an orbital deroofing procedure may be necessary. If the cyst is too large to remove intact, its contents can be aspirated in order to facilitate removal. Recurrence can develop after incomplete excision.

In ruptured cyst:
- Systemic steroid therapy
- Systemic nonsteroidal anti-inflammatory drug (NSAID) therapy (aspirin and ibuprofen)

■ CLASSIFICATION

- Epidermal dermoid cyst—anterior or deep
- Conjuctival dermoid cyst.

Conjunctival Dermoid Cyst

Occasionally, an otherwise typical dermoid cyst is lined by nonkeratinizing epithelium with features of conjunctival epithelium. This is called a conjunctival dermoid cyst.

Incidence

A conjunctival dermoid cyst is lined by conjunctival epithelium. It accounts for about 5% of dermoid cysts that occur in the orbit, with the other 95% being of epidermal origin.

Clinical Features

Conjunctival dermoid cyst is probably congenital but often it is not evident until childhood or sometimes later in life.

It occurs in the superonasal aspect of the orbit usually and presents as firm or fluctuant subcutaneous mass.

Investigation

With CT or MRI, a conjunctival dermoid cyst has features similar to an epidermal dermoid cyst. However, it is more likely to be situated in the orbital soft tissues in the anterior and nasal aspect of the orbit, usually without contact to bone.

Histopathology

Histopathologically, conjunctival dermoid cyst is lined by nonkeratinizing epithelium, which contains goblet cells. Like the epidermoid dermoid cyst, it contains dermal appendages such as hair shafts, sebaceous gland, and occasional sweat glands.

Management

A conjunctival dermoid cyst is usually symptomatic when diagnosed and is best managed by surgical excision.

Either a conjunctival or skin incision superonasally is generally used because it is usually located superonasally in the anterior orbit.

In a skin approach, an eyelid crease incision in the upper eyelid is recommended.

VIVA QUESTIONS

Q.1. What is the epidemiology of dermoid?
Ans. *Epidemiology:*
- Congenital choristoma
- Accounts for 3–8% of orbital tumors in children
- The dermoid cyst becomes the most common noninflammatory space-occupying lesion of the orbit
- In the Wills Eye Hospital pathology series, dermoid cyst accounted for 46% of childhood orbital lesions and for 89% of all cystic lesions.

Q.2. Compare epidermal and conjunctival dermoid cyst?
Ans. See Table 1.

Q.3. Differentiate between anterior and deep dermoid cyst.
Ans. See Table 2.

Q.4. What is choristoma?
Ans. Choristoma is a mass of histologically normal tissue present at abnormal location.

Q.5. What is difference between choristoma and hamartoma?
Ans. While choristoma is a mass of histologically normal tissue present at abnormal location, hamartoma is a mass of neoplastic tissue at abnormal location.

Table 1: Comparison of epidermal and conjunctival dermoid.

Epidermal dermoid	*Conjunctival dermoid*
• *Age of onset:* Anterior dermoids typically present in first decade • It accounts for about 95% of dermoid cysts that occur in the orbit	• *Age of onset:* Deeper dermoids may present in adolescence or adulthood • It accounts for about 5% of dermoid cysts that occur in the orbit
• *Histopathology:* Dermoid cyst is lined by keratinizing stratified epithelium • It contains dermal appendages such as hair shafts, sebaceous gland, and occasional sweat glands	*Histopathology:* Histopathologically, conjunctival dermoid cyst is lined by nonkeratinizing epithelium, which contains goblet cells. Like the epidermoid dermoid cyst, it contains dermal appendages such as hair shafts, sebaceous gland, and occasional sweat glands
Site: Superotemporal usually	*Site:* Superonasal usually
• *Imaging:* On CT, a dermoid typically has a hyperdense wall and a hypodense cavity that remains nonenhancing with contrast. The central cavity may appear heterogeneous as a result of keratin and other cystic debris • An estimated 85% of dermoids are associated with such bony changes as smooth pressure erosion near the affected suture, clefts, and full-thickness bony channels • *On MRI:* Hypointense on T1-weighted imaging; hyperintense on T2-weighted imaging	*Imaging:* With CT or MRI, a conjunctival dermoid cyst has features similar to an epidermal dermoid cyst. However, it is more likely to be situated in the orbital soft tissues in the anterior and nasal aspect of the orbit, usually without contact to bone
Treatment: Anterior orbitotomy (superior eyelid crease incision)	• *Treatment:* Anterior orbitotomy—conjunctival or skin incision superonasally • In a skin approach, an eyelid crease incision in the upper eyelid is recommended

(CT: computed tomography; MRI: magnetic resonance imaging)

Table 2: Differences between anterior and deep dermoid cysts.

Anterior dermoid	Deep dermoid
Age of onset: Anterior dermoids typically present in first decade	*Age of onset:* Deeper dermoids may present in adolescence or adulthood
• *Suture involved:* – *Lateral:* Frontozygomatic suture – *Medial:* Frontoethmoidal or frontolacrimal sutures	*Suture involved:* Sphenozygomatic or sphenoethmoidal suture
Symptoms: Painless fullness of upper eyelid, most commonly at lateral orbital rim	*Symptoms:* Painless, progressive proptosis, diplopia
Signs: Subcutaneous, mobile nodule, most commonly located at frontozygomatic suture	*Signs:* Proptosis, motility deficit, inferior or superior displacement of globe
Treatment: Anterior orbitotomy (superior eyelid crease incision)	*Treatment:* Lateral orbitotomy

Q.6. What is the most common location?

Ans. *Children:*
- The most common location is in the superior temporal aspect of the orbit. The second most common location is in the superior nasal aspect of the orbit.
- Lesions located superotemporally are generally smooth, firm subcutaneous masses attached to the orbital rim in the region of the zygomaticofrontal suture.
- The mass is generally <1 cm in diameter, nontender, and oval in shape. Little displacement of the globe usually occurs.
- Orbital dermoid cysts are not attached to the skin, which helps differentiate them from sebaceous cysts. The cyst usually is tethered to the periosteum of the bone near suture lines, including the sinuses or intracranial cavity.

Adults:
- The cysts are palpated less easily and have more vague borders. They are more likely to displace the globe and may erode their way into adjacent structures.
- *Dystopia:* A larger dermoid cyst can cause downward and medial displacement of the globe.
- Motility deficits
- Diplopia

Anterior lesions: Typically present in the first few years of life as smooth, well-circumscribed, subcutaneous, and painless masses.
- *Site:* The most common location for the anterior dermoid cyst is at the *superolateral* aspect of the orbit *at the frontozygomatic suture*, as seen in the case described here. Medial lesions occur less frequently and often arise from tissue sequestered in the frontoethmoidal or frontolacrimal sutures. If there is no orbital extension, the posterior aspect of the mass may be palpable.
- *Ptosis:* Because of their anterior location, these lesions do not usually cause globe displacement, but they can cause visually significant ptosis if they grow to a large enough size.

Deep lesions are more insidious, and
- *Site:* Often develop at the sphenozygomatic or sphenoethmoidal suture.
- *Proptosis:* Their presence is usually declared by mass effect on surrounding structures. Patients with deep lesions may present in late adolescence or adulthood with painless, progressive proptosis.
- *Dumbbell dermoids:* Dermoids may also straddle the orbital bones (most commonly the lateral orbital wall) such that they have both an anterior lobe and a deeper orbital lobe. These so-called "dumbbell" dermoids must be imaged to assess the extent of the orbital component before excision.

Rupture:
- A dermoid cyst can rupture spontaneously or with trauma, inciting an intense inflammatory response in the orbital soft tissues. This response may be limited to injection of the conjunctiva

or may be severe and mimic orbital cellulitis.
- Occasionally, subconjunctival droplets of fat are seen. In some cases, a secondary fistula between the cyst and the skin may allow the contents of the cyst to drain intermittently.
- While this is rarely the first presenting sign for an anterior dermoid, it may be the first presenting sign of a deep dermoid.

Complications:
- Rupture of the cyst
- Orbital cellulitis
- Recurrent cyst
- Compressive neuropathy
- Amblyopia
- Strabismus

ORBITAL HEMANGIOMA

Aditi Dubey, Sanjana M, Rajesh Pattebahadur

INTRODUCTION

Orbital hemangiomas are of two types—capillary hemangioma and cavernous hemangioma. Capillary hemangioma is the most common primary benign tumor of orbit in children (infancy). Cavernous hemangioma is more common in adults (20-30 years), usually women.[1,2]

CAPILLARY HEMANGIOMA

History

Chief Complaints

Mass over eyelid present since birth or appear in the first few weeks of birth.

History

Usually parents complain of bluish or pink mass over eyelid present since birth with enlarging with age. In addition, there will be a history of increases in size on crying.

Examination

Inspection

Superficial hemangiomas are confined to the dermis, pink-purple mass lesion with mulberry appearance or dimpled texture and increases on crying or Valsalva. Deep orbital lesions may present with axial/nonaxial proptosis.

Palpation

Soft, nontender, nonpulsatile, ill-defined mass over the eyelid which may have an orbital extension.

Auscultation

No bruit or pulsation heard.
Deep orbital lesions may present with hyperopia, optic nerve edema (due to compression), retinal striae, raised intraocular pressure, and strabismus.

Classification

- *Superficial or simple:* Involves the skin and appear as a bright red, soft mass with a dimpled texture.
- *Preseptal or subcutaneous:* Dark blue/purple soft ill-defined nontender mass **(Fig. 1)**. Increases on crying and Valsalva, nonpulsatile no bruit.
- *Deep:* Located deeper within the orbit may present merely as a progressively enlarging mass without any overlying skin change (Differential diagnosis: Rhabdomyosarcoma should be ruled out).

Management

Normally the course of capillary hemangioma is as follows:
- Rapid growth up to 6–12 months
- 30% spontaneous resolution by 3 years
- 70% spontaneous resolution by 7 years.

Oculoplasty

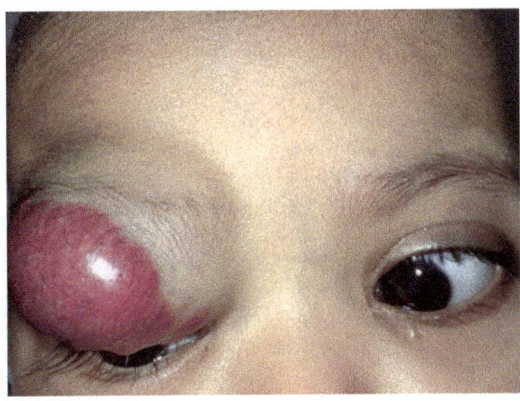

Fig. 1: Capillary hemangioma.

Most lesions will regress spontaneously, therefore; observation, refractive correction and amblyopia therapy are the first line of management. Treatment should be deferred until it is clear that the natural course of the lesion will not lead to the desired result.

Indication for Treatment

- Amblyopia secondary to astigmatism, ptosis, and anisometropia
- Exposure keratopathy
- Optic nerve compression
- Severe disfigurement or cosmetic blemish
- Infection

Modalities of Treatment

- Small lesion <2 mm thickness—laser
- Superficial or preseptal lesion—intralesional steroid [betamethasone (4 mg/mL) 1–2 mL or triamcinolone (40 mg/mL) 1–2 mL at different site repeat after 2 months]. Adverse effects of steroid injection include skin necrosis, subcutaneous fat atrophy, orbital hemorrhage, and rarely central retinal artery occlusion.
- Deep/orbital lesions—systemic steroids
- Systemic beta-blockers (inhibits angiogenesis and acts as vasoconstrictor)
- Surgical excision may be considered for lesions that are smaller, subcutaneous, or refractory to steroids
- Interferon-α (however, it has significant systemic adverse effects and poorly tolerated)

- Radiation therapy has also been used, but it has the potential to cause cataract formation, bone hypoplasia, and future malignancy.

■ CAVERNOUS HEMANGIOMA

Chief Complaints

Cavernous hemangioma—slowly progressive proptosis (growth may accelerate during pregnancy).

History

Cavernous hemangiomas are usually seen in adults presenting as progressive proptosis, sometimes decreased visual acuity may be present due to compressive optic neuropathy.

Examination

Examination is similar to a case of proptosis due to an intraconal tumor. It usually leads to axial proptosis.

Course and Management of Cavernous Hemangioma

- This lesion rarely resolves spontaneously.
- *Observation:* If asymptomatic
- *An indication of treatment:* (1) Symptomatic lesion (lesion compromising ocular function) and (2) gradually enlarging
- *Treatment:* Surgical excision.

VIVA QUESTIONS

Q.1. Classify orbital hemangioma.
Ans.
- Cutaneous
- Purely preseptal
- Preseptal with orbital involvement (extraconal)
- Preseptal with orbital involvement (extraconal + intraconal).

Q.2. What are the risk factors for capillary hemangioma?
Ans. Premature infants and newborns whose mothers had chorionic villus sampling.

Q.3. What is the most common location of hemangioma?

Ans. *Capillary hemangioma:* Predilection for the superonasal quadrant of the orbit and the medial upper eyelid, may involve skin over face, and some patients may have cutaneous and visceral hemangiomas.
Cavernous hemangioma: Extraconal and retrobulbar.

Q.4. Histopathology and imaging in hemangioma?

Ans. Shown in **Table 1**.

Q.5. What are the systemically associated syndromes with capillary hemangioma?

Ans.
- *Kasabach Merritt syndrome:* Triad of hemangioma, decrease coagulation factors, and thrombocytopenia. Associated with rapidly expanding visceral hemangiomas.
- *Maffucci syndrome:* Multiple skin and visceral hemangiomas associated with enchondromas.
- High output heart failure associated with fast growing visceral hemangiomas.
- *PHACES syndrome:* Posterior fossa malformations–hemangiomas–arterial anomalies–cardiac defects–eye abnormalities–sternal cleft and supraumbilical raphe syndrome.

Q.6. What are the other vascular malformations of the orbit?

Ans.
- *Hemangiopericytoma:*
  - The uncommon lesion, well encapsulated, hypervascular, and hypercellular
  - Appear in middle age
  - Resemble cavernous hemangiomas on both CT and MRI, but they appear bluish intraoperatively
  - Histologically composed of plump pericytes that surround a rich capillary network, microscopically "benign" lesions may recur and metastasize, whereas microscopically "malignant" lesions may remain localized
  - Treatment—complete excision because they may recur, undergo malignant degeneration, or metastasize
- *Lymphatic malformation:*
  - Also known as lymphangiomas
  - Due to vascular dysgenesis
  - Become apparent in the first decade of life
  - Occurs in the orbit, conjunctiva, eyelids, oropharynx, or sinuses
  - Contains both venous and lymphatic components

Table 1: Differentiating features between capillary and cavernous hemangioma.

Parameters	Capillary hemangioma	Cavernous hemangioma
Histopathology	Tumor composed of small anastomosing channels without true encapsulation	Lesions are well encapsulated and composed of large, cavernous spaces containing red blood cells with walls of the spaces containing smooth muscle
B scan	For extension of disease and anatomical relations	Well encapsulated mass lesion with cavernous fluid (blood) filled spaces
CT scan	Homogeneous enhancing soft tissue mass ± extraconal extension with fingerlike projections	Homogeneously slowly enhancing, well-encapsulated mass
MRI scan	Fine intralesional vascular channels and high blood flow	Small intralesional vascular channels with slowly flowing blood, that is, flow voids. Chronic lesions may contain radiodense phleboliths

(CT: computed tomography; MRI: magnetic resonance imaging)

- May enlarge during URTIs and present with sudden proptosis caused by spontaneous intralesional hemorrhage
- *Histology:* Characterized by large, not encapsulated, serum-filled channels that are lined by flat endothelial cells
- *MRI:* Pathognomonic features multiple grapes like cystic lesions with a fluid-fluid layering of the serum and red blood cells. Venography shows no arterial or venous connection.
- *Management:* Surgical intervention should be deferred unless vision is affected due to the risk of hemorrhage. A subtotal resection is generally needed to avoid sacrificing important structures. Orbital hemorrhage is allowed to resorb spontaneously; but if optic neuropathy or corneal ulceration threatens vision, aspiration of blood through a hollow-bore needle, or by open surgical exploration can be attempted.

- *Venous malformations:*
  - Also known as *orbital varices*
  - Low-flow vascular lesions due to vascular dysgenesis
  - *Clinical features:* Enophthalmos at rest (when the lesion is not engorged), proptosis when the patient's head is dependent or after a Valsalva maneuver
    - *Diagnosis:* Contrast-enhanced rapid spiral CT during a Valsalva maneuver showing characteristic enlargement of the engorged veins. Phleboliths may be present on imaging.
    - *Treatment:* Conservative
    - *Biopsy:* Avoided because of the risk of hemorrhage
    - *Surgery:* Reserved for the relief of significant pain or for cases in which the venous malformation causes vision-threatening compressive optic neuropathy. Complete surgical excision is difficult. Intraoperative embolization of the lesion may aid surgical removal.

- *Arteriovenous malformations:*
  - High-flow developmental anomalies due to vascular dysgenesis
  - Composed of anastomosing arteries and veins without an intervening capillary bed
  - *Sign:* Dilated corkscrew episcleral vessels
  - *Treatment:* Selective occlusion of the feeding vessels followed by surgical excision of the malformations (complication—arterial hemorrhage).

■ REFERENCES

1. Albert DM, Miller JW, Azar DT. Albert & Jakobiec's Principles and Practice of Ophthalmology, 3rd edition. Philadelphia: Saunders/Elsevier; 2008.
2. Bowling B. Kanski's Clinical Ophthalmology: a systematic approach, 8th edition. Edinburgh: Elsevier; 2015.

COLOBOMA OF EYELID

Shipra Singhi, Anasua Ganguly Kapoor

■ INTRODUCTION

An eyelid coloboma is a full-thickness defect of the eyelid.[1,2] The word coloboma comes from the Greek word that means, "Curtailed." Lid coloboma occurs due to a delayed fusion of mesodermal components of frontonasal and maxillary processes of the face. It is caused by the failure of fusion of the mesodermal lid folds. Although an eyelid coloboma can occur in many locations, the most common position is at the junction of the medial and middle third of the upper lid.[3-5] In examinations, it can be given as a short or spot case.

■ HISTORY

Chief Complaint

A case of coloboma usually presents with cosmetic issues due to the defect (notching) in the eyelid. It can be associated with following:
- Absence of eyeball
- Bluish colored swelling (in case of cryptophthalmos)
- Small size of eyeball
- Drying of eyes
- *Diminution of vision:* Blurring of vision is related to corneal opacity, exposure keratopathy, cataract, and choroidal coloboma. It is usually present since birth which may progress and painless in origin.
- Diplopia due to restriction
- Painless mass (associated limbal dermoid)
- Foreign body sensation/irritation.

Past History

A careful past history should be taken of any:
- Perinatal and pregnancy history
- Family history of congenital eyelid colobomas or other congenital anomalies, especially facial (e.g., cleft lip/palate)
- History of other current birth defects
- Pediatric review of systems, hearing loss, cardiovascular disease, facial asymmetry
- History of progressive corneal problems.

Past Surgical History

Previous history of ocular surgery may or may not be present.

■ EXAMINATION

Systemic Examination

It may be associated with multiple systemic anomalies.
- Cardiovascular abnormalities, facial hemiatrophy, atresia of the external auditory meatus, accessory auricles, nevus flammeus, neurofibromatosis, preauricular appendages, and pretragal fistulas can be there. One-third of cases associated with Goldenhar's syndrome (triad of peribulbar dermoid, preauricular appendages, and pretragal fistulas).
- Facial defects that may be associated with eyelid colobomas, include a less prominent supraorbital margin, and a bifid nose.
- Among the syndromes that may include eyelid, colobomas are Goldenhar, Treacher Collins syndrome, Delleman, Fraser, and nanopalpebral lipoma coloboma syndrome.

Ocular Examination

Visual acuity: Is variably impaired depending on associated abnormalities such as limbal dermoid.

Eyeball: Microphthalmos, anophthalmos, euryblepharon, cryptophthalmos, lagophthalmos, and esotropia can be there.

Extraocular movement: Duane's retraction syndrome may be an associated feature.

Eyebrow: Loss of eyebrow hair may be seen.

Eyelids: Eyelid colobomas have following features:
- Most commonly triangular with the base at the eyelid margin.
- It is usually located on the medial half of the upper eyelid or lateral half of the lower eyelid.
- They are usually unilateral, generally located at the medial one-third of the upper eyelids (90%), and may vary from a small notch to complete defects of the eyelid.
- Upper eyelid coloboma (**Fig. 1**) is more common than lower lid coloboma and may be associated with Goldenhar syndrome.
- *Lower eyelid coloboma:* Lower lid colobomas are more commonly associated with facial clefts. Treacher Collins syndrome is usually associated with this.

Lacrimal system: Obstruction proximal to the lacrimal sac and lacrimal stenosis can be there.

Oculoplasty

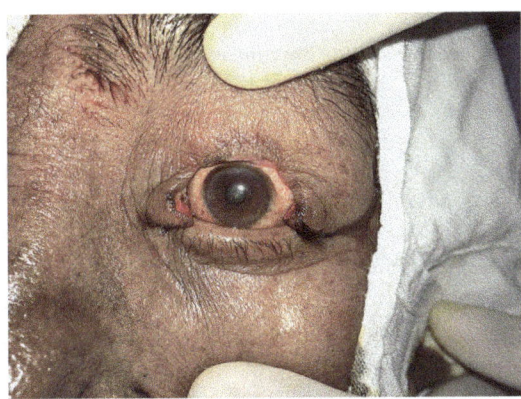

Fig. 1: Surgical eyelid coloboma.

Conjunctiva: Symblepharon, absence of an upper eyelid fornix, and malformation of the caruncle can be seen. Conjunctival traction bands are common (present in a third of eyelid colobomas). These bands are highly amblyogenic owing to strabismus. Forced duction testing (FDT) is often positive in such cases of restriction.

Cornea: Following anomalies can be seen:
- Exposure keratopathy
- Corneal opacities
- *Limbal dermoid:* Yellowish-white, solid, vascularized, elevated nodules straddling the corneal limbus. Size may vary ranging from 2 to 15 mm in diameter. Corneal dermoid occur as single lesions mostly, but may be multiple, and they may be unilateral or bilateral, the former being the more common.
- Dellen formation may occur
- Cicatrization

Lens: Cataract (anterior polar) and subluxation of the lens may be there.

Sclera: Epibulbar dermoid tumor can be there.

Iris: Coloboma (key hole)—may be typical or atypical, complete, or incomplete, partial, or total.

IOP: It is usually normal.

Fundus: There may be choroidal coloboma, retinal detachment due to choroidal coloboma, and hypoplastic disc.

■ CLASSIFICATION

Lid coloboma can be due to following:
- Congenital lid coloboma (isolated or syndromic)
- Acquired lid coloboma (traumatic or postsurgical).

Depending upon the associations, it is classified as discussed here.

Isolated Coloboma

- Coloboma associated with cornea palpebral adhesions:
  – *Complete:* No discernable eyelid differentiation and the eyes are completely covered with skin.
  – *Incomplete:* A skin fold devoid of tarsus covers the medial aspect of the palpebral aperture, significant cornea palpebral adhesions, lower fornix, and lateral upper eyelids usually spared.
  – *Abortive type/congenital symblepharon variant:* True coloboma of variable sizes with a diverse range of cornea palpebral adhesions, lower fornix, and lateral upper eyelids usually spared.
- *Simple coloboma:* Coloboma not associated with cornea palpebral adhesions.

Syndromic Variants

- Fraser syndrome
- Goldenhar syndrome
- *Rare syndromes:* Manitoba oculotrichoanal syndrome, ablepharon-macrostomia syndrome, nasopalpebral lipoma-coloboma syndrome, amniotic band sequence, oculoectodermal syndrome, neurocutaneous syndromes, CHARGE (coloboma, heart defect, atresia choanae, retarded growth and development, genital abnormality, and ear abnormality) syndrome.

■ GRADING

Lid coloboma can be graded as follows (Nouby):[3]
- *Grade 1:* Coloboma without cryptophthalmos
- *Grade 2:* Coloboma with abortive cryptophthalmos

- *Grade 3:* Coloboma with complete cryptophthalmos
- *Grade 4:* Classic cryptophthalmos (absence of all eyelid structures and complete coverage of eye by skin)
- *Grade 5:* Severe cryptophthalmos (with severe deformity of the nose and ectropion of the upper lip).

■ INVESTIGATION

The diagnosis of a lid coloboma requires a direct clinical examination. Specific laboratory studies are generally indicated in associated syndromes that may include following:
- X-ray of spine—for hemivertebra or scoliosis
- Electrocardiography (ECG), echocardiography—for cardiac defect
- MRI of brain
- Complete blood count
- Renal function test
- Audiometry for hearing assessment.

■ MANAGEMENT

Medical Management

Corneal protection is the primary goal in the medical treatment of eyelid colobomas. Medical therapy includes artificial tears and ointment and bedtime patching.

Surgical Management

Indications of surgery include the following:
- Exposure keratitis
- Trichiasis, which may cause corneal lesion
- Cosmesis
- Amblyopia
- Strabismus.

The initial evaluation of an upper eyelid coloboma consists of measuring the size of the eyelid margin defect and comparing it with the overall length of the horizontal palpebral fissure. The surgical procedure used depends on the size and the location of the defect.

Small defects: If the defect in the upper eyelid involves less than one-third of the margin, and well managed with topical lubrication, then surgery may be delayed until later in childhood. This surgery may require a lateral canthotomy and/or superior cantholysis to rotate or advance adjacent tissue to prevent excessive tension on the wound. The edges of the defect are freshened with sharp incisions, and the precise anastomosis is performed. The lid margin is brought together using a 2-layer approximation of the tarsus and the skin. Lateral cantholysis and placement of near-far, far-near sutures may be necessary to minimize horizontal tension.

Moderately sized defects: Larger defects, a Tenzel semicircular rotational flap may be used for defects involving approximately one-third of the eyelid margin.

Large defects: If the defect is larger than one-half of the upper eyelid, other surgical procedures should be used. The various surgeries that can be performed include a free transconjunctival graft from the contralateral upper eyelid can be taken, modified Hughes procedure (for lower lid coloboma), modified Cutler-Beard procedure (upper lid coloboma), and rotational flap from cheek (Mustard's technique).

Prognosis: Prognosis is excellent-to-good in eyelid coloboma, depending on the size of the lesion and the speed of therapy.

Patient education: Genetic consultation is highly recommended, especially for patients with associated syndromes, such as Treacher Collins syndrome, which is autosomal dominant with variable penetrance and expressivity.

VIVA QUESTIONS

Q.1. When should the coloboma of eyelid be repaired?

Ans. This depends on the size of the defect and on the presence of corneal exposure. If the defect of the eyelid is small and not associated with corneal exposure, surgery can be delayed until the age of 3–4 years, when there is an increased amount of eyelid tissue is available for repair. In a case of large defect, surgery should be done as soon as possible to avoid corneal lesions.

Q.2. What is the difference between lower and upper eyelid coloboma?

Ans. See **Table 1**.

Table 1: Difference between upper lid and lower lid coloboma.

Upper eyelid coloboma	Lower eyelid coloboma
More common	Less common
Usually isolated	Usually syndromic association
Occur at the junction of the inner and middle thirds	Occur most frequently at the junction of the middle and lateral thirds
Tend to be full thickness	Tend to be partial thickness involving preferentially the anterior lamella
Have normal adjacent lid margins	Adjacent lid margins may be abnormal
Usually not associated with facial clefts	Usually associated with facial clefts
Often associated with cryptophthalmos	Usually not

Table 2: Treacher Collins syndrome.

Structure affected	Clinical features
Eyes	• Antimangloid slant of palpebral fissures • Coloboma of lower eyelid • Hypoplasia of lower eyelid • Hypertelorism
Ears	• Microtia • Conductive hearing loss • Stenosis or complete atresia • External ear abnormalities
Face	• Hypoplasia of facial bones (mandibular or zygomatic arch) or complete absence of zygomatic arch • Dental malocclusion • Microstomia • High arched palate, cleft palate • Clonal atresia • Nasal dorsus parrot-like shape
Others	• Malformations associated with heart, kidney, vertebral column, and extremities • Obstructive sleep apnea

Q.3. What are the clinical findings in Treacher Collins syndrome?
Ans. *See* **Table 2**.

Q.4. What are the clinical findings in Goldenhar syndrome?
Ans.
- Limbal dermoid (bilateral in 25% of cases)
- Eyelid coloboma
- Preauricular appendages/skin tags
- Microtia or anotia of external ear can be associated with hearing loss with or without middle ear malformation
- Vertebral abnormalities (butterfly vertebrae or hemivertebrae)
- Congenital heart disease (numerous anomalies have been reported)
- Central nervous system abnormalities (hydrocephalus, intracranial lipomas, cranial nerve dysgenesis, and mental retardation have been described).

Q.5. What are the clinical findings in Fraser syndrome?
Ans. *Major characteristics:*
- Cryptophthalmos
- Syndactyly
- Genital anomalies
- Sibling with Fraser syndrome

Minor characteristics:
- Alterations of the nose
- Alterations of the ears
- Alterations of the larynx
- Oral clefts (cleft lip and/or palate)
- Umbilical hernia
- Renal agenesis (unilateral or bilateral)
- Skeletal anomalies.

■ REFERENCES

1. Casey TA. Congenital colobomata of the eyelids. Trans Ophthalmol Soc UK. 1976;96(1):65-8.
2. Collin JR. Congenital upper lid coloboma. Aust NZ J Ophthalmol. 1986;14:313-7.
3. Online Mendelian Inheritance in Man (OMIM) database. [online] Available from http://www.ncbi.nlm.nih.gov/omim [Last accessed Februrary, 2024].
4. Pearson AA. The development of the eyelids. Part I. External features. J Anat. 1980;130(1):33-42.
5. Sevel D. A reappraisal of eyelid development. Eye. 1988;2:123-9.

CHAPTER
2

Cornea and Conjunctiva

LONG CASES

CORNEAL ULCER

Prafulla Kumar Maharana, Shipra Singhi, Ritu Nagpal, Tushar Agarwal, Namrata Sharma

■ INTRODUCTION

Any breach in the continuity of an epithelial surface is called an ulcer. However, a corneal ulcer is better defined as an epithelial defect associated with superficial tissue loss along with variable grades of inflammation. Corneal ulcers often appear as a long case in examinations. A careful history and examination often clinch the diagnosis.

■ HISTORY

Chief Complaints

The common presenting symptoms in a case of corneal ulcer are as follows:
- Pain
- Diminution of vision
- Redness, watering, discharge, and foreign body sensation
- Photophobia
- Swelling of lids

History of Present Illness

The points that must be recorded in history are given in the following text.

Onset and Progression

The onset of corneal ulcer depends on the predisposing factor, the virulence of the organism, and the host immunity. The predisposing factors are summarized in **Table 1**.

Sudden onset and rapid progression are generally associated with bacterial corneal ulcers such as *Staphylococcus aureus*, *Pseudomonas aeruginosa*, and *Pneumococcus* species. Gradual onset and an indolent course are commonly seen in ulcers caused by fungi and parasites (*Acanthamoeba*) and a few bacteria, such as *Moraxella*, coagulase negative *Staphylococcus*, *Nocardia* species, and atypical mycobacteria.

In *Acanthamoeba,* the keratitis course can be variable (gradual or rapid) and it may be associated with a prolonged course with remissions.

Pain

The occurrence of pain in corneal ulcers can be minimal to excruciating. The type of causative organism and depth of the ulcer influence the severity of the pain.
- Superficial corneal ulcers are more painful than deep corneal ulcers due to the rich

Table 1: Predisposing factors in cases of corneal ulcers.	
Predisposing factors	**Examples**
Ocular	• *Trauma:* Mycotic (vegetative) and *Acanthamoeba* keratitis • *Contact lenses:* Pseudomonas (most common) and *Acanthamoeba* keratitis • *Lid and adnexal infections:* Pneumococcus keratitis (dacryocystitis) and *Actinomyces* (canaliculitis) • Abnormality in lids, such as trichiasis, coloboma, ectropion, entropion, lagophthalmos, exophthalmos, proptosis, blepharitis, and meibomitis • Ocular surface disease • Allergic eye disorders • Bullous keratopathy • Topical medications (topical corticosteroids, honey, and prolonged use of topical antibiotics) • Prior ocular surgery (pterygium surgery, keratoplasty, photorefractive keratectomy and LASIK)
Systemic	• Diabetes mellitus • Sjögren's syndrome • Stevens–Johnson syndrome • HIV • Advanced malignancies • Connective tissue disorders • Alcoholics • Extremes of age • Measles • Malnutrition • Smoking
Occupational	Farmers (mycotic keratitis), animal handlers (*Listeria keratitis*), Gardners, fishermen, and swimmers

(HIV: human immunodeficiency virus; LASIK: laser in situ keratomileusis)

sensory nerve supply in the superficial cornea which harbors the sub-basal nerve plexus.
- *Acanthamoeba* keratitis usually presents with excruciating pain due to associated radial keratoneuritis. The pain is usually out of proportion to the objective clinical findings.

  In contrast, the reverse is true for fungal ulcers where pain may be completely absent despite an advanced corneal ulcer.
- A sudden relief in pain in the case of the corneal ulcer may be indicative of perforation of the corneal ulcer.

Redness and Photophobia

A corneal ulcer is usually associated with circumciliary congestion or a combination of conjunctival and circumciliary congestion. Photophobia can be severe due to irritation of the anterior ciliary nerves. Spasm of the ciliary muscles caused due to inflammation also contributes to the pain.

Discharge

Most of the corneal ulcers are associated with discharge, which may be watery (in viral or small bacterial corneal ulcer), mucopurulent, or purulent (bacterial ulcer). Corneal ulcers caused by *Pseudomonas* are associated with a greenish-yellowish discharge. A membranous discharge is seen with keratitis caused by *Corynebacterium diphtheriae*.

Decreased Visual Acuity

Loss of vision depends upon the severity and location of the ulcer. The central corneal ulcers (caused by *Pseudomonas* species, *Staphylococcus aureus*, and *Fusarium* species) are associated with significant loss of visual acuity (VA). The visual acuity may not be severely affected in small and peripheral ulcers (e.g., the early cases of *Acanthamoeba* keratitis where only epithelium is affected).

Other factors that can reduce visual acuity include the presence of associated corneal edema, pupillary membrane, hypopyon, cataract, glaucoma, and endophthalmitis.

History of Past Illness

History of trauma, contact lens (CL) use, allergic eye disorders, topical medication use, prior ocular surgery, or systemic disease **(Table 1)** has to be noted carefully.

Family History

Family history may be present in cases with connective tissue disorders.

Past Surgical History

Recent surgery can be a predisposing factor for infective keratitis **(Table 1)**.

■ EXAMINATION

General Examination/Specific Systemic Examination

A thorough general examination must be carried out to look for the following:
- Potential source of infection
- Connective tissue disorders
- Immunocompromised states

Ocular Examination

- *Visual acuity:* Visual acuity may be reduced in cases where the ulcer is located in the center of the cornea or due to the presence of corneal edema, massive hypopyon, or associated endophthalmitis. The endothelium and associated anterior chamber inflammation (cell, flare, hypopyon, or fibrin) should not be overlooked.
- *Eyeball:* Look for the presence of any lagophthalmos or proptosis/exophthalmos. Blepharophimosis can be there in the presence of severe inflammation. Bell's phenomenon must be checked in all patients with lagophthalmos.
- *Lid:* Look for trichiasis, lid coloboma, entropion, lid lag, ectropion, and blepharitis that may be predisposing factors.
- *Lacrimal sac:* Look for dacryocystitis (can be associated with pneumococcal corneal ulcers) and canaliculitis (associated with *Actinomyces* keratitis). Regurgitation, syringing, and probing must be done in all cases to rule out any potential source of infection.
- *Conjunctiva:* The bulbar conjunctiva and the upper and lower tarsal conjunctiva should be examined for the presence of:
  – Any follicles, papillae, and diseases, such as vernal catarrh and atopic conjunctivitis
  – Discharge
  – Erythema, cicatrization, keratinization, suggestive of poor ocular surface, severe dry eye, and limbal stem cell deficiency
  – *Membrane, pseudomembrane formation:* Membranous conjunctivitis is seen with keratitis caused by *Corynebacterium diphtheriae*. Gonococcal, pneumococcal, and *Haemophilus* keratoconjunctivitis may be associated with pseudomembrane formation.
  – Foreign bodies can be a cause for nonhealing corneal ulcers.
- *Discharge:* Characteristics of discharge can provide a clue about the probable diagnosis, such as:
  – *Watery*—viral or small bacterial corneal ulcer
  – *Mucoid*—bacterial corneal ulcer
  – *Mucopurulent*—*Pseudomonas* and *Gonococcus*
  – *Frankly purulent*—severe bacterial corneal ulcer
  – Corneal ulcers caused by *Pseudomonas* are associated with a greenish–yellowish discharge. A membranous discharge is seen with keratitis caused by *Corynebacterium diphtheriae*.

CORNEA

Ulcer

The following parameters must be noted:
- *Location:* The location of the ulcer gives an indication about the probable cause, visual prognosis, and the initial choice of antibiotics. The location can be:
    - *Central: Staphylococcus aureus* **(Fig. 1)**, *Pseudomonas,* and *Fusarium*
    - *Paracentral: Staphylococcus aureus, Pseudomonas,* and *Fusarium*
    - *Peripheral:* Coagulase-negative *Staphylococcus aureus, Mycobacterium tuberculosis,* and Herpes simplex
    - *Superior:* Ulcer associated with shield ulcer [vernal keratoconjunctivitis (VKC)], foreign body (FB) in sulcus subtarsalis (common in children) or superior limbic keratoconjunctivitis.
    - *Inferior:* Ulcers associated with exposure keratopathy.
- *Size:* Record the size of the ulcer along the two largest meridians (Two axes where the extent is maximum that can be vertical and horizontal or two oblique axes). The illumination beam present in the slit lamp is used to record the size of the corneal ulcer. Other methods that may be used to record the size of an ulcer include a U-shaped tool made by the Schirmer's strips, a Castroviejo Caliper, and/or a Digital Caliper. Recording the baseline size is important as it helps in grading and monitoring of therapy.

The size of the epithelial defect and the size of the infiltration should be measured separately. They should be measured separately as their sizes may not be similar (in corneal abscesses corneal epithelium may be intact). The epithelial defects are best examined using a slit lamp with cobalt blue light after staining the cornea with sodium fluorescein dye.

Infiltration may be single or multiple and may be of varying sizes depending on the organism involved, severity, and duration of the infection. Look for satellite infiltrates in fungal corneal ulcers.

- *Shape:* The shape of the ulcer can give a clue about the probable cause. Examples include:
    - *Dendritic, amoeboid, or a geographic shape:* Viral keratitis
    - *Ring-shaped ulcer: Acanthamoeba* **(Fig. 2)**
    - *Staphylococcus*
    - *Oval:* Neurotrophic ulcer
- *Margins of ulcer:* Margins can be as follows:
    - *Well-defined:* Seen in healing infectious ulcers or sterile ulcers
    - *Punched out:* In cases of neurotrophic ulcers
    - *Indistinct:* Seen in cases of progressive ulcers
    - *Hyphae or feathery:* Characteristic of a fungal corneal ulcer
    - *Overhanging:* Mooren's ulcer
- *Base:* Usually, the base of the ulcer is filled with necrotic slough. A dry-looking ulcer bed suggests a fungal corneal ulcer.

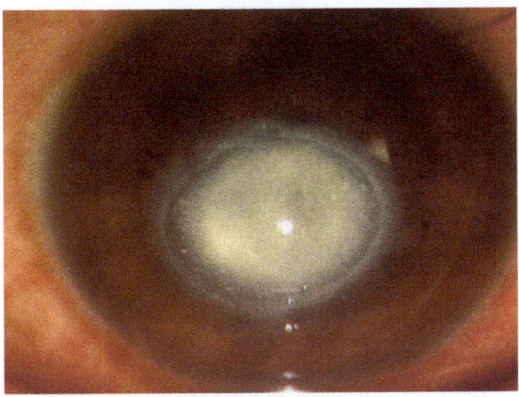

Fig. 1: Central corneal ulcer.

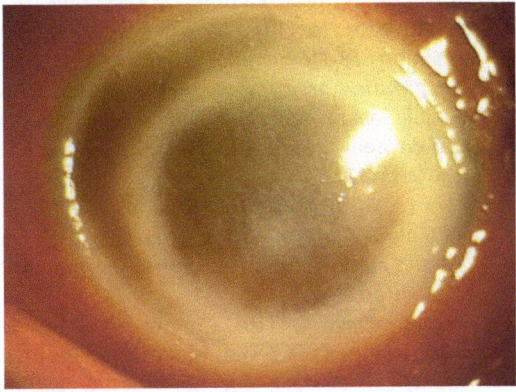

Fig. 2: Ring-shaped ulcer in *Acanthamoeba*.

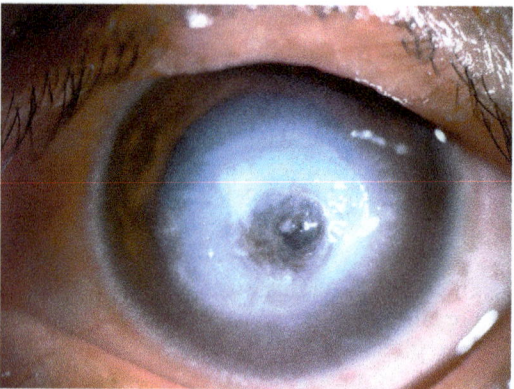

Fig. 3: Descemetocele.

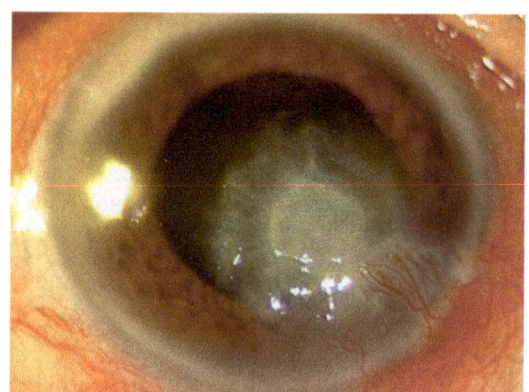

Fig. 5: Appearance of new vessels in a case of healing keratitis.

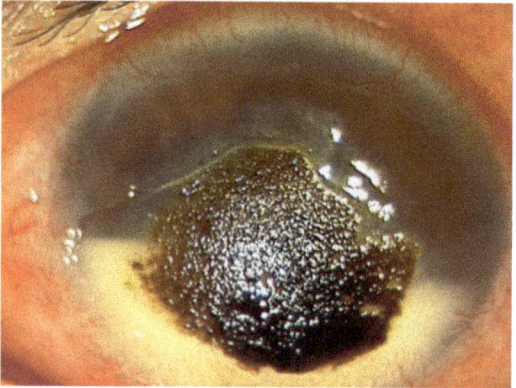

Fig. 4: Corneal ulcer with the pigment production.

- *Depth:* The depth of the ulcer is best measured with the use of a slit lamp. It helps in grading the ulcer and deciding the initial treatment protocol. A deep-seated ulcer (>50%) or descemetocele (**Fig. 3**) may warrant the initiation of systemic antibiotics.
- *Surrounding area:* Look for the presence of satellite lesions (characteristic of fungal ulcer) and corneal scars (ghost scars, in recurrent viral keratitis).
- *Pigmentation:* Pigment-producing fungi such as *Curvularia* and *Alternaria* can give a distinct color to the ulcer due to the pigment production (**Fig. 4**).
- *Vascularization:* The appearance of new vessels (**Fig. 5**) is a sign of healing keratitis. Superficial or deep corneal vascularization of varying extents may be seen in cases of infectious keratitis. A quadrant-wise record of corneal vascularization should be made.

Corneal Sensations

Corneal sensations should be measured with the help of a cotton wisp or esthesiometer (Cochet–Bonnet esthesiometer). In cases of herpetic keratitis, neuropathic keratitis, and cases with diabetes mellitus, the corneal sensations are decreased. It must be made sure that corneal sensations are measured through the normally clear cornea, as corneal sensations would naturally be decreased in areas with scarring.

Surrounding Cornea

The cornea surrounding the lesion may be, clear or hazy due to edema depending on the virulence of the organisms. *Candida* tends to cause localized lesions with distinct borders and minimal surrounding edema. Some organisms like *Pseudomonas* produce ulcers in which the surrounding cornea becomes hazy and grossly edematous appearing like a ground glass. Clearing of the surrounding corneal edema after the initiation of medical therapy is an early sign of the resolution of the ulcer.

Corneal Thinning/Perforation

The ulcer should be closely monitored for the development of corneal thinning, descemetocele, and perforation (**Fig. 6**). In the presence of a

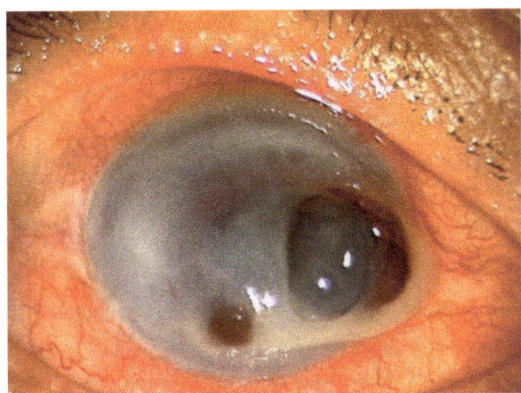

Fig. 6: Perforated corneal ulcer.

shallow anterior chamber and low intraocular pressure (IOP), a *Seidel's* test should be performed in all cases. Severe corneal thinning and perforation warrant immediate surgical therapy (glue or tectonic patch graft).

Other Findings

Look for other findings that may give a clue about the possible cause for the ulcer, such as foreign bodies, exposed or broken sutures, signs of corneal dystrophies, previous corneal inflammation (thinning, scarring, or neovascularization), and signs of previous corneal or refractive surgery.

Fluorescein or rose Bengal staining may provide additional information, such as the presence of dendrites, pseudodendrites, lose or exposed sutures, and epithelial defects.

Documentation

The documentation of the corneal ulcer may be done using color clinical photographs or using detailed schematic and color drawings.

Color Photographs

In all cases of corneal ulcers, a colored photograph of the diffuse and the slit section of the cornea should be taken. Measurements should be made of the maximum diameter of the ulcer and the meridian perpendicular to it. Apart from this infiltrate, the size should also be measured in the same manner.

Schematic Drawings

The following color coding is used to depict a corneal ulcer:
- *Black*—outline of the corneal limbus, indicating scars resulting from keratitis, degeneration, and foreign bodies.
- *Blue*—designates edema, small dots for epithelial edema or circles for lakes of fluid within the stroma, and wavy lines to depict the folds in Descemet's membrane (DM). Omega sign for the presence of bullae.
- *Brown*—indicates melanin or iron pigmentation including pupil and iris.
- *Red*—is used to depict blood vessels and rose Bengal staining. Red wavy lines indicate subepithelial vessels, straight lines indicate deep stromal vessels and dotted lines indicate ghost vessels. The wavy lines of superficial vessels begin outside the limbus circle; whereas, the straight lines of the stromal vessels begin at the margin of the circle. Solid shading depicts hemorrhage, and the red dots indicate an area stained by the rose Bengal.
- *Orange/yellow*—denotes inflammation and the presence of white blood cells, which may be in the following forms—stromal infiltrate, hypopyon, or keratic precipitates (KPs).
- *Green*—indicates fluorescein staining of the cornea and dots represent punctate epithelial keratopathy, small lines depict filaments and a shaded outline demonstrates epithelial defects. The green color is also used to depict the location of the lens and vitreous opacities/hemorrhage, etc.

Clinical features of the specific keratitis have been described in **Table 2**.

Sclera

One should look for scleral inflammation, ulceration, nodules, or ischemia. Any involvement of the sclera should be recorded as this helps in prognosticating the case and in the management protocol. Scleral involvement warrants the use of systemic antimicrobial agents. Sclerokeratitis usually occurs in cases of immunologic disorders and *Acanthamoeba* keratitis.

Table 2: Clinical features of specific keratitis.

Disease-specific	Clinical features
Bacterial keratitis	Well-defined infiltrate with moderate inflammation in the anterior chamber
Fungal keratitis	Dry-looking ulcer with feathery margins, satellite lesions, ring ulcer, endothelial plaque, pigmentation in dematiaceous keratitis
Acanthamoeba keratitis	Epithelial haze with pseudodendrites, radial perineuritis, ring ulcer
Microsporidiosis	Multifocal punctate raised epithelial lesions with clear underlying stroma
Viral keratitis	Dendrites, geographic ulcer, and annular stromal edema with keratic precipitates (KPs)
Pseudomonas keratitis	Rapidly sloughing ulcer, ring ulcer, with evident corneal edema in the uninvolved cornea, and rapid melting with perforation of the cornea
Microsporidiosis	Multifocal punctate raised epithelial lesions with clear underlying stroma
Atypical bacteria	Cracked windshield corneal ulcer, minimal changes in surrounding cornea, and minimal reaction in the anterior chamber
Pythium keratitis	Dense gray–white infiltrate with necrosis, feathery margins, flocculent debris, midstromal tentacle, such as infiltrates, subepithelial expanding dot-like infiltrates, hyphated edges, and peripheral furrowing

Table 3: Characteristics of hypopyon.

Characteristics	Probable diagnosis
Central	Pneumococcal corneal ulcer
Hemorrhagic	Pneumococcal corneal ulcer and herpes simplex viral keratitis
Mobile	Bacterial corneal ulcer
Fixed/immobile	Fungal corneal ulcer
Sterile	Behçet's syndrome

Anterior Chamber

Mild flare to severe hypopyon **(Fig. 7)** formation may be there. The size of the hypopyon should be measured using a slit-lamp micrometer. Hypopyon and its characteristics are helpful in establishing the etiological diagnosis **(Table 3)**. In order to test the mobility of the hypopyon, following a slit-lamp examination, the patient is asked to lie supine for 10 minutes, and a slit-lamp examination is then done. In the case of the fixed hypopyon **(Fig. 8)**, there is no change in the position of the hypopyon as demonstrated by the height of the hypopyon. In the case of the mobile hypopyon, there is an actual movement, and the upper level or height of the hypopyon decreases.

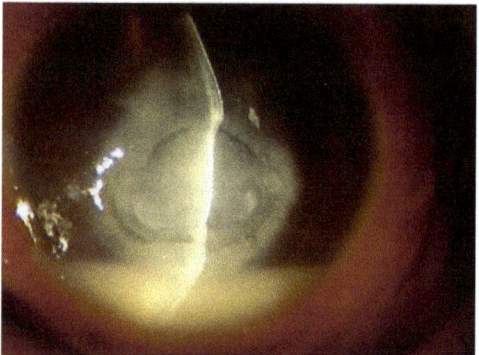

Fig. 7: Hypopyon.

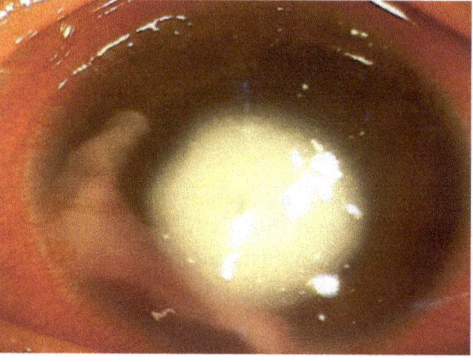

Fig. 8: Fixed hypopyon.

Iris

Variable degrees of uveal inflammation can occur with infectious keratitis. Synechiae formation may be there. The presence of new vessels on the iris (rubeosis iridis) can also be seen in cases of prolonged inflammation. If the ulcer perforates, uveal prolapse may occur and this may later form a corneoiridic scar.

Pupil

Any abnormality in the pupil size, shape, and location should be recorded. In the presence of severe inflammation, the iris may be atonic.

Intraocular Pressure

Digital tonometry in experienced hands is the most practical method of assessing IOP in cases of corneal ulcer. Secondary glaucoma may be present in some cases. Hypotony may be present in the case of corneal perforation.

Lens

Cataract formation may be there, or pigment deposit may be there.

Posterior Segment

Usually, it is not possible to view the vitreous and retina in case of a corneal ulcer due to the presence of a hazy cornea. However, if the ulcer is small and peripheral, slit-lamp biomicroscopy may be done to visualize the anterior one-third of the vitreous. Additionally, an indirect ophthalmoscopy may be performed to check for the involvement of the posterior segment.

Fellow Eye

One should also examine the fellow eye as bilateral involvement may be there (usually in immunological cases).

■ GRADING OF CORNEAL ULCER

Refer to **Table 4**.

■ DIFFERENTIAL DIAGNOSIS

Based on history and clinical examination a provisional diagnosis can be made. The differentiating features are described in **Table 5**.

■ INVESTIGATIONS

Microbiological Diagnosis of Infectious Keratitis

Owing to the considerable overlap in the clinical appearances of corneal ulcers due to various micro-organisms, a standard basic laboratory methodology should encompass techniques that allow for the recognition of as large a number of offending organisms as possible.

Collection of Samples

The samples should be collected at the initial presentation before the start of antimicrobial therapy. The treatment can be initiated based on the results of the smear examination. Samples for diagnosis of corneal ulcer can be the following:
- Eyelid swab—not of much use
- Conjunctival swab—not of much use
- Corneal scraping—most important
- Contact lens, contact lens case, and solution—must in contact lens user

Table 4: Grading of corneal ulcer.

Feature	Mild	Moderate	Severe
Size of ulcer (mm)	<2	2–5	>5
Depth of ulcer (%)	<20	20–50	>50
Infiltrate • Density • Extent	• Dense • Superficial	• Dense • Extension up to mid stroma	• Dense • Deeper than midstroma
Scleral involvement	Not involved	Not involved	May be involved

Table 5: Differential diagnosis of corneal ulcer.

Parameters	Bacterial	Fungal	Viral	Acanthamoeba	Atypical bacteria
Risk factors	Blepharitis, dacryocystitis, trichiasis, contact lens use, and ocular surface disorder	Trauma with vegetative matter, indiscriminate use of topical antibiotic or steroid	Past history of viral infection	Contact lens use and swimming	Prior corneal surgery
Symptoms	Severe symptoms and rapid progression	Indolent course signs more than symptoms	Like bacterial, may be associated with recurrences	Waxing and waning course and severe pain	Indolent course, failure to respond to routine antibiotics
Signs	Epithelial defect, infiltration, mobile hypopyon, anterior chamber reaction, and mucopurulent discharge	Feathery margins/ hyphate edges, rough and dry texture, satellite lesions, gray/brown pigmentation, immune ring of Wessely, collar button configuration, and fixed hypopyon	Epithelial keratitis (punctate, dendritic, geographic, marginal, and neurotrophic), stromal keratitis (immune ring of Wessely, and stromal neovascularization), endotheliitis, uveitis, decreased corneal sensation, and periocular lymphadenopathy	Pseudodendrites, radial keratoneuritis, and ring-shaped infiltrate	Cracked windshield corneal ulcer, minimal changes in surrounding cornea, and minimal reaction in the anterior chamber

- Anterior chamber paracentesis (hypopyon)—deep ulceration or when insufficient material is present.

Corneal Scrapings

Instruments

Kimura's spatula is traditionally used to collect scrapings from a corneal ulcer though Bard–Parker blade number 15, 26G needle, hypodermic needle, and platinum spatula are also used. Cotton swabs are not recommended for the collection of corneal material (may interfere with fungal filament interpretation).

Technique

A topical anesthesia drop (0.5% of proparacaine) is applied. A lid speculum is applied gently to separate the lids. Any slough or mucus debris must be removed gently. Multiple scraping of the ulcer base and margins is done under topical anesthesia (0.5% of proparacaine hydrochloride is proffered since it is the least bactericidal compared to other anesthetic agents like 4% of lignocaine hydrochloride or tetracaine) with the aid of a slit-lamp or operating microscope. Streptococci pneumoniae is more readily found at the edge of the ulcer; whereas *Moraxella* is more likely to be present at the ulcer base hence both the base and margin have to be scrapped. Several scrapings are collected and used in a sequence to prepare smears and inoculate culture media. The blade or spatula may be reused when a sterile medium has been streaked; however, a blade must be changed (spatula should be flamed) when a smear has been made on a slide, which may not be sterile.

More recently, calcium alginate swabs moistened with trypticase soy broth provide another method of collecting corneal specimens for yielding a higher number of bacteria and fungi compared to the platinum spatula. However, one limitation is that the calcium itself may act as an antibacterial agent. Scrapping has to be done with utmost care in cases of severe keratolysis, descemetocele, and deep stromal keratitis.

Inoculation

Solid agar media (**Table 6**) are inoculated on the surface making multiple "C"-shaped marks without cutting the agar. In the liquid media, the spatula or blade is swirled to allow the sample to be transferred. In the case of thioglycollate, broth, and Sabouraud dextrose agar (SDA) deep inoculation of the medium is ensured by transferring the sample to a swab tip and dropping the swab in the tube allowing it to settle at the bottom.

Routine Smears and Stains

Gram stain (most common), Kinyoun stain (cold carbol fuchsin), or Giemsa stain (**Table 7**) are employed to study the corneal material which is spread as a thin layer on several clean glass slides within an area defined with a wax pencil on the reverse. In the preparation of wet mounts such as potassium hydroxide (KOH), lactophenol cotton blue, and calcofluor white (CFW), the scrapings can be placed on the slide in a demarcated area and covered with a drop of the solution followed by a coverslip. Special stains and media may be included whenever usual procedures have yielded negative results.

Interpretation

Staining methods yield a rapid result and help to determine the initial choice of an antimicrobial agent. *Potassium hydroxide wet preparation*—a 10-20% solution of KOH is used to visualize fungal elements in corneal scrapes. Owing to the chitin in their cell wall, fungal filaments, and cysts of *Acanthamoeba* are clearly delineated in a homogeneous background of corneal tissue digested by KOH. Its sensitivity ranges from 90 to 99%. Gram stain is utilized to identify bacteria, fungi, and *Acanthamoeba*. It has been reported to yield an accuracy of 60-75% in identifying

Table 6: Common culture media for various organisms.

Culture medium	Growth	Incubation temperature
Blood agar plate	• Aerobic bacteria • Facultative anaerobic bacteria • Fungi	35°C
Chocolate agar plate	• Aerobic bacteria • Facultative anaerobic bacteria • *Neisseria* • *Haemophilus* • *Moraxella*	35°C
Thioglycollate broth	• Aerobic bacteria • Anaerobic bacteria	35°C
Sabouraud's dextrose agar plate with antibiotic	• Fungi • *Nocardia*	Room temperature
Brain–heart infusion broth plate with antibiotic	• Fungi • *Nocardia*	Room temperature
Cooked meat broth	Anaerobic bacteria	35°C
Thayer–Martin blood agar plate	*Neisseria*	35°C
Lowenstein–Jensen media	*Mycobacteria* species	35°C with 3–10% CO_2
Middlebrook–Cohn agar	• *Mycobacteria* species • *Nocardia*	35°C with 3–10% CO_2

Table 7: Different stains used for smear examination.

Type of stain	Organism visualized	Color of the organism
Gram stain	Bacteria	Gram-positive—purple Gram-negative—pink
Acridine orange	Bacteria, fungi, and *Acanthamoeba*	Yellow-orange
Calcofluor white	Fungi	Bright green
	Acanthamoeba cysts	Bright green
	Acanthamoeba trophozoites	Reddish orange
Acid-fast	Mycobacteria, *Nocardia*, and other atypical mycobacteria	Pink

the responsible organisms. Calcofluor white is a fluorescent brightener with a great affinity for certain polysaccharides such as cellulose and chitin, thus providing the basis for the demonstration of fungal cell walls and cysts of *Acanthamoeba* species. The preparation is viewed under the fluorescence microscope. The cysts of *Acanthamoeba* and fungal filaments appear as a bright green apple in a corneal scraping stained with CFW. *Acanthamoeba* trophozoites and bacteria such as *Nocardia* and *Actinomyces* do not stain with CFW.

Cultures

Identification of the bacteria may be accomplished within 48 hours along with its antibiotic susceptibility pattern. In some cases, the pathogen may be recognized in 12–15 hours. Standardized disk diffusion or dilution techniques should be utilized for antibiotic susceptibility testing of the bacteria. The majority of fungi causing keratitis can be detected on SDA within 72 hours. *Aspergillus* and *Fusarium* species grow on the blood agar, SDA, and brain-heart infusion broth within 48 hours. However, appreciably characteristic colonies develop after 1–2 weeks; hence, culture media should be observed for at least 2 weeks before they are considered negative. Non-nutrient agar (NNA) is the standard medium used with an overlay of *Escherichia coli* for the growth of *Acanthamoeba*. The specimen is simply touched to the surface of the plate without streaking or breaking the surface. Two plates may be inoculated for incubation at 25 and 37°C since some species do not grow at the higher temperature and the plates are examined for trophozoites and cysts directly under the microscope (100X). Trophozoites may be seen in 24–48 hours. They move and cover the entire plate surface on further incubation and turn into cysts. The plates should be observed for at least 7 days.

Special media, selective and nonselective, may be indicated in certain clinical situations. Löwenstein–Jensen medium is used when mycobacterial infection is suspected. *Nocardia* organisms can grow, though slowly, on blood agar and other bacterial media.

Remember: Aerobic cultures of the corneal specimens should be held for 7 days, anaerobic cultures for 7–14 days, and mycobacterial and fungal cultures for 4–6 weeks before being reported as having no growth.

Interpretation of Culture Results

Interpretation of culture results should be made with regard to the clinical situation, the adequacy of the sample, and the possibility of contamination by organisms present on the skin, eyelids, and conjunctiva. Positive culture rates vary from 40 to 73%.

An isolate is more likely to be considered significant if it is consistent with the clinical signs plus:
- The same organism is grown on more than one medium.
- Confluent growth of a known ocular pathogen in one solid medium
  Or

The growth in one medium of an organism with positive smear results or growth of the same organism in a liquid media.

Jones Criteria for Positive Culture

- Clinical signs of infection plus isolation of bacteria (10 or more colonies) on one solid medium and one additional medium, *or*
- Isolation of organism (any detectable growth) on any two solid media, *or*
- Isolation of organisms in one medium in the presence of a positive smear.

When the culture results are negative, antibiotic treatment can be suspended for 24 hours and rescraping is done, following which repeat cultures are sent and examined.

Corneal Biopsy

Corneal biopsy is indicated if infectious keratitis is suspected clinically, and twice repeated microscopic evaluation of smears and culture results are negative and no clinical improvement is noted on the initial broad-spectrum antibiotic therapy. In addition, in certain cases of deep mycotic keratitis and intrastromal abscesses a corneal biopsy is indicated.

A partial-thickness trephination employing a trephine of sufficient size, to guarantee adequate material for the laboratory, is required. Care is taken to avoid the visual axis as far as possible. Biopsy from below a lamellar flap can be considered for a midstromal lesion; such as infectious crystalline keratopathy and a deep stromal lesion, such as fungal keratitis.

Anterior Chamber Paracentesis

This procedure is rarely indicated in the diagnostic evaluation of a patient with a corneal ulcer; however, this procedure may be indicated in the instance where keratomycosis is strongly suspected clinically, yet corneal scrapings and biopsy have been negative, the damage to the cornea is progressive and a hypopyon is present or increasing.

Confocal Microscopy

In vivo, confocal microscopy (IVCM) is a non-invasive in vivo diagnostic method for microbial keratitis. It has been successfully used to distinguish some unusual pathogens, such as *Acanthamoeba* cysts and fungal hyphae. With a new generation, IVCM can help in initiating antifungal therapy and in monitoring the response to therapy.

Newer Methods

The need for rapid diagnosis has led to the modification of various conventional techniques and the introduction of new techniques, such as immunohistochemistry, fluorescent microscopy, enzyme immunoassays, radioimmunoassay, polymerase chain reaction (PCR), and molecular biology. Most ocular infections can now be diagnosed by these modern techniques within 1–6 hours.

Ultrasonography

It is done in cases of corneal haze for fundus evaluation. In cases of perforated corneal ulcer, endophthalmitis, choroidal, and retinal detachment should be excluded.
- Refractive surgery
- Trauma

Anterior Segment Optical Coherence Tomography

Several findings in anterior segment optical coherence tomography (ASOCT) can help in identifying specific features of microbial keratitis which may help in diagnosis and management. In addition, ASOCT is also helpful in identifying cases with stromal lysis/thinning. The anterior segment details can also be imaged. Once the treatment has started, ASOCT helps in monitoring such patients.

■ MANAGEMENT

Management of Bacterial Keratitis

Bacterial keratitis should be treated as an ocular emergency due to its rapid progression and disastrous complications. Initially, an empirical antibiotic therapy (combination therapy) is started to cover for both gram-positive and gram-negative organisms. Standard therapy is a combination of:
- Fortified cefazoline 5% or 10% + tobramycin 1.3%
- Fluoroquinolones (moxifloxacin 0.5% or gatifloxacin 0.3%) + tobramycin 1.3%.

Table 8: Comparison of fluoroquinolones and fortified eye drops.

Fluoroquinolones	Fortified drops
Cheaper	More expensive
Readily available	Need to be prepared
Stable	Preferable to refrigerate
Shelf life of 1 month	Shelf life of 1 week
Less toxic	More toxic
Poor coverage of gram-positive organisms with older generations	Better coverage

Monotherapy can be considered in cases where the ulcer is in the periphery and is small (<3 mm). For monotherapy, fluoroquinolones are preferred (ofloxacin 0.3%, ciprofloxacin 0.3%, gatifloxacin 0.3%, or moxifloxacin 0.5%). A comparison of fluoroquinolones and fortified eye drops is given in **Table 8**.

The frequency of instillation of drops depends upon the severity, but it is usual to start half-hourly drops all through 24 hours for most patients. A loading dose of a drop, every 5 minutes for the first 30 minutes is used in severe ulcers. The frequency is reduced based on the clinical response described further.

Favorable Signs

- Stabilization and no progression and improved symptoms
- Reduced activity at infiltrate margins/blunting of ulcer edges
- Resolution of infiltration
- Progressive healing of the epithelial defect
- Reduction in adjacent stromal inflammatory reaction and anterior chamber reaction
- Reduction in hypopyon
- Vascularization

Unfavorable Signs

Signs that suggest poor response to therapy include the following:
- Deterioration in symptoms
- Increase in size and density of infiltration
- Increase in size of anterior chamber reaction
- Nonhealing of the epithelial defect
- Progressive stromal thinning

The clinical response should be the first guideline of therapy, although, in nonhealing ulcers, in vitro sensitivity should be given due attention. In vitro sensitivity should be correlated with in vivo response before considering a change in therapy as inadequate frequency, poor penetration, stromal lysis, and necrotic debris covering the site of infection can be the causes of the nonresponsiveness of ulcer to therapy.

The aminoglycoside antibiotics used in fortified drops are gentamycin and tobramycin. They give excellent gram-negative coverage and are active against staphylococci and some streptococci but not against pneumococci. The most commonly used cephalosporin in fortified drops is cefazolin. It gives good coverage for nonpenicillinase-producing gram-positive bacteria.

Adjunctive therapy is required to alleviate the symptoms including cycloplegic drugs, antiglaucoma drugs, tear supplements, and topical corticosteroids. Management in specific bacterial keratitis has been described in **Table 9**.

The indications of systemic antibiotics in bacterial keratitis includes the following:
- Perforated/impending perforation in corneal ulcer
- Postperforating injury
- Scleral involvement
- Endophthalmitis
- Highly virulent organisms—*Neisseria* and *Haemophilus*

The steroid for corneal ulcer trial (SCUT) found no significant difference in 3-month best corrected visual acuity (BCVA) between patients receiving topical corticosteroid or placebo as adjunctive therapy in the treatment of bacterial corneal ulcers. No apparent increased risk of corneal perforation was observed with the use of corticosteroids.

Management of Fungal Keratitis

The major group of antifungal agents available includes the following:
- *Polyenes:* Natamycin, nystatin, and amphotericin B
- *Azoles:* Fluconazole, itraconazole, voriconazole, posaconazole, and ravuconazole
- *Fluorinated pyrimidines:* Flucytosine
- *Echinocandins:* Caspofungin and micafungin

Table 9: Management of specific bacterial keratitis.

Organism	Topical	Systemic
Methicillin-resistant *Staphylococcus*	Vancomycin 50 mg/mL	Vancomycin 2 g/day
Severe *Pseudomonas* keratitis	Ceftazidime (50 mg/mL)	Ceftazidime (1–2 g/day IV or IM)
Mycobacterium fortuitum—chelonae	Amikacin 40–100 mg/mL	Clarithromycin 500 mg BD
Nocardia	Amikacin 40–100 mg/mL Or Trimethoprim (16 mg/mL) Sulfamethoxazole (80 mg/mL) injectable	Trimethoprim/sulfamethoxazole (10–20 mg/kg/day) IV
(IM: intramuscular; IV: intravenous)		

Table 10: Sensitivity of different antifungals (MIC values of different genera in microgram/mL).

Fungus	Voriconazole	AMB	Fluconazole	Natamycin
Candida	0.08–0.016	0.25–0.5	0.12–0.5	3.12–12.5
Aspergillus	0.25–0.5	1–2	>256	3.12–25
Fusarium	1–4	1–2	>256	1.56–6.25
(AMB: amphotericin B; MIC: minimum inhibitory concentration)				

The standard treatment followed includes the following step-wise approach:
- *Topical antifungals:* 5% natamycin (drug of choice) is given hourly in the daytime, 2 hourly at bedtime
- Taper after 4–7 days intervals depending upon clinical response.
- Surface debridement helps to remove slough and reduce the load of infection. Benefits are controversial but still preferred by most of the clinicians.
- If worsening (after 14 days of the treatment)— add 0.15% of amphotericin B drops or 1% of voriconazole. Also, review the culture report.
- Therapy duration is 3-4 weeks. Complete resolution often requires 4–8 weeks.

Unlike antibacterials, antifungals suffer from the limitations of poor ocular penetration, poor bioavailability, epithelial toxicity, and poor commercial availability. The sensitivity of currently available antifungals is summarized in **Table 10**. The indications of systemic antifungals in fungal keratitis are as follows:
- Perforated/impending perforation corneal ulcer
- Severe deep ulcer (involving >2/3 of the stromal depth)
- Large ulcer (>6 mm diameter)
- Postpenetrating keratoplasty
- Scleral involvement
- Endophthalmitis

The commonly used systemic antifungals include ketoconazole (200 mg BD), fluconazole (200 mg BD), itraconazole (100 mg BD), and voriconazole (200 mg BD). The systemic antifungals can cause a number of adverse reactions; hence, monitoring of blood glucose, blood pressure, and liver function tests has to be done regularly.

Targeted Drug Delivery

About 20% of fungal ulcers are refractory to medical therapy. In such cases, targeted drug delivery (providing the drug where it is needed the most) is a useful alternative before proceeding with surgery. The different modalities are intracameral, intracorneal, or intrastromal drug delivery. The different agents used are amphotericin B (5–7.5 µg/0.1 mL/5% dextrose) and voriconazole 50–100 µg/0.1 mL.

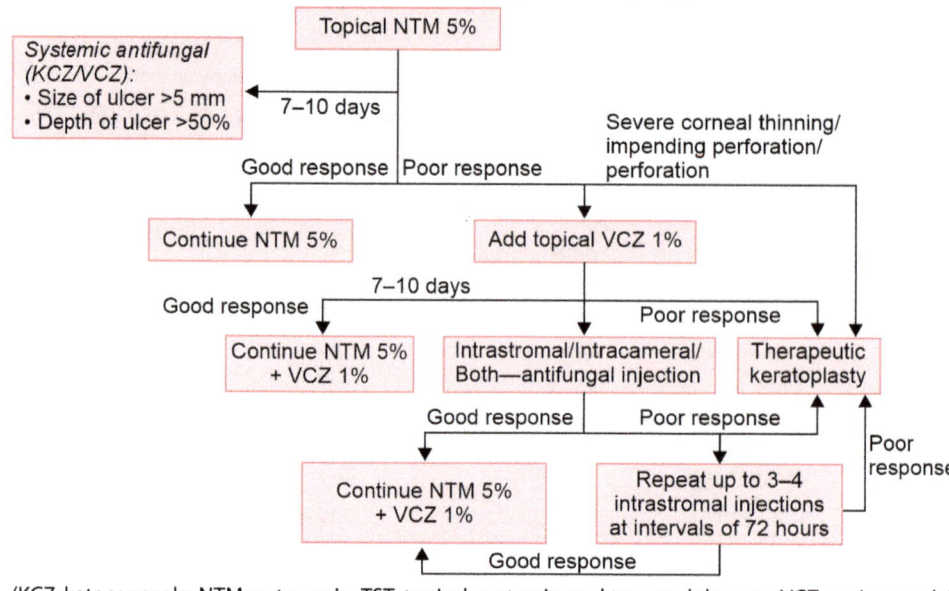

Flowchart 1: Management of fungal keratitis (TST) protocol.

(KCZ: ketoconazole; NTM: natamycin; TST: topical, systemic, and targeted therapy; VCZ: voriconazole)

Algorithm for the Management of Fungal Keratitis [Topical, Systemic, and Targeted Therapy (TST) Protocol]

The topical, systemic, and targeted therapy (TST) protocol provides a comprehensive treatment protocol for the management of fungal keratitis **(Flowchart 1)**.

Management of Viral Keratitis

The different antivirals available include acyclovir 3% ointment, vidarabine 3% ointment, trifluorothymidine (TFT) 1%, and idoxuridine 1%. The dose and duration of antivirals (acyclovir) have been described in **Table 11**. Remember if a true ulceration persists after 14 days of treatment, one must distinguish between a neurotrophic ulcer and persistent infectious epithelial keratitis. A neurotrophic ulcer has smooth borders and lacks the scalloped edges of infectious epithelial keratitis. If the lesion is persistent infectious epithelial keratitis, resistance to the antiviral medication must be considered, and an alternative medication can be initiated. The readers are advised to refer to a standard textbook for treatment of viral keratitis in detail.

Surgical Management

Surgical treatment is indicated in cases of impending perforation, perforated corneal ulcer, and nonhealing corneal ulcer (to reduce microbial load). The decision to surgically intervene in a case of active infectious keratitis should be made after a proper evaluation of the clinical progress. Surgery helps eliminate or reduce the microbial load and in providing tectonic support to the globe where the integrity is threatened, as in cases of thinning or perforation of the cornea. The different surgical options and various modalities of treatment available in such cases are:
- Removal of epithelium and anterior lamellar keratectomy
- Conjunctival flaps (Gunderson's flap)
- Patch graft
- Tissue adhesives with bandage contact lens (BCL) and therapeutic penetrating keratoplasty
- Deep anterior lamellar keratoplasty
- Collagen crosslinking (CXL).

Epithelial Removal and Anterior Lamellar Keratectomy

This is useful in cases of fungal keratitis. Regular debridement of the base of the ulcer helps in the

Table 11: Treatment protocol for viral keratitis.

Type of keratitis	Topical acyclovir 3%	Topical corticosteroids	Oral antivirals	Supportive	Comments
Epithelial keratitis*	• Five times for 1 week • Three times for 2–3 weeks	Contraindicated	• Not required if topical given • Tablet acyclovir 400 mg five times for 1–2 weeks • Tablet valacyclovir 500 mg BD for 1–2 weeks	• Lubricants • Cycloplegics	Debridement in the early stages may also help in a few cases
Epithelial + stromal	• Five times for 1 week • Three times for 2–3 weeks	• After the epithelium heals • Prednisolone acetate 2–4 hourly	• Tablet acyclovir 400 mg five times for 2 weeks, thereafter twice a day • Tablet valacyclovir 500 mg BD for 2 weeks	• Lubricants • Cycloplegics	• Taper both by 6–8 weeks • Tablet acyclovir 400 mg BD (or tablet valacyclovir 500 mg OD) should be continued if there is a history of two or more episodes in the last 1 year
Necrotizing and non-necrotizing stromal herpetic stromal keratitis (HSK)	• Five times for 2–4 weeks • Three times for 2–3 weeks thereafter	Prednisolone acetate 2–4 hourly	• Tablet acyclovir 400 mg five times for 2–4 weeks* • Tablet valacyclovir 500 mg BD for 1–2 weeks	• Lubricants • Cycloplegics	Tablet acyclovir 400 mg BD (or tablet valacyclovir 500 mg OD) should be continued if there is a history of two or more episodes in the last 1 year
Endotheliitis	Not useful	Prednisolone acetate 2–4 hourly	• Tablet acyclovir 400 mg five times for 2–4 weeks* • Tablet valacyclovir 500 mg BD for 1–2 weeks	• Cycloplegics • Antiglaucoma	Tablet acyclovir 400 mg BD or (tablet valacyclovir 500 mg OD) should be continued if there is a history of two or more episodes in the last 1 year

Note:
- Few clinicians including the American Academy of Ophthalmology (AAO) recommend doubling the dose of oral antivirals in cases of geographic ulcer and necrotizing keratitis.
- Prophylactic dose of oral valacyclovir is controversial.
- Ganciclovir ophthalmic gel 0.15% or ointment is an alternative to topical acyclovir and is given five times daily until healing of corneal ulcer occurs, followed by one drop three times a day for 7 days.

elimination of organisms and necrotic material. This procedure facilitates the penetration of antifungal drugs. This can be done under topical anesthesia leaving a margin of 1–2 mm at the limbus with a number 15 Bard–Parker blade. Anterior lamellar keratectomy helps in the removal of the thick mat of the fungal filaments on the cornea and facilitates increased drug penetration in cases of dematiaceous fungal filaments. Anterior stromal corneal infiltrates can also be ablated with the phototherapeutic keratectomy.

Conjunctival Flaps

Conjunctival flaps help in achieving a stable epithelial surface in cases of persistent or recurrent epithelial defects and progressive ulceration, especially in viral keratitis. In advanced cases of corneal ulcer, where the only aim is to save the globe, a Gunderson's flap is done where the entire surface is covered with a conjunctival flap.

Tissue Adhesives

Tissue adhesive (cyanoacrylates) helps in supporting corneal thinning and sealing corneal perforation up to 2–3 mm. In addition, cyanoacrylate adhesive is bacteriostatic for gram-positive bacteria. Necrotic stroma or epithelium and other debris must be removed from the base of the ulcer before the adhesive is applied. A BCL is fitted after the application. The adhesive is left in place until it loosens spontaneously, the bed becomes vascularized, or keratoplasty is performed.

Patch graft: The different types of patch graft that can be done include the following:
- *Tenon's patch graft:* For peripheral ulcers, inexpensive, and seals the defect by the fibroblastic response of the Tenon's tissue.
- *Multilayered amniotic membrane graft (AMG):* In cases of severe thinning or small perforations.
- *Tectonic patch graft:* A small patch of corneal graft, in perforations 3–5 mm in size.

Therapeutic penetrating keratoplasty: A full-thickness graft is performed in perforations ≥5 mm. The results of keratoplasty in acutely infected or inflamed eyes are relatively poor, and the risk of rejection and glaucoma is greater, especially in larger grafts. In all these cases at least 0.5 mm of clear tissue all around the infected area is to be excised to decrease the incidence of recurrence. Postoperative antimicrobial treatment is to be continued. In fungal keratitis, postoperative topical steroids are to be used with caution. Ideally, steroids should be avoided until the culture report (suggesting free margins) is available or at least for 10–14 days. Surgery when performed with 8 mm or smaller diameter donor grafts has better results than larger grafts; hence, penetrating keratoplasty (PKP) is to be considered early when fungal ulcers do not respond to antifungal medication. The results of PKP for *Acanthamoeba* keratitis are poor and surgery is to be considered only in patients with gross corneal thinning or perforation.

CXL: CXL has direct bactericidal activity (by oxidative damage) to the pathogens and also cross-linked corneas become more resistant to degrading enzymes of organisms. Several studies have shown its effectiveness in refractory keratitis.

VIVA QUESTIONS

Q.1. What is the role of hypopyon in the etiological diagnosis of corneal ulcers?
Ans. Already discussed in the text.

Q.2. What are the signs of healing and nonhealing corneal ulcer?
Ans. Already discussed in the text.

Q.3. What is the interpretation of culture results and describe Jones criteria?
Ans. Already discussed in the text.

Q.4. What are the indications of corneal biopsy in the corneal ulcer?
Ans.
- If infectious keratitis is suspected clinically and twice repeated microscopic evaluation of smears and culture results are negative.
- No clinical improvement is noted on the initial broad-spectrum antibiotic therapy.
- Certain cases of deep mycotic keratitis and intrastromal abscesses.

Cornea and Conjunctiva

Q.5. What is the grading of corneal ulcers?
Ans. Already discussed in the text.

Q.6. What does the Herpetic Eye Disease Study (HEDS) recommend about viral keratitis?
Ans. In herpes simplex virus (HSV) stromal keratitis—topical antivirals + steroids are less likely to fail the treatment.
- No beneficial effect of systemic acyclovir is there in HSV stromal keratitis.
- Oral acyclovir is beneficial in the prevention of stromal keratitis/iritis in epithelial HSV keratitis.
- Oral acyclovir is beneficial in preventing the blinding sequelae of HSV iridocyclitis.
- Prophylaxis is beneficial in recurrent ocular HSV or stromal HSV (400 mg BD).

(*Note:* Refer to **Table 12**)

Q.7. What are the indications of systemic therapy in case of corneal ulcer?
Ans. Already discussed in the text.

Q.8. What are the indications of surgical intervention in case of corneal ulcer?
Ans. Already discussed in the text.

Q.9. Different stains used in keratitis.
Ans. A modification of Gömöri's methenamine silver stain may be helpful for the identification of fungal elements and *Acanthamoeba* cysts in corneal scrapings. Fungi and *Acanthamoeba* cysts stain black on a light green background.
- The periodic acid–Schiff (PAS) stain may also be used to visualize fungal elements and *Acanthamoeba,* especially in tissue sections.
- Lactophenol cotton blue stain, which is generally used for the microscopic examination of fungal cultures, has been effectively used for the demonstration of fungal elements and *Acanthamoeba* cysts in corneal scrapings.
- Ziehl–Neelsen stain or its modification (Kinyoun stain) is indicated for the detection of *Mycobacteria* and *Nocardia* species, respectively.

Q.10. Prophylaxis for post-PKP herpetic keratitis.
Ans. Oral acyclovir 400 mg BD for 1 year is prescribed.

Table 12: Herpetic Eye Disease Study (HEDS).

Study group	Intervention	Recommendation
HEDS-1		
Stromal keratitis not on steroids; on TFT	Topical prednisolone phosphate	Faster resolution and fewer treatment failures
Stromal keratitis on steroids and TFT	Oral acyclovir 400 mg five times a day	No added benefit
HSV iridocyclitis on steroids	Oral acyclovir 400 mg five times a day	Fewer patients were recruited but potential benefits noted
HEDS-2		
HSV epithelial keratitis trial	Oral acyclovir 400 mg five times a day for 3 weeks	No benefit in preventing subsequent stromal keratitis/iridocyclitis
Acyclovir prevention trial	Oral acyclovir 400 mg BD	Reduced the risk of any form of ocular herpes by 41% and stromal keratitis by 50%
Ocular HSV recurrence study	Studied the association between psychological and other forms of stress with HSV recurrence	No association noted

(HSV: herpes simplex virus; TFT: trifluorothymidine)

Q.11. Antimicrobials for acanthamoeba keratitis.

Ans.
- *Biguanide:* Polyhexamethylene biguanide (PHMB) 0.02% or chlorhexidine 0.02%
- *Diamidine:* Propamidine 0.1% or hexamidine 0.1%
- *Others:* Miconazole and clotrimazole 1–2% suspension
- Usually, a combination of biguanide and diamidine is used and the treatment has to be continued for at least 6 months.

Q.12. What are the indications of starting systemic antibiotics in a case of infective keratitis?

Ans. Already discussed in the text.

Q.13. What are the specific features of Pythium keratitis?

Ans.
- *Characteristics:*
  - *Pythium* is an oomycete that closely mimics fungal keratitis, hence the name "parafungus" or "fungus-like organism.
  - *Pythium insidiosum* is the most commonly isolated organism causing keratitis.
  - Classical features include patchy reticular dot-like subepithelial and stromal infiltrate, multifocal infiltrates, cotton wool-like stromal infiltrate with hyphated edges, peripheral furrowing, early limbal spread, peripheral corneal thinning with guttering, and tentacular projections.
- *Diagnosis:*
  - 10% KOH wet mount shows the presence of long, sparsely septate hyaline hyphae
  - Gram stain shows thick cell wall, a few septate, and ribbon-like folding patterns of fungal hyphae
  - Confocal microscopy shows thin, hyper-reflective, and occasionally branching structures with varying angles
  - Culture can be done on 5% sheep blood agar and potato dextrose agar (PDA)
  - PCR and deoxyribonucleic acid (DNA) sequencing is done for species identification.
- *Management:*
  - Similar on the line of general principles of keratitis management
  - The most commonly used drugs are 0.2% linezolid and 1% azithromycin hourly, tapered based on the clinical response.
  - Surgical management includes therapeutic keratoplasty and evisceration/enucleation when there is a rapid progression to panophthalmitis.
  - Prognosis is usually poor.

BIBLIOGRAPHY

1. Gupta N, Tandon R. Investigative modalities in infectious keratitis. Indian J Ophthalmol. 2008;56(3):209-13.
2. Gurnani B, Kaur K, Venugopal A, Srinivasan B, Bagga B, Iyer G, et al. Pythium insidiosum keratitis: a review. Indian J Ophthalmol. 2022;70(4):1107-20.
3. Krachmer JH, Mannis MJ, Holland EJ. Cornea, 2nd edition. Philadelphia: Elsevier, Mosby. 2005;1:955.
4. Soliman W, Fathalla AM, El-Sebaity DM, Al-Hussaini AK. Spectral domain anterior segment optical coherence tomography in microbial keratitis. Graefes Arch Clin Exp Ophthalmol. 2013;251(2):549-53.
5. Vajpayee RB, Namrata S. Corneal ulcer: diagnosis and management, 1st edition. New Delhi: Jaypee Brothers Medical Publishers; 2008.

KERATOCONUS

Prafulla Kumar Maharana, Sapna Raghuwanshi, Manasi Tripathi, Ritu Nagpal, Namrata Sharma

■ INTRODUCTION

Keratoconus (KC) is a disorder characterized by progressive corneal steepening (usually asymmetrical noninflammatory), most typically inferior to the center of the cornea, with eventual corneal thinning, induced myopia, and irregular astigmatism. Although keratoconus was previously considered noninflammatory, recent evidence suggests that the underlying inflammation may be there in patients associated with atopy and VKC. It is the most common corneal ectatic disorder seen in clinical practice. In the postgraduate examination, it can be given as a long case.

■ HISTORY

Epidemiology/Demography

The prevalence of keratoconus is about 54.5 cases/100,000.[1-3] Keratoconus occurs in people of all races. There is no significant gender predilection. Keratoconus usually occurs bilaterally but can often be asymmetrical. Unilateral cases can occur but are rare (in the range of 2–4%).[1-3] The age at onset is usually around the age of puberty. It is more prevalent in the Asian countries than in the West. Asian patients present at a younger age compared to the Western world.

Chief Complaints

A case of keratoconus is presented with the following points:
- Progressive blurring and/or distortion of vision due to irregular astigmatism. It may be associated with photophobia, glare, monocular diplopia, and ocular irritation.
- Often manifests during the late teens or early twenties, then progresses slowly for the next decade or two as the cornea scars and becomes more elongated.
- Frequent change of glasses—the irregular astigmatism is often difficult to correct with glasses, hence the patient keeps on visiting different optometrists.
- Patients can come with complaints of acute onset redness, pain, and watering as in the case of keratoconus with acute hydrops.
- A case may present with symptoms of associated diseases, such as recurrent attacks of itching, and eye rubbing (vernal keratoconjunctivitis), and keratoconus is incidentally discovered on examination.

History of Present Illness

The onset and progression of the disease is characteristic. The onset is usually at puberty. The disease has a rapid progression stage until the age of 30 years. The rate of progression plateaus after this. After the age of 40 years, the disease progression usually stops. The onset in Indian eyes may occur earlier, especially in cases with associated VKC. It is important to know whether the keratoconus is progressive or not. In case of progression, the patient can be advised to undergo corneal CXL. The best way to document progression is serial topography and/or tomography, considering the change in keratometry, anterior, and posterior elevation. However, progressive deterioration of BCVA, progressive decrease in corneal thickness, and a previously contact lens-tolerant patient becoming contact lens-intolerant are certain other clinical clues of keratoconus progression.

Past History

The following past history must be recorded carefully.

Contact Lens Wear

If the contact lenses have not been fitted properly, the constant pressure or continual injury can lead to scarring. Its role in keratoconus progression is controversial. In addition, a better BCVA with contact lenses indicates a good prognosis after keratoplasty.

Eye Rubbing

Mechanical epithelial trauma leads to the release of cytokines that have a role in corneal weakening and ectasia. In addition, rubbing can cause mechanical trauma to the keratocytes and increase hydrostatic pressure in the eye. Chronic eye rubbing can lead to orbital fat atrophy which often gives a clue about the cause of keratoconus in cases where a clear-cut history of eye rubbing is not there.

Topography

The patient might have been already a case of diagnosed keratoconus, and the patient might have undergone corneal topography several times. In that case, a serial recording of the keratometry, central corneal thickness (CCT), and thinnest pachymetry must be done. Remember, an increase in keratometry by 1D over a period of 1 year suggests progression and such cases require CXL (few clinicians consider an increase of 0.5D/6 months). A decrease in thinnest pachymetry by 20% over 1 year is also suggestive of progression.

Ocular Surgery

Keratoconus can occur secondary to ocular surgeries, such as laser in situ keratomileusis (LASIK) and radial keratotomy (RK). Hence, any past refractive surgery must be enquired about. In a few cases, a previous history of CXL may be there.

Past Medical History

Keratoconus can be associated with certain ocular and systemic disorders. A careful history must be taken to rule out these disorders.

Ocular Associations

- Floppy eyelid syndrome
- VKC
- Refractive surgery
- Trauma
- Leber's congenital amaurosis
- Retinitis pigmentosa
- Aniridia
- Iridoschisis
- Cone-rod dystrophy
- *Corneal dystrophies:* Posterior polymorphous corneal dystrophy (PPMD), Fuchs' corneal dystrophy, granular, and lattice corneal dystrophy (LCD).

Systemic Associations

- Down syndrome
- Atopy-bronchial asthma and angioneurotic edema

Noninflammatory connective tissue disorders:
- Marfan syndrome
- Ehlers–Danlos syndrome
- Osteogenesis imperfecta
- Congenital hip dysplasia
- Mitral valve prolapse
- Rosacea

Family History

A three-generation pedigree chart must be prepared. An autosomal dominant mode of inheritance with variable expression has been suggested for keratoconus. Between 6 and 18% of patients with keratoconus have a positive family history.[1-3]

■ EXAMINATION

Visual Acuity

Uncorrected visual acuity and BCVA must be assessed in all cases. Refraction must be attempted in all such cases:
- Scissoring of the red reflex on retinoscopy is one of the earliest signs of keratoconus.
- In the presence of irregular astigmatism, visual acuity with rigid gas-permeable (RGP) lenses may provide the BCVA. This is important before surgical planning to know the visual potential.

Facial Appearance/Orbit

Look for signs of orbital fat atrophy/oculodigital sign (Franceschetti–Leber phenomenon) suggestive of chronic eye rubbing.

Eyelid

Look for signs of allergic conjunctivitis. In advanced keratoconus *Munson's sign*, a V-shape deformation of the lower eyelid when the eye is in a downward position can be elicited.

Conjunctiva

Look for the presence of papillae in the tarsal conjunctiva. In India, keratoconus is often associated with VKC or allergic conjunctivitis. Signs of VKC include papillae, Horner-Trantas dots (gelatinous thickening of limbus), limbal nodules, pigmentation, and ropy discharge.

Cornea

The slit-lamp examination reveals the following signs:[1-3]

- *Corneal thinning:* The thinnest part of the cornea is usually located outside the visual axis, and corneal thinning is a common sign preceding ectasia. Thinning is most commonly seen inferiorly **(Fig. 1)** or inferotemporally.
- *Corneal ectasia:* An eccentrically located ectatic protrusion of the cornea is noted in keratoconus. The apex is usually inferior to a horizontal line through the pupillary axis **(Fig. 1)**. Corneal thinning from one-half to one-fifth of the normal thickness is observed in the apex of the protrusion. Three types of cones can be seen in advanced keratoconus. The round or nipple-shaped cone is more common. It is of smaller diameter. The center lies mostly inferonasally. These corneas are more easily fit with contact lenses. The oval or sagging cone is larger and lies predominantly inferotemporally. This cone is more often associated with hydrops, scarring, and contact lens fitting problems. When the ectasia involves >75% of the cornea, it is termed a globus type of cone.
- Corneal scarring **(Fig. 2)**
- Fleischer ring—in moderate and advanced cases of keratoconus, a Fleischer's ring is a partial or complete annular line commonly seen at the base of the cone. This line is nothing, but a hemosiderin (Iron deposits) arc or circle line seen around the cone base. The ring is formed from hemosiderin pigment deposited deep in the epithelium from the tear film onto the cornea as a result of severe corneal curvature changes induced by the disease and/or due to modification of the normal epithelial slide process. This ring is brown in color and best appreciated with the cobalt blue filter using a broad, oblique beam.[1]
- *Vogt's striae:* These are fine vertical lines produced by compression of DM **(Fig. 3)**, which tend to disappear when physical pressure is applied on the cornea digitally or by gas-permeable contact lens wear. The lines are seen in the deep stroma and DM and are parallel to the axis of the cone.

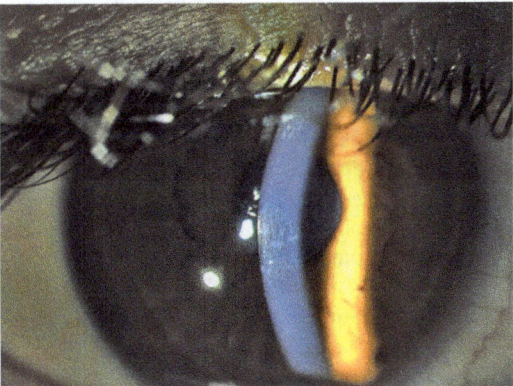

Fig. 2: Corneal scar.

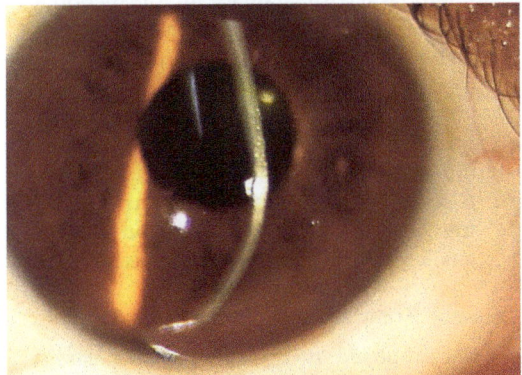

Fig. 1: Ectatic protrusion of the cornea with thinning.

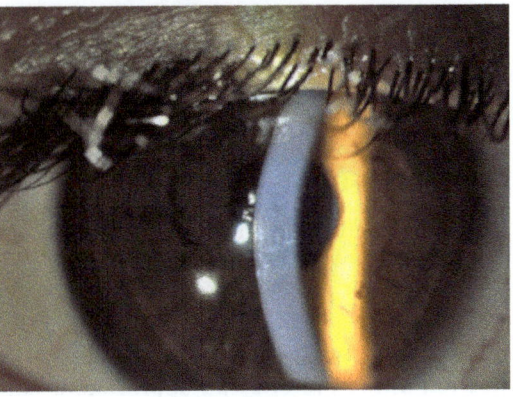

Fig. 3: Vogt's striae.

- *Prominent corneal nerves:* The increased visibility of corneal nerves results from the outward bowing and thinning of the ectatic cornea.
- Superficial and deep corneal opacities.
- *Increased intensity of the corneal endothelial reflex:* An endothelial reflex may appear at the peak of the cone due to the increased concavity of the posterior corneal surface. An annular dark shadow separates the bright reflex of the cone from the reflex of the corneal periphery. This shadow results from total internal light reflection induced by the corneal ectasia. It is best demonstrated using the direct ophthalmoscope in a dilated pupil.
- *Subepithelial fibrillary lines:* Bron et al. have described, white subepithelial fibrillary lines in concentric bundles lying just inside the Fleischer's ring.[1] These are best seen under high magnification with a broad, oblique slit beam. The pattern is characteristic of keratoconus and occurs in approximately one-third of the patients with this disease.[1]
- Corneal hyperesthesia can be detected early in the course of the disease. Later the cone becomes relatively less sensitive.
- *Rizzuti phenomena:* This is demonstrated by a penlight shining on the temporal side of the cornea or parallel to the iris plane. Normally, the light rays illuminate the nasal limbal area. In mild keratoconus, the ectatic cornea focuses the light sharply inside the nasal limbus. In more advanced states, the light is focused at the nasal limbus and beyond. It is important to remember that this response can also be elicited in patients with refractive errors.
- Breaks in DM have been described in severe keratoconus, causing acute stromal edema, known as hydrops (**Fig. 4**), sudden vision loss, and significant pain.

Fundus Examination

Fundus evaluation after mydriasis is essential for any concomitant fundus abnormality.

Charleux Sign

With a dilated pupil and a lens + 6D positioned in front of the eye one can appreciate a dark reflex in the area of the cone with a central bright reflex resembling a drop of honey or oil (sign of "Charleux"), in the reflection of the red reflex from a distant direct ophthalmoscopy. This is one of the earliest signs of keratoconus.

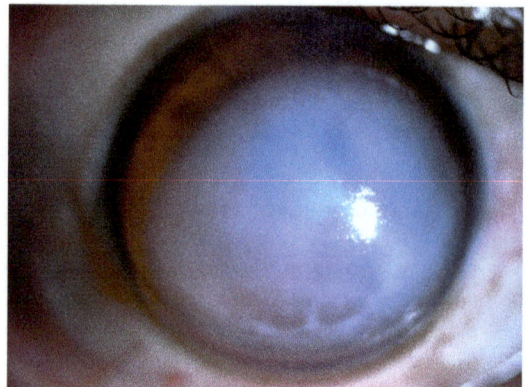

Fig. 4: Corneal hydrops.

■ DIFFERENTIAL DIAGNOSIS

See **Table 1**.

■ CLASSIFICATION

Keratoconus is classified based on morphology, disease evolution, ocular signs, and index-based systems.

Morphology

Classically, keratoconus has been classified into:
- *Nipple:* The cone has a diameter ≤5 mm, round morphology, and is located in the central or paracentral cornea, more commonly in the inferonasal corneal quadrant. Correction with contact lenses is normally relatively easy.
- *Oval:* The cone has a diameter >5 mm and a paracentral to peripheral location, more commonly in the inferotemporal corneal quadrant. Contact lens correction is more difficult.
- *Globus:* The cone is located throughout 75% of the cornea. Contact lens correction is a difficult challenge, except in very limited cases.

Disease Progression

Amsler proposed the first keratoconus classification based on the disease evolution.[2,3] The details of classification are given in **Table 2**.

Table 1: Differential diagnosis of keratoconus.

Characteristics	Keratoconus	PMD	Keratoglobus	TMD
Frequency	Most common	Less common	Rare	Rare
Laterality	Usually, bilateral	Bilateral	Bilateral	Bilateral
Age at onset	Puberty	20–40 years	Usually at birth	Middle-aged to elderly
Thinning	Inferior paracentral	Inferior band 1–2 mm wide	Maximum in periphery	Superior cornea
CCT	Reduced	Usually, normal	May be normal	Usually, normal
Protrusion	Thinnest at apex	Superior to a band of thinning	Generalized	Superior cornea
Rizzuti's phenomenon and Munson's sign	Present	Absent	Present	Absent
Fleischer ring	Present	Sometimes	None	Absent
Scarring	Common	Only after hydrops	Mild	Superior cornea with vascularization, lipid deposition, and inflammation
Vogt's striae	Common	Sometimes	Sometimes	Absent

(CCT: central corneal thickness; PMD: pellucid marginal degeneration; TMD: Terrien's marginal degeneration)

Table 2: Amsler–Krumeich classification of keratoconus.

Stage	Description
1	• Eccentric corneal bulging • Myopia and/or astigmatism <5D • Corneal radius ≤48D • Vogt's striae • No central opacity
2	• Myopia and/or astigmatism >5D but <8D • Corneal radius ≤53D • No central opacity • Pachymetry ≥400 μ
3	• Myopia and/or astigmatism >8D but <10D • Corneal radius >53D • No central corneal opacity • Pachymetry 200–400 μ
4	• Refraction not possible • Corneal steepening >55.00D • Corneal scarring • Pachymetry <200 μ

Curvature

Keratoconus is classified into the following:
- *Mild:* <45D
- *Moderate:* 45–52D
- *Advanced:* >52D
- *Severe:* >62D

The Belin ABCD Grading System

This staging system incorporates anterior and posterior curvature, thinnest pachymetry values, and distance visual acuity **(Table 3)**.

This better reflects the anatomical changes seen in keratoconus.

A = *A*nterior radius of curvature (ARC) 3 mm from the thinnest corneal pachymetry

B = Posterior (*B*ack surface) radius of curvature (PRC) 3 mm from the thinnest corneal pachymetry

C = Thinnest *C*orneal pachymetry

D = Best corrected *D*istance visual acuity (BDVA)

Scarring: (−) Clear cornea, no scarring; (+) scarring present but iris details visible; and (++) scarring present, iris details obscured.

Table 3: Belin ABCD grading system.

ABCD criteria	A	B	C	D	
	ARC (3 mm zone)	PRC (3 mm zone)	Thinnest pachymetry	BDVA	Scarring
Stage 0	>7.25 mm (<46.5D)	>5.90 mm (<57.25D)	>490	=20/20 (=1.0)	–
Stage 1	>7.05 mm (<48D)	>5.70 mm (<59.25D)	>450	<20/20 (<1.0)	–, +, ++
Stage 2	>6.15 mm (<53D)	>5.15 mm (<65.5D)	>400	<20/40 (<0.5)	–, +, ++
Stage 3	>6.15 mm (<55D)	>4.95 mm (<68.5D)	>300	<20/100 (<0.2)	–, +, ++
Stage 4	<6.15 mm (>55D)	<4.95 mm (>68.5D)	<300	<20/400 (<0.05)	–, +, ++

(ARC: anterior average radii of curvature; PRC: posterior average radii of curvature)

Table 4: ASOCT classification of keratoconus.

Stage	Features
Stage 1	Thinning of epithelial and stromal layers at the cone
Stage 2	Hyperreflective anomalies occurring at Bowman's layer with epithelial thickening and stromal thinning
Stage 3	Posterior displacement of the hyperreflective structures occurring at the Bowman's layer with epithelial thickening and stromal thinning
Stage 4	Pan-stromal scar
Stage 5	Hydrops

Anterior Segment Optical Coherence Tomography-based Classification

See **Table 4**.

INVESTIGATIONS

Keratometry

Keratometry mires in keratoconus are commonly steep, highly astigmatic, irregular, and often appear egg-shaped (rather than circular or oval). The inability to superimpose the central keratometric rings suggests irregular corneal astigmatism, a hallmark of keratoconus. In early cases, keratometry may be normal. Some patients with keratoconus do not exhibit these signs. The disadvantages of keratometry in keratoconus are, that it provides information about the central 3 mm of cornea only, and it is not useful in irregular astigmatism. Few clinicians perform central keratometry, followed by keratometry with the patient in upward gaze, to identify the steepening in the inferior cornea but it is often difficult and inconclusive.

Videokeratography

This is based on the Placido disk principle. It provides qualitative contour information. In early cases, there will be an isolated area of smaller ring spacing and distortion. As the keratoconus worsens, the cornea becomes steeper; the ring spacing decreases overall and becomes increasingly irregular. Its disadvantage is it does not give accurate information about posterior curvature (cannot detect early keratoconus) and corneal thickness.

Orbscan

It uses the principle of scanning slit combined with a Placido system. It provides reliable data on anterior and posterior elevation best-fit spheres and a corneal pachymetry map. However, the posterior curvature maps are based on assumptions and may not be 100% accurate. In addition, it requires patient fixation for the accuracy of data which is difficult at times, and data of the central cornea (near the point of fixation) is not accurate.

Pentacam

This device uses a rotating Scheimpflug camera. It provides reliable measurement of anterior and posterior corneal elevation and accurate measurement of corneal thickness. Pentacam differs fundamentally from the Orbscan by the way in which it takes image slices of the cornea. The Orbscan takes vertical image slices that are separated from one another and have no common point. Thus, the Orbscan cannot reregister for any eye movement that occurs while it is capturing the images. The Pentacam maintains the central point (the thinnest point) of each meridian. Thus, during the examination, the software can reregister these central points and eliminate eye movement. This single feature makes the Pentacam's measurements 10 times more accurate. Thus, it is largely independent of patient fixation with better repeatability than Orbscan. In addition, the central corneal curvature can be measured more accurately compared to Orbscan.

Early Diagnostic Features on Pentacam

Pachymetry: Both ultrasonic and optical-based devices (ASOCT) can be used to measure the pachymetry. Measurement of corneal thickness is useful for diagnosis, documenting progression, and planning treatment (*see* treatment section).

Ocular response analyzer: The ocular response analyzer allows keratoconus diagnosis and classification by assessing corneal hysteresis and resistance.

Corvis-ST: Corvis ST is a new investigative modality that measures the biomechanical properties of the cornea. It uses a high-speed Scheimpflug camera and a noncontact tonometer to assess the same.

■ MANAGEMENT

The treatment of keratoconus varies depending on the disease severity. Early cases are managed with spectacles, mild to moderate cases are managed with contact lenses, and severe cases can be treated with keratoplasty. Other surgical treatment options include intracorneal ring segments, corneal cross-linking, intraocular lens implants, or a combination of these.[4-6]

Nonsurgical Management

- *Spectacles:* Spectacles are normally used in early cases of keratoconus only. As the disease progresses, irregular astigmatism develops, and adequate visual acuity cannot be achieved with this type of visual correction.
- *Contact lens:* Different contact lenses used for the treatment of keratoconus are soft toric lenses, standard bicurved hard lenses, custom-back toric lenses, piggyback systems, hybrid lenses (made of the combined hard lens with a soft skirt), scleral lenses, and miniscleral lenses.
  - *RGP lenses:* RGP corneal lenses are the lenses of the first choice for correcting irregular astigmatism. The aim is to provide the best vision possible with maximum comfort so that the lenses can be worn for a long period. The different fitting strategies of gas-permeable contact lenses are as follows:
    * *Apical clearance:* In apical clearance fitting there is no bearing or touch in the apical area and the lens bearing is in the periphery. The advantages are reduced risk of scarring, whorl keratopathy, and erosions; the limitation is that tightening at the periphery can hamper tear exchange and the edge of the lens can come into the visual axis, especially in cases with advanced ectasia. This strategy is very rarely used nowadays.
    * Apical touch fitting technique is characterized by providing primary lens support on the apex of the cornea, in which the central optic zone of the lens actually touches or "bears on" the central cornea. The advantage is better quality of vision, but the problem is there can be heavy bearing on the cornea resulting in corneal scarring and intolerance over long-term use.
    * The three-point touch fitting technique is the most popular technique. In three-point touch fitting the lens bearing is shared between the apex and the mid-peripheral cornea that minimizes the risk of apical scarring. These lenses provide good vision, better comfort, and prolonged wearing time and are hence the most preferred type of lenses.
- *Piggyback systems:* Consisting of fitting an RGP on top of a soft contact lens. The soft contact lens is used to improve wearing comfort

and provide a more regular area for the gas-permeable contact lenses to sit, whereas the gas-permeable contact lens is primarily used for providing adequate visual acuity.

- *Hybrid contact lenses (such as softperm, Solotica, and SynergEyes):* Hybrid contact lenses contain an RGP center with a soft skirt. New-generation hybrid contact lens provides higher oxygen permeability and greater strength of the RGP/hydrogel junction. These lenses are fitted with no or minimal apical touch in the central cornea. The lenses can be fitted on cones of any severity but the problem with these lenses is they can cause hypoxia-related changes, such as vascularization and central corneal clouding. However, these lenses have not been widely accepted as the current designs, because they are generally more expensive than the permeable gas lenses, and do not normally provide improved visual correction and wearing comfort in comparison with gas-permeable contact lenses.
- Rose K lenses (Rose K, Rose K2 XL, and Rose K2 IC) are multicurve lenses with a small optical zone that snugly fits over the cone. The Rose-K contact lens provides greater comfort, and better quality of vision and requires less chair time in cases with keratoconus. The Rose K2 IC is a large-diameter, intralimbal lens that can be used for large or oval cones.
- *Scleral lenses:* These lenses rest on the sclera and do not touch the cornea and limbus, leaving a clear area between the contact lens and the cornea. The advantages are good centration, stability, and improved VA. The PROSE is a nonfenestrated scleral contact lens that is filled with fluid before insertion in the eye. Treatment has a high success rate when measured by the ability to achieve satisfactory fit and impact on VA. PROSE treatment can be an alternative to PKP for patients with corneal ectasia who are contact lens intolerant. The Boston ocular surface prosthesis (BOSP) is a fluid-filled scleral contact lens. These lenses rest on the sclera and do not touch the cornea. There is a constant pool of tears over the cornea, which acts as a liquid corneal bandage and avoids any friction between the posterior surface of the contact lens and the corneal apex. In addition, these lenses mask corneal surface astigmatism and improve best-corrected VA. Thus, these lenses are extremely useful in patients with advanced ectasia where the patients are intolerant to contact lenses, or immediate surgery is not possible, or when the patient refuses surgery. The limitations of the use of scleral lenses are high cost, reduced tear exchange, and difficult insertion-removal, which require considerable practice. Overall, studies have shown a good outcome with these lenses.[2,3]

Surgical Management

Current surgical options include:
- *Corneal transplantation:* Bowman membrane transplant, deep anterior lamellar keratoplasty, and penetrating keratoplasty.
- *Intrastromal corneal lenticule*
- *Intracorneal ring segment insert:* Intacs and Ferrara Rings.
- Ultraviolet A (UVA)/riboflavin corneal collagen cross-linking with riboflavin (C3R).
- Thermokeratoplasty
- *Lenticular refractive surgery:* Refractive lens exchange with toric intraocular lenses, and toric phakic intraocular lenses.

Penetrating Keratoplasty

Penetrating keratoplasty in keratoconus in comparison to other indications is considered low risk in terms of graft rejection, graft survival, and postoperative complications. The success rate is 90–95%. Visual recovery takes several weeks/months, with full stabilization not occurring until a year, after which time the sutures can be removed.

Deep Anterior Lamellar Keratoplasty

Deep anterior lamellar keratoplasty (DALK) has several advantages over PKP **(Table 5)**. In keratoconic eyes, the corneal endothelium is usually intact; with good cell counts even after cases of acute hydrops; hence, DALK is the procedure of choice. The major disadvantage is corneal stromal rejection and migration of host keratocytes to replace donor keratocytes resulting in recurrence of the disease in graft. However, stromal rejection can never lead to graft failure and recurrence in the graft is extremely rare.

Table 5: Comparison of deep anterior lamellar keratoplasty (DALK) and penetrating keratoplasty (PKP).

Parameter	DALK	PKP
Indication	Stromal opacification with healthy endothelium	Both endothelial failure and stromal opacification
Visual rehabilitation	Early	Delayed
Quality of vision	Poor than PKP	Best
Interface haze	Affects vision	None
Higher order aberrations	More	Less
Postoperative astigmatism	Less	More
Wound strength	Better	Poor
Open sky procedure	None	Risk of expulsive hemorrhage
Intraocular surgery	None	Complications can occur
Tensile strength	Better	Poor
Steroid use	Early taper	Prolonged
Donor criteria	Not stringent even nonoptical grades can be used	Only optical grade
Single donor multiple-use	Possible	Not possible
Graft rejection	Low-risk	High-risk
Technique	Difficult	Easy
Learning curve	Steep	Less steep

The goal of DALK is to achieve a depth of dissection as close as possible to DM. Various agents have been used to create a plane of separation between DM and the deep stromal layers. These include air, fluid, viscoelastic, microkeratome, and a femtosecond laser (FSL). The common techniques of DALK are described further.

Layer-by-layer manual dissection: In this technique, after an initial partial trephination of variable depth ranging from 50 to 70% of corneal thickness, the stroma is removed using either a crescent knife or various types of lamellar dissectors. This is followed by layer-by-layer stromal removal, which is repeated multiple times to reach as close as possible to the DM. The major limitations of this technique are poor visual outcomes due to residual stroma and interface haze. In addition, it is a very time-consuming process.[7]

Air-assisted deep anterior lamellar keratoplasty: Air-assisted lamellar keratoplasty involves the injection of air into the corneal stroma that helps to achieve dissection as close as possible to DM.

Archila first described the technique of air-assisted deep lamellar keratoplasty. Over a period of time, many modifications of air-assisted DALK were tried. The big-bubble technique was described by Anwar and Teichmann and it is the most widely used technique of DALK.[7]

Big bubble DALK: The basic step of this technique involves injecting air into the corneal stroma deep into a groove, which is created by trephining 60–80% of the stromal thickness. The air infiltrates the potential space between the deep stromal layer and DM. The air anterior to DM creates a dome-shaped detachment of DM, which is then identified by a ring visible with the microscope. Once a plane of separation is achieved, the stromal tissue can be easily excised. The main advantage of this technique is that the quality of vision achieved is as good as PK. However, the learning curve associated with this technique is very steep. Often its repeatability is uncertain even with the most experienced surgeons. Inadvertent DM perforation can occur at any stage of the surgery.[7]

Types of bubbles:
- *Viscoelastic-assisted DALK:* Melles et al. described a technique that uses a viscoelastic injection rather than air to achieve a cleavage plane between DM from stroma. The depth of stromal dissection is guided by the "air to endothelium" interface which is seen by a specular light reflex localized at the tip of the blade. Once the plane is achieved, the superficial stroma is removed using trephine and lamellar dissection.[7]
- *Hydrodelamination:* This technique was described by Sujita et al. In this technique, saline solution is injected into the cornea, which enhances the identification and removal of the deep stromal fibers. An initial partial thickness corneal trephination is done up to approximately two-thirds of the thickness using vacuum trephines. However, it is difficult to achieve an actual cleavage plane over DM by hydrodelamination.[7]

Femtosecond-assisted DALK: The FSL computer-guided cuts allow precise, accurate, and reproducible placement of incisions at desired depths in the corneal stroma. Hence, it can be used to create the initial cut at the desired depth to inject air for the successful formation of big bubbles. In addition, it can be used to create corneal incisions with customized graft edges and lamellar planes for both donor and recipient corneas. Thus, FSL can be utilized for creating customized graft host interfaces, such as mushroom and zigzag-shaped DALK. The greatest advantages are its accuracy of forming the bubble at the desired corneal depth and its positive refractive outcomes due to the successful alignment of the donor and recipient zigzag or mushroom configurations. However, the major limitations are the cost and availability.[7]

Diamond knife-assisted DALK: Vajpayee et al. have described a new technique of DALK that is easy to perform, provides visual outcomes comparable to those of big-bubble DALK, and can be performed in cases of extreme corneal thinning or corneal scars. The essential steps of this technique involve the use of a diamond knife set at a depth of 30 μ less than the pachymetry reading, to make a 2.0 mm incision at the 11–12 o'clock position. This incision is then extended circumferentially and centripetally to take out the anterior stromal lamella, leaving a thin stromal bed. The authors found comparable outcomes to the big bubble DALK.[4,7]

Epikeratophakia: It involves removing the corneal epithelium from the host and then sewing onto the corneal stromal bed a previously cryolathed lenticule of the donor cornea. The procedure has generally resulted in less favorable outcomes than PKP with reports of failure of reepithelialization, poor BSCVA, stromal and lenticule inflammation and opacification, and interface haze. It is rarely performed nowadays.

Intracorneal ring segment inserts (intacs and Ferrara rings): The technique consists of the implantation of one or two polymethyl methacrylate segments in the corneal stroma to flatten the central cornea and improve visual acuity, contact lens tolerance, and delay the need for corneal graft. It acts by its arc-shortening effect. It is commonly used to treat mild to moderate cases of keratoconus, as normal corneal transparency and a minimum corneal thickness of 450 μm at the site of the incision is required.

Three types of rings are available: Intacs® which have a hexagonal cross-section and are placed more peripheral than Ferrara rings which are triangular/prismatic in shape. Recently, Intacs® SK (SK—severe keratoconus) has been introduced for use in more severe forms of corneal ectasia. It has two significant design modifications, i.e. (1) a smaller inner diameter of 6.0 mm compared with 6.8 mm of the standard Intacs® and (2) an elliptical cross section compared with a hexagonal cross section of the standard Intacs®.

The rings are inserted into the posterior stroma (about 75% of the corneal depth at the incision site) in a quick outpatient technique performed under topical anesthesia. The circular intralamellar pockets for the rings are created either using a specially designed vacuum lamellar dissector or with the FSL. It is assumed that they push out against the ectatic curvature peripherally flattening the peak of the cone centrally and returning the cornea to a more spherical shape. Intracorneal ring technology does not offer a cure for the condition but can very often produce a marked improvement in unaided and BCVA and allow eyes to be corrected with spectacles and/or soft rather than rigid lenses.

Corneal CXL with riboflavin (C3R) or corneal cross linkage: CXL using riboflavin (vitamin B_2)/UVA (370 nm) light is a therapeutic modality that can halt and stabilize the keratoconic process. It increases corneal rigidity and biomechanical stability. The success rate varies between studies but overall, 60–70% of cases show some stabilization after CXL.[2,4] The procedure involves removing the corneal epithelium in a 6–7 mm diameter central zone followed by riboflavin 0.1% of solution application and corneal radiation with UVA light at 370 nm. UVA light radiation activates riboflavin generating reactive oxygen species that induce covalent bonds between collagen fibrils in the corneal stroma. The irradiation level at the corneal endothelium, lens, and retina is significantly smaller than the damage threshold. It has been recommended not to perform this technique in corneas thinner than 400 μm as toxic reactions could take place in the corneal endothelium. In such cases, hypotonic CXL has been tried with variable success. Other contraindications of CXL include high preoperative keratometry (>58 km), age >35–40 years (as the disease tends to stabilize by this age, BCVA > 20/25, history of viral keratitis (risk of reactivation), central corneal opacity, and history of incisional refractive surgery.

The conventional CXL is contraindicated for corneas thinner than 400 μm due to the potential risk of damage to the endothelium by ultraviolet (UV) rays. However, certain medications have been described to overcome this. These include use of hypoosmolar riboflavin (0.1% riboflavin + 0.9% normal saline) instead of iso-osmolar, transepithelial techniques, small incision lenticule extraction (SMILE) lenticule-assisted CXL, customized pachymetric-guided epithelial debridement [topographic photorefractive keratectomy (PRK) + CXL], using riboflavin soaked BCL and CXL using adapted fluence.

Corneal crosslinking is largely safe except for the risk of post-CXL keratitis. No long-term problems in terms of loss of transparency of the cornea or lens have occurred and endothelial counts have been unchanged postoperatively. In addition, this technique has been successfully used in combination with other surgery techniques, such as corneal ring segments and corneal lenticule-assisted CXL.

Refractive lens exchange: Refractive lens exchange or toric phakic intraocular lens insertion may be of some benefit in correcting myopia and astigmatism in selected eyes with early/mild/stable disease with good spectacle-corrected visual acuity.

VIVA QUESTIONS

Q.1. Discuss about refractive surgery in keratoconus.

Ans. Keratoconus as a contraindication to corneal surgical procedures, such as LASIK, photorefractive keratectomy (PRK), laser epithelial keratomileusis (LASEK), and excimer laser phototherapeutic keratectomy (PTK).

Q.2. What are the complications associated with keratoconus?

Ans. Complications of keratoconus include corneal hydrops and corneal perforation. Corneal hydrops are characterized by corneal edema due to seepage of aqueous humor through a tear in the DM. Corneal hydrops have also been reported with PMD, TMD, keratoglobus, and post-LASIK ectasia. If not treated, resolution usually takes a long time and occurs by endothelial sliding over a period of 2–4 months. Medical management consists of topical hypertonic drops, topical steroids, prophylactic antibiotic drops, and antiglaucoma medications. However, persistent edema can cause complications, such as corneal neovascularization, infection, and corneal perforation. Surgical intervention is often performed to shorten the duration of the disease. Intracameral injection of air/isoexpansile gases (C3F8/SF6) is the most commonly performed procedure. In the presence of a large DM detachment or stromal clefts, ASOCT-guided intrastromal drainage with stab incisions; compressive sutures, and even PKP may have to be performed.

Q.3. What is Munson's sign?
Ans. *See* text.

Q.4. What is Rizzuti's sign?
Ans. *See* text.

Q.5. What is posterior keratoconus?

Ans. Posterior keratoconus refers to a congenital corneal anomaly in which the posterior corneal surface protrudes into the stroma. It usually occurs in a localized area but may be more diffuse. It is usually sporadic, unilateral, and nonprogressive. Bilateral and familial cases do occur but are less frequent. The anterior corneal contour is usually unaffected. Frequently, scarring occurs in the stroma anterior to Descemet's bulge. Scarring at the level of Bowman's membrane and thinning of DM with excrescences has been reported on histopathology. It is considered a variant of corneal mesenchymal dysgenesis. Treatment usually is not necessary, although occasionally keratoplasty is indicated.

Q.6. Discuss about forme fruste keratoconus (FFKC).

Ans. FFKC is an ill-defined term as the criteria of diagnosis differ; however, it is largely accepted that FFKC is a normal cornea with the fellow eye having keratoconus. It is a subclinical disease and is not a variant of KC. Cornea specialists define FFKC in two ways:
1. FFKC is *a normal cornea* with the fellow eye having keratoconic or there is a family history of KC.
2. Subclinical keratoconus is *an abnormal cornea*. Corneal topography or corneal hysteresis [ocular response analyzer (ORA)] or both are abnormal but there are no obvious clinical signs of keratoconus.

Q.7. Discuss about hypotonic CXL.

Ans. It has the following features:
- Used for thin corneas <400 µ (320–400 µ)
- Iso-osmolar uses riboflavin 0.1% solution in 20% dextran while hypo-osmolar uses riboflavin 0.1% solution in 0.9% NaCl
- Corneal thickness increases (hypotonic solution) thus allowing for safe CXL
- Results variable.

Q.8. What is the difference between PMD and keratoconus?

Ans. *See* **Table 1**.

Q.9. Explain systemic association and keratoconus.

Ans. *See* the discussion part.

Q.10. Give Amsler–Krumeich classification.

Ans. *See* **Table 2**.

Q.11. Discuss topographic patterns in the normal cornea.

Ans. The topographic patterns of both the eyes of an individual often show mirror-image symmetry. This phenomenon is called enantiomorphism. Topographic patterns seen in a normal eye are following: round, oval, superior steepening, inferior steepening, symmetric bow tie, symmetric bow tie with skewed axes, asymmetric bow tie with inferior steepening, asymmetric bow tie with superior steepening, and asymmetric bow tie (AB) with skewed radial axes (SRAX) and irregular. Skewing of >30° is described as significantly abnormal.

Q.12. What is the keratoconus percentage index (KISA) index?

Ans. Rabinowitz/Rasheed described KISA% to diagnose keratoconus. The KISA% index is usually applied to the axial map. It uses four indices on the topography. It is calculated as:

$$KISA\% = \frac{(K) \times (I-S) \times (AST) \times (SRAX) \times 100}{300}$$

- K-central keratometric value in excess of 47.2 D (i.e., K-47.2). If the value is ≤47.2, it is replaced by 1.
- I-S or inferior-superior asymmetry
- AST calculated from (Sim K1-Sim K2)
- SRAX is calculated from 180°—the angle between two steep axes above and below the horizontal meridian (smaller of the two angles). To amplify any abnormality, the value 1 was substituted in the equation whenever a calculated index has a value of <1

KISA% > 100% is considered as highly suggestive of keratoconus.

REFERENCES

1. Krachmer JH, Feder RS, Belin MW. Keratoconus and related noninflammatory corneal thinning disorders. Surv Ophthalmol. 1984;28(4):293-322.
2. Mannis MJ, Hooland EJ. In: Krachmer JH, Mannis MJ, Holland EJ (Eds). Cornea, 2nd edition. Philadelphia: Elsevier, Mosby; 2005. pp. 955.
3. Maharana PK, Dubey A, Jhanji V, Sharma N, Das S, Vajpayee RB. Management of advanced corneal ectasias. Br J Ophthalmol. 2016;100(1):34-40.
4. American Academy of Optometry. Keratoconus. 2008. pp. 1-13.
5. Espandar L, Meyer J. Keratoconus: Overview and update on treatment. Middle East Afr J Ophthalmol. 2010;17(1):15-20.
6. Romero-Jiménez M, Santodomingo-Rubido J, Wolffsohn JS. Keratoconus: A review. Cont Lens Anterior Eye. 2010;33(4):157-66.
7. Maharana PK, Agarwal K, Jhanji V, Vajpayee RB. Deep anterior lamellar keratoplasty for keratoconus: a review. Eye Contact Lens. 2014;40(6):382-9.

CORNEAL STROMAL DYSTROPHY

Shipra Singhi, Divya Agarwal, Prafulla Kumar Maharana

INTRODUCTION

The corneal dystrophies are a group of noninflammatory, inherited, and bilateral disorders of the cornea characterized by pathognomonic patterns of corneal deposition and morphological changes that are slowly progressive and not related to environmental or systemic factors. The stromal corneal dystrophies primarily affect the stroma. Over time, they often extend into the anterior corneal layers, and some may affect DM and the endothelium. In examinations, corneal dystrophy can be given as both long and short case.[1-3]

HISTORY

Demography

Usually, the patients are young adults, typically <45 years of age. The disease is usually bilateral; however, the presentation may be unilateral.[1-3]

Chief Complaints

The patient presents with the following complaints:
- *Blurring of vision:* Blurring of vision is rare before the fifth decade of life in the case of granular corneal dystrophy type 1 (GCD1). It appears as early as 3 years of age in the case of GCD2 and between 3 and 9 years of age in the case of macular corneal dystrophy (MCD). Lattice dystrophy may present as progressive loss of vision in the first decade in LCD1 and in the third or fourth decade in LCD2. Schnyder's crystalline dystrophy (SCD) is rare before the fourth decade.
- *Photophobia:* Photophobia is mild in the case of GCD1. More in the case of GCD2 and macular dystrophy.
- *Glare:* Due to diffraction of light by the opacities.
- *Foreign body sensation:* Due to recurrent erosion or lesions extending up to epithelium.
- *Color haloes:* Due to the deposits and corneal edema.
- *Recurrent corneal erosion:* Presents with mild to extreme irritation, and discomfort that is worse in the morning. It may be associated with severe pain due to epithelial defect and fluctuating vision or blurred vision due to irregular astigmatism (uneven surface). These are uncommon with GCD, common with MCD, and frequent with LCD.
- *Systemic features:* Rarely, especially in cases with LCD2, the patient may be referred by a physician with systemic symptoms. The various systemic symptoms include dry, itchy skin, laxity of the facial skin, edema over feet, breathlessness, severe mask-like facial paresis with gradual onset of facial drooping, protruding lips, and pendulous ears (due to amyloid deposition and secondary muscular dysfunction).

- Usually asymptomatic in the early stage and may be detected accidentally.

History of Present Illness

Points mentioned further must be noted in the present illness.

Age of Onset

- *Blurring of vision* is rare before the fifth decade of life in the case of GCD1. It appears as early as 3 years of age in the case of GCD2 and between 3 and 9 years of age in the case of MCD. Lattice dystrophy may present as progressive loss of vision in the first decade in LCD1 and in the third or fourth decade in LCD2. The onset of visual loss is insidious and progressive in all types of stromal dystrophy.
- *Recurrent erosion can occur* in all types of stromal dystrophy, but it is most commonly seen in LCD. The onset of recurrent corneal erosions (RCEs) is in the first to second decade in cases of LCD, in cases of GCD can occur in the early stages but episodes are usually mild and rare (more patients with GCD2 or Avellino corneal dystrophy experience recurring erosions than patients with typical GCD1). MCD usually presents with blurring of vision but RCE can occur in the second to third decade.
- *Corneal opacities* in MCD usually first appear in adolescence but may become apparent anytime from early infancy to the sixth decade of life. Affected individuals usually experience severe visual impairment before the fifth decade of life, usually in the second to third decade, once opacities have coalesced and the entire stroma becomes cloudy. The onset of corneal changes in lattice corneal dystrophy type I (LCD1) usually occurs in the first decade of life, although patients may remain asymptomatic for years. Signs of lattice dystrophy most often appear in early childhood and become more prominent in the second and third decades. In the case of GCD, the opacities usually appear in the first to second decade but become symptomatic only in the third to fourth decade.

Progression: Stromal dystrophies are progressive diseases. To begin with, the lesions are localized to the stroma. With time the lesions progressively involve the other layers too. The progression is relatively faster in MCD followed by LCD when compared to GCD.

Past History

Similar episodes of recurrent corneal erosion associated with pain and redness in the past may be there.

Past Surgical History

History of prior surgery such as PTK, PKP, and DALK must be recorded carefully.

Past Medical History

A careful systemic history is required to rule out hypertension, diabetes and cardiac abnormality, renal failure, skin disease, and neuropathy. Multiple systems may be affected in LCD2.

Family History

A pedigree chart should be drawn to know the hereditary pattern. Autosomal dominant pattern is found in LCD and GCD and autosomal recessive in MCD.

■ EXAMINATION

Systemic Examination

Systemic features associated with LCD2 are as follows:
- Dry and itchy skin
- Laxity of the facial skin
- Intermittent proteinuria (nephrotic syndromes)
- Severe mask, such as facial paresis with gradual onset of facial drooping, protruding lips, and pendulous ears (due to amyloid deposition and secondary muscular dysfunction)
- Cranial and peripheral neuropathy
- Peripheral polyneuropathy affects mainly senses of vibration and touch
- Carpal tunnel syndrome
- Autonomic disturbance includes orthostatic hypotension, cardiac conduction abnormalities, and dysfunction of perspiration.

Ocular Examination

Visual Acuity

Uncorrected as well as corrected visual acuity must be recorded in all cases. This is important for planning treatment.

Eyeball

Lagophthalmos can be present in LCD2.

Lids

Dermatochalasis can be present in LCD2.

Conjunctiva

Usually, normal.

Cornea

On slit-lamp biomicroscopy, the following signs must be noted:
- *Corneal size:* Usually normal
- *Corneal shape:* Keratoconus can be found in Avellino and granular dystrophy is otherwise normal.
- *Corneal opacity.*
- *Epithelium/anterior cornea:* Shows atrophy and degeneration of basal epithelial cells and focal thinning or loss of Bowman layer
- *Stroma*

Granular Corneal Dystrophy Type 1

In the early stage of the disease fine dots and radial lines are seen in the anterior stroma; these dots are opaque on focal illumination and translucent on retroillumination **(Figs. 1 and 2)**. Opacities are usually grouped into three basic morphologic types, i.e., (1) drop-shaped, (2) crumb-shaped, and (3) ring-shaped. The deposits can resemble crushed breadcrumbs snowflakes or popcorn or Christmas trees. The overall pattern is ray- or disk-shaped. The granules are primarily located in the central cornea. Initially, the stroma between the opacities remains clear **(Fig. 3)**. As the disease progresses individual lesions increase in size and number and coalesce. Lesions extend into the deeper and more peripheral stroma but 2–3 mm of the peripheral cornea usually remain free of deposits. In more advanced diseases, the

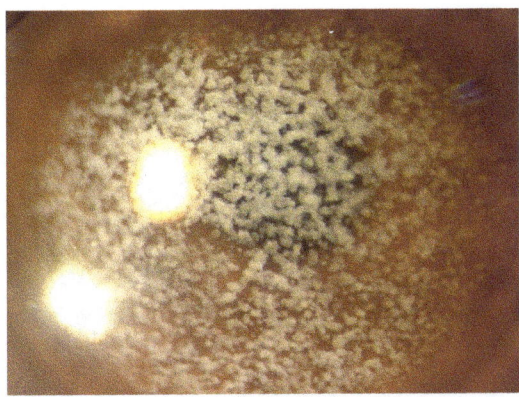

Fig. 1: Multiple opacities resembling popcorn with clear intervening cornea in a case of granular dystrophy.

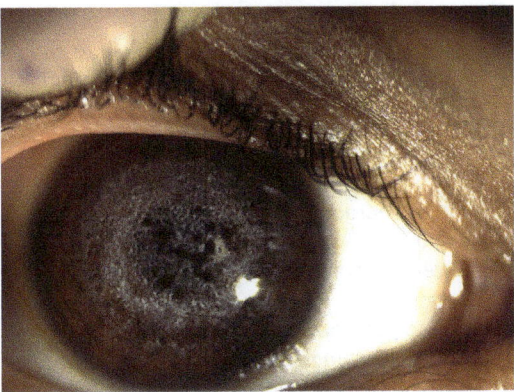

Fig. 2: Multiple opacities resembling crushed breadcrumbs with clear intervening cornea in a case of granular dystrophy.

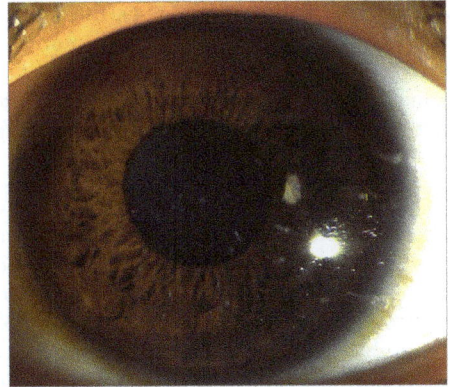

Fig. 3: Multiple scattered opacities with the clear intervening cornea in a case of early granular dystrophy.

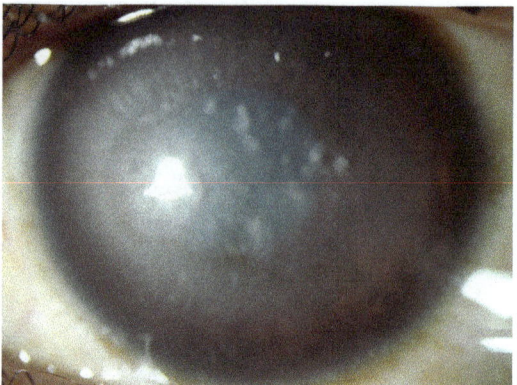

Fig. 4: Pleomorphic opacities with hazy intervening area between the opacities giving a ground-glass appearance in a case of macular dystrophy.

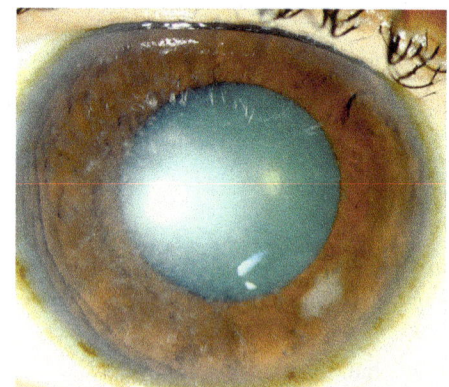

Fig. 5: Multiple anterior stromal white dots and small filamentary lines in a case of lattice dystrophy.

intervening cornea develops a diffuse, ground-glass appearance. The corneal sensation is variably affected.

Granular Corneal Dystrophy Type 2

The three characteristic clinical signs of Avellino corneal dystrophy must be noted:
1. Anterior, stromal, discrete gray–white granular deposits
2. Mid to posterior stromal lattice lesions
3. Anterior stromal haze

Lattice lesions develop after the granular deposits appear. With increasing age, the granular lesions become larger and more prominent and often coalesce to form linear opacities, especially in the inferior cornea. The lattice lesions also become more prominent with age (**Fig. 4**). Initially, they are found in the mid and deep stroma and later involve the entire stroma. The stromal haze is seen only in patients with advanced granular and lattice opacities and becomes more prominent with age.

MCD

In the early stages of the disease, a ground-glass-like haze in the central and superficial stroma is seen. The epithelium is usually spared. With progression, small, multiple, gray–white, pleomorphic opacities with irregular borders are seen (**Fig. 5**). The opacities are more superficial and prominent in the central cornea and are deeper and more discrete in the periphery. The intervening area between the opacities is hazy and gives a ground-glass appearance. In later stages, the stroma is diffusely involved, DM takes on a gray appearance and careful slit-lamp examination may show deposits over DM. When the opacities grow anteriorly, the corneal surface becomes irregular and can lead to RCE, glare, and photophobia. There can be associated guttae. This opacification usually involves the entire thickness of the cornea by the second decade of life. The corneal thickness is reduced.

LCD1

In the early stages of the disease discrete ovoid or round subepithelial opacities, anterior stromal white dots, and small refractile filamentary lines may appear (**Fig. 6**). With progression of the disease the lesions can appear as small nodules, dots, and threadlike spicules, or thicker, radially-oriented branching lines. The lines can extend into deep stroma and may opacify. The lattice lines are typically refractile with a double contour and a clear core on retroillumination (**Fig. 7**). The filaments are opaque with irregular margins. They are radially oriented with dichotomous branching near their central terminations. The lines overlap one another, creating a latticework pattern. The stroma between the lines and dots is clear initially. In extreme cases, vascularization may be present. Central corneal sensitivity also can be decreased. In more advanced stages, the lattice depositions may also exhibit *autofluorescence* with slit-lamp

Cornea and Conjunctiva

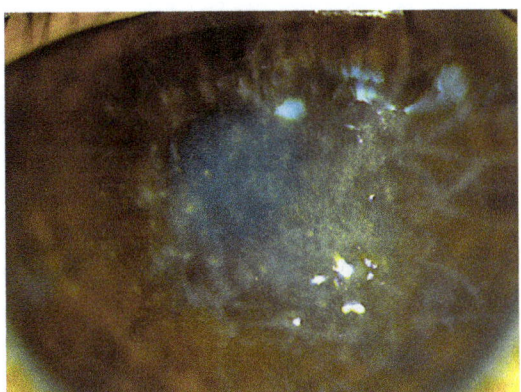

Fig. 6: Lattice lesions along with granular deposits in a case of Avellino corneal dystrophy.

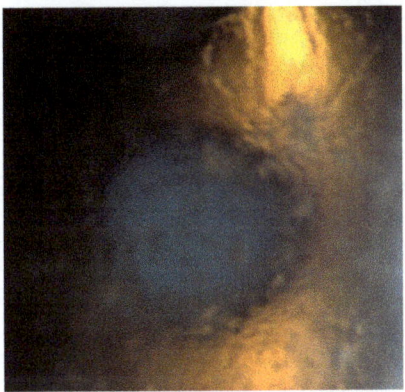

Fig. 7: Lattice lines are typically refractile with a double contour and a clear core on retroillumination.

illumination using the cobalt-blue filter. In LCD2 the fine lattice lines extend to the limbus. In LCD3 the lattice lines appear thick and ropy and without any RCE. Lattice dystrophy type IIIA has been described with similar corneal changes but with recurrent erosions. A late-onset lattice dystrophy, type IV, with deep stromal opacities has also been described.
- *DM/endothelium:*
    - Unaffected in GCD and LCD.
    - In the advanced stage of MCD DM gets opacified and endothelial guttate changes occur.
- *Corneal sensations:* Corneal sensations are *reduced* in LCD and MCD and in advanced cases of GCD

- *Corneal vascularization:* It can occur in advanced cases of LCD.
- *Corneal thickness:* It is normal in GCD and LCD. Reduction of corneal thickness occurs in MCD.

The rest of the anterior segment is usually normal.

Tonometry

Increased IOP can be seen in the case of LCD2 which may be associated with POAG.

Posterior Segment

Usually, normal. In case of media haze due to corneal opacity, USG is done to evaluate the posterior segment.

Examination of Fellow Eye is Important

Dystrophy is a bilateral disease.

■ INVESTIGATIONS

- *Axial length (AL), keratometry (Km):* All these cases may undergo keratoplasty and cataract extraction with intraocular lens implantation may be required at a later date. Thus, AL and Km must be done in all these cases.
- *CCT:* It is reduced in cases of MCD.
- *Anterior segment optical coherence tomography (ASOCT):* The depth of the lesions can be determined by ASOCT. This is extremely important for planning of surgery. ASOCT can also provide details about the anterior segment structure and corneal thickness.
- *Specular microscopy:* It is done to evaluate corneal endothelium in cases of MCD. A healthy endothelium is necessary for any lamellar keratoplasty. Involvement of endothelium requires a full-thickness graft.
- *Confocal microscopy:*
    - *GCD1:* Hyper-reflective opacities.
    - *GCD2:* Findings are a combination of GCD1 and LCD. Reflective, breadcrumb-like round deposits with well-delineated borders or highly reflective, irregular trapezoidal deposits are present in the anterior stroma (similar to GCD1). Linear and branching deposits with changing reflectivity are observed (similar to LCD).

- *MCD:* Blurred limited accumulations of light-reflective material are located in the anterior part of the corneal stroma.
- *LCD1:* Linear and branching structures in the stroma with changing reflectivity and poorly demarcated margins. Lines must be differentiated from other similar images.
- *LCD2:* Prominent deposits, presumably amyloid, are seen contiguous to basal epithelial cells and stromal nerves. In severely affected corneas, sub-basal, and stromal nerves are reduced or absent. Anterior stroma shows fibrosis and abnormal extracellular matrix. Thick anterior and midstromal filaments corresponding to lattice lines and thin undulating structures are visible.

- *Corneal biopsy:* When a corneal transplant is performed, the specimen is submitted for histopathology evaluation. Corneal biopsy is the gold standard for confirming the diagnosis. Various histochemical stains are specific for stromal dystrophies such as:
  - *LCD:* Congo red-pink to orange staining. DICHROISM-alternating red and green color when viewed in green light through a polarized filter. Birefringence-yellow green color against black background viewed through two rotating filters.
  - *MCD:* Stained with PAS, colloidal iron, and Alcian blue. Colloidal iron stain shows an abnormal aggregation of *glycosaminoglycan* at subepithelial Bowman's and endothelial layer.
  - *GCD: Amorphous hyaline* deposits stains with Masson trichrome as bright red deposits. Congo red may show some foci of amyloid in GCD2.
- *Genetic analysis:* It is not required routinely (kindly see the Viva section for details).
- Polymorphic amyloid degeneration (LCD2).

DIFFERENTIAL DIAGNOSIS

The differentiating features are summarized in **Table 1**.

CLASSIFICATION OF CORNEAL DYSTROPHY

The corneal dystrophies are classified further:[2-5]

IC3D Classification (C = Category)(Weiss et al. Cornea. 2015)[5]

- *Epithelial and subepithelial dystrophies:*
  - Epithelial basement membrane dystrophy (EBMD) is majority degenerative, and rarely category 1 (C1)
  - Epithelial recurrent erosion dystrophies (EREDs):
    * Franceschetti corneal dystrophy (FRCD) C3
    * Dystrophia Smolandiensis (DS) C3
    * Dystrophia Helsinglandica (DH) C3
  - Subepithelial mucinous corneal dystrophy (SMCD) C4
  - Meesmann corneal dystrophy (MECD) C1
  - Lisch epithelial corneal dystrophy (LECD) C2
  - Gelatinous drop-like corneal dystrophy (GDLD) C1
- Epithelial-stromal TGFBI dystrophies:
  - Reis–Bücklers corneal dystrophy (RBCD) C1
  - Thielz–Behnke corneal dystrophy (TBCD) C1
  - LCD1 C1—variants (III, IIIA, I/IIIA, and IV) of LCD C1 **(Table 2)**
  - GCD1 C1
  - GCD2 C1
- *Stromal dystrophies*:
  - MCD C1
  - SCD C1
  - Congenital stromal corneal dystrophy (CSCD) C1
  - Fleck corneal dystrophy (FCD) C1
  - Posterior amorphous corneal dystrophy (PACD) C1
  - Central cloudy dystrophy of François (CCDF) C4
  - Pre-Descemet corneal dystrophy (PDCD) C1 or C4
- *Endothelial dystrophies:*
  - Fuchs endothelial corneal dystrophy (FECD) C1, C2, or C3
  - Posterior polymorphous corneal dystrophy (PPCD) C1 or C2
  - Congenital hereditary endothelial dystrophy (CHED) C1
  - X-linked endothelial corneal dystrophy (XECD) C2

Table 1: Differential diagnosis of corneal stromal dystrophy.

Features	Granular dystrophy	Macular dystrophy	Lattice dystrophy
Age of onset of lesions	First decade	First decade	First decade
Age at presentation (years)	30–40	3–9	10–20
Common presentation	Loss of vision in advanced cases (40–50 years)	MC loss of vision (10–30 years) and erosion	MC recurrent erosion (10–20 years) and loss of vision (20–30 years)
Heredity	Autosomal dominant	Autosomal recessive	Autosomal dominant
Opacity	Breadcrumbs or snowflakes or popcorn opacities with a sharp border	Small, multiple, gray–white, pleomorphic opacities with irregular borders	• Lattice lines-refractile with a double contour and a clear core on retroillumination • Refractile tiny lines and dots, and subepithelial spots in early stages
Intervening stroma	Clear	Hazy	Hazy
Deeper extension	DM, endothelium free	DM and endothelium involved	DM and endothelium-free
Extension to limbus	Usually, absent	Present	Usually, absent
Corneal sensation	Reduced in late stages	Reduced early	Reduced early
Corneal thickness	Normal	Thinned	Normal
Characteristic histochemical stains	Masson trichrome	Periodic acid–Schiff, colloidal iron, Alcian blue, and metachromatic dyes	Periodic acid–Schiff, Congo red, thioflavin T (fluorescence), crystal violet (metachromasia), positive birefringence, and dichroism
Material accumulated	Hyaline	Glycosaminoglycans	Amyloid

(DM: Descemet's membrane; MC: most common)

Removed Dystrophies

Grayson–Wilbrandt corneal dystrophy (GWCD) C4.

Evidential Categories for IC3D Classification

- *Category 1 (C1):* A well-defined corneal dystrophy in which the gene has been mapped and identified and specific mutations are known.
- *Category 2 (C2):* A well-defined corneal dystrophy that has been mapped to one or more specific chromosomal loci, but the gene(s) remains to be identified.
- *Category 3 (C3):* A clinically well-defined corneal dystrophy in which the disorder has not yet been mapped to a chromosomal locus.
- *Category 4 (C4):* This category is reserved for a suspected new or previously documented corneal dystrophy, where the evidence for it being a distinct entity is not yet convincing.

TREATMENT

Medical Management

Medical management consists of the following:
- *Photophobia:* Tinted cosmetic lenses for photophobia.

Table 2: Differentiating features between LCD1, LCD2, and LCD3.

Features	Type I	Type II (Meretoja)	Type III
Inheritance	AD	AD	AR
Age of onset	<10 years	20–35 years	>40 years
Visual acuity	Poor after the age of 40 years	Good until the age of 65 years	Impaired after the age of 60 years
Recurrent erosions	Frequent	Infrequent	None
Cornea	• Numerous delicate lines • Many amorphous deposits • Periphery clear	• Few thick lines • Few amorphous deposits • Extend to the periphery	Thick lines
Systemic involvement	None	Systemic amyloidosis (skin, arteries, and other organs)	None
Face	Normal	Facial paresis and blepharochalasis after the age of 40 years	Normal

(AD: autosomal dominant; AR: autosomal recessive; LCD: lattice corneal dystrophy)

- *Recurrent corneal erosion:* Patching, hypertonic agents, artificial tears, or a therapeutic contact lens.

Surgical Management

It depends on the depth of the opacities **(Table 3)** and is described further.

Superficial Opacities

For superficial opacity following options are available:
- Epithelial scraping
- Superficial keratectomy
- Lamellar keratoplasty
- PTK with the argon-fluoride excimer laser

Deep Stromal Lesions and Significant Visual Loss

DALK or penetrating keratoplasty. The comparison between the two techniques has been described in **Table 3**.

Macular Corneal Dystrophy

- Keratoplasty is required earlier in MCD.
- DALK carries a higher risk of failure due to endothelial involvement (often there is subclinical involvement of endothelium without any clinical evidence). Hence, few surgeons prefer PKP to DALK.
- The recurrence is less common and appears 1.5–11 years after the surgery. The earliest site of recurrence is the graft host junction.

Granular Corneal Dystrophy

- *PTK:* Used for superficial lesions and recurrence
- Endothelium is usually uninvolved hence; DALK is preferred over PKP in deeper involvement. The success rate for PKP is around 85% at 1 year.
- The recurrence rate is higher than MCD and can recur between 1 and 19 years.

Lattice Corneal Dystrophy

- Endothelium is usually uninvolved hence; DALK is preferred over PKP in deeper involvement.
- Recurrence is very common and usually occurs 2–14 years after surgery.

VIVA QUESTIONS

Q.1. Differentiate between LCD1, LCD2, and LCD3.
Ans. *See* **Table 2**.

Q.2. Describe different types of histochemical stains.
Ans. *See* the investigation section.

Table 3: Comparison of deep anterior lamellar keratoplasty (DALK) and penetrating keratoplasty (PKP).

Parameter	DALK	PKP
Indication	Stromal opacification with healthy endothelium	Both endothelial failure and stromal opacification
Visual rehabilitation	Early	Delayed
Quality of vision	Poor than PKP	Best
Interface haze	Affects vision	None
Higher order aberrations	More	Less
Postoperative astigmatism	Less	More
Wound strength	Better	Poor
Open sky procedure	None	Risk of expulsive hemorrhage
Intraocular surgery	None	Complications can occur
Globe strength	Better	Poor
Steroid use	Early taper	Prolonged
Donor criteria	Not stringent even nonoptical grades can be used	Only optical grade
Single donor multiple-use	Possible	Not possible
Graft rejection	Low-risk	High-risk
Technique	Difficult	Easy
Learning curve	Steep	Less steep

Q.3. Differentiate between GCD, MCD, and LCD.

Ans. *See* **Table 1**.

Q.4. Differentiate between dystrophy and degeneration.

Ans. The difference between dystrophy and degeneration is enumerated in **Table 4**.

Q.5. What is the *BIGH3* gene?

Ans. Keratoepithelin (transforming growth factor, beta-induced, and 68kDa) is a protein that in humans is encoded by the *TGFBI* gene (initially called *BIGH3* and *BIG-H3*), locus 5q31. Keratoepithelin is produced in superficial epithelial cells, and it has a role in modulating cell adhesion. Mutation of this gene causes accumulation of this product in abnormal deposits. This is associated with several corneal dystrophies; such as *GCD1*, *Lattice dystrophy*, *Avellino*, and *Reis–Bucklers* (remember the mnemonic GLARe).

Q.6. Classify MCD.

Ans. MCD is classified into three phenotypic variants based on the reactivity of the serum and corneal tissue to an antibody that recognizes sulfated epitopes on antigenic keratan sulfate (AgKS).

- Type I has no detectable antigenic keratan sulfate
- Type IA the serum lacks detectable antigenic keratan sulfate, but the keratocytes react with antibodies to keratan sulfate.
- *Type II*: All the abnormal accumulations react positively with AgKS and the serum has normal or lower levels of AgKS.
- Clinically they are indistinguishable from each other.

Table 4: Difference between dystrophy and degeneration.

Dystrophy	Degeneration
A condition where cells have some inborn defects due to which pathological changes may occur during the passage of time	A condition where normal cells of tissue undergo some pathological changes under the influence of some abnormal circumstances
Family history positive	Family history absent
Hereditary (except Cogan's)	No inheritance patterns
Usually bilateral and symmetrical	Usually unilateral; if bilateral asymmetrical
Onset—early life and slowly progressive	Onset—middle life or later and progressive
Located centrally	Located peripherally or at least eccentrically
To begin with, affects a particular layer of the cornea	Usually not restricted to a single layer
No vascularization (except LCD)	May be accompanied by vascularization
No role of environmental factors	Environmental factors have a role in pathogenesis
Usually not associated with any ocular disease	May be secondary to some ocular disease
Not associated with systemic disease	May be associated with systemic disease
Examples—Meesmann dystrophy, lattice dystrophy, and Fuchs' dystrophy	Examples—BSK, SND, and spheroidal degeneration

(BSK: band-shaped keratopathy; LCD: lattice corneal dystrophy; SND: Salzmann nodular degeneration)

Q.7. What are the associated ocular and systemic findings with LCD2?

Ans. *Ocular:*
- Corneal hypothesia
- Dermatochalasis (due to amyloid deposition and secondary muscular dysfunction)
- Lagophthalmos
- POAG

Systemic:
- Dry, itchy skin
- Laxity of the facial skin
- Intermittent proteinuria (nephrotic syndromes)
- Cardiac conduction abnormalities, orthostatic hypotension, and perspiration dysfunctions
- Severe mask-like facial paresis with gradual onset of facial drooping, protruding lips, and pendulous ears (due to amyloid deposition and secondary muscular dysfunction).

Q.8. What are the advantages of the lamellar keratoplasty over full-thickness penetrating keratoplasty?

Ans. *See* **Table 3**.

Q.9. Discuss the different techniques of DALK.

Ans. The goal of DALK is to achieve a depth of dissection as close as possible to DM. Various agents have been used to create a plane of separation between DM and the deep stromal layers. These include air, fluid, viscoelastic, microkeratome, and FSL. The common techniques of DALK are described here:[6]

- *Layer-by-layer manual dissection:* In this technique, after an initial partial trephination of variable depth ranging from 50 to 70% of corneal thickness, the stroma is removed using either a crescent knife or various types of lamellar dissectors. This is followed by layer-by-layer stromal removal, which is repeated multiple times to reach

DM as close as possible. The major limitations of this technique are poor visual outcomes due to residual stroma and interface haze. In addition, it is a very time-consuming process.
- *Air-assisted DALK:* Air-assisted lamellar keratoplasty involves the injection of air into the corneal stroma that helps to achieve dissection as close as possible to DM. *Archila* first described the technique of air-assisted deep lamellar keratoplasty. Over a period of time, many modifications of air-assisted DALK were tried. The big-bubble technique was by *Anwar and Teichmann* and it is the most widely used technique of DALK.
- *Big bubble DALK:* The basic step of this technique involves injecting air into the corneal stroma deep into a groove, which is created by trephining 60–80% of the stromal thickness. The air infiltrates the potential space between the deep stromal layer and DM. The air anterior to DM creates a dome-shaped detachment of DM, which is then identified by a ring visible with the microscope. Once a plane of separation is achieved, the stromal tissue can be easily excised. The main advantage of this technique is that the quality of vision achieved is as good as PK. However, the learning curve associated with this technique is very steep. Often its repeatability is uncertain even with the most experienced surgeons. Inadvertent DM perforation can occur at any stage of the surgery.
- *Viscoelastic-assisted DALK:* Melles et al. described a technique that uses a viscoelastic injection rather than air to achieve a cleavage plane between DM from stroma. The depth of stromal dissection is guided by the "air to endothelium" interface which is seen by a specular light reflex localized at the tip of the blade. Once the plane is achieved, the superficial stroma is removed using trephine and lamellar dissection.
- *Hydrodelamination:* This technique was described by Sujita et al. In this technique, saline solution is injected into the cornea, which enhances the identification and removal of the deep stromal fibers. An initial partial thickness corneal trephination is done up to approximately two-thirds of the thickness using vacuum trephines. However, it is difficult to achieve an actual cleavage plane over DM by hydrodelamination.
- *Femtosecond-assisted DALK:* The FSL computer-guided cuts allow precise, accurate, and reproducible placement of incisions at desired depths in the corneal stroma. Hence, it can be used to create the initial cut at the desired depth to inject air for the successful formation of big bubbles. In addition, it can be used to create corneal incisions with customized graft edges and lamellar planes for both donor and recipient corneas. Thus, FSL can be utilized for creating customized graft host interfaces, such as mushroom and zigzag-shaped DALK. The greatest advantages are its accuracy of forming the bubble at the desired corneal depth and its positive refractive outcomes due to the successful alignment of the donor and recipient zigzag or mushroom configurations. However, the major limitations are the cost and availability.
- *Diamond-knife assisted DALK:* Vajpayee et al. have described a new technique of DALK that is easy to perform, provides visual outcomes comparable to those of big-bubble DALK, and can be performed in cases of extreme corneal thinning or corneal scars. The essential steps of this technique involve the use of a diamond knife set at a depth of 30 µ less than the pachymetry reading, to make a 2.0 mm incision at the 11–12 o'clock position. This incision is then extended circumferentially and centripetally to take out the anterior stromal lamella, leaving a thin stromal bed. The authors found comparable outcomes to the big bubble DALK.

Q.10. What are the genetics of the stromal dystrophies?

Ans.
- *Granular dystrophy-AD* TGFBI (5q31) corneal dystrophy.
- *Macular dystrophy (MCD):* Autosomal recessive, chromosome 16 (16q22.1), a mutation in a new carbohydrate sulfotransferase gene (*CHST6*) has been identified as the cause of macular dystrophy.
- *Lattice dystrophy:* TGFBI gene-related dystrophy with two different types, both representing C1.

Lattice corneal dystrophy type II (LCD2) is not a true corneal dystrophy. It is part of the systemic *disorder familial amyloid polyneuropathy type IV (Finnish type), also known as Meretoja's syndrome.* Nearly all cases are bilateral, progressive, and usually inherited as an autosomal dominant trait and it is due to a single amino acid substitution in the plasma protein *gelsolin*, the consequence of a single nucleotide guanine to adenine change on chromosome 9q 32–34. *Lattice corneal dystrophy type III (LCD3)* is an autosomal recessive disorder. The gene has not yet been mapped. *LCD3A*—has an autosomal dominant pattern, and the clinical findings are due to a mutation at 5q31(Pro501Thr, Ala622His, and His626Ala). The lattice corneal dystrophy type IV (LCD4) is associated with a Leu527Arg mutation in the βig-H3 and is a dominant form of late-onset, deep lattice dystrophy.[3-5]

Q.11. Discuss the dystrophies associated with keratoconus.

Ans. Keratoconus[7] associated with other corneal dystrophies.

In a study by Cremona et al., 51 patients manifested typical signs and topographic evidence of keratoconus associated with another corneal dystrophy.[7] These dystrophies were as follows:
- Fuchs dystrophy (most common)—52.9%
- Anterior basement membrane dystrophy—25.5%
- Posterior polymorphous dystrophy—13.8%
- Combination of Fuchs dystrophy and anterior basement membrane dystrophy—5.8%
- Granular dystrophy—2%

Few case reports have reported keratoconus in association with macular dystrophy and Avellino dystrophy also.

Q.12. What is the best treatment option for MCD?

Ans. As per the recent consensus, most corneal surgeons believe that in MCD PKP is the preferred procedure since endothelial involvement is almost universal. However, in the Indian setup, patients' age, socioeconomic status, and follow-up compliance must be considered for planning and often DALK is the preferred choice.

REFERENCES

1. Brad Bowling. Kanski's Clinical Ophthalmology: A Systematic Approach, 8th edition. Edinburgh: Elsevier; 2015.
2. De Sousa LB, Mannis MJ. The Stromal Dystrophies. In: Krachmer JH, Mannis MJ, Holland EJ (Eds). Cornea, 2nd edition. Philadelphia: Elsevier Mosby; 2005.
3. Dighiero P, Niel F, Ellies P, D'Hermies F, Savoldelli M, Renard G, et al. Histologic phenotype-genotype correlation of corneal dystrophies associated with eight distinct mutations in the *TGFBI* gene. Ophthalmology. 2001;108(4):818-23.
4. Dighiero P, Drunat S, D'Hermies F, Renard G, Delpech M, Valleix S. A novel variant of granular corneal dystrophy caused by the association of 2 mutations in the TGFBI gene-R124L and DeltaT125-DeltaE126. Arch Ophthalmol. 2000;118(6):814-8.
5. Weiss JS, Møller HU, Aldave AJ, Seitz B, Bredrup C, Kivelä T, et al. IC3D classification of corneal dystrophies--edition 2. Cornea. 2015;34(2):117-59.
6. Maharana PK, Agarwal K, Jhanji V, Vajpayee RB. Deep anterior lamellar keratoplasty for keratoconus: a review. Eye Contact Lens. 2014;40(6):382-9.
7. Cremona FA, Ghosheh FR, Rapuano CJ, Eagle RC Jr, Hammersmith KM, et al. Keratoconus is associated with other corneal dystrophies. Cornea. 2009;28(2):127-35.

FUCHS' ENDOTHELIAL CORNEAL DYSTROPHY

Prafulla Kumar Maharana, Sapna Raghuwanshi, Manasi Tripathi, Ritu Nagpal, Namrata Sharma

■ INTRODUCTION

Fuchs' endothelial corneal dystrophy (FECD) is the most common corneal endothelial dystrophy seen in clinical practice. It is characterized by bilateral, noninflammatory, progressive loss of corneal endothelium that ultimately results in corneal decompensation and loss of vision. In examinations, it is given as a long case. Most of the time it may be a case of corneal decompensation following cataract surgery with evidence of FECD in the other eye or it may be a case of operated corneal graft in one eye for corneal decompensation with evidence of FECD in the other eye.

■ HISTORY

Demography

The FECD is a slowly progressive disease affecting persons between the fifth and seventh decade. The onset of the disease occurs around one decade earlier in Asian countries compared to the Western world. Females are affected more than males (corneal guttae 2.5 times and corneal edema 5.7 times more than males; overall 4:1 ratio).[1]

Chief Complaints

Presenting features may depend upon the stage of the disease. Patients may present with the following complaints:
- *Early stage:* Blurring of vision (initially in the morning gradually improving as the day passes)
- *As the disease progresses:* Mild blurring due to stromal edema, glare, and colored halos around lights (due to corneal edema) can occur.
- *Late stages:* Loss of vision, recurrent attacks of redness, pain due to epithelial edema, and bullae rupture.
- *Advanced stages:* Loss of vision but without any pain or photophobia due to corneal scarring.

History of Present Illness

The natural course of the disease is quite characteristic. The onset is gradual. In the early stages, there is a blurring of vision in the morning that gradually improves as the day passes. As the disease progresses the blurring of vision becomes persistent and symptoms of pain, photophobia, and watering may appear due to epithelial edema. There may be repeated exacerbations of the symptoms associated with episodes of epithelial bullae formation-rupture-healing cycle. In advanced cases a pannus or fibrosis forms that leads to the resolution of symptoms.

Past History

Past medical history must include diseases, such as diabetes mellitus, hypertension, tuberculosis, and bronchial asthma. These diseases may not be related directly to FECD but are important for surgical planning.

Past Surgical History

Quite often a case may present with persistent corneal edema following cataract surgery and a careful examination of the other eye reveals signs of FECD. Thus, a history of any recent intraocular surgery must be noted. In addition, the postoperative BCVA is an important parameter when considering keratoplasty and its visual prognosis.

■ EXAMINATION

General Examination

A thorough general examination must be carried out to look for any systemic condition that may need attention before surgical planning.

Ocular Examination

- *Visual acuity:* It depends on the stage of the disease and severity of corneal edema (*See* Chief Complaint).

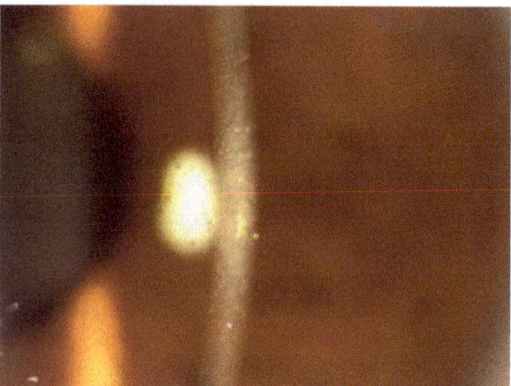

Fig. 1: Central corneal guttae in stage 1 of FECD.

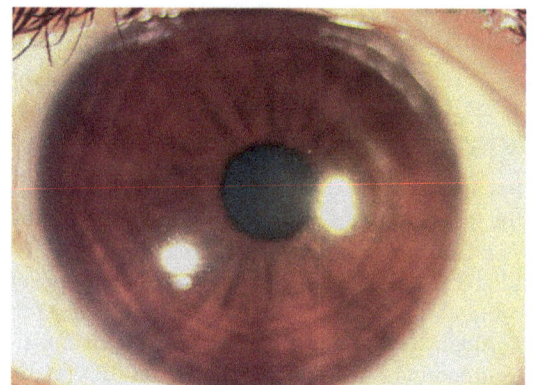

Fig. 2: Progressive stromal edema with ground-glass opacification in FECD stage 2.

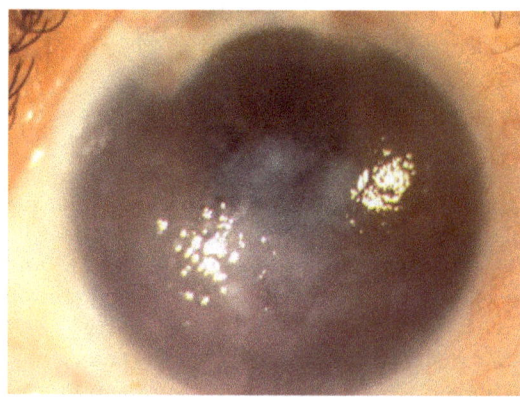

Fig. 3: Bullae formation and progressive stromal edema in stage 3 FECD.

- *Eyeball:* Usually normal.
- *Eyelid:* Usually normal. There may be blepharospasm in the presence of corneal epithelial defect as a consequence of ruptured bullae.
- *Conjunctiva:* Conjunctival congestion and watery discharge can be there in the presence of epithelial defect.
- *Cornea:* The findings in cornea depend upon the stage of the disease.
  – Stage 1 (stage of corneal guttae):
    - *Central corneal guttae:* They appear as tiny dark spots **(Fig. 1)** on the posterior corneal surface on direct illumination. Specular reflection also reveals dark spots and disruption of regular endothelial mosaic. In retroillumination, the guttae appear as dewdrops.
    - As the disease progresses, guttae spread peripherally and coalesce centrally along with pigment dusting on the endothelium. This characteristically gives the appearance of a "beaten metal appearance."
    - As the disease progresses the DM becomes thickened and irregular.
  – Stage 2 (stage of corneal stromal edema):
    - Corneal edema initially appears in the posterior stroma, which is best seen with sclerotic scatter as a fine gray haze.
    - Vertical wrinkles or striae in DM appear due to the swelling of the corneal stroma.
    - Progressive stromal edema results in a ground-glass opacification with marked thickening of the central cornea **(Fig. 2)**.
  – Stage 3 (stage of corneal epithelial edema):
    - Multiple epithelial microcysts that may coalesce to form bullae **(Fig. 3)**.
    - Rupture of bullae leads to epithelial erosions and fingerprint lines following the healing of such lesions.
  – Stage 4 (stage of scarring):
    - Avascular subepithelial fibrous scarring occurs between the epithelium and Bowman's membrane. Scarring leads to the resolution of symptoms but visual acuity further deteriorates due to the irregularity of the corneal surface **(Fig. 4)**.
    - Peripheral superficial corneal neovascularization.

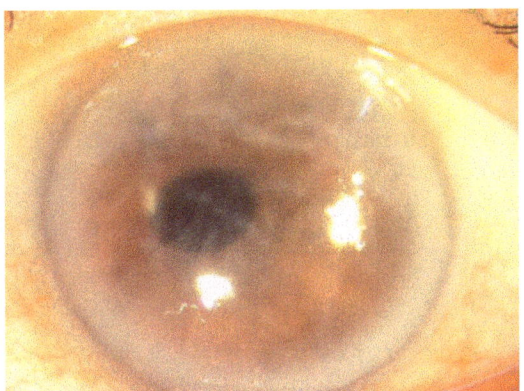

Fig. 4: Stromal scarring in stage 4 FECD.

The anterior chamber/sclera/iris/pupil/fundus are usually within normal limit. Shallow AC with angle closure glaucoma has been reported in a few cases.
- *Lens:* Carefully examine the lens for the presence of a cataract. Detection of a cataract is important for the management of FECD.

■ DIFFERENTIAL DIAGNOSIS

A case of FECD must be differentiated from the following:
- Hassall–Henle bodies
- Central herpetic disciform keratitis-KP present
- Aphakic or pseudophakic bullous keratopathy
- Congenital hereditary endothelial dystrophy (CHED)
- Iridocorneal endothelial syndrome (Chandler's syndrome) (ICE)
- Posterior polymorphous corneal dystrophy (PPCD)

Hassall–Henle Bodies

They are present in 70% of the population over 40 years old. It resembles guttae of FECD but are located only in the peripheral cornea and are not associated with progressive visual loss or corneal edema.

Central Herpetic Disciform Keratitis

Differentiating features are as follows:
- Presence of KPs
- Respond to steroids
- Presence of scarring (herpetic footprints)

Aphakic or Pseudophakic Bullous Keratopathy

The following are the differential features:
- History of cataract surgery often with signs of complicated surgery
- Another eye will be normal

Congenital Hereditary Endothelial Dystrophy/Iridocorneal Endothelial Dystrophy/Posterior Polymorphous Corneal Dystrophy

Differential diagnosis of FECD is enumerated in **Table 1**.

Pseudoguttae

These are associated with trauma, intraocular inflammation, infection, or toxins. Pseudoguttae are transient in nature and disappear with a resolution of an underlying condition. Diagnosis is confirmed on the serial examination.

■ INVESTIGATION

- *Specular microscopy:* Specular microscopy can reveal the following changes
  – Qualitative parameters—pleomorphism (variation in shape, indicates disruption in the regular hexagonal pattern of the endothelium) and polymegathism (variation in size, indicates injury to endothelium)
  – Quantitative parameters:
    ♦ Reduced endothelial cell density in mm^2
    ♦ Increased coefficient of variation (CV)—CV represents the degree of variation in the sizes of the endothelial cells (polymegethism), CV values between 0.22 and 0.31 are considered normal. CV values from 0.32 to 0.40 are elevated, and CV values above 0.40 are abnormal
    ♦ Percentage of hexagonal cells (HEXs)—in a normal endothelium, >60% of the endothelial cells are hexagonal. In FECD it is <60%

Table 1: Differential diagnosis of FECD.

Parameters	FECD	PPMD	CHED	ICE
Age of onset	40–50s	Teens to 20s	Birth to 10 years	Young adult
Laterality	Bilateral	Bilateral	Bilateral	Unilateral
Sex predilection	F > M	F = M	F = M	F > M
Heredity	AD	AD	AD	No
Basic defect	Attenuation and reduced number of endothelial cells	Epithelialization of endothelium	Mutation of solute carrier family 4 and sodium borate transporter member 11–SLC4A11	Abnormal proliferation of endothelium
Corneal findings	Guttae, stromal thickening, epithelial edema, and subepithelial fibrosis	Vesicles, bands, diffuse opacities, and plaques at Descemet's membrane	Marked corneal thickening, opacification, and endothelium are rarely visible	Fine, guttae-like changes, and "hammered silver"
Other ocular abnormalities	Increased intraocular pressure and narrow angles	Iris atrophy/corectopia, broad-peripheral synechiae, and glaucoma 25%	Usually none	Iris atrophy, iris nodules, and glaucoma in 80–100%
Progression	Progressive	Minimal	Progressive	Relentless
Specular microscopy	• Polymorphism • Polymegathism • Decreased endothelial cell count	Focal change and endothelial cells usually enlarged but count is usually normal	Not possible	Diffuse changes, ICE cell

(CHED: congenital hereditary endothelial dystrophy; FECD: Fuchs' endothelial corneal dystrophy; ICE: iridocorneal endothelial dystrophy; PPCD: posterior polymorphous corneal dystrophy)

- *Corneal pachymetry:* Measurement of CCT is important for diagnosis (in doubtful and early cases) and planning of treatment.
- *Confocal microscopy:* In the presence of corneal edema, confocal microscopy is the best technique for the evaluation of corneal endothelium.
- *ASOCT:* It can provide the details of the anterior chamber in the presence of an edematous cornea. In addition, corneal thickness and level of scarring can also be detected.
- *Ultrasonography (USG):* USG is done to rule out any posterior segment pathology before proceeding with keratoplasty.

■ MANAGEMENT

The management of FECD is given further.[2,3]

Medical Management

- *Corneal edema:*
  - *Topical hypertonic saline solutions and ointments:* They artificially raise the osmolality of the tear film and dehydrate the cornea by drawing fluid from the epithelium and anterior stroma.
  - Dehydration of the cornea by a blow dryer in the morning or throughout the day can decrease the symptoms in the early stages.
  - Cycloplegics and nonsteroidal anti-inflammatory agents are useful in diminishing corneal pain from bullous keratopathy.
  - *Reduction of IOP:* Use of IOP-lowering medications may reduce corneal edema in patients with elevated or even normal IOP.

- *Recurrent erosion:*
  - *BCL:* The use of therapeutic contact lenses helps in relieving the pain from recurrent epithelial erosions while decreasing irregular astigmatism in cases that have progressed to bullous keratopathy.
  - Anterior stromal puncture/AMG/ phototherapeutic keratectomy/anterior stromal puncture/conjunctival flaps have been described for symptomatic relief of bullous keratopathy when the visual prognosis is poor. However, these procedures are rarely required in FECD, where the visual potential is often good.

Surgical Management

The different surgical options in the case of FECD are described further.

Endothelial Keratoplasty

Currently the treatment of choice. The different techniques of endothelial keratoplasty are as follows:
- *Descemet's stripping endothelial keratoplasty (DSEK):* The donor tissue (consisting of DM-endothelium complex and some stroma) is prepared using a manual technique.
- *Descemet's stripping automated endothelial keratoplasty (DSAEK):* Similar to DSEK except the donor tissue is prepared using a microkeratome.
- *DM endothelial keratoplasty (DMEK):* Donor tissue consists of only DM-endothelium complex and no stroma. Technically difficult than DSAEK but visual results are better than DSAEK.

Penetrating Keratoplasty

A full-thickness graft is indicated in the presence of a corneal scar, or the surgeon lacks the expertise.

FECD with cataract: Senile cataract is commonly seen in cases of FECD due to the common age group affected. It is often a dilemma to decide if only cataract surgery is enough or if the patient needs a triple procedure. Although there are no universal guidelines, most corneal surgeons follow the following approach:
- *Only cataract with IOL:*
  - Specular count >1,000 cells/mm^2
  - CCT < 600 µm
  - Good corneal clarity to allow cataract surgery
- *Triple procedure:*
  - Specular count <800 cells/mm^2
  - CCT >640 µm
  - Corneal clarity is not enough to allow cataract surgery
- *Staged EK before cataract surgery:*
  - Age <50 years with visually significant FECD and a clear presbyopic lens with a deep anterior chamber
  - Advantage—the ability to optimize keratometry and improve the accuracy of IOL power selection

In cases where the values of CCT and endothelial counts are in between, the decision is individualized and based on the surgeon's experience.

Choice of IOL: Monofocal, hydrophobic, and aspheric preferably with a larger optic diameter. If endothelial decompensation is anticipated, keep target refraction at –0.75 to –1.25 D. If planning for DSAEK/DSEK and around –0.5 if one is planning for DMEK. This is to compensate for the hyperopic shift that follows endothelial keratoplasty.

Descemetorhexis

Descemetorhexis without endothelial keratoplasty (DWEK) or Descemet's stripping only (DSO) DWEK or DSO is a procedure where the central afflicted 4–5 mm of the central DM is excised without any graft. The rationale is the healthy peripheral endothelial cells will migrate centrally and restore the pump function. Thus, it is useful only in early cases and when patients have central corneal guttae with relatively unaffected peripheral endothelium. The procedure can be combined with the simultaneous use of Rho kinase (ROCK) inhibitor inhibitors (ripasudil and netarsudil) that promote endothelial migration and survival.[4,5]

However, the results are unpredictable and need specialized instruments; visual rehabilitation requires a prolonged time and if done inappropriately can lead to scarring.

VIVA QUESTIONS

Q.1. Discuss the association of FECD.
Ans. FECD has been associated with the following:
- Axial hypermetropia, shallow anterior chamber, and angle closure glaucoma
  - Keratoconus
  - Increased prevalence of age-related macular degeneration (controversial)
  - Increased rate of cardiovascular disease (controversial)

Q.2. What are the causes of corneal guttae?
Ans. Corneal guttae may be seen in the following cases:
- *Interstitial keratitis:* Focal gutta formation without corneal edema
- Macular dystrophy
- Posterior polymorphous dystrophy
- Pseudoguttae (appears as gutta but these are transient, due to edema of the endothelial cells, and disappear with a resolution of the underlying condition)
  - Trauma, intraocular inflammation, infection, toxins, and thermo-keratoplasty

Q.3. What is the difference between early and late-onset FECD?
Ans. *See* **Table 2**.

Q.4. What is normal endothelial cell count and discuss the rate of endothelial loss.
Ans. The normal endothelial cell count as per age is as follows:
- At birth: 4000–5000
- 10–19 years: 2,900–3,500 cells/mm^2
- 20–29 years: 2,600–3,400 cells/mm^2
- 30–39 years: 2,400–3,200 cells/mm^2
- 40–49 years: 2,300–3,100 cells/mm^2
- 50–59 years: 2,100–2,900 cells/mm^2
- 60–69 years: 2,000–2,800 cells/mm^2
- 70–79 years: 1,800–2,600 cells/mm^2
- 80–89 years: 1,500–2,300 cells/mm^2

The normal rate of endothelial loss is approximately 0.6%/year.

Q.5. Discuss the comparison between DSAEK and PKP.
Ans. The comparison between DSAEK and PKP is enumerated in **Table 3**.

Table 2: Early and late-onset FECD.

	Early FECD	*Late FECD*
ICD category	Category 1	Category 2/3
Genetics	Mutation in the gene for the alpha 2 chain of collagen VIII (COL8A2-Q455K) on chromosome 1 p34.3-p32	AD, many with no inheritance pattern 13pTel-13q12.13/18q21.2-q21.32/ possible SLC4A11
Onset	First decade	Fourth to fifth
Retroillumination	Fine, patchy distribution of corneal guttae	Coarse and distinct corneal guttae
Specular microscopy	Small, shallow guttae	Larger guttae
DM	Considerably thicker than late	—
Sex distribution	F = M	F > M

(AD: autosomal dominant; DM: Descemet's membrane; F: female; FECD: Fuchs' endothelial corneal dystrophy; M: male)

Table 3: Comparison between DSAEK and PKP.

Parameter	DSAEK	PKP
Indication	High astigmatism, and significant corneal haze, are relative contraindications	This can be done in all cases
Visual rehabilitation	Early	Delayed
Quality of vision	Poor than PKP	Best
Interface haze	Affects vision	None
Suture-related problems	Absent	Present
Higher order aberrations	More	Less
Postoperative astigmatism	None	Yes
Wound strength	Better	Poor
Open sky procedure	None	Risk of expulsive hemorrhage
Globe strength	Better	Poor
Steroid use	Early taper	Prolonged
Donor criteria	Stringent	Only optical grade
Single donor multiple-use	Possible	Not possible
Graft rejection	Low-risk	High-risk
Technique	Difficult	Easy
Learning curve	Steep	Less steep

Q.6. What is the comparison between DSAEK and DMEK?
Ans: *See* **Table 4**.

Table 4: Comparison between DSAEK and DMEK.

Parameters	DSEK/DSAEK	DMEK
Indication	Can be performed in difficult cases, such as iris defect, corneal haze, and aphakia	Difficult in cases, such as iris defect, corneal haze, and aphakia
Donor selection	Young donor age is not a barrier but an advantage, due to a greater number of endothelial cells	Older (>50 years) donors are preferred (as the DM is relatively firmly attached to the Dua's layer in young corneas)
Learning curve	Easy	Difficult
Need for microkeratome	Yes (DSAEK)	No
Graft size	At least 3 mm less than the recipient cornea diameter (to prevent closure of the AC angle)	8–8.5 mm (larger graft can be taken)
Amount of manipulation required during graft placement	Less	More
Visual outcomes (contrast visual acuity and aberrations)	Poorer (transplant of additional stroma and consequent hyperopic shift)	Better (only DM is grafted, with no hyperopic shift)
Final visual acuity	Around 6/12	6/9–6/6

Contd...

Contd...

Parameters	DSEK/DSAEK	DMEK
Percentage (%) of cases with 20/20 vision	Less	More
Postoperative graft detachment	Lower	Higher
Hyperopic shift	Present	Absent
Endothelial cell loss	Little lower	Higher
Graft detachment	Lower	Higher
Graft rejection	Higher (12–15%)	Lower (<1%)
Primary graft failure	Lower rate of primary graft failure	Higher rates of primary graft failure than DSEK (6–8%)

■ REFERENCES

1. Albert DM, Miller JW, Azar DT. Albert and Jakobiec's Principles and Practice of Ophthalmology; 2008.
2. Bowling B. Kanski's Clinical Ophthalmology: A Systematic Approach, 8th edition. Edinburgh: Elsevier; 2015.
3. Weisenthal RW, Streeten BW. Descemet's Membrane and Endothelial Dystrophies. In: Krachmer JH, Mannis MJ, Holland EJ (Eds). Cornea Volume II: Cornea and External Disease, Clinical Diagnosis and Management. Mo. Mosby: St Louis; 2011.
4. Maharana PK, Sahay P, Singhal D, Garg I, Titiyal JS, Sharma N. Component corneal surgery: An update. Indian J Ophthalmol. 2017;65(8):658-72.
5. Sharma N, Maharana PK, Singhi S, Aron N, Patil M. Descemet stripping automated endothelial keratoplasty. Indian J Ophthalmol. 2017;65(3):198-209.

ACUTE GRAFT REJECTION

Ritu Nagpal, Vaishali Ghanshyam Rai, Prafulla Kumar Maharana

■ INTRODUCTION

Corneal graft rejection can be defined as the development of graft edema in conjunction with inflammatory signs in a graft that has been clear for at least 2 weeks in a primary graft and 1 week in a regraft. It is an immunological response of the host to the donor corneal tissue without regard to the effect of the response on graft survival. Immune rejection of the transplanted cornea is the major cause of graft failure in the intermediate and late postoperative period. It is primarily of three types: (1) Epithelial, (2) stromal, and (3) endothelial rejection. Endothelial rejection is the most common and clinically important type of rejection. Approximately 30% of the eyes with PKP experience at least one episode of graft rejection and about 5-7% lead to eventual graft failure. Around 12% of graft rejection cases in patients with good prognostic keratoplasty and 40% in complicated cases have been reported that lead to subsequent graft failure.[1-3]

■ HISTORY

Demography

Several clinical series have shown that a younger recipient conferred a higher risk of rejection probably due to a robust immune system. Recipients younger than 40 years are at a higher risk for graft rejection.

Chief Complaints

A case of acute graft rejection presents with the following symptoms:
- Redness
- Sensitivity to light

- *V*ision loss
- *P*ain

These characteristic symptoms are present in approximately 70% of the cases while 30% of the cases are asymptomatic and diagnosed during routine follow-up.

History of Present Illness

- The onset is usually acute and progresses if not treated. Graft rejection after PKP usually occurs after an average period of 8 months. Most cases occur within 1 year. If the symptoms are there from day one, it may be a case of primary graft failure.
- It is important to enquire about the best vision gained after the corneal graft. This helps in deciding on a regraft at a later date.

Past History

A careful past history must be taken to rule out the risk factors responsible for graft rejection. The following history is important in a case of graft rejection:
- History of ocular surface diseases and treatment should be asked of the patient, e.g., ocular surface diseases, such as severe dry eye, severe chemical burns, radiation burns, ocular pemphigoid, Stevens–Johnson syndrome, and neuroparalytic disease.
- Past history of herpes simplex keratitis and recurrent episodes should be asked.
- Past history of any ocular surgery, e.g., penetrating keratoplasty, excimer laser phototherapeutic keratectomy (can also trigger a corneal graft rejection episode).
- Past history of glaucoma and antiglaucoma medications are taken.
- History of a previous graft failure, especially if the failure was a result of an allograft rejection. One study demonstrated that the rate of graft failure secondary to allograft rejection increased from 8% in patients with no history of previous transplantation to 40% in patients with two or more previous grafts.
- *Details of the surgery*: Look for the following if the detailed record of the surgery is available
  – Presence of corneal vascularization at the time of surgery—puts the graft at high risk for graft failure
  – Concomitant vitrectomy with PKP—a twofold increased risk of graft failure
  – Concurrent intraocular inflammation
  – Donor endothelial count
  – Presence of anterior synechiae in host.

All these factors are risk factors for graft rejection and subsequent graft failure.

Past Medical History

A case of acute graft rejection needs aggressive steroid therapy. Hence any systemic history that is a contraindication for systemic therapy must be ruled out. A careful history of diabetes mellitus, hypertension, peptic ulcer disease, tuberculosis, osteoporosis, and any neuropsychiatric disorder must be ruled out.

■ EXAMINATION

General/Systemic Examination

Carefully look for any systemic contraindication for steroid therapy.

Ocular Examination

- *Visual acuity:* BCVA must be recorded at the baseline. Monitoring BCVA on a daily basis can indicate the response to pulse steroid therapy.
- *Eyeball/eyelids* look normal. However, lid edema can be there in an acutely inflamed eye. Also look for any findings such as ectropion, entropion, meibomian disease, and trichiasis that may put graft at risk.
- *Conjunctiva:* Circumciliary congestion is characteristically seen in corneal graft rejection. Often, it is the earliest sign of rejection reaction and can occur before the clinical appearance of cellular infiltrates in the cornea or the anterior chamber.
- *Cornea:*
  – Cellular infiltration of the cornea as discrete subepithelial infiltrates reminiscent of those seen in epidemic keratoconjunctivitis. These small (0.2–0.5 mm), hazy infiltrates are usually scattered in the central cornea and occur exclusively in the donor tissue but not the peripheral recipient tissue.
  – An epithelial rejection line, also known as Krachmer's line, in the graft from the host graft junction without edema and KPs/

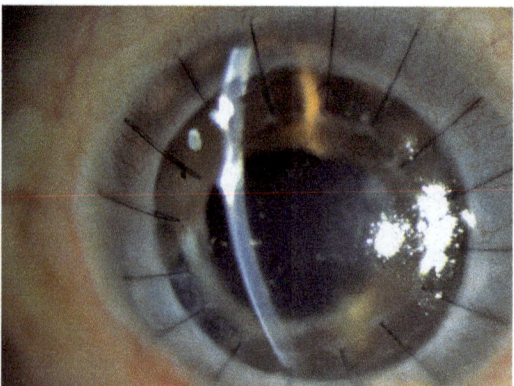

Fig. 1: Khodadoust line on the endothelium in a case of acute graft rejection following penetrating keratoplasty.

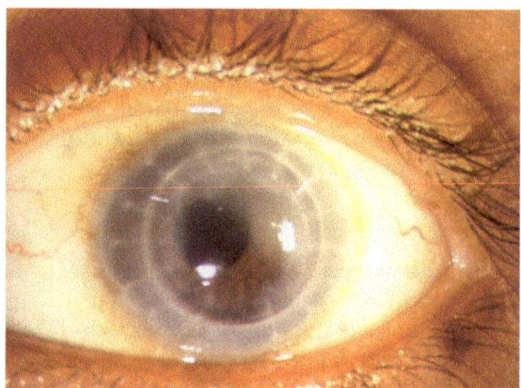

Fig. 2: Differential stromal edema in a case of acute graft rejection.

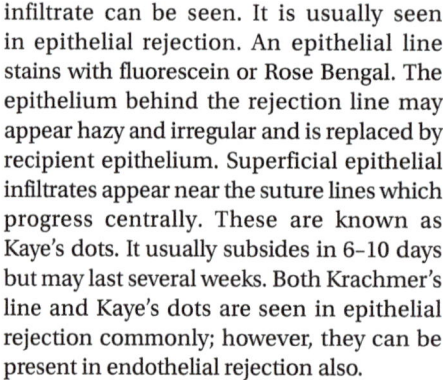

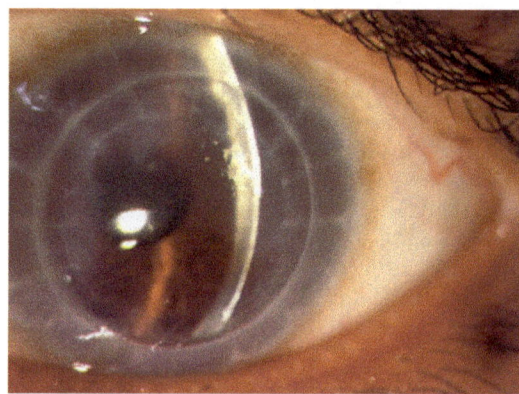

Fig. 3: Acute graft rejection with stromal thickening and edema.

infiltrate can be seen. It is usually seen in epithelial rejection. An epithelial line stains with fluorescein or Rose Bengal. The epithelium behind the rejection line may appear hazy and irregular and is replaced by recipient epithelium. Superficial epithelial infiltrates appear near the suture lines which progress centrally. These are known as Kaye's dots. It usually subsides in 6–10 days but may last several weeks. Both Krachmer's line and Kaye's dots are seen in epithelial rejection commonly; however, they can be present in endothelial rejection also.

- *KPs:* They can appear as scattered deposits or can form a distinct line known as the Khodadoust line **(Fig. 1)**. This line tends to migrate from the peripheral cornea to the central cornea and many times its origin can be traced to a loose suture or donor corneal vessel. The Khodadoust line is the hallmark of graft rejection.
- *Differential edema:* Endothelial rejection is often associated with stromal edema overlying the areas that have been traversed by the endothelial rejection line while the areas ahead of the line are clear **(Figs. 2 and 3)**.
- Deep corneal vascularization should be noted.
- *Staining:* The cornea must be stained to look for the presence of an epithelial defect or recurrence of herpetic keratitis.
- In delayed presentation the entire graft becomes edematous **(Fig. 4)** with significantly increased graft thickness **(Fig. 5)**.
- *Anterior chamber (AC):* AC flares and cells can be noted which indicates elevated levels of protein in the aqueous humor due to leakage from the uveal vasculature.
- *IOP* raised IOP can both be a consequence and cause for corneal graft rejection. In edematous cornea, IOP may be falsely low with Goldmann applanation tonometry. A Mackay-Marg principle-based tonometer (Tonopen) can give more reliable values.

Cornea and Conjunctiva

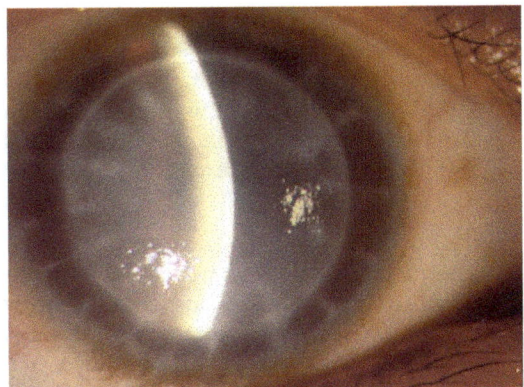

Fig. 4: Failed graft after an episode of acute graft rejection.

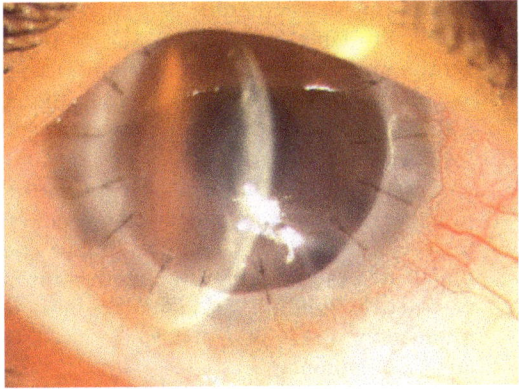

Fig. 5: Decompensated corneal graft with stromal thickening after acute graft rejection.

■ DIFFERENTIAL DIAGNOSIS

A case of acute corneal graft rejection must be differentiated from graft failure, sterile/infectious endophthalmitis, epithelial down growth, and recurrent herpetic keratitis. The differentiating points are summarized in **Table 1**.

■ INVESTIGATIONS

Pachymetry

Increased CCT is often the first indicator of endothelial dysfunction. Central corneal thickness can be measured with the help of an ultrasonic pachymeter, Orbscan, Pentacam, or anterior segment OCT (ASOCT). Serial monitoring of CCT is important for monitoring the response to steroid therapy.

Table 1: Differential diagnosis of acute corneal graft rejection.

Condition	Features
Late graft failure	• Gradual onset of graft edema • Not associated with signs of inflammation such as AC cells/flare or keratic precipitates • No Khodadoust line or differential edema
Sterile/infectious endophthalmitis	• Inflammatory signs are severe • Presence of hypopyon • Presence of infiltrates in vitreous
Epithelial down growth	• Clumps of cells-like material in the anterior chamber • Cells larger than that of cells of inflammation • These cells do not respond to corticosteroid therapy • Presence of white membrane over the anterior surface of the iris • Associated increased intraocular pressure that is unresponsive to medical therapy
Recurrent herpetic keratatis	• KPs are restricted to host cornea only • History of previous herpetic keratitis • Absence of Khodadoust line • Characteristic shape • Response to topical antiviral therapy

Specular Microscopy

It can reveal the reduced endothelial cell count that further reduces each episode of graft rejection.

Confocal Microscopy

In the presence of a severe graft edema, where specular microscopy is not possible, confocal microscopy can reveal endothelial changes.

Ultrasonography

In the presence of a severe corneal edema, USG is helpful in ruling out sterile endophthalmitis.

MANAGEMENT

Most episodes of allograft rejection can be reversed if prompt and aggressive treatment is initiated. The treatment of choice is steroids.

Steroids

Topical Steroids

A case of acute graft rejection can be managed on an outpatient basis but admission to the hospital for the first few days of treatment is helpful in monitoring compliance. Aggressive administration of potent topical corticosteroids with good intraocular penetration (such as prednisolone acetate 1% and prednisolone phosphate 1% eye drop) aborts most attacks of acute graft rejection. The commonly used treatment regime is given as follows:
- 1 hourly—3 days
- Second hourly—15 days
- Four times—2 months
- Three times—2 months
- Two times—3 months
- Once-4 months

The topical steroids are effective in epithelial rejection, stromal rejection, and mild-moderate endothelial rejection.

Systemic Steroids

- Severe episodes of endothelial rejection need systemic steroid therapy.
- Pulse steroid therapy is more effective than oral steroids for the treatment of a rejection episode. A single pulse [500 mg intravenous (IV) methylprednisolone] in a single dose is more effective and better tolerated than daily oral prednisolone. Repeating the dose at 24 or 48 hours after the initial dose does not add any advantage.
- IV dexamethasone (100–200 mg) single dose has been found to be equally efficacious as methylprednisolone and thus may be used as an alternative in patients who are nonaffording.
- In severe cases of rejection, topical prednisolone acetate at 1% hourly, one dose of pulsed IV methylprednisolone (500 mg), and oral prednisone at 1 mg/kg/day for 5 days is recommended.
- The IV steroid therapy beyond 8 days of the onset of symptoms may not add any benefit to intense topical steroid therapy. In a study by Hills et al. when patients were treated within 8 days of the onset of symptoms, the survival rate of grafts was 92% versus 55%.

Supportive Therapy

Antiglaucoma medications have to be given when IOP is raised. Cycloplegics can reduce pain by relieving ciliary spasms. Topical lubricating drops are useful in the presence of sutures and associated epithelial defects.

Immunosuppressive Therapy

Immunosuppressive therapy is not required routinely. Probable indications include high-risk grafts and cases where long-term steroid use is contraindicated or causes complications. Following immunosuppressive therapy has been tried with variable success.
- *Cyclosporine A (CsA):* CsA is a powerful immunosuppressive agent that binds to an intracellular protein called cyclophilin and inactivates calcineurin. The inactivation of calcineurin inhibits IL-2 and lymphokine production, thus limiting the activity of CD4+ and CD8+ lymphocytes.
    - *Topical CsA* is available as 2% in castor oil or 1% in artificial tears four times daily
    - *Systemic:*
        * Recommended dosage is 15 mg/kg/day for 2 days followed by 7.5 mg/kg/day for 2 days then adjusted to maintain trough blood levels of 100–200 mg/L for 6 months after reversal of acute rejection episode
        * Close monitoring of blood pressure, renal function including serum creatinine, and liver function test

    Recently studies suggested topical CsA and oral CsA have not been found to reduce the risk of allograft rejection.
- *Mycophenolate mofetil (MMF):*
    - MMF acts by inhibiting inosine monophosphate dehydrogenase required for the proliferation of T- and B-lymphocytes
    - Dose 750 mg BD

- Renal, hepatic, and bone marrow function must be monitored
- Recent studies suggest that oral MMF is effective in the prevention of allograft rejection in high-risk keratoplasties
- Unlike CsA, therapeutic drug monitoring is not required which significantly reduces the cost of treatment
- *Azathioprine:*
  - 1–2 mg/kg/day orally
  - It reduces the need for systemic corticosteroids; and thus, reduces the systemic complications expected by high-dose corticosteroids.
  - Renal, hepatic, and bone marrow function must be monitored.
- *Tacrolimus (FK-506):*
  - Macrolide immunosuppressant with a mechanism of action similar to CsA, but 10–100 times more potent than the latter. It inhibits calcineurin by binding to immunophilin or FK-506 binding protein (FKBP). Topical (ointment 67 or drops) as well as systemic tacrolimus has shown to be promising as a prophylactic agent against corneal graft rejection.
  - A dose of 0.16 mg/kg/day.
  - Renal function must be monitored.
- *Other agents:* Rapamycin/sirolimus and antilymphocyte monoclonal antibodies have been tried with variable success.

VIVA QUESTIONS

Q.1. What are the risk factors for acute corneal graft rejection?

Ans.
- *Donor factors:*
  - The method and duration of storage of the donor cornea and nature of donor button cutting.
  - Pretreatment of donor tissue with UV radiation may reduce the chances of development of rejection.
- *Host factors:*
  - *Vascularization of the host cornea:* Deep stromal vascularization of the host cornea of two or more quadrants classifies as a high-risk cornea. CCTS has defined vascularization of the host bed in two or more quadrants extending at least 2 mm into the stroma as a risk factor-associated highly with the rejection of the corneal grafts.
  - *Regraft:* A cornea with a previously failed graft due to any cause is considered to be at a high risk.
  - *HSV keratitis:* Active or healed HSV keratitis is considered as a high risk for graft rejection. The increase in risk is due to the vascularization associated with HSV keratitis.
  - Ocular surface diseases such as severe dry eye, severe chemical burns, radiation burns, ocular pemphigoid, Stevens–Johnson syndrome, and neuroparalytic disease are also associated with poor prognosis for corneal graft.
  - Young patients and bilateral grafts have more chances of graft rejection due to an active immune system.
  - *Pediatric patients:* The immune system of children is more active than that of adults and due to rapid wound healing suture becomes loose early, both these factors along with the inability of the child to communicate timely lead to an increased risk of rejection. These eyes are more prone to rejection.
- *Intraoperative factors:*
  - *Large graft:* Graft is nearer to limbal vessels
  - *Eccentric graft:* Proximity to limbal vessels
  - *Small graft:* Less endothelial cells transferred
  - *Iris adhesion at graft host junction:* Immune cells through iris vasculature get exposed to antigens
  - *Recent anterior segment surgery:* Associated inflammation brings more immune cells
  - Anterior vitrectomy
  - Full thickness graft > lamellar graft

- *Postoperative factors:*
  - Corneal epithelial breach
  - *Exposed suture knots, loose suture:* By inciting vascularization
  - Postoperative uveitis
  - Postoperative glaucoma
  - Synechiae between iris and graft host junction.

Q.2. What are the measures you can take to prevent graft rejection?

Ans.
- *Preoperative measures:* Reducing the antigenic load of donor tissue.
  - Use the central corneal graft
  - Removal of the donor epithelium
  - Exposure to UV light
  - Depletion of local macrophages—subconjunctival injection of clodronate liposomes which alters delayed-type hypersensitivity
  - Pretreatment of the graft with hyperbaric oxygen and use of heterologous antibody-treated corneal button.
- *Intraoperative factors:* Meticulous surgical technique, including of avoiding decentration of the recipient bed cut, optimal suturing, and good graft-host apposition
- *Postoperative measures:* Controlling or alleviating the host's immune response to the foreign donor tissue. Steroids are the best option for prophylaxis against graft rejection. Long-term (12–18 months) of topical steroids have a better rejection-free graft survival.

Q.3. What is the relation between corneal vascularity and graft rejection?

Ans.
- Low risk—avascular
- *Medium risk:* Vascularization in one to two quadrants
- *High risk:* Vascularization of three or more quadrants.

Q.4. Write a note on graft rejection following endothelial keratoplasty.

Ans. Graft rejection in EK differs from rejection following PKP in the following ways:
- Lower rates of rejection compared to cases with PKP are probably due to the lower antigenic load.
- The incidence of graft rejection is around 7.5%.
- Rejection episodes are less severe with high rates of reversibility and low rates of graft failure
- One-third of the patients with graft rejection after endothelial keratoplasty are asymptomatic
- Presenting symptoms are minimal, such as mild irritation, photophobia, and rarely mild blurring of vision

Q.5. What are the unusual manifestations of graft rejection?

Ans.
- Rarely acute graft rejection can present with the following (without the characteristic presentation described in the history section).
- Raised IOP due to engorgement and or edema of TM.
- Acute epithelial defect along with ocular inflammation. This type of unusual presentation is usually seen in young patients.

■ **REFERENCES**

1. Hill JC. High risk corneal grafting. Br J Ophthalmol. 2002;86(9):945.
2. Hill JC, Ivey A. Corticosteroids in corneal graft rejection: Double versus single pulse therapy. Cornea. 1994;13(5):383-8.
3. Panda A, Vanathi M, Kumar A, Dash Y, Priya S. Corneal Graft Rejection. Surv Ophthalmol. 2007;52(4):375-96.

SHORT CASES

PTERYGIUM

Aafreen Bari, Ritu Nagpal

■ INTRODUCTION

Pterygium is a triangular wing-shaped mass of fibrovascular conjunctival degenerative growth that encroaches on to the cornea with time. It is usually present in the interpalpebral fissure nasally; however, they may even be temporal or even double-headed. It may be unilateral or bilateral with variable grade of pterygium in both the eyes. The prevalence may vary from 3 to 20% in general population.[1,2]

■ HISTORY

Chief Complaints

A patient may present with following complaints:
- Whitish mass over the cornea
- *Blurred vision:* Blurring vision could be due to mass encroaching the visual axis or irregular astigmatism
- Watering/irritation/foreign body sensation
- Acute onset of pain, redness, and watering in case of an inflamed pterygium
- Diplopia or restriction of movement if extraocular muscles are involved

History of Present Illness

A careful history must be recorded to document onset and progression of the pterygium. Frequent episodes of inflammation may warrant surgery.

Other Relevant History

A meticulous history such as profession, demography, and proximity to equator must be recorded to identify the possible risk factors.

■ EXAMINATION

Ocular Examination

Visual acuity: A good refraction is mandatory in all cases of pterygium. Often, it decides whether to go for surgery. Pterygium induces with-the-rule corneal astigmatism and corneal irregularity. Trefoils, horizontal coma, and quatrefoils are the common higher order aberrations (HOAs) induced by the pterygium.

Always rule out cataract before concluding that pterygium is the sole reason for loss of vision.

The ocular examination includes:
- *Eyeball:* Usually normal
- *Eyelids:* Usually normal
- *Conjunctiva:* Wing-shaped fibrovascular proliferation of conjunctiva over the cornea
- *Cornea:* Variable involvement may be seen based on grade of pterygium:
  – Classic wedge-shaped involvement with variable vascularity and may include cystic degenerative changes
  – *Three parts:* Cap/head and tail **(Fig. 1)**
  – Cap is flat gray zone in the cornea consisting of fibroblasts that may invade Bowman layer; head is whitish thickened vascular area firmly attached to cornea, just behind the cap; tail is fleshy mobile vascular area on conjunctiva with distinct edges. It is important landmark for surgical correction.
  – Pigmented epithelial iron line (Stocker's line) may be present—suggestive of chronic involvement.

■ GRADING OF PTERYGIUM

1. *Based on extent of pterygium:*
   – *Grade 1:* Between limbus and mid-way between limbus and pupillary area
   – *Grade 2:* Extends up to pupillary margin
   – *Grade 3:* Extends beyond pupillary margin
2. *Based on Clinical grading (Tan et al):*[1]
   – *T1 (Atrophic):* Episcleral vessels unobscured and clearly distinguished. It has least rate of recurrence
   – *T2 (Intermediate):* Episcleral vessels indistinctly seen/partially obscured

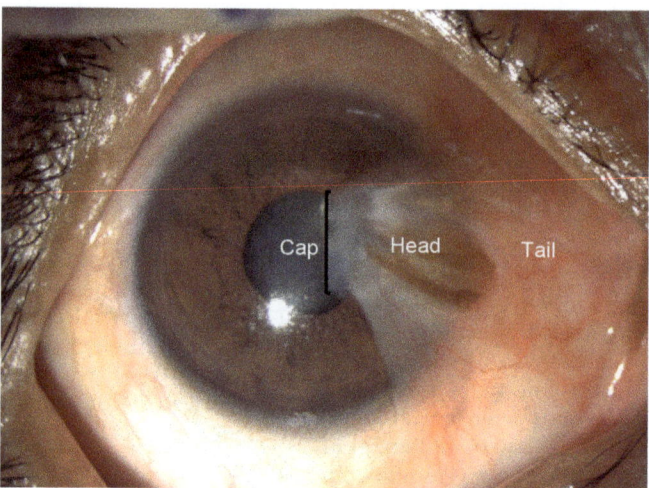

Fig. 1: Three parts of pterygium—head, neck, and body.

Table 1: Differences between pterygium and pseudopterygium.

Features	Pterygium	Pseudopterygium
Age	Elder age group (>40 years)	Any age
Gender	Male	Male = Females
Etiology	Sun damage, dry humid conditions	Post-traumatic, postchemical injury, postinfective
Site	Interpalpebral area, nasal most common	Any site
Progress	May progress based on grade of pterygium	Stationary
Probe test	Negative	Positive

- *T3 (Fleshy):* Episcleral vessels are totally obscured. These cases have highest recurrence.

DIFFERENTIAL DIAGNOSIS

- *Pseudopterygium:* A pterygium must be differentiated from pseudopterygium based on features as discussed in **Table 1**.
- *Pinguecula:* Localized, no corneal encroachment
- *Pannus:* No definite mass/growth
- *Conjunctival intraepithelial neoplasia or ocular surface squamous neoplasia (OSSN):* Feeder vessels, gelatinous look, and diffuse network of microvasculature on the surface points toward OSSN. However, in case of confusion, an impression cytology must be ordered.

INVESTIGATIONS

- *Corneal tomography/video keratography/keratometry:* To assess the astigmatism caused due to pterygium
- *Anterior segment optical coherence tomography (AS-OCT):* May be used to differentiate malignancy from pterygium. Pterygium may have normal epithelial thickness with underlying subepithelial fibrosis. Malignant lesions may have thickened hyper-reflective epithelium with abrupt transition between normal and abnormal zone.

MANAGEMENT

Management options include observation, conservative management, surgical excision with

Table 2: Advantages and disadvantages of common surgical methods in pterygium.

Techniques	Advantages	Disadvantages	Recurrence
Bare sclera technique	Easy	• Recurrence is common • *Risk of complications*: Scleral necrosis, symblepharon, infectious scleritis	24–89%
Excision with primary conjunctival closure	Easy	Higher recurrence than autograft	• Simple closure—37% • Rotational flap—29%
Pterygium excision with conjunctival autograft	Lowest recurrence	Technically challenging in larger defects	• With fibrin glue—0–9% • With suture—9–16% • With intraop MMC—0–16%
Pterygium excision with AMG	Useful in large recurrent pterygium with large defects	Availability	• Isolated 7–41% • With intraoperative MMC—16%

(AMG: amniotic membrane grafting; MMC: mitomycin-C)

conjunctival autograft, use of antiproliferative drugs, and use of amniotic membrane graft.
- *Conservative management:* It includes use of topical lubricants and vasoconstrictors. For an inflamed pterygium, a short course of steroid must be given. Sun protection must be advised including hats and sunglasses.
- *Surgical management*: Indications for surgical management are as follows:
    – Cosmetic
    – Causing visual disturbances
    – Recurrent inflammatory attacks
    – Interference with contact lens use
    – Degenerative changes
    – Restriction of ocular movements

Advantages and disadvantages of various surgical methods are summarized in **Table 2**.

VIVA QUESTIONS

Q.1. Name few adjuvants used in pterygium surgery.
Ans. Mitomycin-C (MMC), 5-fluorouracil, polytetrafluoroethylene (PTFE), and bevacizumab are few adjuvants used in pterygium surgery to decrease recurrence rate.

Q.2. How do we plan management in cases of pterygium with cataract?
Ans. Any pterygium with extension >2 mm into the cornea or astigmatism of 1.8 D, pterygium excision should be performed first. Cataract surgery can be performed after 8–12 weeks. If pterygium is <2 mm into cornea or causing astigmatism <1.8 D, a combined or only cataract surgery can be done. Note, few surgeons take 1.5 D as the cutoff ton decide between single stage versus combined surgery.

Q.3. What refractive error is expected in cases of pterygium?
Ans. Pterygium typically causes flattening of the cornea along horizontal meridian causing with-the-rule astigmatism. Grade 3 pterygium may cause irregular astigmatism.
It is important to remember that the area of pterygium is the most important factor correlating with amount of astigmatism. The thickness of pterygium has very minimal impact on the amount of astigmatism it causes.

Q.4. What is surgery-induced scleral necrosis following pterygium surgery?
Ans. Surgery-induced scleral necrosis is one of the known complications following

pterygium surgery. It is believed to be due to type IV hypersensitivity reaction. It presents as focal thinning and melt of the sclera; it may even be associated with uveal tissue prolapse in extremes of situations. The underlying risk factors include use of MMC and systemic autoimmune or connective tissue disorder. The treatment includes use of topical and oral steroids and immunomodulators such as cyclophosphamide, azathioprine, and tacrolimus. In treatment-resistant cases, surgical options such as amniotic membrane graft, conjunctival advancement, and patch graft may be planned.

Q.5. What is the use, dose, duration, advantages, and complications of MMC use in pterygium?

Ans. Mitomycin-C is an alkylating agent that inhibits fibroblast proliferation and thus reduces the chances of pterygium recurrence. It is used locally intraoperatively 0.002% to 0.4% for 30 seconds to 5 minutes. The most commonly used dose is local application in concentration of 0.02% for 2 minutes. It has also been described as topical drops to prevent recurrence. Increased concentration and duration of MMC application is associated with complications such as limbal stem cell deficiency, necrotizing scleritis, corneal dellen, ulceration, edema, iritis, glaucoma, cataract, hypotony by injury of the ciliary body, and damage to the corneal epithelium and endothelium.

Q.6. What surgical options have been described for management of recurrent pterygium?

Ans. In cases of recurrent pterygium, following techniques have been described:
- Pterygium excision with conjunctival autograft (CAG)
- Pterygium Extended Removal Followed by Extended Conjunctival Transplantation (P.E.R.F.E.C.T) technique
- Pterygium excision with use of antifibrotic agents such as MMC and anti-vascular endothelial growth factors (VEGFs)
- Use of Ologen implant
- Use of amniotic membrane graft
- Excision with simple limbal epithelial transplant
- Excision followed by lamellar keratoplasty if there is severe corneal thinning following excision of the pterygium

Q.7. Enumerate the complications of pterygium surgery.

Ans. Complications of pterygium surgery are as follows:

Intraoperative complications:
- Intraoperative hemorrhage
- Corneal thinning
- Corneal perforation
- Scleral thinning
- Scleral perforation
- Extraocular muscle disinsertion
- Reversal of autograft
- Autograft damage/button hole

Postoperative complications:
- *Immediate postoperative:*
  - Subconjunctival hemorrhage
  - Conjunctival autograft edema
  - Conjunctival chemosis
  - Conjunctival recession
  - Graft displacement
- *Late postoperative:*
  - Corneal scar
  - Corneal persistent epithelial defect
  - Corneal dellen
  - Pterygium recurrence
  - Suture-related inflammation
  - Tenon's cyst
  - Diplopia and strabismus
  - Scleral necrosis
  - Scleral perforation

Q.8. Pathogenesis of pterygium.

Ans. Various etiologies have been proposed in pathogenesis of pterygium as follows:
- UV exposure: It causes—
  - Direct damage to conjunctival epithelial cells

- Damage to limbal stem cells causing activation of fibroblasts through transforming growth factor (TGF)-beta and fibroblast growth factor (FGF)-dependent pathways
- Direct damage to endothelial cells may alter metabolism of stromal fibroblasts by alteration of collagen and elastin fibers.
- **Chronic ocular irritation:** It may be due to hot weather, wind, or dust allergies, hence termed "Surfer's disease."
- **Hereditary factors:** Matrix metalloproteinase (MMP) 1 has been predisposed to be associated with familial pterygiums.
- **Viral etiologies:** Human papillomavirus virus (HPV) and herpes simplex virus (HSV) have been associated with "second-hit hypothesis" where oncogenic viral infections stimulate pterygium formation.

Q.9. What is an inflamed pterygium and how do you manage it?

Ans. Patient with inflamed pterygium usually presents with redness, watering, and foreign body sensation. The appearance is classically described as "Fish-flesh appearance." The treatment involves a short course of topical steroids along with topical vasoconstrictor drops and lubricants.

■ REFERENCES

1. Tan DT, Chee SP, Dear KB, Lim AS. Effect of pterygium morphology on pterygium recurrence in a controlled trial comparing conjunctival autografting with bare sclera excision. Arch Ophthalmol. 1997;115(10): 1235-40.
2. Shahraki T, Arabi A, Feizi S. Pterygium: an update on pathophysiology, clinical features, and management. Ther Adv Ophthalmol. 2021;13:25158414211020152.

KERATOGLOBUS

Prafulla Kumar Maharana, Sapna Raghuwanshi, Aafreen Bari

■ INTRODUCTION

Keratoglobus is a rare noninflammatory corneal thinning disorder characterized by generalized thinning and globular protrusion of the cornea (**Fig. 1**). Nearly all cases are bilateral. The onset is often at birth with minimal or no progression. However, both congenital and acquired forms have been reported and may be associated with various other ocular and systemic syndromes including the connective tissue disorders. In examinations, it is given as a short case.

■ HISTORY

Chief Complaints

A patient may present with following complaints:
- Blurring of vision due to irregular astigmatism (most common presentation)
- Itching, watering [if associated with atopy, vernal keratoconjunctivitis (VKC)]
- Corneal perforation, either spontaneous or following minimal trauma
- At times diagnosed incidentally and may be completely asymptomatic

Rarely, a case may present with sudden loss of vision, pain, conjunctival injection, photophobia, and glare, typically in cases of acute hydrops.

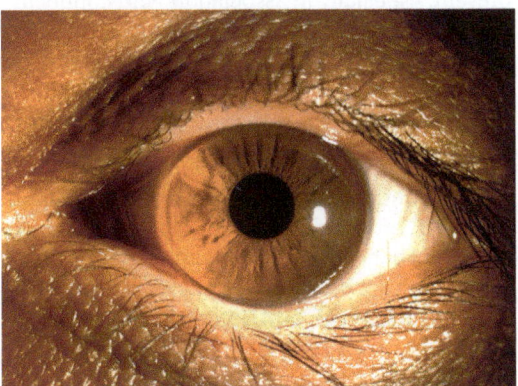

Fig. 1: Globular corneal protrusion and corneal thinning in a case of keratoglobus.

Table 1: Associations of keratoglobus.	
Connective tissue disorders	• Ehlers–Danlos syndrome type VI • Marfan syndrome • Rubinstein–Taybi syndrome • Osteogenesis imperfecta
Hereditary ocular disorders	• Leber congenital amaurosis • Posterior polymorphous dystrophy
Acquired ocular disorders	• Vernal keratoconjunctivitis • Chronic marginal blepharitis • Idiopathic orbital inflammation • Post-traumatic

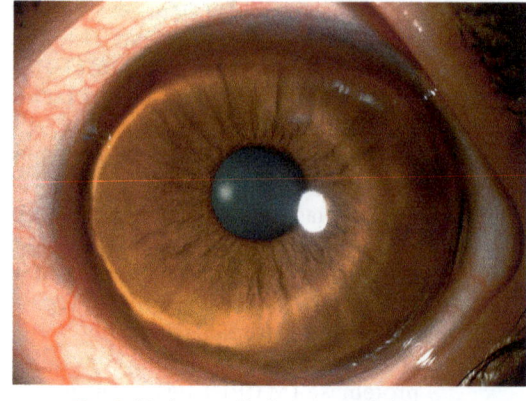

Fig. 2: Limbus-to-limbus corneal thinning.

■ EXAMINATION

Systemic Examination

Keratoglobus can be associated with connective tissue disorders; hence, a thorough systemic examination must be carried out (especially look for blue sclera, joint hypermobility, skeletal abnormalities, hearing loss, abnormal dentition, and high-arched palate). The diseases that have been reported to be associated with keratoglobus are described in **Table 1**.

Ocular Examination

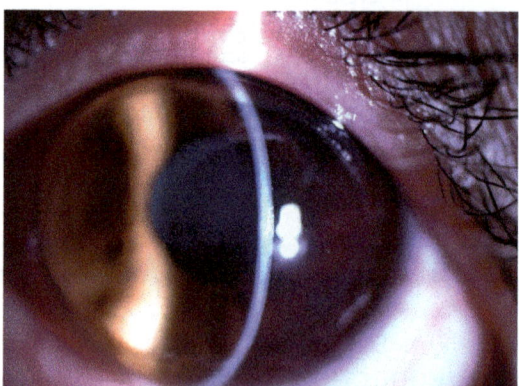

Fig. 3: Globular corneal protrusion with normal corneal diameter.

The ocular examination includes following:
- *Eyeball:* Usually normal
- *Eyelid:* Usually normal
- *Conjunctiva:* Usually normal, however signs of VKC can be there
- *Cornea:* Corneal thinning is characterized by the presence of limbus-to-limbus corneal thinning **(Fig. 2)** with globular corneal protrusion **(Fig. 3)**. Usually the thinning is greatest in the corneal periphery or midperiphery initially but with progression, limbus-to-limbus thinning occurs.

Prominent folds and areas of thickening may be present in Descemet membrane. Other corneal parameters, however, are normal, including a normal corneal diameter that is an important criterion in differentiating it from conditions such as buphthalmos.

Sclera: Usually scleral thinning or "blue sclera" is present, especially in association with connective tissue disorders and is most apparent over the ciliary body. It creates a "blue halo" around the limbus.

Anterior chamber (AC): It is usually deep.

Iris/pupil/lens/fundus/intraocular pressure (IOP): All these findings are usually within normal limits. However, retinal changes of associated diseases such as Leber congenital amaurosis may be there.

■ DIFFERENTIAL DIAGNOSIS

The differentiating features from other corneal ectatic disorders are summarized in **Table 2**. In addition, it must be differentiated from the diagnoses as discussed here.

Table 2: Differential diagnosis.

Parameters	Keratoconus	Pellucid marginal degeneration	Keratoglobus	Terrien's marginal degeneration
Frequency	Most common	Less common	Rare	Less common
Laterality	Usually bilateral	Bilateral	Bilateral	Bilateral
Age at onset	Puberty	20–40 years	Usually at birth	20–40 years
Thinning	Inferior	Paracentral	Inferior band 1–2 mm wide, greatest in periphery	Usually starts superiorly then progress circumferentially
Protrusion	Thinning at apex	Superior to band of thinning	Generalized	
Iron line	Fleischer ring	Sometimes	None	None
Scarring	Common	Only after hydrops	Mild	Only after hydrops
Striae	Common	Sometimes	Sometimes	Sometimes

Megalocornea

It is nonprogressive symmetric enlargement of the cornea (>12.5 mm in horizontal diameter) without a significant change in corneal thickness or contour unlike keratoglobus where corneal diameter is normal but thickness is reduced.

Congenital Glaucoma

It is associated with elevated intraocular pressure, a cloudy cornea, changes in the optic disc, or generalized enlargement of the eye that are absent in keratoglobus.

■ INVESTIGATIONS

The diagnosis of keratoglobus is essentially a clinical one owing to the characteristic clinical findings. The investigations done in a case of keratoglobus if the diagnosis is doubtful and while planning treatment are discussed here.

Ultrasonic Pachymetry

It would show reduced corneal thickness.

Corneal Topography (Orbscan/ Videokeratography/Pentacam)

It shows diffuse thinning and irregular astigmatism with irregular power distribution. In advanced cases, it is often difficult to perform corneal topography.

■ MANAGEMENT

Conservative Management

Often the patient maintains a good visual acuity till late. Thus, observation is the rule in early cases. These patients are advised to use protective eye wear (e.g., polycarbonate glasses) and avoid contact sports owing to the high risk of perforation even with trivial trauma. Visual rehabilitation is achieved through refractive correction for high myopia. Spectacles are normally used in early cases of keratoglobus only. The disease is potentially blinding in children owing to timely adequate refractive correction at proper age.

As the disease progresses, irregular astigmatism develops and adequate visual acuity cannot be achieved with this type of visual correction.

Contact Lens

Various types of contact lenses (CL) are available for treatment of keratoglobus such as scleral lenses, rigid gas permeable (RGP) lenses, reverse geometry hydrogel lenses, and large diameter inverse geometry RGP lenses.

Table 3: Treatment options for keratoglobus.

Surgical procedure	Advantage	Disadvantage
Large diameter (limbus-to-limbus) PKP	Covers the thinned part and suturing is easy	• Increased rejection due to proximity of limbal vasculature • Limbal stem cell damage • Damage to angle structure
Epikeratoplasty	• Good tectonic stability • Corneal flattening effect	• Limbal stem cell disruption • Persistent epithelial defect
Epikeratoplasty with 360 host peripheral intrastromal tucking	• No limbal stem cell disruption • No angle structure disruption	Poor visual outcome due to interface opacities and intraepithelial cysts
Tuck-in lamellar keratoplasty	• Good tectonic stability • No limbal stem cell disruption • No angle structure disruption	• Technically difficult • Interface haze
Pentacam-based deep anterior LK	Advantages of lamellar graft	Technically demanding
Corneoscleral rim (Buttress over thinned corneal periphery for tectonic stability)	• Technically easy • Allows for delay in further surgical intervention	Temporary measure
Epikeratoplasty/tectonic LK followed by 2nd stage PKP	Better visual outcome	• Two-stage procedure • Two donor corneas required

(LK: lamellar keratoplasty; PKP: penetrating keratoplasty)

Surgical Management

Surgery in keratoglobus is difficult because of the following reasons:
- Large graft is required to include the thinned periphery and large graft as such is a risk factor for graft rejection.
- Owing to the fragility of the thinned cornea at periphery, placement of sutures is difficult and often leads to cut through or "cheese-wire."
- Proximity of the graft to limbus can lead to increased chance of graft rejection.
- Higher chance of perforation while performing lamellar graft due to limbus-to-limbus thinning.

The various treatment options for keratoglobus are summarized in **Table 3**.[1]

VIVA QUESTIONS

Q.1. Difference between congenital and acquired keratoglobus.

Ans. Remember keratoglobus is almost always a congenital disease. Recently, it has been reported to be associated with few acquired diseases **(Table 1)**. The acquired types are more severe with a higher chance of perforation from trivial trauma. Few authors consider these acquired forms as nothing but severe variants of keratoconus only.

Q.2. What is the role of corneal collagen cross-linking in cases of keratoglobus?

Ans. Collagen cross-linking (CXL) is assumed to have a limited role in cases of keratoglobus due to paucity of literature on same. There are only few case reports which have described the sub400 epithelium-off CXL protocol using individualized fluence for arrest of disease progression.

■ REFERENCE

1. Wallang BS, Das S. Keratoglobus. Eye. 2013;27(9):1004-12.

PELLUCID MARGINAL DEGENERATION

Aafreen Bari, Sapna Raghuwanshi, Namrata Sharma

■ INTRODUCTION

Pellucid marginal corneal degeneration (PMCD) is a bilateral, peripheral corneal ectatic disorder characterized by a band of thinning 1–2 mm in diameter extending from 4 o'clock to 8 o'clock position in the inferior cornea. The area of thinning is separated from limbus by a 1–2 mm width of normal thickness cornea. Atypical cases can present with superior thinning or thinning beyond 4 o'clock to 8 o'clock hour, but these cases are rare. In examinations, PMCD can be given as a short case.

■ HISTORY

Demography

The disease is almost always bilateral without any gender predilection. The onset is often between second to fifth decade of life.

Chief Complaints

A patient may present with following symptoms:
- Blurring of vision due to marked against-the-rule astigmatism (most common presentation)
- Frequent changes of glasses
- Rarely a case may present with sudden loss of vision, pain, conjunctival injection, photophobia, and glare typically in cases of acute hydrops.

Past History

Past history of spectacle or CL use must be noted carefully.

■ EXAMINATION

Ocular Examination

Eyeball/eyelid/conjunctiva is usually within normal limits.

Cornea: On slit lamp biomicroscopy, following signs may be present:
- *Corneal thinning:* A band of thinning 1–2 mm in width, typically in the inferior cornea, extending from the 4 o'clock to 8 o'clock position is present **(Figs. 1 and 2)**. Between the area of thinning and limbus, there is usually a 1–2 mm width of the cornea with normal thickness. Unlike Terrien marginal degeneration, there is no scarring, lipid deposition, or vascularization.
- *Corneal protrusion:* The area of ectasia is just superior to the area of thinning **(Fig. 3)**.

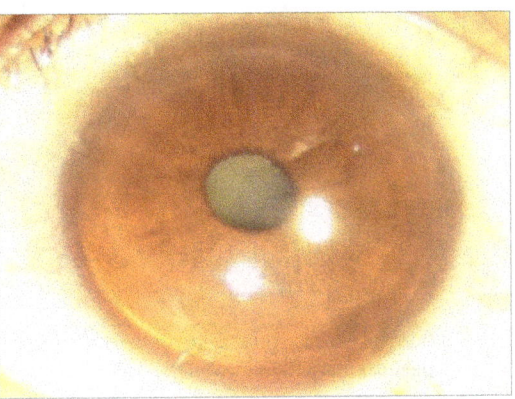

Fig. 1: Inferior corneal thinning extending from the 4 o'clock to 8 o'clock position.

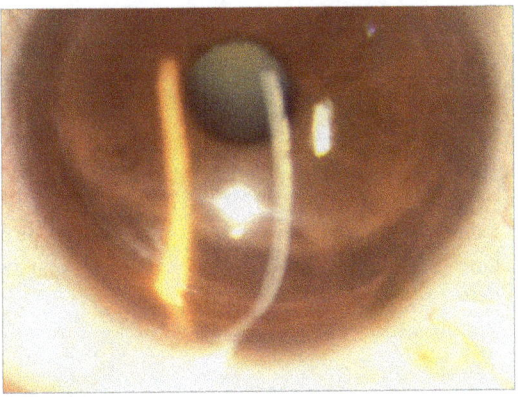

Fig. 2: Inferior corneal thinning extending from the 4 o'clock to 8 o'clock position with a 1–2 mm width of corneal with normal thickness between the area of thinning and limbus.

Unlike keratoconus, the protruding cornea is of normal thickness. When viewed from the side, the inferior-central cornea in PMD typically shows the side-profile contour of a "beer belly."
- *Stromal scars:* Scarring can be present at the superior aspect of the thinned area and can extend into the mid stroma.
- *Descemet folds:* These are occasionally seen concentric to the inferior limbus and may disappear with external pressure.

- *Bowman layer:* It may be normal or focal disruption within the area of corneal thinning can be there.
- In case of previous attack of hydrops, corneal scarring and vascularization of the inferior cornea can be seen.

Other ocular findings are usually within normal limits.

■ DIFFERENTIAL DIAGNOSIS

A case of PMCD must be differentiated from peripheral corneal thinning disorders such as Terrien marginal degeneration, Mooren ulcer, and Furrow degeneration. The differentiating features are summarized in **Table 1**. Advanced keratoconus and rarely keratoglobus can also be confused with PMCD. The differentiating features are summarized in **Table 2**.

■ INVESTIGATIONS

Corneal Topography

Topography characteristically shows inferior peripheral steepening extending into the midperiphery, inferior oblique corneal meridians in a classic "crab-claw," "butterfly,"

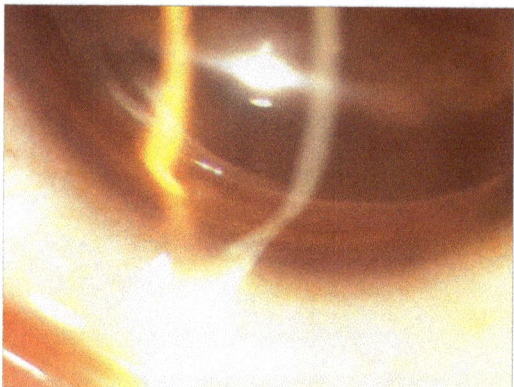

Fig. 3: Corneal ectasia superior to area of thinning in pellucid marginal degeneration (PMD).

Table 1: Differential diagnosis of pellucid marginal corneal degeneration.

Features	Pellucid marginal corneal degeneration	Terrien marginal corneal degeneration	Mooren ulcer	Senile furrow degeneration
Age at onset	Second to fifth decade	Middle-aged to elderly	Adult to elderly	Elderly
Laterality	Bilateral	Bilateral	Either	Bilateral
Gender	M = F	M > F	M > F	M = F
Astigmatism	Common	Common	Sometimes	Absent
Thinning	Inferior band 1–2 mm wide	Superior cornea	Starts within lid fissure	Occurs within arcus
Inflammation	Absent	May be present	Present	Absent
Epithelial defect	Absent	Usually absent	Present	Absent
Vascularization	Absent	Crosses area of thinning	Peripheral edge of thinning	Absent
Lipid deposition	Absent	Common; central to thinning	Rarely	Absent
Perforation	Can occur	Can occur	Can occur	Never

(F: female; M: male)

Table 2: Differential diagnosis of pellucid marginal degeneration (PMD).

Characteristics	Keratoconus	PMD	Keratoglobus
Frequency	Most common	Less common	Rare
Laterality	Usually bilateral	Bilateral	Bilateral
Age at onset	Puberty	20–40 years	Usually at birth
Thinning	Inferior paracentral	Inferior band 1–2 mm wide	Maximum in periphery
CCT	Reduced	Usually normal	May be normal
Protrusion	Thinnest at apex	Superior to band of thinning	Generalized
Rizzuti phenomenon and Munson sign	Present	Absent	Present
Fleischer ring	Present	Sometimes	None
Scarring	Common	Only after hydrops	Mild
Striae	Common	Sometimes	Sometimes

(CCT: central corneal thickness)

or "kissing doves" appearance. It shows the presence of superior flattening with against-the-rule astigmatism superiorly and with-the-rule astigmatism inferiorly.

■ MANAGEMENT

Spectacles: Spectacles are normally used in early cases of PMD only. As the disease progresses, irregular astigmatism develops and adequate visual acuity cannot be achieved with this type of visual correction.

CL: Newer generation CL such as ROSE K, scleral lenses [Prosthetic Replacement of the Ocular Surface Ecosystem (PROSE) and Boston ocular surface prosthesis (BOSP)] and hybrid lenses (such as the Soft Perm-gas-permeable lens center and a hydrogel skirt) have shown promise in PMCD in early studies. These lenses offer improvements in the VA and good stability so they could be an option for patients who have failed conventional treatments before considering surgery.

Surgical Treatment

- *Large diameter or eccentric penetrating keratoplasty (PKP):* A large diameter PKP is done so as to include the thinned out periphery. The problems with such grafts are an increased risk of rejection due to proximity to the limbus and severe postoperative astigmatism associated with a decentered graft.
- *Combined lamellar keratoplasty (LK) with PKP:* LK with PKP can be done in the same setting or as a two-stage procedure (LK followed by PKP 6 months later). The large diameter lamellar graft provides the tectonic support to the weakened peripheral host cornea while a central small diameter full thickness graft can provide excellent visual outcome.
- *Crescentic LK:* A "match and patch" lamellar graft procedure is done. Precise lamellar dissection of the recipient bed is done to achieve vertical margins and an even stromal bed depth. A lamellar donor undersized by 0.25–0.5 mm is then sutured to the recipient bed that results in flattening and reduction of ectasia.
- *Crescentic or wedge excision:* This technique is useful when the ectasia is confined to a small sector of periphery. It has several advantages over a corneal graft such as preservation of normal central cornea, no risk of rejection or interface haze, better wound strength, and shorter visual rehabilitation period. However, postoperative unstable astigmatism is an issue due to persistent tension at the sutured wound. Various modifications have been described to improve the outcome of wedge resection, such as wedge resection followed

by complete (limbus-to-limbus) or partial host lamellar dissection and corneal wedge resection combined with paired, opposed clear corneal penetrating relaxing incisions. The relaxing incisions prevent the astigmatic drift seen following wedge resection.

VIVA QUESTIONS

Q.1. What are typical described signs of PMCD?
Ans. PMCD is known to have typical inferior peripheral band of corneal thinning from 4 o'clock to 8 o' clock with steepening above the area of thinning. Clinically it is known to have "beer belly" appearance. On corneal topography, there is "classic butterfly," "crab claw," and "kissing doves" appearance. On pachymetry, there is reversal of typical pattern, center being thicker. On Orbscan, the "kissing birds" sign has been described.

Q.2. What refractive error has been described in PMCD?
Ans. PMCD cases are typically known to have against-the-rule astigmatism and irregular astigmatism in severe cases.

Q.3. What is the role of collagen CXL in PMCD?
Ans. A customized collagen CXL with irradiation to inferior periphery of cornea has been described in cases of PMCD. These have shown its effectivity in terms of arrest of progression of PMCD with relative flattening of inferior cornea, thus decreasing the need for keratoplasty in these cases.

Q.4. How to differentiate between keratoconus and PMCD?
Ans. *See* **Table 1**.

Q.5. How to differentiate between PMCD and TMCD?
Ans. *See* **Table 2**.

Q.6. What are the difficulties in performing PKP in PMCD?
Ans. There are the following challenges in performing PKP cases of PMCD:
- Due to involvement of paracentral and peripheral cornea, a large graft with increased proximity to limbus is required that increases the chances of graft rejection.
- Extreme corneal thinning makes suturing difficult and increases the chances of intraoperative DM perforation.

◼ BIBLIOGRAPHY

1. Feder RS, Gan TJ. Noninflammatory ectatic disorders. In: Krachmer JH, Mannis MJ, Holland EJ (Eds). Cornea. St. Louis, MO: Mosby; 2011.
2. Jinabhai A, Radhakrishnan H, O'Donnell C. Pellucid corneal marginal degeneration: A review. Cont Lens Anterior Eye. 2011;34(2):56-63.
3. Maharana PK, Dubey A, Jhanji V, Sharma N, Das S, Vajpayee RB. Management of advanced corneal ectasias. Br J Ophthalmol. 2016;100(1):34-40.

BAND-SHAPED KERATOPATHY

Manpreet Kaur, Sapna Raghuwanshi, Ritu Nagpal

◼ INTRODUCTION

Band-shaped keratopathy (BSK) is a slowly progressive, usually painless, corneal degeneration characterized by deposition of calcium across the cornea at the level of Bowman membrane, epithelial basement membrane, and stroma. BSK is divided into two forms calcific and noncalcific form.

Its examination is especially important as it is given as short case in examination.

◼ HISTORY

Chief Complaints

Patients present with following complaints:
Early stage: Usually asymptomatic
Late stage: May present with the following symptoms:
- Blurring of vision
- Foreign body sensation
- Tearing
- Photophobia

Table 1: Associations of band-shaped keratopathy.

Ocular disease	Hypercalcemia	Systemic diseases	Chemicals	Familial
• Chronic uveitis • Phthisis bulbi • Long-standing glaucoma • Interstitial keratitis • Dry eye and corneal exposure syndromes • Spheroidal keratopathy • Keratoprosthesis • Trachoma • Viscoelastics	• Hyperparathyroidism • Hypophosphatasia • Sarcoidosis • Renal failure (e.g., Fanconi syndrome) • Excessive vitamin D (e.g., oral intake, sarcoidosis, and osteoporosis) • Multiple myeloma • Milk alkali syndrome • Metastatic carcinoma to bone • Idiopathic • Paget disease	• Discoid lupus • Gout • Tuberous sclerosis • Norrie disease • Congenital band keratopathy • Still disease • Uremia	• Mercury fumes • Phosphate containing drops • Intraocular silicone oil • Viscoelastic • Thiazides • Lithium • Vitamin D toxicity	• Fanconi's disease • Ichthyosis • CHED

(CHED: congenital hereditary endothelial dystrophy)

Past History

Band-shaped keratopathy may be associated with several diseases **(Table 1)**, hence a thorough history must be taken to rule out these disorders.

■ EXAMINATION

Systemic Examination

A careful systemic examination is carried out to rule out any systemic association **(Table 1)**.

Ocular Examination

Eye ball: It is usually normal. Blepharophimosis may be present in cases of epithelial erosion or elevated nodules associated with inflammation.

Eyelid: Lid edema may be present if BSK is associated with ocular inflammation.

Conjunctiva: It may be normal or signs of previous disease may be present. Ciliary as well as conjunctival congestion can be there in presence of epithelial defect.

Cornea: On slit lamp examination, following signs must be noted:
- Most of the times, the opacity begins in the form of peripheral interpalpebral calcification at the 3 and 9 o'clock positions **(Fig. 1)**.
- In the peripheral form, sharply demarcated peripheral edge of the opacities separated from

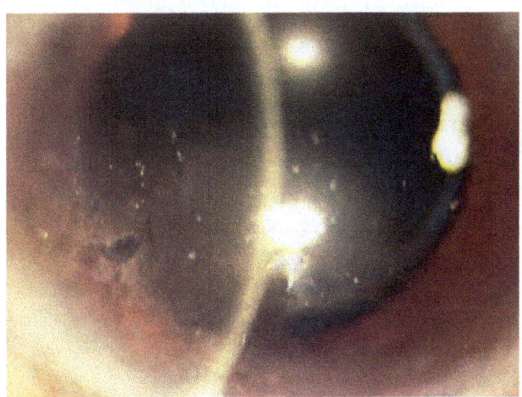

Fig. 1: Interpalpebral calcification.

the limbus by a lucent zone is seen. This zone is either due to the lack of Bowman layer at the periphery or from the buffering capacity of the limbal vessels, which prevent precipitation of calcium.
- In chronic ocular inflammation, the band may start centrally.
- Gradual central spread to form a complete limbus-to-limbus band-like chalky plaque containing the small lucent holes representing penetrating corneal nerves is seen in late stage.
- Advanced lesion may become nodular and elevated which may lead to epithelial breakdown **(Fig. 2)**.

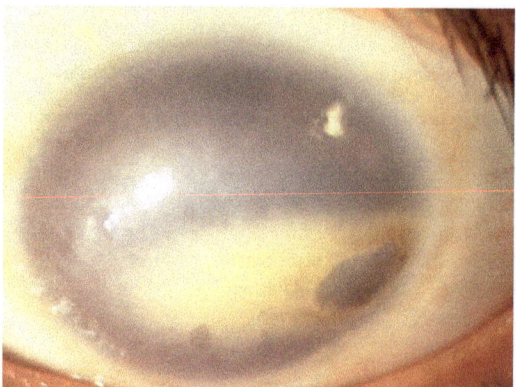

Fig. 2: Band-shaped keratopathy (BSK) in congenital hereditary endothelial dystrophy (CHED).

Iris: Festooned pupil, muddy iris, and posterior synechiae may be present in case of uveitis.

AC: Emulsified silicon oil may be present in AC.

Lens: Complicated cataract may be present in case of uveitis.

Other findings are usually within normal limits.

■ INVESTIGATION

Following investigations should be done in BSK to rule out underlying systemic disorders that affect the calcium homeostasis:
- Serum calcium
- Serum phosphorus
- Serum uric acid
- Renal function measurements
- Parathyroid hormone (PTH)
- Angiotensin-converting enzyme (ACE) levels

Anterior segment optical coherence tomography (OCT) is similar to in vivo histology, which helps to delineate the calcium deposits around Bowman membrane.

■ MANAGEMENT

The most important part is to recognize and treat the underlying causes. The indications for corneal intervention in a case of BSK are:
- Central band keratopathy contributing to reduced vision
- Mechanical irritation because of calcific deposits causing discomfort and foreign body sensation

Following are the surgical options for BSK:
- *Mechanical debridement:* If calcium plaque is thick, it is scraped off the cornea with forceps.
- *Superficial keratectomy:* Superficial calcium is scraped off the corneal surface with a no. 15 scalpel blade until a sufficiently clear cornea can be observed.
- *Chelation:* After application of topical anesthesia and placement of an eyelid speculum, all the epithelium overlying the calcium deposits is removed with a sponge or a no. 15 blade to allow penetration of the ethylenediaminetetraacetic acid (EDTA). EDTA (0.05 mol/L) is applied to the subepithelial calcification by surgical sponges or directly using a corneal trephine as a well. The chemical reaction takes several minutes to occur (5–30 minutes depending on the severity). Then all of the calcium can be removed using blunt dissection with cellulose sponges or with gentle scraping using a blunt spatula.
- *Phototherapeutic keratectomy (PTK):* The basic steps of PTK include removal of corneal epithelium with hockey stick spatula, ablation of superficial corneal tissue with excimer laser and placement of bandage contact lens. The complications of PTK include hyperopic shift, cornel haze, glare, and myopic shift.
- *Anterior LK (ALK):* When the opacities extend into deeper stroma and the visual potential is good, ALK is performed. Visual prognosis is generally good after ALK.
- *Amniotic membrane transplantation (AMT):* AMT is used as an adjunct to augment conventional surgical and chemical removal of band keratopathy by replacing the damaged basement membrane. It facilitates healing and provides long-term stability to the corneal epithelium.

VIVA QUESTIONS

Q.1. What is Still's syndrome?
Ans. Still's disease is also known as systemic-onset juvenile idiopathic arthritis. Still's triad consists of complicated cataract, glaucoma, and BSK. It is characterized by high spiking fevers, salmon-colored rash that comes and goes, arthritis, and hepatosplenomegaly.

Q.2. Pathogenesis of BSK.

Ans. Following mechanisms are involved in the deposition of calcium in cornea:
- Corneal exposure-calcium deposition occurs primarily in the exposed part of cornea due to precipitation left as tears evaporate
- Alteration of tear film osmolarity
- Elevation of pH due to corneal tissue metabolism
- Increase in concentration of calcium and phosphate

Q.3. Histopathology of BSK.

Ans. Calcium is deposited as the hydroxyapatite salt in the epithelial basement membrane, basal epithelium, and Bowman membrane. The deposits are usually extracellular, although hypercalcemia may cause intracellular epithelial accumulation.

■ BIBLIOGRAPHY

1. Albert DM, Miller JW, Azar DT. Albert & Jakobiec's Principles and Practice of Ophthalmology, 3rd edition. Philadelphia: Saunders/Elsevier; 2008.

SPHEROIDAL DEGENERATION

Sapna Raghuwanshi, Aafreen Bari, Ritu Nagpal

■ INTRODUCTION

Spheroidal degeneration (SD) is a corneal degeneration characterized by the appearance in the cornea, and sometimes in the conjunctiva, of translucent, golden brown, spheroid deposits in the superficial stroma. It is known by many different names including Bietti nodular corneal degeneration, Labrador keratopathy, climatic droplet keratopathy, degeneration corneae sphaerularis elaioides, corneal elastosis, Fisherman's keratitis, keratinoid corneal degeneration, Eskimo corneal degeneration, blindness of Dahalach, superficial central primary degeneration of Oleogutta, and chronic actinic keratopathy. SD and climatic droplet keratopathy (CDK) are the most commonly used terms.

■ HISTORY

Epidemiology/Demography

Spheroidal degeneration is commonly seen in cases associated with high UV exposure and/or reflected light such as observed in desert, ocean, and snow-covered regions. Thus, it is more common in males and persons involved in outdoor activities. It is a disease of elderly and the incidence rises with age.

Chief Complaints

The presenting features depend upon the severity of the disease:

- *Grade 1 (nodules in periphery):* Usually asymptomatic (diagnosed incidentally during routine corneal examination)
- *Grade 2 (nodules encroaching pupillary axis):* Blurring of vision (6/30)
- *Grade 3 (involvement of visual axis):* Blurring of vision (<6/60)
- *Grade 4 (raised elevated nodules):* Pain, photophobia, redness, and foreign body sensation. CDK is slowly progressive, painless, asymmetric, may be unilateral or bilateral, and is more common in males.

Past History

A careful past history can identify the predisposing factor. Most cases are idiopathic and following are the risk factors for secondary spheroidal degeneration:
- Ultraviolet light exposure
- Drying of the cornea and repeated corneal trauma
- Corneal scars after keratitis, trachomatous keratopathy, or trauma
- Lattice corneal dystrophy
- Glaucoma
- Microtrauma including sand, dust, wind, and drying
- Herpes keratopathy

EXAMINATION

Systemic Examination

One must look for chronic signs of sun damage on the skin in addition to routine systemic examination.

Ocular Examination

Eye ball: It is usually normal.

Eyelid: If it is associated with inflammation, lid edema may be present. Features of associated disease such as trichiasis (trachoma) may also be there.

Conjunctiva: Signs of chronic sun exposure such as keratinization, pigmentation, pinguecula, or pterygium can be there. In addition, findings of related disease such as conjunctival scar, Herbert's pits must be looked for. If the nodules involve the conjunctiva (type 3), clear to yellow-gold spherules are seen interpalpebrally in the 3 o'clock and 9 o'clock positions. The spherules are generally smaller and less numerous. They may be found in association with pinguecula. The spherules darken with age, progressing from a lighter yellow to a brownish-yellow color.

Cornea: On slit lamp biomicroscopy, following signs must be noted:
- Clear to yellow-gold spherules seen in the subepithelium, within Bowman, or in the superficial corneal stroma. The droplets appear oily **(Fig. 1)**.
- Initially the spherules appear at the limbus in the interpalpebral zone at 3 o'clock and 9 o'clock. Following grades of the primary form have been noted:
  - *Grade I:* Initially SD begins as a gray haze in the superficial cornea, close to the nasal and temporal margins of the cornea but usually separated from them by a clear zone. On retroillumination, the haze can be resolved into small gray deposits, which look like "droplets," immediately beneath the epithelium. The deposits are restricted to a nasal and temporal strip in each cornea but must be present at both margins of the corneas.
  - *Grade II:* As the disease progresses, the deposits extend toward central cornea into the optical axis. The disease is restricted to the interpalpebral area of cornea.
  - *Grade III:* Characterized by central involvement over the pupil, sufficiently dense to reduce vision to any degree. In this stage, exposed band of the cornea appears as ground glass.
  - *Grade IV:* In this stage, the droplets coalesce to form large corneal nodules **(Fig. 2)**. These nodules may cause corneal epithelial defect.
- In type 2, the spherules may be diffuse or begin centrally. There can be associated corneal scarring and neovascularization. A clear interval is observed between the spherules and neovascularization.

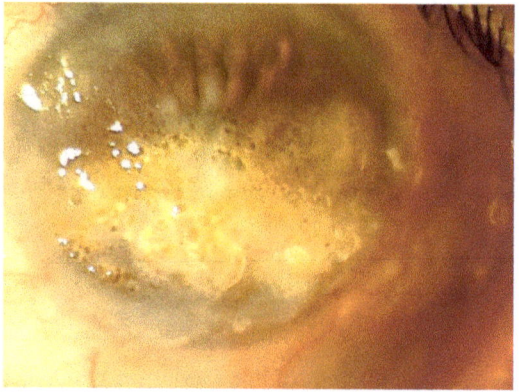

Fig. 1: Yellow-gold spherules in spheroidal degeneration.

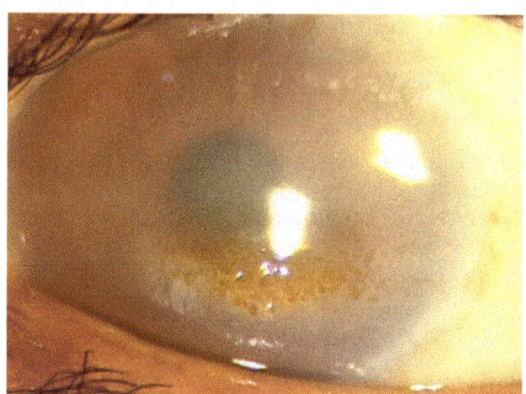

Fig. 2: Coalescence of droplets to form corneal nodules.

Sclera/AC/iris: All these structures are usually within normal limits.

Lens: As the age groups as well as the risk factors are similar to that of senile cataract, these cases are often associated with cataract.

Fundus: The fundus may be normal or signs of age-related macular degeneration may be seen.

In addition, careful examination must be done to rule out any complication such as:
- Sterile ulceration, descemetocele, or perforation
- Corneal scar, macular or leukomatous
- Recurrent corneal epithelial defect

■ CLASSIFICATION

Climatic droplet keratopathy is classified into three basic types:
1. *Type 1 or primary form:* It is usually bilateral, not associated with other ocular pathology.
2. *Type 2 or secondary spheroidal degeneration:* It may be unilateral or bilateral and is associated with other ocular pathology.
3. *Type 3:* It is usually bilateral, involves the conjunctiva too and may associated with type 1.

■ MANAGEMENT

The management of CDK is discussed here.

Medical Management

It consists of artificial tear substitute, both in the form of drops and ointments. In presence of inflammation, topical steroid can be added. Central nodules with recurrent erosion can benefit from application of bandaged contact lens (BCL).

Surgical Management

The surgical management consists of following options:

Conjunctival lesions: These nodules can be directly excised.

Central corneal lesions: These lesions can be managed in following ways:
- *Superficial keratectomy with or without amniotic membrane grafting (AMG):* Superficial keratectomy can be done using a simple no. 15 blade or a crescent knife. After keratectomy, a BCL is placed until the epithelium heals. Application of AMG improves healing and decreases scarring and vascularization.
- *Excimer laser PTK:* If the nodules cannot be removed completely by superficial keratectomy or surface irregularity persists after keratectomy, then PTK has to be done. PTK is useful only for lesions extending up to 100 μm depth. Preoperative corneal thickness must be done before proceeding with PTK. Postoperative corneal haze and hyperopic shift are the major complications associated with PTK.
- *LK/anterior lamellar therapeutic keratoplasty (ALTK):* LK is done in cases where there is A corneal scar and visual potential is good.
- *PKP:* PKP is rarely required in cases of CDK.

VIVA QUESTIONS

Q.1. Histopathology of spheroidal degeneration.

Ans. In SD, deposits appear as extracellular mauve-colored amorphous globules, which may coalesce to form larger masses in Bowman membrane. The globules are often confluent. These globules are made up of a protein material with elastotic features. Histopathology—it is very easy to confuse these globules with calcification especially when they are in the cornea near Bowman layer. However, careful examination shows that they lack the granular quality and deep purple color of calcium crystals but rather are amorphous centrally homogeneous deposits.

Q.2. What are the other names of spheroidal degeneration?

Ans. Already given in Introduction section.

■ BIBLIOGRAPHY

1. Chang RI, Ching S. Corneal and conjunctival degenerations. In: Krachmer JH, Mannis MJ, Holland EJ (Eds). Cornea, 2nd edition. Volume 1. Philadelphia: Elsevier Mosby; 2005. p. 955.

CONGENITAL HEREDITARY ENDOTHELIAL DYSTROPHY

Prafulla Kumar Maharana, Vaishali Ghanshyam Rai

■ INTRODUCTION

Congenital hereditary endothelial dystrophy (CHED) is a corneal endothelial dystrophy. CHED is a disorder characterized by bilateral, symmetric, noninflammatory corneal clouding that is usually present at birth. There are traditionally two forms of CHED—type 1 and 2. However, the International Committee for Classification of Corneal Dystrophies (IC3D) has eliminated CHED 1 and included it in the spectrum of PPCD. CHED 2 has thereafter been termed as simply "CHED."

It is given as short case in postgraduate/DNB/Diploma examination.

■ HISTORY

Chief Complaints

Presenting complaints depend on the type of CHED.

Child's parents present with the following complaints:
- Corneal clouding
- Blurring of vision
- Nystagmus
- Blurring of vision

Age at onset is extremely important. It is usually bilateral, asymmetric, and slowly progressive. CHED is usually evident *at birth or within the early postnatal period*. The course of disease is usually stationary with little to no progression.

■ EXAMINATION

Systemic Examination

A complete examination is a must, preferably by a pediatrician.

Ocular Examination

Visual acuity: Often difficult to record, preferential looking test should be performed whenever possible.

Eyeball: Usually the size of eyeball is normal but if it is associated with glaucoma, then the size of eyeball is increased.

Eyelid: Usually normal. In presence of corneal edema, blepharophimosis may be there.

Conjunctiva: Usually normal, but if it is associated with glaucoma then congestion may be present.

Cornea: On slit lamp biomicroscopy, following signs may be present:
- Initially corneal clouding is seen **(Fig. 1)**
- Diffuse gray-blue ground-glass appearance of cornea **(Fig. 2)**. The corneal opacification extends to the limbus without any clear zones.

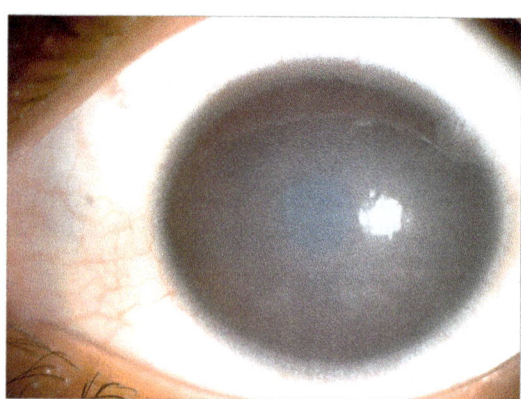

Fig. 1: Corneal clouding in congenital hereditary endothelial dystrophy (CHED).

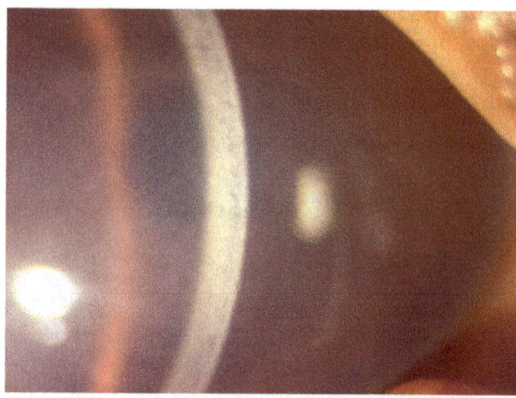

Fig. 2: Diffuse gray-blue ground-glass appearance of cornea in congenital hereditary endothelial dystrophy (CHED)

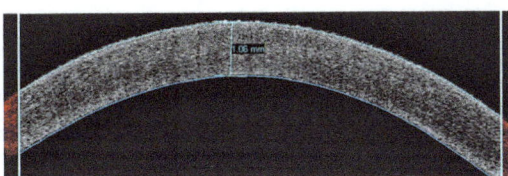

Fig. 3: Increased corneal thickness (>1 mm) in congenital hereditary endothelial dystrophy (CHED).

- Corneal thickness is increased *two to three times than normal* and often >1 mm centrally **(Fig. 3)**.
- Epithelial surface is irregular.
- Discrete white dots may also be seen in the stroma.
- In some areas where stromal opacification is less dense, Descemet membrane appears gray and on specular reflection may have a *peau d'orange* texture.
- A fine corneal pannus may be seen.
  Other ocular findings are usually within normal limits.

■ DIFFERENTIAL DIAGNOSIS

The differential diagnosis of both types of CHED is summarized below.

Congenital Hereditary Endothelial Dystrophy

Congenital glaucoma:
- Congenital rubella
- Forceps injury
- Peters' anomaly (PA)
- Mucopolysaccharidoses
- Congenital rubella
- PPCD
- Fuchs endothelial corneal dystrophy (FECD)
- Iridocorneal endothelial (ICE) syndrome

Mucopolysaccharidoses: Following features differentiate it from CHED:
- Corneal clouding is not present at birth and usually develops within the first few years of life
- Cornea is not thickened
- Systemic stigmata of MPS are typically present.
  A urinalysis or corneal biopsy will usually identify the abnormal metabolic product to confirm the diagnosis.

Congenital glaucoma:
- Increased intraocular pressure in glaucoma
- Increase in corneal diameter
- Haab's striae
- Buphthalmos
  All these features are absent in CHED.

Congenital rubella: In contrast to CHED, there is episcleral injection, nuclear cataract, raised IOP, posterior synechiae, miosis, and chorioretinopathy.

Forceps injury: Edema is transient, localized, overlying the break in Descemet membrane and unilateral in contrast to CHED. A double linear scar in Descemet membrane at the rupture edges can be seen once the edema resolves.

PA: Other associated anterior segment abnormalities would be there.

Congenital hereditary stromal dystrophy (CHSD):
- Normal corneal thickness
- No edema but opacity that is full thickness with feathery clouding of the stroma.

PPCD, ICE, and early-onset FECD: Especially when the patient presents late; the differentiating features are summarized in **Table 1**.

■ INVESTIGATIONS

- *Visually evoked response:* For visual potential assessment
- *Pachymetry:* Corneal thickness increases 2–3 times
- *Ultrasonography:* For posterior segment evaluation
- *Specular/confocal:* Difficult to perform

■ MANAGEMENT

- *PKP* **(Fig. 4)**:
  – Success rate 40–75%
  – Later the onset, better the prognosis
  – Most commonly done procedure
- *Descemet-stripping automated endothelial keratoplasty (DSAEK)* **(Fig. 5)**: Compared to PK, DSEK offers the following advantages:
  – Faster visual recovery
  – No risk of complications of open globe surgery such as expulsive hemorrhage
  – Less corneal astigmatism, less aberration

Table 1: Differences between PPCD, ICE, FECD, and CHED.

Parameters	PPCD	FECD	CHED	ICE
Onset	Teens to 20s	40–50, early onset in 1st–3rd decade	1st decade (at birth)	Young adults
Hereditary	AD	AD	AR	No
Corneal findings	• Vesicles bands • Diffuse opacities • Corneal steepening (rare)	• Guttae stromal thickening • Epithelial edema • Subepithelial fibrosis	• Marked corneal thickening and opacification • Rarely secondary subepithelial band keratopathy	Fine, guttae-like changes, hammered silver appearance
Other ocular abnormalities	Broad peripheral synechiae	Narrow angles	–	Glaucoma iris atrophy/ corectopia
Specular microscopy	• Vesicles, bands, mosaic • Endothelial cells usually enlarged but count may be normal	• Polymorphism • Polymegathism • Decreased endothelial cell count	Often not possible	Diffuse changes, ICE cell

(AD: autosomal dominant; CHED: congenital hereditary endothelial dystrophy; FECD: Fuchs endothelial corneal dystrophy; ICE: iridocorneal endothelial dystrophy; PPCD: posterior polymorphous corneal dystrophy)

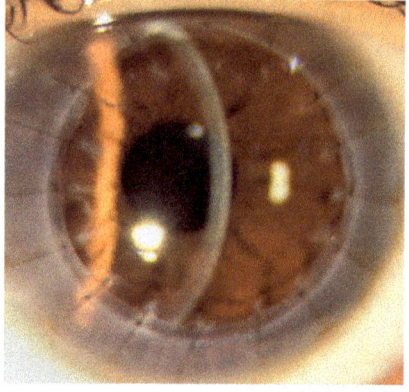

Fig. 4: Penetrating keratoplasty in congenital hereditary endothelial dystrophy (CHED).

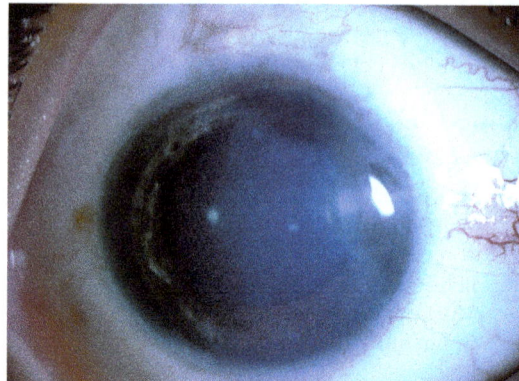

Fig. 5: Descemet stripping automated endothelial keratoplasty (DSAEK) in congenital hereditary endothelial dystrophy (CHED).

– Relatively less chance of graft rejection (although controversial)
– Preservation of corneal tectonic stability

Disadvantages:
- Poor visibility
- Risk of clear lens damage in phakic eye
- DM scoring is difficult

If patients maintain good fixation with normal alignment, surgery may be delayed; loss of fixation or development of nystagmus should lead to prompt intervention.

- *CHED associated with glaucoma:*
  – Trabeculotomy
  – Combined trabeculectomy with trabeculectomy
  – Combined trabeculectomy with trabeculectomy with subconjunctival collagen matrix

VIVA QUESTIONS

Q.1. Pathogenesis.
Ans. Mutations in the *SLC4A11* (solute carrier family 4, sodium borate transporter, member 11) gene is seen in CHED, which encodes a membrane-bound sodium borate cotransporter. The transporter regulates intracellular boron concentration, regulate the growth and terminal differentiation of neural crest cells. Loss of function of this transporter may affect the normal restrictive pattern of corneal endothelial synthesis and secretion that leads to failure of growth regulation during the terminal differentiation and reorganization of the endothelium. Subsequent endothelial cell death may lead to loss of barrier function and progressive corneal edema.

Q.2. Complication of CHED.
Ans.
- Subepithelial fibrosis/corneal pannus
- Amblyopia
- Glaucoma
- BSK

Q.3. What is Harboyan syndrome?
Ans. It is an autosomal recessive disease with CHED and progressive postlingual sensorineural deafness (CDPD).

■ BIBLIOGRAPHY

1. Weisenthal RW, Streeten BW. Descemet's membrane and endothelial dystrophies. In: Krachmer JH, Mannis MJ, Holland EJ (Eds). Cornea. St. Louis, MO: Mosby; 2011.

IRIDOCORNEAL ENDOTHELIAL SYNDROME

Vaishali Ghanshyam Rai, Neelima Aron, Prafulla Kumar Maharana

■ INTRODUCTION

The ICE syndrome describes a group of disorders characterized by abnormal corneal endothelium that is responsible for variable degrees of iris atrophy, secondary angle-closure glaucoma in association with characteristic peripheral anterior synechiae (PAS), and corneal edema. It can be given as a short case in postgraduate examinations.

The following three clinical variations within the ICE syndrome have been distinguished primarily on the basis of changes in the iris **(Table 1)**:
1. Progressive essential iris atrophy
2. Chandler syndrome
3. Cogan–Reese syndrome

Table 1: Iridocorneal endothelial syndrome: Variants.[1]

Parameters	Progressive (essential) iris atrophy	Chandler's syndrome	Cogan–Reese syndrome
Corneal endothelium abnormal (slit lamp or specular microscopy)	Yes, may be subclinical	Yes	Yes
Corneal edema	Variable—late	Present—early	Present
Peripheral anterior synechiae beyond Schwalbe's line	Present	Present	Present
Iris surface change	Present	Present	Present
Iris atrophy	Marked	Minimal	Variable
Iris nodules	Appears late	Appears late	Appears early
Ectropion uveae	Present	Rare	Present
Glaucoma	Present	Present	Present

HISTORY

Epidemiology/Demography

The syndrome affects individuals between 20 and 50 years of age. It occurs more often in women and is almost always unilateral. Glaucoma is present in approximately half of all cases.

Chief Complaints

The ICE syndrome can present in following ways:
- Most common presentation is unilateral pain and decrease in vision (DOV), which may be worse in the morning and improves later in the day.
- In the advanced stages of the syndrome, symptoms of blurred vision and pain may persist throughout the day.
- Patients also may present with a chief complaint of an irregular shape or position of the pupil (corectopia), or they may describe a dark spot in the eye.

EXAMINATION

Cornea

- Corneal edema **(Fig. 1)** with abnormal corneal endothelium may be seen on specular reflection.
- A *fine hammered-silver or beaten metal appearance* on posterior surface of cornea **(Fig. 2)** can be seen, similar to that of Fuchs dystrophy.

Iris

- *Chandler syndrome* usually presents with *corneal edema* and minimal iris alterations like iris stromal atrophy **(Fig. 3)** and corectopia.
- *Progressive iris atrophy* is characterized by marked atrophy of the iris, associated with variable degrees of corectopia and ectropion uveae. The hallmark of progressive iris atrophy is hole formation in the iris, which occurs in two forms—stretch holes and melting holes.
- *Cogan–Reese syndrome* is characterized by any degree of iris atrophy, but the predominant feature is the presence of multiple, pigmented, pedunculated *iris nodules*.

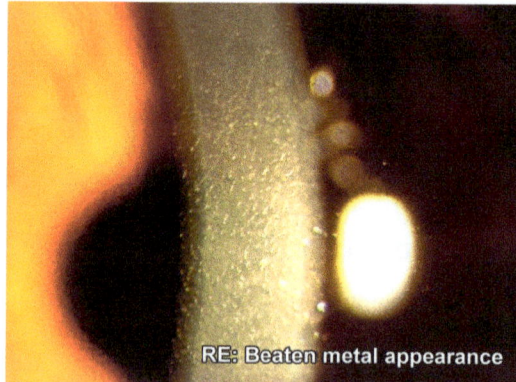

Fig. 2: Hammered-silver appearance on posterior surface of the cornea.

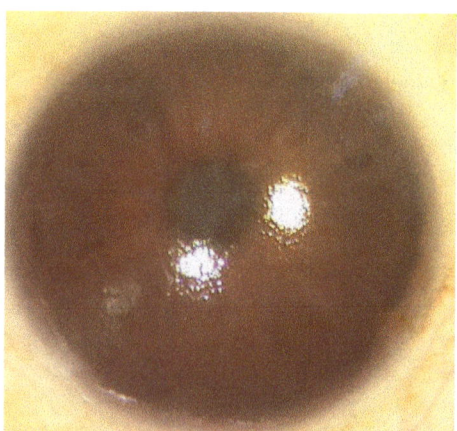

Fig. 1: Corneal edema in iridocorneal endothelial (ICE) syndrome.

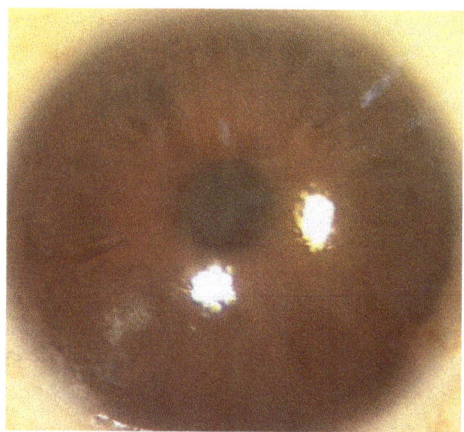

Fig. 3: Iris atrophy in iridocorneal endothelial (ICE) syndrome.

Intraocular Pressure

In early stage, IOP may be in normal range with minimal corneal edema. But in late stage, high IOP with marked corneal edema can be noted.

Gonioscopy

Peripheral anterior synechia on gonioscopy, usually extending to or beyond Schwalbe's line, is another clinical feature common to all variations of the ICE syndrome.

Other ocular structures are usually within normal limits.

■ DIFFERENTIAL DIAGNOSIS

Corneal Disorders

The two main differential diagnoses for corneal endothelial disorders are posterior polymorphous dystrophy (PPMD) and Fuchs endothelial dystrophy (**Table 1**).
1. *PPMD* is a bilateral disorder with autosomal dominant inheritance. Specular microscopic findings are different in two entities.
2. *Fuchs endothelial dystrophy* does not have the AC angle or iris features seen in ICE syndrome. Specular microscopic findings are similar in both conditions.

Iris Disorders

Iris disorders that could be confused with ICE syndrome include Axenfeld-Rieger syndrome, aniridia and iris melanosis.
- *Axenfeld-Rieger syndrome* has clinical and histopathologic similarities to ICE syndrome but differs in being *bilateral* and *congenital*. The iris and angle alterations in Axenfeld-Rieger syndrome are due to retention and contraction of a primordial endothelial layer, whereas changes in ICE syndrome are secondary to migration and subsequent contraction of abnormal corneal endothelial cells.
- *Aniridia* is usually bilateral and congenital absence of the iris tissue.
- *Iris melanosis* should be differentiated from Cogan-Reese syndrome. Iris melanosis is typically bilateral and familial. Glaucoma is uncommon.

■ INVESTIGATIONS

Specular Biomicroscopy
- Specular microscopic appearance of corneal endothelial cells in the ICE syndrome demonstrates the pleomorphism in size and shape, dark areas within the cells, and loss of clear hexagonal margins.
- Endothelial changes studied by specular microscopy are typical: in early stages, a rounding off of cell angles and intracellular blackout areas can be seen; in former stages, black out areas increase and there is a disruption of the regular mosaic.
- Fellow eye specular microscopy is important, which is normal in ICE syndrome whereas abnormal or similar to other eye in Fuchs dystrophy.
- Less role in ICE syndrome with marked corneal edema.
- ICE cells—in which the hexagonal borders are lost, a light or dark area is seen within, and reversal of the usual normal light/dark pattern occurs. Although it is characteristic but not necessary for the diagnosis.

Pachymetry

Increased central corneal thickness (CCT) in involved eye due to corneal edema whereas normal in fellow eye.

Confocal Microscopy
- Important diagnostic tool in case of corneal edema to study corneal endothelium morphology
- Confocal microscopy may be used to diagnose the ICE syndrome by demonstrating epithelial-like endothelial cells with hyperreflective nuclei. Normal in fellow eye.

■ TREATMENT
- *Medical treatment:* Aqueous suppressant medications are effective in controlling the IOP. Corneal edema may often be controlled using hypertonic saline solutions.
- *Surgical treatment:* If the IOP level remains uncontrolled despite medical treatment, filtration surgery is indicated.

VIVA QUESTIONS

Q.1. Clinical variants of ICE.
Ans. *See* Table 1.

Q.2. What is an ICE cell?
Ans. The endothelial mosaic, on specular microscopy, may contain a typical ICE cell in which the hexagonal borders are lost, a light or dark area is seen within, and reversal of the usual normal light/dark pattern occurs. Oval dark and light bodies within cell boundaries and smaller round structures with either a bright or dark appearance near cell centers are thought to be endothelial cell nuclei and blebs of the apical cell membrane. Epithelialization of the endothelial cells are thought to be the histological correlate of the ICE cell seen on specular microscopy. These cells are usually seen in Chandler's syndrome.

Q.3. What is iris nevus syndrome?
Ans. It is considered to be a variant of Cogan-Reese syndrome. It is characterized by loss of surface architecture of the iris resulting in a matted appearance, ectropion uvea, heterochromia, PAS, corneal edema, and unilateral glaucoma.

■ REFERENCE

1. Carpel EF. Iridocorneal endothelial syndrome. In: Krachmer JH, Mannis MJ, Holland EJ (Eds). Cornea. St. Louis, MO: Mosby; 2011.

PETERS' ANOMALY

Shipra Singhi, Neelima Aron, Manpreet Kaur

■ INTRODUCTION

Peters' anomaly is a developmental abnormality of the cornea, usually present at birth and is characterized by a central white opacity (leukoma) with a lucent periphery. Most cases are sporadic and bilateral in 80% of cases. It is associated with glaucoma, presumably due to abnormal development of aqueous humor drainage structures. Approximately 50–70% of the patients with PA will develop glaucoma, which is frequently present at birth.

In examinations, it can be given as a short case.

■ HISTORY

Chief Complaints

- Parents may complain of unilateral or bilateral white opacity or hazy eyes of the child since birth.
- Photosensitivity or lacrimation since birth may be there.
- Infant with cardiac disease or neurological anomaly may be referred by pediatrician to ophthalmologist to rule out PA (Peters' plus syndrome).

Perinatal History

A detailed antenatal history, history of delayed development milestones and history of cardiac disease, central nervous system anomalies, or deafness should be asked as there are many systemic associations with PA.

History of Present Illness

Corneal edema may be present early in the course of the disease and may persist or recur in the face of elevated IOP0. The edema may progressively resolve as peripheral endothelial cells migrate over the posterior defect, leaving an overlying corneal scar. Corneal edema may recur later in life secondary to the natural attrition of already compromised endothelial cells. Glaucoma develops in approximately 50–70% of patients and can present at any time. However, most commonly it develops soon after birth.

■ EXAMINATION

General Examination

Detailed systemic examination of a child is required to rule out any cardiac disease, central nervous system anomaly, deafness, or delayed development. Peters' plus syndrome refers to patients with PA associated with cleft lip and palate, short stature, abnormal ears, and mental retardation. General examination must be done carefully to rule out all these associations.

Ocular Examination

Most of the time the examination has to be done under general anesthesia.

Visual acuity: Child may have poor fixation to light and may resist occlusion of better eye.

Eye ball: Microphthalmos is common with PA.

Cornea: Following findings can be there:
- Bilateral central leukomatous corneal opacity (CO) with lucent periphery is characteristic. Look for central or paracentral corneal edema or central or paracentral CO with a lucent periphery. The size and density of the central defect is variable. It can range from a small, faint opacity to a dense leukoma precluding visualization of the AC.
- *AC:* AC depth may be shallow or irregular.
- *Iris:* Iris strands arising from collarette attached to periphery of CO is an important sign. Iris coloboma can be seen.
- *Lens:* Look for lenticular adhesion to posterior corneal surface which is a sign of type II PA.

Look for presence of cataract that is frequently seen in cases of PA. Cataract can be from a primary lens anomaly or due to a secondary change as the lens is pushed forward against the cornea. The lens may touch or be adherent to the cornea, but can also be in its normal position and yet be cataractous.

Gonioscopy: Using direct gonioscopy, look for PAS or angle anomalies, which is the main cause of glaucoma in PA.

IOP: Raised IOP may be there when associated glaucoma is there. Glaucoma is seen in 50–70% of the cases. Glaucoma in PA can appear at any age, but it is most commonly seen soon after birth.

Posterior segment: Look for choroidal coloboma, persistent hyperplastic primary vitreous, and optic nerve hypoplasia, which can be seen in cases of PA, although rarely.

■ DIFFERENTIAL DIAGNOSIS

Other causes of central corneal opacities in infants **(Table 1 and Box 1)** and the differentiating points **(Table 2)** are summarized below:
- *Congenital glaucoma:* Breaks in Descemet membrane (Haab's striae) as well as buphthalmos are common.

Table 1: Causes of congenital corneal opacities—*STUMPED* classification.

Category	Disease	Subcategories
S	Sclerocornea	
T	Tears in Descemet membrane	• Congenital glaucoma • Birth trauma
U	Ulcer	• Herpes simplex virus • Bacterial • Neurotropic
M	Metabolic (Rarely present at birth)	• Mucopolysaccharidoses • Mucolipidoses • Tyrosinosis
P	Posterior corneal defect	• Peters' anomaly • Posterior keratoconus • Staphyloma
E	Endothelial dystrophy	• Congenital hereditary • Posterior polymorphous corneal dystrophy • Congenital stromal corneal dystrophy
D	Dermoids	• Limbal dermoid

Table 2: Differential diagnosis of congenital corneal opacity.

Peters' anomaly	Sclerocornea	Dermoids	CHED	PPCD
Central leukomatous opacity with normal peripheral cornea	• Diffuse full-thickness corneal opacity, encroaching from periphery • Center relatively clear	Yellowish-white vascularized elevated nodules that may contain hair follicles, sebaceous and sweat glands, smooth and skeletal muscle, nerves, blood vessels, bone, cartilage, and teeth	Diffuse corneal edema	Diffuse corneal edema (less than CHED)
Lens normal or abnormal	Usually normal	Usually normal	Usually normal	Usually normal
Bilateral	Bilateral but asymmetric	Unilateral	Bilateral	Bilateral

(CHED: congenital hereditary endothelial dystrophy; PPCD: posterior polymorphous corneal dystrophy)

- *Birth trauma:* Birth trauma is usually unilateral and should demonstrate breaks in Descemet membrane. Only corneal edema will be there without any opacity characteristic of PA.
- *Mucopolysaccharidoses:* The cornea is usually diffusely hazy with no stromal thickening as opposed to centrally hazy with stromal edema and clear periphery in case of PA. The urinalysis shows the abnormal metabolic product. Systemic features of the underlying cause will be there.
- *CHED:* The cornea is usually diffusely hazy as opposed to centrally hazy in PA. Corneal thickness is 2–3 times increased as compared to PA.

■ CLASSIFICATION

- *Type I:* Consists of a central or paracentral CO with iris strands that arise from the collarette and attach to the periphery of the opacity.
- *Type II:* It has lens adherence to the posterior cornea. Type I usually is unilateral, while type II frequently is bilateral.
- *Peters plus syndrome:* Characterized by PA in association with cleft lip/palate, short stature, abnormal ears, and mental retardation.

■ MANAGEMENT

Treatment of Corneal Opacity

It depends upon the location and size of corneal opacity. In addition, the presence of glaucoma also need to be considered.

Box 1: Congenital corneal opacity.

Neonatal corneal opacification: Primary
- Congenital hereditary endothelial dystrophy
- Congenital hereditary stromal dystrophy
- Posterior polymorphous dystrophy
- CYP1B1 mutation
- Limbal dermoid
- Sclerocornea

Neonatal corneal opacification: Secondary

A. *Congenital:*
- Kerato-irido-lenticular dysgenesis
  - Peters' anomaly
  - Anterior segment dysgenesis
- Iridotrabecular dysgenesis
  - Congenital glaucoma
  - Intracorneal cyst

B. *Acquired:*
- Traumatic
  - Penetrating trauma with scarring
  - Corneoscleral laceration
  - Corneal blood staining
- Infection
  - Infectious keratitis
  - Postinfectious scars
- Metabolic
- Others
  - Keratomalacia

- *Small central opacity and a clear lens:* A large peripheral iridectomy (optical iridectomy)

may permit a formed retinal image. Mydriatic therapy in cases where the opacity is not large can be considered in an effort to reduce the likelihood of amblyopia, while awaiting a more definitive procedure.
- *Large central corneal opacity and a clear lens:* PKP may be required to clear the visual axis.
- *Corneal opacity with cataract:* A triple procedure or a cataract surgery with IOL with pupilloplasty (when CO is small) can be done in such cases. The success rate of penetrating keratoplasty in PA is between 22% and 83%. Prognosis is poor in presence of glaucoma and in type 2 PA.

Treatment of Glaucoma

- Topical antiglaucoma medications and oral carbonic anhydrase inhibitors are effective in few cases. Most cases require surgery for IOP control.
- Surgical treatment such as trabeculectomy, tube-shunt procedures, or cyclodestructive procedures are done in cases of glaucoma refractory to medical management.

VIVA QUESTIONS

Q.1. Ocular anomalies associated with PA.
Ans. Chorioretinal coloboma, iris coloboma, persistent hyperplastic primary vitreous, microphthalmos, and optic nerve hypoplasia.

Q.2. Systemic associations with PA.
Ans.
- *Krause–Kivlin syndrome (inheritance is autosomal recessive):* The systemic associations of PA include short stature, facial dysmorphism, developmental delay, and delayed skeletal maturation.
- *The Peters'-plus syndrome* consists of PA cleft lip and palate, short stature, abnormal ears, and mental retardation.

Q.3. Histopathological findings of cornea in PA.
Ans. There are abnormalities in all layers of the cornea which include:
- Disorganized epithelium
- Loss of Bowman layer
- Stromal edema at the affected area
- An abrupt absence or marked attenuation of the endothelium and Descemet membrane underlying the corneal opacity. Peripheral to the opacity, the endothelium is normal.

Q.4. What are the risk factors for graft rejection in PKP in cases of PA?
Ans. Anterior synechiae, coexisting glaucoma, large corneal grafts, and central nervous system abnormalities.

Q.5. Genetics of PA.
Ans. Most cases are sporadic; however, autosomal recessive and autosomal dominant pedigrees have also been reported rarely. Genetic mutations in four genes have been described in PA. These are as follows:
1. *PAX6* gene associated with aniridia
2. *PITX2* gene associated with Axenfeld–Rieger syndrome
3. *FOXC1* gene associated with Axenfeld–Rieger syndrome
4. *CYP1B1* gene associated with primary congenital glaucoma

■ BIBLIOGRAPHY

1. Parikh M, Alward WLM. Axenfeld-Rieger syndrome and Peters' anomaly. In: Krachmer JH, Mannis MJ, Holland EJ (Eds). Cornea. St. Louis, MO: Mosby; 2011.

LIMBAL DERMOID

Prafulla Kumar Maharana, Deepali Singhal, Aafreen Bari

■ INTRODUCTION

Limbal dermoids are benign congenital tumors that contain choristomatous tissue (tissue not found normally at that site). They appear most frequently at the inferior temporal quadrant of the corneal limbus. Epibulbar choristomas are thought to arise from an early embryological anomaly (occurring at 5–10 weeks' gestation) resulting in metaplastic transformation of the mesoblast between the rim of the optic nerve and surface ectoderm. However, they may occasionally present entirely within the cornea or may be confined to the conjunctiva. They may contain a variety of histologically aberrant tissues, including epidermal appendages **(Fig. 1)**, connective tissue, skin, fat, sweat gland, lacrimal gland, muscle, teeth, cartilage, bone, vascular structures, and neurologic tissue, including the brain. Malignant degeneration is extremely rare. It can be given as a short case or spot case in examination.

■ HISTORY

Chief Complaints

In adults, dermoids may become symptomatic for the first time and grow considerably over a year. Based on this fact, some conclude that these lesions may be dormant for many years or have intermittent growth.

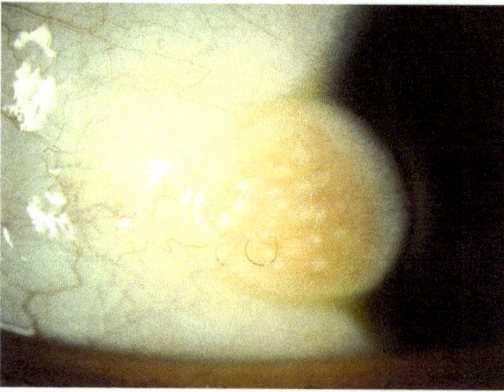

Fig. 1: Limbal dermoid with epidermal appendages such as hair.

- Painless mass (cosmetic deformity)
- Foreign body sensation/irritation
- Drying of eyes
- *Diminution of vision:* Blurring of vision is related to size, astigmatism, and involvement of visual axis. It is usually progressive and painless.
- Diplopia due to mechanical restriction of ocular movements.

Past History

A careful past history should be taken of the following:
- Mass
- Facial asymmetry
- Hearing loss
- Cardiovascular disease
- Infection
- Trauma
- Ocular inflammatory diseases

Past Surgical History

Previous history of intraocular surgery may or may not be present.

■ EXAMINATION

Systemic Examination

Cardiovascular abnormalities, facial hemiatrophy, atresia of the external auditory meatus, accessory auricles, nevus flammeus, neurofibromatosis. preauricular appendages, and pretragal fistulas should be examined if present.

One-third of the cases are associated with Goldenhar syndrome. It is a nonfamilial syndrome that presents with a classic triad of epibulbar dermoids, preauricular appendages, and pretragal fistulas.

Ocular Examination

Visual acuity: It is variably impaired depending on the site of involvement, pupil encroachment size, and astigmatism.

Cycloplegic refraction: Irregular astigmatism—compound hypermetropic

Amblyopia:
- Anisometropic or strabismic amblyopia
- Stimulation deprivation amblyopia.

Eye ball:
- Microphthalmos
- Anophthalmos
- Upper eyelid coloboma
- Lower eyelid coloboma

Lacrimal system: Lacrimal stenosis

Extraocular movement: Duane's retraction syndrome

Slit Lamp Biomicroscopy

Anterior Segment

- *Limbal dermoid:* Yellowish-white, solid, vascularized, elevated nodules straddling the corneal limbus **(Fig. 2)**. Size may vary ranging from 2 mm to 15 mm in diameter. Corneal dermoids occur as single lesions mostly but may be multiple, and they may be unilateral or bilateral, the former being the more common. Dermoids can be central and often appear to have satellite lesions.
- Dellen formation may occur.
- Anterior staphyloma can be present.
- Aniridia may be present.
- Anterior segment dysgenesis—may be present in severe cases.

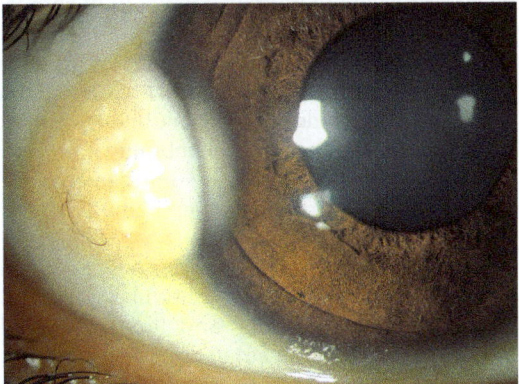

Fig. 2: Limbal dermoid.

- Lens involvement can occur. Congenital cataract or aphakia may be there.
- Neuroparalytic keratitis can occur.

Tonometry
IOP is usually normal.

Gonioscopy
Posterior corneal protrusion, synechiae or pigmentation, and dermoid involving ciliary body.

Fundus: There may be:
- Iridofundal coloboma
- Hypoplastic disc

Complications
- Recurrent dermoid
- Dellen formation
- Amblyopia
- Strabismus

■ DIFFERENTIAL DIAGNOSIS

Differential diagnosis of dermoids is discussed in **Table 1**.

Others
- Ectopic lacrimal gland
- Lymphoma
- Dermolipoma
- Corneal scar (infection or trauma)
- Pterygium, atypical
- Foreign body granuloma
- Epibulbar dermoid
- Episcleral osteoma
- Juvenile xanthogranuloma

■ INVESTIGATIONS

The diagnosis of a limbal dermoid requires a direct clinical examination. Specific laboratory studies are generally not necessary.

Imaging Studies
- *Magentic resonance imaging (MRI):*
    - Some dermoids may appear to extend into the conjunctival fornix or lateral canthus.
    - These lesions may contain connective tissue that entangles with the orbital fat and

Table 1: Differential diagnosis of dermoids.

Dermoids	Corneal keloids	CHED	Peters' anomaly	Sclerocornea
Yellowish-white vascularized elevated nodules	Chalky white solid masses with glistening gelatinous texture	Diffuse corneal edema bilaterally; cornea is not vascularized; there are never hair follicles present	Corneal opacity + iridocorneal adhesions with or without lens abnormality (position or transparency)	Loss of transition between cornea and sclera
Inferotemporal at the limbus junction	Secondary to trauma, surgery, or insult	Inheritance may be recessive or dominant	Denser corneal opacity	Cornea plana commonly associated
May contain hair follicles, sebaceous and sweat glands, smooth and skeletal muscle, nerves, blood vessels, bone, cartilage, and teeth			Most frequently bilateral	Peripheral cornea more opacified than central cornea
Usually unilateral				Surface vascularization
Can be central but do not involve the most peripheral cornea (leaving a definite sclerocorneal junction) and often appear to have satellite lesions				

(CHED: congenital hereditary endothelial dystrophy)

muscle tissue belonging to the extraocular muscles.
- Radiologic imaging with an MRI can be useful in identifying such lesions, especially if surgical management is being considered.
- Biopsy is not necessary except in rare instances when the diagnosis is doubtful.
• *Ultrasound biomicroscopy (UBM):* To determine the depth of the corneal tissue involvement.
  - Ultrasound biomicroscopy may serve as a useful diagnostic adjunct for limbal dermoids. Additionally, it may be helpful in delineating the extent of these lesions.
  - Clinical examination may be done under general anesthesia in pediatric along with an anterior segment high resolution B-scan (UBM) to assess for involvement of Descemet membrane. These steps are necessary in order to plan for the appropriate surgical approach. Meticulous biomicroscopic ultrasound examination is needed to improve the depth of corneal penetration for sound waves as studies have demonstrated that dermoids produce strong sound attenuation, reducing the visibility of deep corneal structures and in particular Descemet membrane.
• *Anterior segment OCT:* Anterior segment OCT is done to determine the depth and posterior extension of the lesion.
• *Histologic findings:* Limbal dermoids contain choristomatous tissue, including epidermal appendages, adipose and lacrimal gland tissue, smooth and striated muscle, cartilage, brain, teeth, and bone. Lymphoid nodules and vascular elements also have been reported.

The surface of the dermoids consists of corneal or conjunctival epithelium. The lesion may be cystic or solid.

Systemic Workup

- X-ray of spine for hemivertebra or scoliosis
- Electrocardiography (ECG)
- Echocardiography—for cardiac defect
- MRI of brain
- Complete blood count
- Renal function test
- Audiometry for hearing assessment

■ MANAGEMENT

Indications for Surgery

- Cosmetic deformity
- Involvement of the visual axis
- Regular or irregular astigmatism
- Amblyopia
- Strabismus
- Dellen formation
- When the lesion becomes progressive and starts to increase in size or cause irritative symptoms.

In a small, asymptomatic orbital epidermal dermoid cyst, no immediate treatment is required.

Medical Management

- Medical management is generally reserved for grade I dermoids, which are smaller lesions in terms of diameter and height
- Inducing only mild astigmatism of <1 D with minimal surface irregularity
- Parents report relatively good compliance with spectacle correction. Essentially small asymptomatic grade I limbal dermoids should not be removed because they may lead to postoperative scarring and development of pseudopterygium. It is recommended that these children undergo close clinical observation with serial examinations in the office, not only to monitor stability but also to provide reassurance for parents.
- Occlusion therapy

Surgical Management

- Shave and excision
- Shave and excision with LK
- Shave and excision with patch graft
- Shave and excision PKP with relaxing corneal incisions
- Shave and excision with corneal-limbal scleral donor graft transplantation
- Shave and excision with amniotic membrane graft/limbal stem cell allograft/pericardial graft—improves postoperative re-epithelialization, prevents postoperative scarring, and protects the limbal stem cells.
- Use of mitomycin C may improve the results.
- It can reduce recurrences by the inhibition of fibroblast proliferation at the level of the episclera. Therefore, the use of mitomycin C can be beneficial in the treatment of limbal dermoids in matters of postoperative complications such as formation of pseudopterygium.
- *Management of amblyopia:* Occlusion treatment, chemical penalization with/without spectacle wear/CL (in unilateral cases) must be continued after surgical excision to obtain optimal results if the surgery is done at a younger age.

Prognosis of Surgical Outcome

Grade	Depth of involve-ment %	Extent of corneal involve-ment from limbus (mm)	Surgery to be planned	Prog-nosis
I	<50	<3	Excision (Ex)	Excellent
II	<50 >50	3–5 <3	Excision+ lamellar kerato-plasty (LK)	Good
III	<50 >50	5.1–7 3–5	Excision/ Ex+LK	Fair
IV	<50 >50	>7 5.1–7	Excision +LK Excision +LK	Guarded
V	>50	>7	Excision +LK	Poor

Complications of Surgery

- Residual vascularization
- Corneal scar
- Persistent epithelial defect
- Pseudopterygium formation
- Ocular perforation
- Recurrent dermoid

Corneal Choristoma Classification—Stargardt Scheme

- *Grade I:* Microphthalmos, no involvement of lens
- *Grade II:* Lens involvement
- *Grade III:* Cornea only
- *Grade IV:* Limbal dermoid

Corneal Choristoma Classification—Mann's Scheme

- *Grade I:* Limbal or epibulbar dermoid
- *Grade II:* Superficial
- *Grade III:* SAnterior segment involvement with or without microphthalmos

■ CLASSIFICATION

Grading of Dermoids

Grade 1 (limbal or epibulbar)	Grade 2	Grade 3
Most frequent type	Much larger	Most severe type
Small (5 mm in diameter)	Covers part or entire central corneal surface	Very rare
Single	Variable depth of stromal extension	Entire anterior segment is involved
Inferotemporal limbus	Does not involve Descemet's membrane or the corneal endothelium	*Associated abnormalities:* Microphthalmos, posterior segment abnormalities

Contd...

Contd...

Grade 1 (limbal or epibulbar)	Grade 2	Grade 3
It may enlarge (especially at puberty)		
Superficial		
One-third of cases associated with Goldenhar's syndrome: Nonfamilial; triad of epibulbar dermoids, preauricular appendages, and pretragal fistulas		
Other abnormalities: Coloboma of the lids, aniridia, microphthalmos, anophthalmos, neuroparalytic keratitis, lacrimal stenosis, Duane's syndrome, cardiovascular abnormalities, facial hemiatrophy, atresia of the external auditory meatus, accessory auricles, nevus flammeus, and neurofibromatosis		

VIVA QUESTIONS

Q.1. What is the epidemiology of dermoid?
Ans. Epidemiology:
- Congenital choristoma
- Account for 3–8% of orbital tumors in children
- The dermoid cyst becomes the most common noninflammatory space-occupying lesion of the orbit.

- In the Wills Eye Hospital pathology series, dermoid cysts accounted for 46% of childhood orbital lesions and for 89% of all cystic lesions.

Q.2. What are the common variants of ocular dermoids?

Ans. There are two main dermoid types that occur on or around the eyes. First, an orbital dermoid is typically found in association with the bones of the eye socket (closure of embryonic sutures). Second, an epibulbar dermoid is found on the surface of the eye. There are two typical locations for an epibulbar dermoid. One of the locations is at the junction of the cornea and sclera (limbal dermoid). The second location of an epibulbar dermoid is on the surface of the eye where the lids meet in the temporal corner (toward the ear).

Q.3. What is the inheritance pattern and site of involvement of ocular epibulbar dermoids?

Ans. A study by Nevares et al. indicated that the majority (76%) of ocular dermoids occur at the inferotemporal bulbar location of the eye, with the other 22% reported to occur superotemporally. In a study by the Armed Forces Institute of Pathology, 75 of 1016 such lesions were documented to be epibulbar choristomas, with >80% of lesions noted to be located temporally and inferiorly. In another study at the Wilmer Eye Institute of Pathology, choristomas comprised 33% of all epibulbar lesions

Table 2: Goldenhar syndrome.

Epidemiology	Signs
• Sporadic, no documented inheritance pattern • No proven environmental insult during pregnancy (medication, infection, or otherwise) • Males affected 2:1 compared to females • Incidence between 1 in 3,000 and 5,600 live births	• Limbal dermoids (bilateral in 25% of cases) • Eyelid colobomas • Preauricular appendages/skin tags • Microtia or anotia of external ear can be associated with hearing loss with or without middle ear malformation • Vertebral abnormalities (butterfly vertebrae or hemivertebrae) • Congenital heart disease (numerous anomalies have been reported) • Central nervous system abnormalities (hydrocephalus, intracranial lipomas, cranial nerve dysgenesis, and mental retardation have been described)
The syndrome is almost always diagnosed early in life before there is any complaint of symptoms by the infant patient. Symptoms could include: • Double vision (motility restriction or strabismus) • Dry eye (exposure due to coloboma or large dermoid)	• Large eyelid colobomas resulting in exposure keratopathy may require surgical repair • Spectacle • Superficial keratectomy may be required to excise large limbal dermoids causing occlusive or astigmatic amblyopia or exposure • Cleft lip and palate will require surgical repair if present • Severe underdevelopment of the mandible may require reconstruction, perhaps with the aid of a bone graft (i.e., from the rib) • In cases of microtia or other ear defect, external ear reconstruction is generally done between 6 and 8 years of age and is a multistage process • Further facial reconstruction may be required • Cardiac defects (ventricular or atrial septal defect, other) are treated accordingly • If the facial or tongue malformation is severe, speech therapy may be indicated

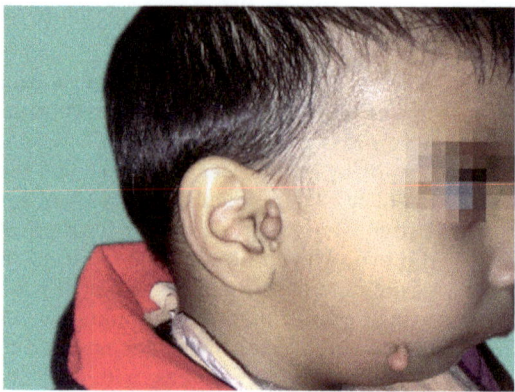

Fig. 3: Limbal dermoid with preauricular tags.

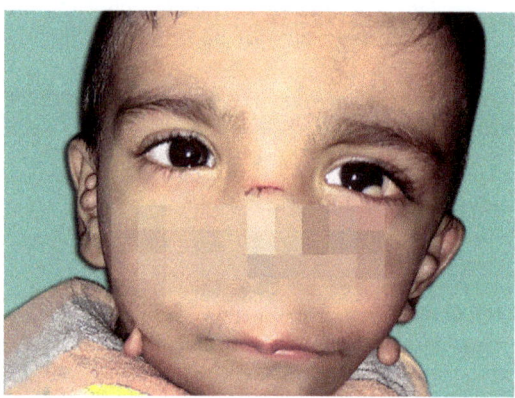

Fig. 4: Goldenhar syndrome with limbal dermoid and ear anomalies.

in individuals younger than 16 years of age. This study showed that these lesions may sometimes be associated with other ocular findings, including scleral/corneal staphyloma, aniridia, congenital aphakia, cataract, and microphthalmia.

The pattern of inheritance is quite variable in epibulbar choristomas. They can be autosomal dominant, recessive, X-linked, or multifactorial.

Q.4. What is Goldenhar syndrome?
Ans. The characteristic features of Goldenhar syndrome (also known as oculo-auriculo-vertebral spectrum, craniofacial dysostosis, or first and second branchial arch syndrome) are summarized in **Table 2, Figures 3 and 4.**

Differential diagnoses for Goldenhar syndrome (especially the facial abnormalities) are as follows:

- Treacher Collins syndrome
- Romberg disease (hemifacial atrophy) seen later in life could have a similar appearance to hemifacial microsomia
- Craniosynostosis
- Hemifacial microsomia

■ BIBLIOGRAPHY

1. American Academy of Ophthalmology. Basic and Clinical Science Course (Series 6). Amercian Academy of Opthalmology; 2012.
2. Ash JE. Epibulbar tumors. Am J Ophthalmol. 1950;33(8):1203-19.
3. Bayraktar S, Bayraktar ST, Ataoglu E, Ayaz A, Elveli M. Goldenhar's syndrome associated with multiple congenital abnormalites. J Trop Pediatr. 2005;51(6):377-9.
4. Beck AE, Hudgins L, Hoyme HE. Autosomal dominant microtia and ocular coloboma: new syndrome or an extension of the oculo-auriculo-vertebral spectrum? Am J Med Genet A. 2005;1;134(4):359-62.
5. Burillon C, Duran L. Solid dermoids of the limbus and the cornea. Ophthalmologica. 1997;211(6):367-72.
6. Cohen J, Schanen NC. Branchial cleft anomaly, congenital heart disease, and biliary atresia: Goldenhar complex or Lambert syndrome? Genet Couns. 2000;11(2):153-6.
7. Goldenhar M. Associations malformatives de l'oeil et l'oreille, en particulier le syndrome dermoide épibulbaire-appendices auriculaires-fistula auris congenita et ses relations avec la dysostose mandibulo-faciale. J Genet Hum. 1952;1:243-82.
8. Gorlin RJ, Jue KL, Jacobsen U, Goldschmidt E. Oculoauriculovertebral dysplasia. J Pediatr. 1963;63:991-9.
9. Grossniklaus HE, Green WR, Luckenbach M, Chan CC. Conjunctival lesions in adults. A clinical and histopathologic review. Cornea. 1987;6(2):78-116.
10. Mann I. Developmental abnormalities of the eye. Cambridge, UK: Cambridge University Press; 1937.

11. Mann I (Ed). Developmental abnormalities of the eye, 2nd edition. Philadelphia, PA: Lippincott; 1957.
12. Mansour AM, Barber JC, Reinecke RD, Wang FM. Ocular choristomas. Surv Ophthalmol. 1989;33(5):339-58.
13. Mattos J, Contreras F, O'Donnell FE. Ring dermoid syndrome. A new syndrome of autosomal dominantly inherited, bilateral, annual limbal dermoids with corneal and conjunctival extension. Arch Ophthalmol.1980;98(6):1059-61.
14. Mohan M, Mukherjee G, Panda A. Clinical evaluation and surgical intervention of limbal dermoid. Indian J Ophthalmol. 1981;299(2):69-73.
15. Nevares RL, Mulliken JB, Robb RM. Ocular dermoids. Plast Reconstr Surg. 1988;82(6):959-64.
16. Oculoauriculovertebral dysplasia. Online mendelian inheritance in man. www.ncbi.nlm.nih.gov/entrez/dispomim.cgi?id=164210.
17. Schaefer, Bradley G, Olney A, Kolodziej P. Oculoauriculo-vertebral spectrum. Ear Nose Throat J. 1998;77:17-8.
18. Singer SL, Haan E, Slee J, Goldblatt J. Familial hemifacial microsomia due to autosomal dominant inheritance. Case reports. Aust Dent J. 1994;39(5):287-91.
19. Stoll C, Viville B, Treisser A, Gasser B. A family with dominant oculoauriculovertebral spectrum. Am J Med Genet. 1998;78(4):345-9.

CHAPTER 3

Glaucoma

LONG CASES

PRIMARY ANGLE CLOSURE GLAUCOMA

Vaishali Ghanshyam Rai, Talvir Sidhu, Dewang Angmo

■ INTRODUCTION

Primary angle closure glaucoma (PACG) is usually allotted in practical examination as a long case. Primary angle closure (PAC) is appositional or synechial closure of the anterior chamber angle caused by pupillary block. The angle closure may or may not be associated with elevated intraocular pressure (IOP) or glaucomatous optic neuropathy and may occur in either an acute or chronic form. This entity does not include secondary forms of angle closure induced by other causes, for example, subluxed lens.

■ HISTORY

Chief Complaints

A case of PACG can present in following ways:
- Majority of patients with ACG are asymptomatic
- Blurred vision or smoke-filled room
- Some patients present acutely with color halos around lights due to corneal edema, aching eye, or brow pain, and/or eye redness
- Patients with acute angle closure attack present usually with unilateral diminution of vision with redness in the eye with severe eye pain associated with ipsilateral headache with nausea and vomiting.

History of Present Illness

Following points must be enquired:
- History of symptoms precipitated by watching television, darkened room, reading, and pharmacological mydriasis
- Brief history of patient's previous records to get baseline IOP
- Patient who is already on treatment for glaucoma is important to know how many medications he/she is using and whether this treatment has sufficiently controlled IOP and visual field loss
- Patient's previous visual fields record should be checked to know the progression of glaucoma.

History of Past Illness

Ask for previous use of glasses. Hypermetropic patients are at a higher risk to develop PACG.

History of Systemic Illness

- Diabetic or hypertensive patients who need frequent dilated fundus examination need special attention to rule out PAC or PACG as shallow anterior chamber depth may develop acute angle closer attack on dilation of the pupil.

- It is very important to ask about cardiovascular disease, renal diseases, and bronchial asthma before deciding on antiglaucoma treatment.

Family History

Relatives of PACG patients are at a higher risk for developing glaucoma. The severity and outcome of glaucoma in family members, including history of visual loss from glaucoma is also important.

Drug History

- History of use of ocular and systemic medications
- Known local or systemic intolerance to ocular or systemic medications
- History of drugs that induce angle closure attack needs to be asked. Such drugs include the following:
    - Anticholinergic agents (topical, e.g., atropine, cyclopentolate, and tropicamide; or systemic, e.g., antihistamine, antipsychotic, especially antidepressants, anti-Parkinsonian, atropine, and gastrointestinal spasmolytic drugs)
    - Adrenergic agents (topical, e.g., epinephrine and phenylephrine; or systemic, e.g., vasoconstrictors, central nervous system stimulants, bronchodilators, appetite depressants, and hallucinogenic agents)
- Specific questioning includes asking about the use of topical or systemic medication (e.g., sulfonamides, topiramate, phenothiazines) that may induce angle narrowing and subsequent symptoms that suggest intermittent angle closure attacks should be enquired.

Surgical History

History of previous ocular surgery such as trabeculectomy or any eye laser like iridotomy must be asked for.

■ EXAMINATION

General examination/specific systemic examination is carried out to look for any contraindication to antiglaucoma medications.

Ocular Examination

- *Eyeball:* Usually looks normal; small eyeball in case of hypermetropia
- *Lids:* Usually normal; in a patient who is already on antiglaucoma medications such as prostaglandin analogs, look for hyperpigmentation of lid margin and long eyelashes.
- *Conjunctiva:*
    - In case of acute angle closure attack, marked circumciliary congestion can be noted.
    - Patients of chronic ACG who are already on antiglaucoma treatment, always look for conjunctival congestion as all antiglaucoma medications can cause some form of conjunctival toxicity. This congestion is more in inferior quadrant.
- *Cornea:* Following signs can be seen—
    - In acute angle closure attack, unilateral epithelial and stromal cornea edema due to raised intraocular pressure (IOP)
    - In chronic cases, Krukenberg spindle (pigment distribution over the inferior corneal endothelium)
- *Anterior chamber:*
    - Anterior chamber is shallow (**Fig. 1**). The Van Herick technique is useful for estimating the peripheral anterior chamber depth. In PACG cases, peripheral anterior chamber is shallow that can be graded by Van Herick technique (**Flowchart 1**) (discussed later in viva questions). When the peripheral anterior

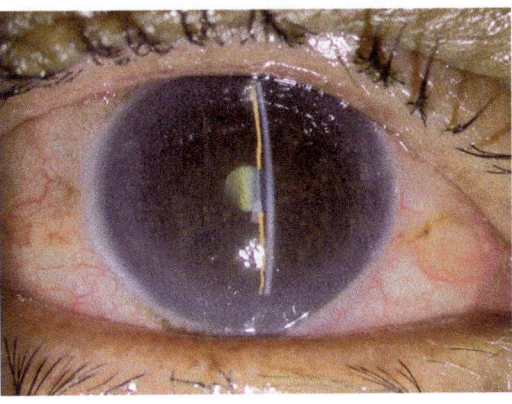

Fig. 1: Shallow anterior chamber.

Flowchart 1: Classification of PACD.

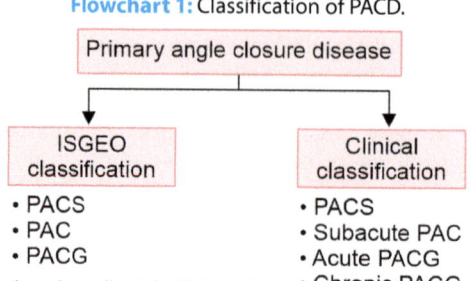

(PAC: primary angle closure; PACD: primary angle closure disease; PACG: primary angle closure glaucoma; PACS: primary angle closure suspect; ISGEO: International Society of Geographical and Epidemiological Ophthalmology)

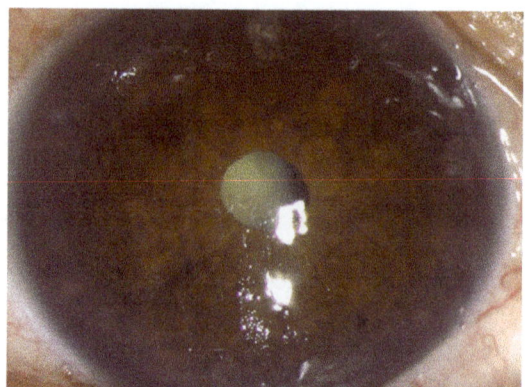

Fig. 2: Patchy iris stromal atrophy.

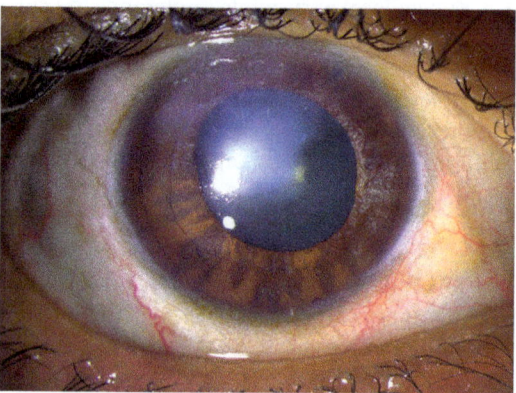

Fig. 3: Segmental iris atrophy.

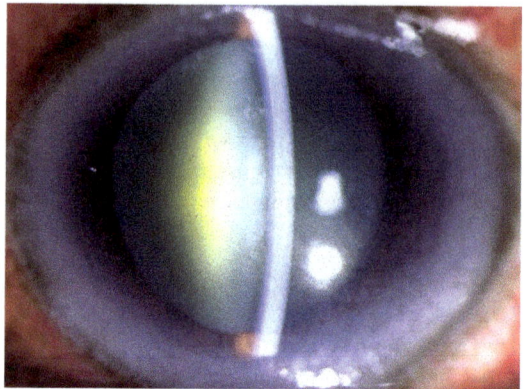

Fig. 4: Glaukomflecken.

chamber depth is less than one-fourth of the corneal thickness, the anterior chamber angle may be potentially occludable.
  – Anterior chamber inflammation suggestive of a recent or current attack.
- *Iris:* Following points must be looked for—
  – In acute attack, iris bombe is usually present due to pupillary block.
  – In recent PACG attack, iris whorling (sectoral infarction of the iris sphincter) or patchy iris stromal atrophy is usually present **(Fig. 2)**.
  – Mid-dilated pupil is common in acute or recent PACG attack.
  – Signs of previous angle closure attacks are peripheral anterior synechiae (PAS), segmental iris atrophy **(Fig. 3)**, posterior synechiae, and irregular pupil.
- *Lens:* In previous angle closure attack, look for Glaukomflecken [small gray-white anterior subcapsular or capsular opacities **(Fig. 4)** in the pupillary zone, due to infarction of lens fibers]. Lens thickness might be increased. An intumescent lens can be there in angle closure attack. Vogt's triad: Sectoral iris atrophy, Krukenberg spindle, and Glaukomflecken are characteristic of PACG.
- *Intraocular pressure:*
  – IOP is measured in each eye, preferably using a contact applanation method (typically a Goldmann tonometer) before performing gonioscopy.
  – During an acute attack of PACG, avoid measuring the IOP by Goldmann

applanation tonometer as due to raised IOP, corneal edema is present and it can cause fallacious recording of IOP due to increased corneal thickness along with rupture of bullae.
- In acute attack, IOP is usually very high (50–100 mm Hg).
- In chronic PACG, IOP elevation may be intermittent.

- *Gonioscopy:*
  - Gonioscopy of both eyes should be performed on all patients in whom angle closure is suspected.
  - This is best performed using first a two-mirror Gonio lens (e.g., Goldmann) to avoid artifactual distortion of the angle caused by inadvertent pressure on the cornea.
  - This is required to evaluate the angle anatomy, appositional closure, and presence of PAC (PAS) **(Fig. 5)**.
  - Compression (indentation) gonioscopy with a four-mirror or similar lens is particularly helpful to evaluate for appositional closure versus synechial angle closure and for extent of PAS.
  - Various grading systems including Scheie, Shaffer, and Spaeth have been proposed for the recording of gonioscopic findings. These gonioscopic grades provide an index of the likelihood of angle closure.

- *Fundus examination:*
  - For patients with PAC or narrow angle who are not in an acute attack, pupil dilation is contraindicated until iridotomies have been performed.
  - Although a dilated examination may not be advisable in patients with anatomic narrow angles or angle closure, an attempt should be made to evaluate the fundus and optic nerve using the direct ophthalmoscope or biomicroscope with +78D or +90D.
  - In acute attack, optic nerve head may look hyperemic and edematous in early stage, the disc then became pale and glaucomatous cupping can be observed after 9 to 10 days.

DIFFERENTIAL DIAGNOSIS

As primary narrow angles and PAC tend to be bilateral, the observation of a wide-open angle in the fellow eye suggests a diagnosis other than PAC.

- *Plateau iris syndrome:*
  - The peripheral iris is forced into the angle by anterior rotation of the ciliary body or anteriorly positioned ciliary processes.
  - Angle closure attack may be precipitated after dilatation of pupil even in presence of patent peripheral iridotomy.
- *Neovascular glaucoma:*
  - Neovascularization of iris or angles is a hallmark sign
- Inflammatory causes of angle closure (e.g., posterior synechiae, iris bombe)
- Iridocorneal endothelial (ICE) syndrome
- Ciliary body engorgement or suprachoroidal effusion caused by systemic medications (e.g., topiramate, sulfonamides, phenothiazines)
- Ciliary body engorgement associated with retinal vascular occlusion or scatter (panretinal) photocoagulation
- Anterior suprachoroidal effusions (e.g., congestion, edema, displacement)
- Aqueous misdirection (ciliary block) syndrome after incisional or laser surgery (e.g., following peripheral iridectomy):
  - May be differentiated clinically with acute attack of PACG
  - In aqueous misdirection, both central and peripheral shallowing of anterior chamber are seen. (Must rule out choroidal detachment or suprachoroidal

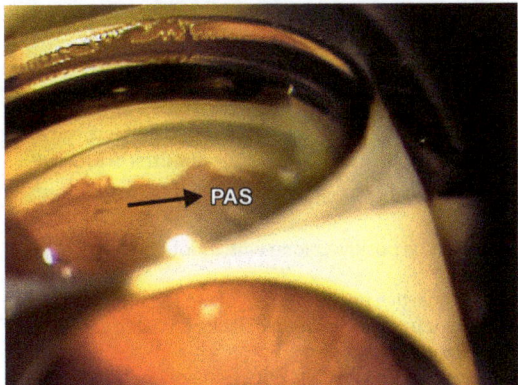

Fig. 5: Gonioscopy shows presence of PAS.

hemorrhage as a cause for this kind of shallowing of anterior chamber.)
– Whereas in acute attack of PACG, typically there is peripheral shallowing of anterior chamber due to iris bombe.
- Lens-induced angle closure (e.g., phacomorphic or subluxed):
  – Will have intumescent lens causing pupillary block (phacomorphic)
  – Will have anterior subluxation or complete dislocation of lens causing blockage of anterior chamber angles (phacotopic glaucoma)
- Developmental disorders (e.g., nanophthalmos, retinopathy of prematurity, persistent hyperplastic primary vitreous)
- Iris or ciliary body mass lesions or cysts.
  – Can be visualized using ultrasound biomicroscopy (UBM).

CLASSIFICATION

Recently angle closure glaucoma has been classified into three categories by the International Society of Geographical and Epidemiological Ophthalmology (ISGEO)(**Table 1**): (1) PAC; (2) PACG; (3) PACS; depending upon the presence of following:

- Iridotrabecular contact (>180°)
- Elevated IOP
- Peripheral anterior synechiae (PAS)
- Glaucomatous optic neuropathy
- *ISGEO classification:* The classification is described in **Table 1**.
- *Clinical classification:*
  – *PACS:* Appositional angle closure with normal gonioscopy and optic nerve (Similar to PACS as in ISGEO classification)
  – *Subacute PAC:* A rise in IOP occurs for a short period of time like minutes to some hours followed by spontaneous resolution of pupillary block.
    • Patient can have unilateral headache with blurring of vision with colored halos during the subacute attack.
  – *Acute ACG:* Acute/congestive ACG caused by sudden rise of high IOP most likely due to sudden occlusion of the angle.
    • Patient will complain of severe diminution of vision, headache with nausea and vomiting, pain, and redness of eye.
    • On clinical examination, typically there will be corneal edema, iris bombe,

Table 1: Classification and management of angle closure glaucoma.

Characteristics	PACS	PAC*	PACG†
Iridotrabecular contact (>180°)	+	+	+
Elevated IOP	–	+/–	+/–
PAS	–	+/–	+/–
Glaucomatous optic neuropathy	–	–	+
Treatment	Close observation with serial gonioscopy or LPI‡	LPI+ medical or surgical therapies to control IOP	LPI+ medical or surgical therapies to control IOP

*For a diagnosis PAC either elevated IOP or PAS, one of them must be positive, along with iridotrabecular contact (>180°).
†For a diagnosis of PACG either elevated IOP or PAS, one of them must be positive, along with iridotrabecular contact (>180°) and optic nerve damage.
‡LPI should be considered taken into consideration of symptoms suggestive of intermittent angle closure, systemic medications that may predispose to pupillary block, need for frequent pupillary dilation or lack of reliable access to healthcare.
(IOP: intraocular pressure; LPI: laser peripheral iridotomy; PAC: primary angle closure; PACG: primary angle closure glaucoma; PACS: primary angle closure suspect; PAS: peripheral anterior synechiae)

ciliary and conjunctival congestion, and vertically oval mid-dilated pupil.
- *Chronic PACG:* IOP is chronically raised leading to synechial angle closure.
  - Patients may be asymptomatic and have gradual diminution of vision.

INVESTIGATION

- Visual field analysis by automated perimetry to document visual field loss.
- *UBM:* It can help to elucidate the underlying mechanism of angle closure in most cases, including plateau iris syndrome and iridociliary cysts, thereby allowing the appropriate treatment to be given.
  - Can especially assess the angle structures in cases of corneal edema where gonioscopy and anterior segment optical coherence tomography (AS-OCT) are not useful.
- *AS-OCT:* It can detect angle closure but has a high rate of false positives when assessed against gonioscopy. ASOCT has not replaced gonioscopy yet.

MANAGEMENT

Medical Management

Management of acute angle closure attack includes the following:
- Acetazolamide (250–500 mg) oral stat, then 125–250 mg tid/qid until symptoms subside or IV mannitol 1.5 g/kg of body weight of 20% 200 mL over 30 minutes, followed by oral acetazolamide 250 mg qid
- Topical pilocarpine 2% stat, then qid can be given but after inflammation control
- Analgesics and antiemetic as required
- Topical beta-blockers eye drop BD
- Topical steroids qid
- Preventive laser peripheral iridotomy (LPI) should be done in fellow eye as early as possible
- Once IOP is controlled and corneal edema clears, an LPI should be performed.

Management of Primary Angle Closure Suspect

Management options include LPI or close observations with regular follow-ups for IOP checking, gonioscopy, and disc evaluation. Indication for LPI in PACS includes the following:
- Patients who needs frequent dilatation, for example, diabetics, hypertensive age-related macular degeneration (ARMD)
- Patients who had previous angle closure attack in one eye. A prophylactic peripheral iridotomy (PI) for fellow eye is advised.
- Hyperopic patient
- Patient who is unlikely to come for regular follow-up
- Family history of glaucoma.

Surgical Treatment

A patient whose IOP does not come under control with PI and medications, and those with fairly advanced disease will require filtering surgery. The application of antifibrotic agents such as 5-fluorouracil (5-FU) and mitomycin C (MMC) results in greater success and lowers IOP following trabeculectomy.

VIVA QUESTIONS

Q.1. How do you grade peripheral anterior chamber depth (PACD) on slit lamp?
Ans. *By Van Herick method:*
- *Grade 0:* Iridocorneal contact
- *Grade 1:* PACD <1/4 corneal thickness
- *Grade 2:* PACD = 1/4 corneal thickness
- *Grade 3:* PAC = 1/4–1/2 corneal thickness
- *Grade 4:* PACD ≥1 corneal thickness
  Grade 0, 1, and 2—suspicious of angle closure

Q.2. Which are the risk factors for developing PACG?
Ans. *Following are risk factors for PACG:*
- *Patient factors:*
  - Advancing age
  - Female gender
  - Asian or Inuit descent
  - Family history of angle closure
- *Ocular factors:*
  - Shallow anterior chamber
  - Narrow angle
  - Relative anterior location of iris-lens diaphragm
  - Hyperopia [increased lens thickness, small corneal diameters, and short axial length (AL)]

Q.3. What are the mechanisms of angle closure?

Ans.
- Pupil block (most common)
  - *Abnormalities anterior to iris:*
    - PAS
    - ICE syndrome
    - Neovascular glaucoma
  - *Abnormalities of iris and ciliary body:*
    - Thick peripheral iris, cysts of iris, or ciliary body
    - Peripheral iris roll
  - *Abnormalities of lens:*
    - Thick intumescent lens
    - Subluxated lens
  - *Abnormalities posterior to lens:* Malignant glaucoma

Q.4. What are the indications for laser peripheral iridotomy in PACS?

Ans.
- Patient who needs frequent dilatation, for example, diabetic, hypertensive, ARMD
- Patient who had previous angle closure attack in one eye, prophylactic PI for fellow eye
- Hyperopic patient
- Patient who is unlikely to come for regular follow-up
- Patient who has a family history of glaucoma

Q.5. Explain the technique to perform LPI.

Ans. The procedure of LPI involves the following:
- *Before LPI:* Pilocarpine (1%) eyedrops, then anesthetize the eye with 0.5% proparacaine
- *LPI:* Abraham's type of contact lens is applied. This lens has a +55 D, peripheral button over a routine contact lens. This lens helps in the following ways:
  - It stabilizes the eye and prevents undue movements.
  - It helps to open the eye and keep the lids retracted during the procedure.
  - It smoothens out the corneal surface.
  - It provides peripheral view, which is highly magnified.
  - It helps to reduce the axial expansion of plasma, which reduces the unnecessary spread of the damage.
  - It increases the power density of the spot.
  - Gives pressure to prevent the bleed from increasing.
- *Site of LPI:* The iridotomy site should be in the peripheral third of the iris, just anterior to the arcus. A crypt or a thinned area of the iris is recommended. Most ophthalmologists place the iridotomy between 11 o'clock and 1 o'clock, where the lids superiorly cover it.
- *Size of LPI:* Iridotomy be at least 200 μm in size. The preferable size is 500 μm in diameter.
- *End point*: Once the iridotomy is complete, one can notice a sudden gush of aqueous or outflowing of the pigment from the posterior to the anterior chamber along with sudden deepening of the anterior chamber. (The presence of retroillumination may be looked for after a few weeks of laser iridotomy; however, it is not a sure sign of total penetration. Visualization of the anterior lens capsule confirms LPI. AS-OCT can also be performed on follow up to look for patency of iridotomy).
- *Parameters for LPI*: In Indian patients with brown irides, LPI can be performed with a neodymium: yttrium-aluminum-garnet (Nd:YAG) laser, using the following settings:
  - *Power:* 4–8 mJ
  - *Pulses/burst:* 1–3
  - *Spot size:* Fixed
- *Monitoring and follow-up post LPI:* At 1 hour after completion of LPI, the IOP should be checked to make sure that it did not increase significantly (i.e., IOP has not increased by ≥8 mm Hg and that IOP does not exceed 30 mm Hg). Topical prednisolone acetate 1% is given four times a day for 5–7 days. Topical beta-blocker is added in cases of PACS or continue antiglaucoma medications if patient is already on antiglaucoma medications. At 1 week, the patient is seen to monitor IOP, to confirm the patency of the iridotomy site, and to check for any significant intraocular inflammation.

Q.6. What are the complications of LPI?
Ans. *Common complications are as follows:*
- Postoperative intraocular pressure spike
- Anterior uveitis
- Iris bleeding and hyphema
- Focal cataract
- Posterior synechiae
- Visual symptoms
- Corneal decompensation

Rare complications of LPI are as follows:
- Aqueous misdirection
- Recurrent herpetic keratouveitis
- Retinal and subhyaloid hemorrhage
- Choroidal and retinal detachment after argon LPI
- Stage I macular hole

Q.7. Risk of progression of PACS to PAC/PACG.
Ans. Over 5 years, PACS has 6% risk of progression to PAC/PACG.

Q.8. The International Society of Geographical and Epidemiology of Ophthalmology classification of ACG.
Ans. The International Society of Geographical and Epidemiology of Ophthalmology classified PAC disease into PACS, PAC, and PACG based on IOP, gonioscopy findings, and disc and visual field examination.

Q.9. Is there a role of LPI in PAC disease in a pseudophakic patient?
Ans. No, in case the patient is pseudophakic, there is no role of LPI in PAC disease.

Q.10. Methods to prevent or manage bleeding during LPI procedure.
Ans.
- With the use of Abraham's lens during the procedure, can apply pressure on the eye for some time till bleeding stops.
- Immediately abandon the procedure in case of bleeding causing media haze and poor visibility.
- Always ask history of the patient taking anticoagulants, as this can lead to severe bleeding during iridotomy. This can be easily prevented by adjusting the dose of anticoagulants before LPI.

Q.11. Points to note while performing gonioscopy.
Ans.
- Posterior most structure visible
- Angle structure visible after manipulative gonioscopy
- Pigmentation of angle
- Insertion of iris
- Presence of iris processes, goniosynechiae, PAS
- Presence of neovascularization
- Presence of blood in Schelmm's canal

Q.12. What are the inclination of mirrors for Goldmann gonioprisms?
Ans.
- *Goldmann single mirror:* Mirror is inclined at 62° for gonioscopy
- *Goldmann three mirror:* One mirror inclined at 59° for visualizing the angle, the other mirror is inclined at 67° to visualize the ora serrata, and the third is inclined at 73° to visualize the equator.

BIBLIOGRAPHY

1. Emanuel ME, Parrish RK 2nd, Gedde SJ. Evidence-based management of primary angle closure glaucoma. Curr Opin Ophthalmol. 2014;25(2):89-92.
2. Kashiwagi K, Abe K, Tsukahara S. Quantitative evaluation of changes in anterior segment biometry by peripheral laser iridotomy using newly developed scanning peripheral anterior chamber depth analyzer. Br J Ophthalmol. 2004;88(8):1036-41.
3. Zhang Y, Thomas R, Zhang Q, Li SZ, Wang NL. Progression of primary angle closure suspect to primary angle closure and associated risk factors: The Handan Eye Study. Invest Ophthalmol Vis Sci. 2021;62(7):2.

SHORT CASES

STURGE–WEBER SYNDROME

Vaishali Ghanshyam Rai, Aditi Dubey, Ritika Mukhija, Dewang Angmo

■ INTRODUCTION

Sturge–Weber syndrome (SWS) is a rare congenital neuro-oculocutaneous disorder present at birth. It is also known as encephalotrigeminal angiomatosis. It is characterized as a part of the neuroectodermal dysplasias, also known as phakomatoses. Unlike other phakomatoses, SWS is not hereditary. The incidence has been reported to be 1 per 50,000 live births and no racial or sex predilection has been found.[1-7] The ocular component manifests as glaucoma and vascular malformations of the conjunctiva, episclera, choroid, and retina. The hamartoma occurring in SWS arises from vascular tissue and produces a characteristic ipsilateral port-wine hemangioma of the skin along the trigeminal distribution. Classic SWS comprises the triad of port-wine facial telangiectasia (nevus flammeus) in the distribution of the trigeminal nerve that respects the vertical midline, ipsilateral glaucoma, and intracranial angiomata.[1-3] Glaucoma occurs in approximately one half of the cases (30–70%) in which the port-wine stain involves the ophthalmic and maxillary divisions of the trigeminal nerve.[4-6]

■ HISTORY

Chief Complaints

A case of SWS can present with the following:
- Commonly referred to an ophthalmologist from general practitioner or neurologist to rule out ocular manifestation of SWS
- Heaviness and dull aching pain around eye
- Progressive peripheral visual field loss.

History

Parents usually give history of presence of unilateral port-wine hemangioma of skin along the trigeminal distribution since birth. The angiomata are present at birth and are usually unilateral, although bilateral cases also occur. History of seizures generally in infancy is usually present.

■ EXAMINATION

Systemic Examination

Sturge–Weber syndrome can involve central nervous system (CNS) as well skin, hence a thorough examination of both the systems is required. SWS is called trisymptomatic when the skin, eye, and CNS involvement is there. Similarly, it is called bisymptomatic when the skin and CNS or the skin and eyes are affected; and monosymptomatic when the skin or the CNS is affected.[4]

Specific examination to rule out nervous system involvement such as hemispheric motor or sensory defects and intellectual deficiency has to be done. Dermatological examination may reveal a characteristic port-wine hemangioma (dilated, telangiectatic cutaneous capillaries) of the skin along the trigeminal distribution (**Fig. 1**).

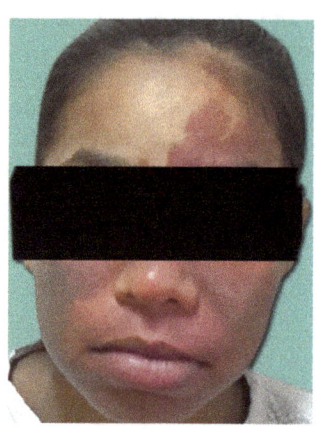

Fig. 1: Bilateral facial angiomatosis.

Ocular Examination

Eyeball: Usually normal

Eyelids: A unilateral port-wine hemangioma of the lid skin long the trigeminal distribution (maxillary and/or ophthalmic division) can be seen.

Conjunctiva: A dense episcleral vascular plexus and occasional ampulliform dilatation of conjunctival vessels is common on the site of cutaneous lesion.

Cornea: Usually normal. Corneal edema can be there in presence of high intraocular pressure (IOP).

Anterior chamber (AC): When the glaucoma is congenital, *abnormalities of the chamber angle* similar to other forms of congenital glaucoma can be there. When glaucoma occurs later in life, at that time, it is associated with a more normal-appearing AC angle.

Fundus: Good indirect ophthalmoscopy should be performed to look for choroidal hemangiomas (increases the chances of choroidal effusion and hemorrhage in surgical cases). Also, look for retinal edema and retinal detachment (RD), which are usually associated with choroidal hemangiomas. A 90 D stereoscopic disc evaluation should be performed to document cup-to-disc ratio (CDR), neuroretinal rim status, and any retinal nerve fiber layer (RNFL) defect.

IOP: In unilateral cases, IOP is >21 mm Hg in ipsilateral eye in around 50% of patients with facial port-wine stain and normal in contralateral eye.[1-3] While in bilateral facial port-wine stain, IOP is >21 mm Hg in both eyes.

Gonioscopy: In infants, look for developmental anomalies or neovascularization of the angle (NVA) of AC. In adults, usually angles of AC look normal.

■ INVESTIGATIONS

Visual fields: A standard automated perimetry to document visual field defect should be performed. Neurological visual field defects such as homonymous hemianopia can be seen in cases of leptomeningeal hemangiomas compressing the optic pathway or occipital lobe.

Pre-perimetric test: Optical coherence tomography (OCT), GDx VCC, or Heidelberg retina tomography (HRT) to document any early glaucomatous damage of RNFL is advisable in cases of SWS with borderline IOP and no evidence of glaucoma.

B-scan: To look for choroidal hemangiomas

Magnetic resonance imaging (MRI) brain/computed tomography (CT) head: To look for cortical calcifications, which can be appreciated as *double densities or railroad tracks*.

■ MANAGEMENT

The treatment is discussed here.

Medical Treatment

Antiglaucoma agents may suffice to control the glaucoma that occurs in later life, whereas the infantile form usually requires surgical intervention. Beta-blockers, alpha-adrenergic agonists, or carbonic anhydrase inhibitors can be used as monotherapy or in combination to achieve target IOP. One should *avoid prostaglandin analogs* in cases of SWS (where episcleral venous pressure is already raised) as it can cause anterior uveal effusion.

Surgical Treatment

In case of failure of medical management, surgical management is considered based on the age of onset. Congenital and infantile cases respond well to angle surgeries. However, in older children, adolescents, or adult cases or in cases of failed angle surgery, trabeculectomy with anti-scarring agents or glaucoma drainage device (GDD) should be considered.

The surgical options include the following:

Goniotomy: It is the first choice as chance of intraoperative choroidal effusion is not associated with goniotomy.

Combined trabeculotomy and trabeculectomy: Trabeculectomy may improve the chances of success by treating both possible sources of elevated IOP that is AC angle anomaly as well as elevated episcleral venous pressure.

Trabeculectomy: Chances of intraoperative choroidal effusion and expulsive choroidal hemorrhage are more with trabeculectomy. It is preferable to perform one or more sclerotomy before trabeculectomy to reduce chances of intraoperative complications.

GDD: Another surgical approach to reduce pressure in these patients while minimizing intraocular complications.

Cyclophotocoagulation: Performed in patients with refractory glaucoma or in patients with high risk of intraoperative or postoperative complications (choroidal expulsive hemorrhage or choroidal detachment) after glaucoma filtration surgery and when the visual potential is poor.

VIVA QUESTIONS

Q.1. What is the cause of glaucoma in SWS?
Ans. The cause differs according to the age of onset.
- In infants or children (approximately 60% of the cases), cause of raised IOP is anomalies of AC angles.
- In late-onset glaucoma (approximately 40% of the cases), raised IOP is due to increased episcleral venous pressure.
- Remember, the incidence of glaucoma increases when the port-wine stain involves the eyelid. It is usually ipsilateral to the lesion but can also manifest bilaterally.[5,6]

Q.2. How to differentiate between congenital glaucoma and glaucoma due to SWS?
Ans. See Table 1.

Q.3. What are the measures to decrease choroidal effusion and expulsive hemorrhage during glaucoma surgeries in patients of SWS?
Ans. The measures are as follows:
- Perioperative oral propranolol (2 mg/kg/day) to reduce the size of choroidal hemangioma
- Posterior sclerotomies just before performing trabeculectomy.

Q.4. Explain portwine stain (PWS).
Ans. Following points must be remembered about PWS:
- It is a well-delineated red macule present at birth.
- With increasing age, it gets darker and thicker and many small and large dark nodules can grow on the surface, resembling pyogenic granulomas.
- It typically presents in the V1 and V2 distributions of the trigeminal nerve.
- The upper eyelid is more frequently affected than the lower.
- In cases where PWS is present bilaterally, the likelihood of having glaucoma due to SWS is higher than unilateral cases.
- Rarely ipsilateral nasal and buccal mucosa may also be involved on the side of PWS.
- The severity of associated neurological deficits and glaucoma is often correlated with the distribution of PWS along various branches of the trigeminal nerve. Involvement of both V1 and V2 carries the highest risk of glaucoma while involvement of only V2 distribution carries the lowest risk.
- The treatment of PWS is pulsed dye laser photocoagulation, which causes irreversible damage to blood vessels but spares other components of the skin. Multiple treatment sessions may be required. The side effects are minimal. However, 100% clearance of the skin discoloration is not possible.

Table 1: Differentiating features between congenital glaucoma and glaucoma due to Sturge–Weber syndrome (SWS).

Congenital glaucoma	Glaucoma due to SWS
Bilateral	Usually unilateral, rarely bilateral
Absence of port-wine stain	Ipsilateral port-wine stain
Other systemic involvement rare	Neurological (seizures) involvement common

REFERENCES

1. Phelps CD. The pathogenesis of glaucoma in Sturge-Weber syndrome. Ophthalmology. 1978; 85(3):276-86.
2. Board RJ, Shields MB. Combined trabeculotomy-trabeculectomy for the management of glaucoma associated with Sturge-Weber syndrome. Ophthalmic Surg. 1981;12(11):813-7.
3. Agarwal HC, Sandramouli S, Sihota R, Sood NN. Sturge-Weber syndrome: management of glaucoma with combined trabeculotomy—trabeculectomy. Ophthalmic Surg. 1993;24(6): 399-402.

4. Awad AH, Mullaney PB, Al-Mesfer S, Zwaan JT. Glaucoma in Sturge-Weber syndrome. J AAPOS. 1999;3(1):40-5.
5. van Emelen C, Goethals M, Dralands L, Casteels I. Treatment of glaucoma in children with Sturge-Weber syndrome. J Pediatr Ophthalmol Strabismus. 2000;37(1):29-34.
6. Amirikia A, Scott IU, Murray TG. Bilateral diffuse choroidal hemangiomas with unilateral facial nevus flammeus in Sturge-Weber syndrome. Am J Ophthalmol. 2000;130(3):362-4.
7. Thomas-Sohl KA, Vaslow DF, Maria BL. Sturge-Weber syndrome: a review. Pediatr Neurol 2004;30(5):303-10.

BUPHTHALMOS

Vaishali Ghanshyam Rai, Aditi Dubey, Nitika Beri

INTRODUCTION

Buphthalmos (OX eye) is generalized ocular enlargement caused by elevated eye due to any cause in infancy is believed to be due to scleral and corneal collagen immaturity. Thus, it can be said that buphthalmos is a term that is applied to congenital glaucomas with enlargement of globe that appears during the first 3 years of life. The incidence of buphthalmos is 1:3,300 in India and 1:10,000 to 1:20,000 in the western world.[1,2] It is bilateral in up to 65–80% of cases. Around 90% of cases appear to be sporadic and 10% of cases appear to be a strong familial component.[1,2] Sometimes, the term hydrophthalmia is used, which refers to the high fluid content of buphthalmic eyes.

HISTORY

Chief Complaints

- The infant is usually referred to an ophthalmologist from a pediatrician due to corneal cloudiness or enlarged eyeball.
- Parents of the infant may complain of large eye ball, lacrimation, or blepharospasm.
- Triad of epiphora, photophobia, and blepharospasm is the most common presentation.

Family History

Similar complaint in other offspring is important due to familial inheritance. The chance of a second child having the disease is approximately 3%, and it may be as high as 25% if two children have the disease.

OCULAR EXAMINATION

- *Visual acuity:* Child may have severe photophobia due to corneal edema and breaks in the Descemet membrane (DM) with torch light while checking fixating and following light. The enlargement of the globe with elevated IOP during the first 3 years of life creates a myopic shift in the refractive error.
- *Eyeball:* Enlarged eyeball is common **(Fig. 1)**, which occurs because the immature and growing collagen that constitutes the cornea and sclera in the young eye still responds to increased IOP by stretching.
- *Sclera:* Bluish discoloration of sclera due to stretching can be seen.
- *Limbus:* Stretching of limbus is characteristic.
- *Cornea:* Increase in corneal diameter **(Fig. 2)**. A horizontal corneal diameter >12 mm gives a high index of suspicion for the disease. Corneal edema with horizontal breaks in DM, that is, Haab's striae should be noted. In severe cases, acute hydrops may be seen. Due to break in DM, there can be subsequent influx

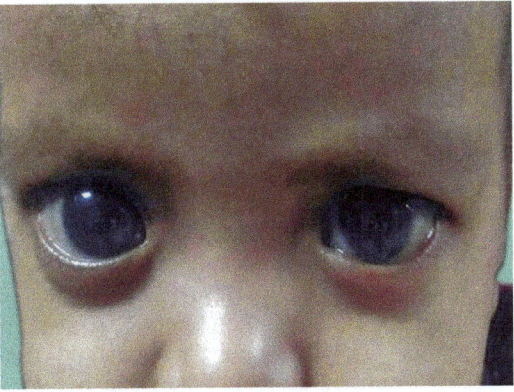

Fig. 1: Clinical photograph of a case of congenital glaucoma showing bilateral buphthalmos.

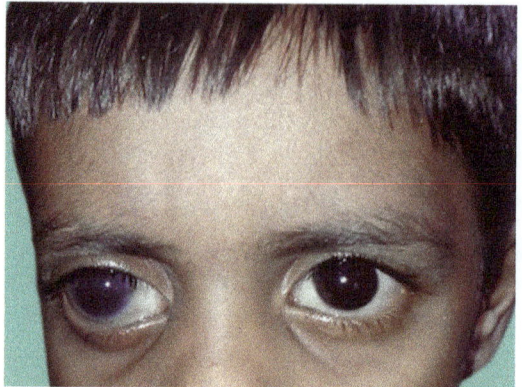

Fig. 2: Clinical photograph of a case showing right eye buphthalmos.

of aqueous in cornea resulting in localized or diffuse edema that appear as glassy parallel ridges ("railroad tracks") on the posterior cornea. These can be better visualized on retroillumination.
- *AC:* Usually deep
- *Iris:* Usually normal, although it may have stromal hypoplasia with loss of the crypts.
- *Lens:* Stretching and ruptures of the zonules can cause lens subluxation in extreme cases.
- *Posterior segment:* Examination of the optic nerve head is important to look for asymmetric cupping between two eyes or >0.3 CDR. Optic nerve cupping decreases greatly in size with IOP reduction and increases again if control of IOP is lost. In contrast, optic nerve damage, which may result from chronic or severe IOP elevation, is irreversible. The cupping appears to be caused by incomplete development of connective tissue in the lamina cribrosa, which allows compression or posterior movement of the optic disc tissue in response to elevated IOP, with an elastic return to normal when the pressure is lowered.

■ INVESTIGATIONS

- *IOP:* The IOP in normal infants is in the range of 11–14 mm Hg using Tono-Pen or handheld Goldmann tonometer (e.g., Perkins tonometer), IOP >14 mm Hg in bilateral cases or >5 mm Hg difference between two eyes in unilateral or asymmetric case should be considered for diagnosis of buphthalmos.

- *Gonioscopy:* Evaluation of the AC angle is essential for the accurate diagnosis of congenital glaucoma. It is done under anesthesia using an infant Koeppe goniolens. The iris inserts anteriorly compared to the normal infant angle. The stroma of the peripheral iris is hypoplastic, unpigmented, and has a scalloped appearance. Indirect gonioscopy with a Zeiss or Sussman gonioprism proves simple to perform at the slit-lamp in the older child, whereas Koeppe (direct) gonioscopy is useful for infants and in the operating room
- *Barkan's membrane:* It refers to a membrane formed due to incomplete resorption of mesodermal tissue across the AC angle, referred to as the Barkan's membrane. Although its existence is controversial, it forms the basis of the surgical procedure of goniotomy, which results in cleaving of the membrane to increase aqueous flow.[1,2]
- *Monster vessels:* Normally, the angle is usually devoid of blood vessels. In congenital glaucoma, loops of blood vessels from the major arterial circle may be seen above the iris surface and referred as monster vessels and this phenomenon is called Loch Ness Monster phenomenon.[1,2]

■ TREATMENT

Treatment of buphthalmos is mainly surgical.
- *Goniotomy:* It is the surgical choice where cornea is clear so that angle of AC can be visualized clearly.
- *Trabeculotomy:* Where cornea is hazy, trabeculotomy is the surgical procedure of choice.
- *Filtration surgery:* Cases where goniotomy and trabeculotomy failed, filtration surgery trabeculectomy or drainage implant is an option. It is usually combined with trabeculotomy (Trab+Trab).
- *Cycloablative procedures:* Cases in which conventional glaucoma surgery has failed to control IOP cycloablative procedures, for example, cyclocryotherapy or laser cyclophotocoagulation may lower the IOP profoundly.
- *Penetrating keratoplasty:* Permanent corneal scarring may persist after normalization of the

IOP, in those cases penetrating keratoplasty can be indicated.
- *Endothelial keratoplasty:* Recently Descemet stripping automated endothelial keratoplasty has gained popularity for treatment of endothelial dysfunction associated with buphthalmos.
  - *Tube surgery:* Initial results are encouraging.
  - *Nonpenetrating Sx:* Rarely done.

VIVA QUESTIONS

Q.1. What is normal corneal diameter in infants and when would you suspect buphthalmos?

Ans. Normal horizontal corneal diameter in infants is 10–10.5 mm, increases from 0.5 to 1.0 mm during the first year of life. A horizontal corneal diameter >12 mm gives a high index of suspicion for the disease.

Q.2. What is differential diagnosis of buphthalmos?

Ans. Differential diagnosis of buphthalmos depending on ocular signs are:
- Corneal edema or clouding:
  - Congenital hereditary endothelial dystrophy—cornea thickness increased two/three times normal and corneal enlargement is typically absent. Corneal clouding is often symmetrical with no Descemet breaks or corneal scarring.[1]
  - Mucopolysaccharidoses—absence of elevation of IOP and corneal enlargement.
  - Sclerocornea—the opaque corneal tissue extends onto the cornea.
  - Obstetric birth trauma ("forceps injury")—See **Table 1**.
- Epiphora and/or red eye:
  - Nasolacrimal duct obstruction
  - Ophthalmia neonatorum/conjunctivitis (viral, chlamydial, bacterial)
  - Corneal epithelial defect and abrasion
- Photophobia:
  - Conjunctivitis
  - Uveitis

Table 1: Differentiation of birth trauma and congenital glaucoma.

Features	Birth trauma	Congenital glaucoma
Corneal diameter	Normal	Large (buphthalmos)
IOP	Normal	High
Photophobia	No	Yes
Onset of corneal edema after birth	Immediate	Weeks to months later
Clearing of edema	Spontaneous	After reducing IOP
Tears in Descemet membrane	Vertical or oblique	Horizontal or concentric to the limbus
Eye affected	Left more	Equal
Soft tissue injuries	May be there	Absent

(IOP: intraocular pressure)

- Corneal enlargement:
  - Axial myopia
  - Megalocornea (X-linked or sporadic)
  - Microphthalmic fellow eye
- Conditions with actual or "pseudo" optic nerve cupping:
  - Physiologically large optic nerve cup
  - Coloboma or pit of the optic nerve
  - Optic nerve malformations or hypoplastic nerve
  - Atrophic optic nerve (with substance loss)

Q.3. How to differentiate between Haab's striae and forceps-related birth injury?

Ans. In case of forceps injury, DM tears are usually vertical or oblique, but these tears are horizontal in congenital glaucoma (i.e., Haab's striae) (*See* **Table 1**).

Q.4. Is buphthalmos reversible?

Ans. Cupping of the optic nerve head proceeds more rapidly in infants than in adults and is more likely to be reversible if the pressure is lowered early enough. The cupping appears to be caused by incomplete development of connective tissue in the lamina cribrosa, which allows compression or posterior movement of the optic disc tissue in response to elevated IOP, with an

Table 2: Hoskins' anatomic classification of the developmental glaucoma.

Group	Major category	Sub-category	Variants	Examples
I	*Isolated trabeculodysgenesis:* Malformation of trabecular meshwork in absence of iris or corneal anomalies	Flat iris insertion	• Anterior insertion • Posterior insertion • Mixed insertion	
		Concave (wraparound) iris insertion		
		Unclassified		
II	*Iridotrabeculodysgenesis:* Trabeculodysgenesis with iris anomalies	Anterior stromal defects of the iris	Hypoplasia	Can be seen in Axenfeld, Rieger, and Peters anomalies
			Hyperplasia	SWS with glaucoma
		Anomalous iris vessels	• Persistence of tunica vasculosa lentis • Anomalous superficial vessels	
		Structural anomalies	• Holes • Colobomas • Aniridia	
III	*Corneotrabeculodysgenesis:* Trabeculodysgenesis with congenital corneal defects. Usually associated with iris anomalies	Peripheral corneal defects		Axenfeld anomaly
		Midperipheral corneal defects		Rieger anomaly
		Central corneal defects		Peters anomaly
		Abnormalities of corneal size		Microcornea or megalocornea and their associations

elastic return to normal when the pressure is lowered. However, optic atrophy, that is, loss of NFL if sets in is irreversible.

Q.5. Write about classification of congenital glaucoma.

Ans.
- Primary:
  - Congenital
  - Infantile
  - Juvenile
- Secondary:
  - Systemic disorders:
    ♦ Chromosomal abnormalities
    ♦ Metabolic disorders (Lowe syndrome, Zellweger syndrome)
    ♦ Phakomatoses (SWS)
  - Ocular developmental disorders:
    ♦ Anterior segment dysgenesis
    ♦ Aniridia
    ♦ Congenital ectropion uvea
    ♦ Nanophthalmos
  - Ocular diseases—retinoblastoma, retinopathy of prematurity (ROP), persistent hyperplastic primary vitreous (PHPV), trauma, and uveitis

Q.6. What are the issues in management of congenital glaucoma?

Ans. Following are the issues in management of congenital glaucoma:
- Assessing etiology and inheritance of congenital glaucoma

- Managing systemic problems of secondary congenital glaucoma
- Deciding type of surgery:
  - Goniotomy–clear cornea
  - Trabeculotomy or trabeculotomy + trabeculectomy
  - Valve implant
- Managing associated ocular problems—refractive errors, corneal opacity, cataract, squint, and amblyopia
- Counseling of parents

Q.7. Give details of Hoskin's anatomic classification of the developmental glaucoma.

Ans. *See* **Table 2**. Developmental anomalies of anterior segment are the hallmark of congenital glaucoma. It may involve one or more of the angle structures such as the trabecular meshwork (TM), the iris, and/or the cornea. Hoskin's classification is based on this. It is very useful for planning the treatment as well as prognostication of the cases.[3]

Q.8. What are the clinically differentiating features between advanced and moderate cases?

Ans. In advanced cases, dense opacification of the corneal stroma may persist despite IOP reduction, whereas in moderate cases IOP elevation insufficient to produce noticeable corneal opacity gradually enlarges the infant's corneas, sometimes proceeding unnoticed. So, at times, the moderate cases become more advanced due to the subtle signs that go unnoticed while severe cases present early.

Q.9. Which antiglaucoma medication is contraindicated in children?

Ans. **Brimonidine tartrate.**

Q.10. Give details of tests performed in EUA in a case of buphthalmos?

Ans.
- External examination (brief)
- Anterior segment examination
- Tonometry (Tono-Pen/iCare/Perkins)
- Corneal diameter measurement (calipers used)
- Intraoperative gonioscopy
- Fundus examination
- Pachymetry (central corneal thickness)
- Ultrasound to measure axial length and/or B-scan if indicated
- Refraction
- **Ultrasound biomicroscopy (UBM) if cornea hazy to visualize the angle**

■ REFERENCES

1. Moore DB, Tomkins O, Ben-Zion I. A review of primary congenital glaucoma in the developing world. Surv Ophthalmol. 2013;58(3):278-85.
2. Krishnadas R, Ramakrishnan R. Congenital glaucoma—A brief review. J Curr Glaucoma Prac. 2008;2(2):17-25.
3. Hoskins HD Jr, Shaffer RN, Hetherington J Jr. Anatomical classification of the developmental glaucomas. Arch Ophthalmol. 1984;102(9):1331-6.

NEOVASCULAR GLAUCOMA

Jennil Shetty, Talvir Sidhu, Anu Malik

■ INTRODUCTION

Neovascular glaucoma (NVG) is a severe form of secondary glaucoma characterized by proliferation of fibrovascular tissue in the AC such as iris and angles. It is a potentially blinding clinical condition where delayed diagnosis or poor management can result in severe loss of vision. The treatment involves management of both the elevated IOP and the underlying cause of disease.[1,2] Most of the cases are preceded by the hypoxic damage to retina such as central retinal vein occlusion (CRVO), diabetic retinopathy (DR), branch retinal vein occlusion (BRVO), and carotid ischemic diseases. Central retinal artery occlusion (CRAO) or branch retinal artery occlusion (BRAO) are less likely to cause NVG. There is production of vascular endothelial growth factor (VEGF) from the Müller cells in response to retinal ischemia and capillary compromise, which diffuses anteriorly resulting in iris and angle neovascularization.

HISTORY

Chief complaints: A case of NVG usually presents with:
- Pain, redness, and decrease of vision in the affected eye (at times decreased vision can precede the redness and pain in setting of retinal vascular disorders)
- Watering or increased lacrimation or photophobia
- Depending on the cause of the neovascularization, patient may give a history of diminution of vision preceding pain and redness for few weeks or months.

History of Present Illness

Diminution of vision may precede the history of pain and redness by few weeks to months depending on the cause of the neovascularization. Usually, the loss of vision in the affected eye is of sudden onset but may be of gradual onset as well depending on the underlying cause. At the time of presentation, patient may or may not have regained the lost vision.

History of Past Illness

Neovascular glaucoma can be associated with recurrent attacks of angle closure glaucoma, hence similar episodes of diminution of vision in the past may be present.

Past Surgical History

- Patients may have history of cataract surgery. More often, it is associated with complicated cataract surgeries resulting in posterior capsular dehiscence or leaving the patient aphakic.
- Common in post-vitrectomized eyes of proliferative DR, especially if the eye is having untreated RD.

EXAMINATION

Systemic Examination

The underlying cause of retinal ischemia is associated with several systemic diseases such as diabetes, hypertension, and carotid ischemic diseases. A thorough systemic examination is carried out to look for signs or complications of these diseases.

Ocular Examination

Lid: Normal or edematous if there is acute rise of IOP in the affected eye as in angle closure glaucoma stage.

Conjunctiva: May be congested, circumciliary congestion is more marked if IOP is grossly raised.

Cornea: Clear or hazy due to epithelial edema depending on the IOP.

Iris: Presence of neovascularization can be seen (**Fig. 1**). A careful examination of the iris and angle of the AC is essential before the pupil is dilated and any drops are put in the eye. Slit-lamp examination under high magnification to look for neovascularization of the iris (NVI) or neovascularization of the angle (NVA); these are fine vessels over iris or angle resembling knuckles. Once the pupil is dilated, it may not be easy to find the NV.[1] During the early stages, NVI is essentially at the pupil margin and is very fine and delicate in character (**Fig. 1**). At times, new vessels may be seen in angles (NVA) on gonioscopy, while NVI is yet to appear; so it is essential to carry out gonioscopy in all such cases before pupillary dilatation (**Fig. 2**). These vessels in early stage are very fragile and can collapse by pressure of gonioprism. If the disease is caught at this stage, then development to NVG can be prevented by treating the underlying cause.

AC: The AC often shows the presence of flare and sometimes a few cells in the acute angle closure stage. There may be presence of hyphema also.

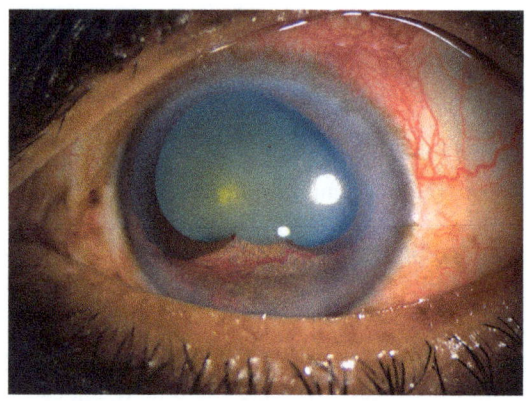

Fig. 1: Neovascularization of the iris.

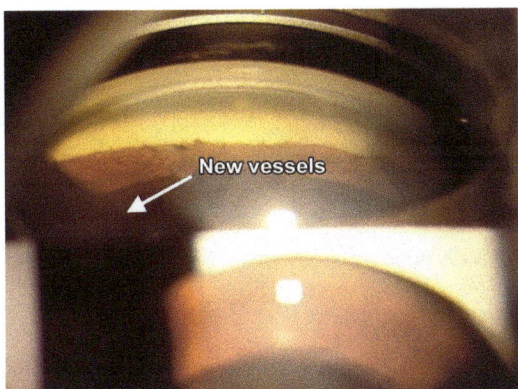

Fig. 2: Neovascularization of the angle.

Pupil: Following signs can be seen:
- Fine randomly oriented superficial vessels near pupillary margin in the initial stage
- Presence of ectropion uveae (in cases of progressive synechial angle closure)
- Pupillary reaction may be sluggish or absent or there may be relative afferent pathway defect (RAPD) depending upon the extent of optic nerve damage.

IOP: Markedly raised in angle closure stage.

Lens: Pseudophakia with or without posterior capsular dehiscence or aphakia are risk factors for NVI.

Fundus: Evidence of retinal ischemia in the form of CRVO, proliferative DR (PDR), BRAO, etc., maybe there.

Optic nerve head (ONH) damage depends upon the duration and severity of raised IOP.

It is important to remember that the disease process progresses through four stages and the symptoms and signs depend upon the stage at which the patient presents. The stages and the associated symptoms and signs have been described in **Table 1**.

■ DIFFERENTIAL DIAGNOSIS

Normal iris vessels: In some eyes, normal iris vessels are seen easily, particularly in blue eyes that may be mistaken for NVI or even NVA when the vessels are seen near the root of the iris.[1] Following points may help in differentiating:

- Iris vessels are present in stroma but new vessels are superficial.
- Iris vessels are radial in arrangement, unlike irregularly arranged new vessels.
- Sizes of iris vessels are uniform, new vessels are of varying sizes.
- Branching of new vessels is absent in iris vessels.
- New vessels are leaky as is found in fluorescein angiography or fluorophotometry.

In the *open angle stage*, NVG may have to be differentiated from other glaucoma of acute onset such as angle closure glaucoma and glaucoma with uveitis. NVG can be differentiated easily by the presence of rubeosis iridis in spite of the fact that eyes with uveitis may have dilated iris vessels.

In *angle closure stage*, when new vessels are less apparent, the condition has to be differentiated from other causes of iris distortion and peripheral anterior synechia, for example, old trauma or iridocorneal endothelial (ICE) syndrome.

■ MANAGEMENT

The treatment of NVG includes identifying the underlying etiology and its timely and adequate treatment to prevent the development and progression of NVG. Once NVG develops and IOP is high, the target is to control high IOP and prevent optic nerve damage in addition to treatment of underlying etiology.

Prophylactic Treatment

Panretinal photocoagulation (PRP): Mechanism is uncertain, but probably it acts by reducing oxygen demand. PRP is able to reverse IOP elevation in the open angle glaucoma stage and in early angle closure stage where synechial angle closure is not more than 270° yet.

Transscleral panretinal cryotherapy or anterior retinal cryopexy (ARC): When cloudy media preclude PRP.

Anti-VEGF agents: As an adjunctive treatment with PRP to reduce the VEGF load but has short lived effect and is not definitive.

Medical Management

Medical management consists of following:

Antiglaucoma drugs: Mainstay of medical treatment is to reduce aqueous production with

Table 1: Stages of neovascular glaucoma.

Stage	Characteristic	NVI/NVA	Symptoms	Other signs	IOP	Gonioscopy
Prerubeosis stage	Predisposing ocular/extraocular condition is present	Absent	Absent	Laser photometry or fluorescein iris angiography is helpful in detecting early leakage of iris vessels	Normal	Open angle
Preglaucoma stage	Rubeosis iridis stage	Present	Absent	Usually none	Normal	Open angle with early NVA
Open angle glaucoma stage	Florid rubeosis with leaky vessels	Florid	Present	Cells, flare, hyphema	Elevated	Open angle with florid NVA
Angle closure glaucoma stage	Contraction of fibrovascular membrane in the angle	New vessels become less apparent	Present	• Loss of visual acuity Ectropion uveae, flat smooth, glistening appearance of the iris • Conjunctival congestion • Corneal edema • Cells, flare, hyphae • Optic disc changes	Persistently high (>60 mm)	Variable PAS Sometime complete angle closure

(IOP: intraocular pressure; NVA: neovascularization of the angle; NVI: neovascularization of the iris; PAS: peripheral anterior synechiae)

topical beta-blockers, alpha-2 agonists, and with topical and/or oral carbonic anhydrase inhibitors. Mannitol (hyperosmotic agents) may also be required in cases of acute rise in IOP. Topical prostaglandin analogs and miotics are better avoided as they may increase ocular inflammation.

Anti-inflammatory drugs: Topical steroids and cycloplegics are recommended to reduce the inflammation that is often present.

Antiangiogenic drugs: Several studies propose the usefulness of anti-VEGF agents as an adjunct to traditional treatments such as PRP and additional surgery. Anti-VEGF agents (intracameral or intravitreal, or both simultaneously) have been used in following circumstances:
- As an adjunct to PRP or bevacizumab alone when visibility of the posterior segment is difficult due to opacities of the media (e.g., hemorrhage).
- Intracameral injection of bevacizumab may provide additional strategy for treating rubeosis iridis in NVG. Bevacizumab is well tolerated, effectively stabilizes NVI, and controls IOP when used alone and at an early open angle stage of NVG.
- In advanced cases of NVG, it can be used as a therapeutic window before PRP or surgical intervention (usually 1 week before but can be used within 14–48 hours also). It decreases the risk of failure, hemorrhage, and inflammation.
- In cases where PRP is not possible due to poor retinal view, intravitreal bevacizumab can be given followed by trabeculectomy with mitomycin C (MMC).

Remember
- Bevacizumab (most reported anti-VEGF in NVG) causes regression of the NVI within 24–48 hours following intravitreal injection whereas NVI starts regressing post PRP by 2 weeks and is complete by 4–6 weeks.[3]
- Most studies report similar dose for intravitreal and intracameral use (1.25 mg/0.05 mL).
- Medical management with anti-VEGF along with retinal ablation can control the IOP in the open angle stage of NVG only; in advanced

stage with synechial angle closure surgical intervention for IOP lowering is often required.

Surgical Management

The type of surgery depends upon level of IOP, presence of active or regressed NVI, prior laser or anti-VEGF treatment, prior intraocular surgeries, degree of inflammation, stage of disease, degree of angle closure, severity of glaucomatous optic neuropathy, and visual potential.[3] Following options are available:

- *Filtration surgery:* Success rate of trabeculectomy is poor if performed alone. It is usually combined with use of intraoperative MMC. Chance of success increases significantly when combined with preoperative bevacizumab and/or PRP (success rate may improve up to 95%).[3]
- *GDD surgery:* GDDs are often considered as a primary surgical procedure in the management of NVG where there is a high risk for failure of conventional filtering surgery. Various drainage devices such as Molteno implant, Baerveldt implant, and Ahmed glaucoma valve have been used in management of NVG and shown comparable results to trabeculectomy.
- *Cyclodestructive procedure:* These procedures are indicated in cases with refractory NVG with poor visual prognosis. Transscleral cyclophotocoagulation (TSCPC) with noncontact neodymium:yttrium-aluminum-garnet (Nd:YAG) or semiconductor diode laser cyclophotocoagulation (DLCP) have proven useful in treatment of such cases. Repeat treatment may be required to maintain good control of IOP.[3]
- *Other surgeries:* Endoscopic cyclophotocoagulation, intravitreal injection crystalline triamcinolone acetonide, and injection of silicon oil during revision of vitrectomy after unsuccessful vitreous surgery in diabetics.

VIVA QUESTIONS

Q.1. Name important causes of neovascular glaucoma.
Ans.
- *DR:* Most common cause of NVI. In fact, one-third of rubeotic cases have DR.
- *Retinal vascular occlusive diseases:* Second most common cause—ischemic CRVO, CRAO, BRVO, BRAO, sickle cell retinopathy
- *Extraocular diseases:* Carotid artery disease, ocular ischemia, giant cell arteritis, pulseless disease, and carotid-cavernous fistula
- *Assorted retinal diseases:* ROP, RD, Eale's disease, Coat's disease, PHPV, Norrie disease
- Trauma
- *Ocular neoplasms*: Malignant melanoma, retinoblastoma, and optic nerve glioma
- *Ocular inflammatory diseases:* Chronic uveitis, endophthalmitis, sympathetic ophthalmia, and Vogt-Koyanagi-Harada (VKH) disease
- *Ocular surgery:* Cataract extraction especially in diabetics, vitrectomy, and RD surgery

Note: Of all these causes, three most common causes are DR, ischemic CRVO, and ocular ischemic syndrome. In Indian set-up, chronic angle closure glaucoma is also an important cause of NVG.

Q.2. Where does neovascularization start?
Ans. At pupillary margin from capillaries of minor arterial circle.

Q.3. In what percentage of cases of NVG, NVA may be found in absence of NVI at the pupillary margin?
Ans. In approximately 12%.[1,3]

Q.4. How can we differentiate between normal iris vessels and new vessels?
Ans. Following points helps:
- Iris vessels are present in stromal, but new vessels are superficial.
- Iris vessels are radial in arrangement, unlike irregularly arranged new vessels.
- Sizes of iris vessels are uniform, new vessels are of varying sizes.
- Branching of new vessels is absent in iris vessels.
- New vessels are leaky as is found in fluorescein angiography or fluorophotometry.

Q.5. How do you identify NVA on gonioscopy?
Ans. New vessels extend from iris root across the ciliary body and sclera spur; arborize over the TM.

Q.6. What is hundred-day glaucoma?
Ans. NVG occurring after 3 months following CRVO.

Q.7. Describe the stages of NVG.
Ans. Stages of NVG are as follows (*See* **Table 1**)
- *Prerubeotic stage:* In patients with PDR and ischemic CRVO, neovascularization must be looked for carefully under high magnification on the iris and in the angle of the AC (NVA) at every visit. The iris should be examined before dilatation of the pupil and pupillary margins and margins of iridotomy should be carefully looked for new vessels.
- *Preglaucoma stage/rubeosis iridis:* Variable amounts of neovascularization (rubeosis) can be found at pupillary margin, iris surface, and in the angle. Characteristic features of this stage are normal IOP, unless pre-existing concomitant primary open-angle glaucoma (POAG)/primary angle-closure glaucoma (PACG) is present. Patients are usually asymptomatic at this stage unless the underlying condition produces symptoms like field loss due to CRVO or decreased vision due to vitreous hemorrhage or macular ischemia in DR.
- *Open angle glaucoma stage:* New vessels spreading and fibrovascular tissue covering angle. At this stage, IOP begins to rise and stays elevated. In some cases, the IOP may rise suddenly resulting in acute-onset glaucoma. Rubeosis iridis in this stage is more florid and is often associated with anterior chamber inflammatory reaction. Due to fragile nature of the new vessels, a hyphema can also present at this stage sometimes. Gonioscopy shows an open angle but with more intense neovascularization.
- *Angle-closure glaucoma stage:* Heavy neovascularization and extensive peripheral anterior synechia. Most patients present or are detected at this stage. In this stage, the contraction of fibrovascular membrane in the angle leads to progressive synechial angle closure, ectropion uveae, and flat, smooth, glistening appearance of the iris. Gonioscopy reveals varying degrees of peripheral anterior synechiae or complete angle closure may be present at this stage. The IOP is usually very high and can go up to 60 mm Hg. Conjunctival congestion and corneal edema are frequently present. Glaucomatous optic nerve damage is often moderate to advance. Visual acuity may also be severely affected.

Few authors include a regression stage characterized by total synechial angle closure and less visible vessels.

Q.8. How does surgery influence the occurrence of neovascularization?
Ans. Crystalline lens, posterior capsule, vitreous all act as mechanical barriers for angiogenic factors liberated by ischemic retina to reach anterior chamber. Vitrectomy, cataract surgery especially with disruption of posterior capsule removes this mechanical barrier and an increased risk of NVG.

Q.9. What are the theories behind neovasculogenesis in NVG?
Ans. Following factors play an important role in NVG:
- *Retinal hypoxia:* Stimulus for release of angiogenic factors
- *Angiogenesis factors:* VEGF with its several isoforms, angiogenin, and platelet-derived endothelial growth factor, transforming growth factor (TGF)-beta, tumor necrosis factor (TNF) alpha, and VEGF
- *Vasoinhibitory factors:* Vitreous and lens may be potential source of these factors; explains why NVG is more common following lensectomy and vitrectomy.

Q.10. What is the treatment for painful blind eye?
Ans. Cyclodestructive procedure (cryo or laser) if not relived then retrobulbar absolute alcohol injection, and if everything fails then enucleation.

REFERENCES

1. Hayreh SS. Neovascular Glaucoma. Prog Retin Eye Res. 2007;26(5):470-85.
2. Saito Y, Higashide T, Takeda H, Ohkubo S, Sugiyama K. Beneficial effects of preoperative intravitreal bevacizumab on trabeculectomy outcomes in neovascular glaucoma. Acta Ophthalmol. 2010;88(1):96-102.
3. Sharma P, Agarwal N, Choudhry RM. Neovascular glaucoma: a review. Delhi J Ophthalmol. 2016;26:170-5.

ANGLE RECESSION GLAUCOMA

Prakhar Goyal, Nitika Beri, Divya Agarwal, Talvir Sidhu

INTRODUCTION

Angle recession glaucoma is a secondary open angle glaucoma that is associated with blunt trauma to the eye. Angle recession is a tear between the longitudinal and circular muscles of the ciliary body. It is a gonioscopy diagnosis. Post-traumatic hyphema is strongly associated with angle recession (60–90%).[1,2]

HISTORY

Chief Complaints

The patient may present with following complaints:
- Deep set pain, redness, and gradually diminishing vision for distance (when associated with glaucoma)
- Onset can be immediately after injury or months to years after blunt trauma
- May be completely asymptomatic.

History of Past Illness

Patients presenting late with complaints of deep-seated ocular pain or other symptoms of raised IOP will give past history of trauma weeks or months back. The case may present years after the trauma when glaucoma occurs. Although eye trauma invariably occurs before angle recession, it is common to have forgotten details of the injury or even the entire episode after a number of years have passed.

EXAMINATION

General Examination/Specific Systemic Examination

Look for any signs of trauma especially scars around the eye.

Ocular Examination

Examination will show features of trauma along with angle recession which is diagnosed on gonioscopy.

Eyeball: Look for any associated signs of trauma such as orbital fracture, enophthalmos, and periocular scars.

Lid: In case of early presentation, lid edema or lid laceration may be present due to blunt trauma. Those presenting late may show scar of eyelid repair.

Conjunctiva: May be normal in delayed presentation. Presence of subconjunctival hemorrhage can be seen in acute cases.

Cornea: Following points must be noted:
- Stromal edema and pigment deposition on the endothelium and blood staining of the endothelium may be there in early onset cases.
- Long-standing cases, no abnormality can be seen.

Sclera: Partial or complete scleral tear may be associated in early presentation.

AC: Following points must be noted:
- Deep and irregular AC depth may be seen
- Hyphema in early onset

Iris: Look for other manifestations of blunt trauma such as:
- Iridodialysis (D-shaped pupil)/cyclodialysis
- Iris sphincter tears
- Iridoschisis

Pupil: Signs of trauma such as corectopia and traumatic mydriasis can be there.

IOP: IOP is raised when presents with glaucoma. A reduced IOP may be seen in early cases due to ciliary shock/ciliary shutdown.

Lens: Look for previous signs of trauma such as:
- Subluxated or dislocated lens
- Cataract may be present in some cases due to associated trauma
- Vossius ring

Vitreous: Vitreous hemorrhage may be present as a consequence of trauma.

Fundus: Following signs of trauma must be looked for:
- Retinal dialysis, RD, and subretinal hemorrhages
- Patients with long-standing raised IOP will show glaucomatous optic nerve changes and other features as seen in POAG.

Gonioscopy: In acute cases, gonioscopy examination should be deferred for at least 4–6 weeks after acute injury. Gonioscopy signs are as follows:
- Gonioscopy examination using 4-mirror Gonio lens shows asymmetry of angle recess if compared to nontraumatized eye or to other quadrants of same eye. Simultaneous, bilateral Koeppe gonioscopy is the most useful technique to detect subtle angle recession.
- Widening of the ciliary body band due to retrodisplacement of iris root is the most important gonioscopic findings of angle recession **(Fig. 1)**.
- Prominent scleral spur
- Irregular and darker pigmentation of angle
- Peripheral anterior synechiae.

■ DIFFERENTIAL DIAGNOSIS

Although diagnosis of angle recession glaucoma is evident on gonioscopy and optic disc examination, other differential diagnosis of *unilateral glaucoma* should be considered like:
- Pseudoexfoliation glaucoma (PXG)
- NVG
- Lens particle and phacolytic glaucoma should be considered and differentiated from angle recession.

■ MANAGEMENT

The treatment of angle recession glaucoma is discussed here.

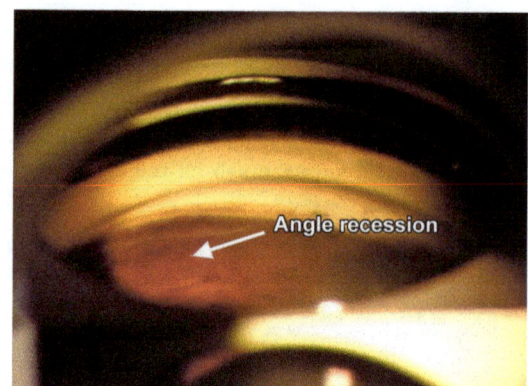

Fig. 1: Widening of the ciliary body band due to retrodisplacement of iris root.

Medical Management

In acute cases, treatment should be directed at lowering IOP and reducing inflammation by use of aqueous suppressants like topical beta-blockers such as timolol (0.5%) BD and/or alpha-2 agonists such as apraclonidine or brimonidine (0.2%). Topical cycloplegics such as atropine and steroids should be given for relief of pain and to reduce inflammation and possibly risk of secondary hemorrhage.

Laser Trabeculoplasty

It has found to be *ineffective* in angle in most cases due to distortion of angle anatomy and TM scarring. Nd:YAG laser trabeculopuncture has been found to be effective in some cases as shown in some studies where TM was intact on gonioscopy.

Filtration Surgeries

Trabeculectomy is effective in controlling IOP when used with antimetabolites; however, success rate is lower as compared to POAG. Use of glaucoma drainage devices has also limited benefits in angle recession glaucoma.

VIVA QUESTIONS

Q.1. What is the incidence of angle recession after blunt trauma?

Ans. Angle recession is reported to occur in 20–94% of eyes after blunt trauma. It is often masked initially due to the presence of concomitant hyphema, which results from shearing of the anterior ciliary arteries.[1]

Q.2. What are the chances of getting angle recession in a case of traumatic hyphema?

Ans. Angle recession may occur in 85% (range 71 to 100% of eyes) of the patients with traumatic hyphema.[1,2]

Q.3. What is the mechanism of angle recession?

Ans. Close globe injury causes anteroposterior globe compression with equatorial scleral expansion, limbal stretching, and posterior displacement of the lens/iris diaphragm. This may lead to the angle recession.

Q.4. What is the mechanism of glaucoma in angle recession?

Ans. Mainly due to trabecular damage and not the recession itself.

Q.5. What are the sources of traumatic hyphema?

Ans.
- Major arterial circle and branches of the ciliary body (most common, >90% cases)
- Choroidal arteries (rare)
- Ciliary body veins (very rare)
- Iris vessels at the pupillary margin or in the angle (very rare)

Q.6. What are the 7 rings of trauma?

Ans. This often refers to the seven commonly injured intraocular structures following contusion injury:
- Iris sphincter tear
- Iridodialysis
- Angle recession
- Cyclodialysis
- Tear in TM
- Zonular dialysis, subluxation, or dislocation of lens
- Retinal dialysis or tears

Q.7. What is the risk of glaucoma in angle recession?

Ans.
- Glaucoma is seen in only 5.5% (7 to 10%) of patients with angle recession.[1-3]
- An increased risk of glaucoma development was found if the angle recession exceeded 180°.
- Two peaks in incidences of glaucoma are seen, <1 year and at least 10 years after trauma. A 3.4% incidence of glaucoma after ocular contusion has been reported during a 6-month follow-up and up to 10% during the 10 years after trauma.[1,2]

Q.8. How to differentiate angle recession from cyclodialysis?

Ans. Ciliary muscle is torn between the longitudinal and circular layers in angle recession. The longitudinal or meridional ciliary muscle remains attached. This distinguishes recession from cyclodialysis, where the entire ciliary body including the longitudinal muscle is detached.

Q.9. What are the causes for early rise of IOP after blunt trauma?

Ans.
- Hyphema
- Inflammation
- Lens dislocation
- Uveal effusion
- Vitreous filling the anterior chamber
- Schwartz–Matsuo syndrome

REFERENCES

1. Girkin CA, McGwin G Jr, Long C, Morris R, Kuhn F. Glaucoma after ocular contusion: a cohort study of the United States eye injury registry. J Glaucoma. 2005;14(6):470-3.
2. Kaufman JH, Tolpin DW. Glaucoma after traumatic angle recession: a ten-year prospective study. Am J Ophthalmol. 1974;78(4):648-54.
3. Sihota R, Sood NN, Agarwal HC. Traumatic glaucoma. Acta Ophthalmol Scand. 1995;73(3):252-4.

STEROID-INDUCED GLAUCOMA

Vaishali Ghanshyam Rai, Talvir Sidhu, Nitika Beri

■ INTRODUCTION

A certain percentage of the general population responds to repeated instillation of topical corticosteroids with a variable increase in the IOP. Certain people do manifest this response to chronic steroid therapy, whether given by the topical, systemic, or periocular route, and the IOP elevation can lead to glaucomatous optic atrophy and loss of vision. Such a condition is referred to as steroid-induced glaucoma. Following 4–6 weeks of topical steroid administration, about 5% of the population will demonstrate a rise in IOP of >16 mm Hg and 30% will demonstrate a rise of 6–15 mm Hg.[1]

■ HISTORY

Chief Complaints

The clinical presentation and onset are highly variable. A patient may present with pain and gradually diminishing vision for distance or may be completely asymptomatic.

Past History

A patient may give history of long-term use of corticosteroids in any form such as topical, systemic, or local applications in the past. History of intravitreal triamcinolone acetonide (IVTA) or slow release intravitreal implant of dexamethasone such as Ozurdex is also important.

Risk factors for steroid-induced glaucoma include:
- Patients with POAG
- Family history of POAG
- Children below 10 years
- High myopia
- Diabetes mellitus
- Connective tissue disorder, for example, rheumatoid arthritis.

■ EXAMINATION

Ocular examination:
- Eyeball—normal
- Eyelids—usually normal, or may show eyelid skin atropy or ptosis with topical steroids
- Conjunctiva and sclera—usually normal
- Cornea—long-term topical steroid may cause increased corneal thickness or corneal ulcers
- Angle of anterior chamber—normal depth and contents
- Pupil—topical steroids use can cause mydriasis
- Lens—usually appears normal or may show posterior subcapsular cataract that is also a side effect long-term use corticosteroid
- Vitreous—normal
- Fundus—glaucomatous cupping of optic nerve
- IOP—with Goldmann's applanation tonometer may be normal due to discontinuation of steroid therapy in the past. IOP may be high in cases of intravitreal steroid implants or patient currently on any steroid medication.
- Gonioscopy with four mirror Gonio lens reveals open angles in all quadrants.

■ DIFFERENTIAL DIAGNOSIS

Primary Open-Angle Glaucoma

- Usually bilateral with high IOP. Steroid-induced glaucoma can be unilateral or bilateral depending upon steroids used with normal or high IOP.
- History of steroid intake:
  – Uveitic glaucoma
  – Normal tension glaucoma—usually bilateral with thin cornea with normal IOP
  – Glaucomatocyclytic crisis—usually unilateral with other uveitis signs such as circumciliary congestion, keratic precipitates on corneal endothelium, and AC reaction with raised IOP
  – Primary juvenile open-angle glaucoma.

■ MANAGEMENT

- Stop the responsible steroid medication, in majority of cases raised IOP comes to normal levels within few weeks to months.
- In refractory cases with advanced glaucomatous optic nerve, damage management

- would be cessation of steroids and starting antiglaucoma medication to reduce IOP.
- Glaucoma following IVTA needs to be managed with antiglaucoma medication till the intravitreal steroid crystals resolve, that is, 6 months.
- Intractable glaucoma following intravitreal steroid depot may be treated by removal of depot through pars plana vitrectomy combined with trabeculectomy.
- Substitute potent steroid with lower potency steroid where complete cessation of steroid for medical condition is not possible. Lower potency steroids such as phosphate form prednisolone and dexamethasone, rimexolone, and loteprednol etabonate or fluorometholone can be used to substitute potent steroids.
- Steroids can also be substituted with nonsteroidal anti-inflammatory drugs such as diclofenac, nepafenac, or ketorolac.
- Other steroid-sparing agents are immunosuppressants such as tacrolimus ointment or cyclosporine for vernal keratoconjunctivitis or methotrexate can be used in uveitis or systemic conditions.
- *Laser trabeculoplasty:* Argon laser trabeculoplasty or selective laser trabeculoplasty can be considered where medical treatment failed to control the IOP or patient is intolerant to medical treatment or in cases where filtering surgery is precluded due to systemic condition.
- *Trabeculectomy:* With or without antimetabolites is indicated in patients whom both medical and laser treatments fail to control IOP.
- Prevention of steroid-induced glaucoma:
  - By regular monitoring of patients on steroids for IOP, check every 2 weeks.
  - Avoid topical steroids wherever possible by using alternatives.
  - Use of lower potent steroids such as fluorometholone or loteprednol.

VIVA QUESTIONS

Q.1. Define steroid-induced glaucoma.
Ans. Steroid-induced glaucoma is a form of open angle glaucoma occurring as an adverse effect exogenous corticosteroid therapy or excess endogenous production of glucocorticoids.

Q.2. What is the average time taken for IOP rise in different routes of steroid administration?
Ans. *See* **Table 1**.

Q.3. Explain the mechanism of steroid-induced glaucoma.
Ans. Corticosteroids cause IOP elevation by increasing the outflow resistance and thereby decreasing the facility of aqueous outflow. The main mechanisms of steroid-induced glaucoma are as follows:
- Stabilization of lysosomal membranes, leading to accumulation of polymerized glycosaminoglycan (GAG).
- Alteration of the composition of the extracellular matrix through which aqueous flows, thereby increasing resistance to outflow.
- Increased production of collagen, elastin, laminin, and fibronectin within TM and resulting in increased in TM resistance.
- Inhibition of phagocytosis activity of endothelial cells lining the TM and leading to accumulation of debris in the TM.
- Decreased production of extracellular proteinase such as fibrinolytic enzymes, stromolysin, and matrix metalloproteinases.
- Inhibition of the production of outflow-enhancing prostaglandins such as PGF2α.

Q.4. Name the gene associated with steroid-induced glaucoma.
Ans. Many genes associated with steroid-induced glaucoma are myocin, optineurin, antichymotrypsin, pigment epithelium-derived factor, cornea-derived transcript 6, prostaglandin D2 synthase, decorin, insulin-like growth factor binding protein 2, ferritin light chain, and fibulin-1C. Myocilin gene (previously known as the TM inducible glucocorticoid response or *TIGR* gene) is the most studied among these.[1,2]

Table 1: Average time taken for intraocular pressure (IOP) rise in different routes of steroid administration.

Route	Average dose	Average time taken for IOP rise
Oral	25 mg hydrocortisone/day 50 mg prednisolone/day	1 year 2–15 months
Inhalational	Most of steroid inhalers	3 months
Pulse steroids	140 mg repeated 4 weekly	6 months
Dermatological	Betamethasone cream 0.1%	3 months
Topical	QID doses of potent steroid	2–6 weeks
IVTA	4 mg	4–8 week
Posterior subtenon	40 mg of triamcinolone acetonide	5–9 weeks

(IVTA: intravitreal triamcinolone acetonide)

Table 2: Becker and Armaly studies.

Parameters	Becker	Armaly
Frequency	QID	TDS
Duration	6 weeks	4 weeks
Parameter	Final IOP	IOP change
Type of responder		
Low	<20 mm Hg	<6 mm Hg
Intermediate	20–30 mm Hg	6–15 mm Hg
High	>31 mm Hg	>15 mm Hg

(IOP: intraocular pressure)

Table 3: Intraocular pressure elevation in different type of steroids.

Type of steroid	Mean intraocular pressure rise (in mm Hg)
Dexamethasone 0.1%	22
Prednisolone 1.0%	10
Dexamethasone 0.005%	8
Fluorometholone 0.1%	6
Hydrocortisone 0.5%	3
Tetrahydrotriamcinolone 0.25%	2

Q.5. Name two landmark studies done on steroid-induced glaucoma. What findings were demonstrated in those studies?

Ans. Becker and Armaly studies. The findings have been described in **Table 2**.

Q.6. Low-potency steroid and risk of glaucoma.

Ans. Different low potency steroids are phosphate forms prednisolone 0.1% and rimexolone 1%, loteprednol etabonate 0.5%, or fluorometholone 0.1%. Risk of glaucoma after use of low-potency steroid has not been studied in detail. However, the general agreement is that the risk is very less.

Q.7. IOP elevation in different types of steroids.

Ans. See **Table 3**.[2]

■ **REFERENCES**

1. Jones R 3rd, Rhee DJ. Corticosteroid-induced ocular hypertension and glaucoma: a brief review and update of the literature. Curr Opin Ophthalmol. 2006;17(2):163-7.
2. Kersey JP, Broadway DC. Corticosteroid-induced glaucoma: a review of the literature. Eye (Lond). 2006;20(4):407-16.

PSEUDOEXFOLIATION GLAUCOMA

Ashi Gupta, Vaishali Ghanshyam Rai, Dewang Angmo

■ INTRODUCTION

Pseudoexfoliative syndrome (PXF) is a systemic condition characterized by the deposition of white powdery or fluffy material within the anterior segment of the eye including lens, angle, pupil, and cornea. The deposits are most notable on the anterior lens capsule. PXF can cause secondary open angle glaucoma, which is more aggressive in its clinical course with high IOP at onset, progresses at a faster rate, and responds poorly to medical therapy, compared to POAG. PXG is seen in up to 50% of eyes with PXF.[1,2]

Capsular delamination or true exfoliation is the separation of superficial layers of lens capsule from the deeper capsular layers to form scroll-like margins, which occasionally float in the AC as thin, clear membranes. This condition was described in glassblowers as a result of excessive infrared radiation.

■ HISTORY

Epidemiology

Pseudoexfoliative syndrome is seen worldwide with a high prevalence in Scandinavian countries. Incidence varies between 1.5 and 27%. Its incidence increases with age. It is commonly seen after the age of 40 years. Few studies suggest a female preponderance, however it is still debated.[1,2]

Chief Complaints

Patient may present with the following complaints:
- Pain and redness usually unilateral
- Gradually diminishing vision for distance
- Patient may be completely asymptomatic. The majority of patients are asymptomatic, and PXF is often an incidental finding.

■ EXAMINATION

Ocular Examination

- Eyeball—usually normal or may be deep seated as patients with pseudoexfoliation are usually present in 7–8th decade. Relative anterior microphthalmos (normal axial length but anterior segment is smaller) may also be there.
- Eyelid—normal
- Conjunctiva—may be normal or ciliary congestion can be there in presence of raised IOP
- Cornea—small whitish powdery flakes or clumps may be found on corneal endothelium. Early corneal endothelial decompensation is common with PXF syndrome (*Fuchs like keratopathy*). Corneal guttata may also be found; the exact cause of which is not known. Pigment can be observed dispersed on the endothelium. The pigment is believed to arise from disruption of iris pigment epithelium secondary to frictional interaction with PXF material on the lens capsule.[2]
- *AC*: AC may be shallow in pseudoexfoliation syndrome. Small pigments can be appreciated floating in AC. PXF syndrome has been associated with a disrupted blood-aqueous barrier. Testing with a flare meter demonstrated markedly increased flare in comparison with POAG.[2] The zonulopathy can also lead to anterior displacement of the lens, that is, a phacomorphic narrowing, with intermittent pupillary block.
- *Iris and pupil:* Iris and pupil examination can reveal following signs:
  - Small flecks of PXF material "(dandruff like)" deposits can be seen on the pupillary margin, which is a hallmark of PXF syndrome.
  - There may be flakes deposits on iris crypts and folds.
  - Transillumination defect can be appreciated in the pupillary margin resulting from atrophic and/or fibrotic changes in the iris sphincter muscle. The pupillary margin of the iris is also affected with loss of the pupillary ruff. These changes collectively result in what is described as a "moth eaten" pupil margin.[2]

- Look for iridodonesis, which is common in PXF syndrome.
- Sphincter muscle degeneration and posterior synechiae are also seen.
- *Pupil:* Usually poor mydriasis (atrophic and/or fibrotic changes in the iris sphincter muscle) and asymmetric pupil is seen in PXF.
- *Lens:* Following signs can be seen:
  - Whitish powdery ring deposit on anterior lens capsule is more consistent and diagnostic sign of PXF **(Fig. 1)**.
  - *Target sign:* The deposition is observed in three distinct zones—a central zone of material deposition, clear intermediate zone (secondary to iris excursion rubbing the PXF material off), and a peripheral zone of PXF material **(Figs. 2 and 3)** outside of this intermediate zone. The central zone may be absent in 20% of cases of PXF and the peripheral granular zone can only be observed with dilation.[2] Clinically, three distinct zones can be found on the anterior lens capsule on dilated pupil and two concentric rings of powdery deposits with central translucent zone.
  - Cataractous lens, nuclear sclerosis is more common with PXF. Asymmetric nuclear cataract formation can be there.
  - Look for phacodonesis.
  - Often associated with hard nuclear cataracts.
  - In advanced stage, there can be subluxated or dislocated cataractous lens due to weak zonules.
- *Fundus:* Unilateral glaucomatous cupping of optic disc with diffuse neuroretinal rim damage if media is clear. In cases of mature cataract, needs to get B-scan to see optic nerve head and retina status.
- *IOP:* Measured with Goldmann applanation tonometer shows >21 mm Hg. Usually mean IOP in a PXF patient is more than that of POAG cases. 40% of pseudoexfoliation syndrome patients will develop glaucoma or ocular hypertension.
- *Gonioscopy:* Shows characteristic increased pigmentation of TM, more prominent in superior quadrant, and usually unilateral. Dark, dense, and uneven wavy pigmentation

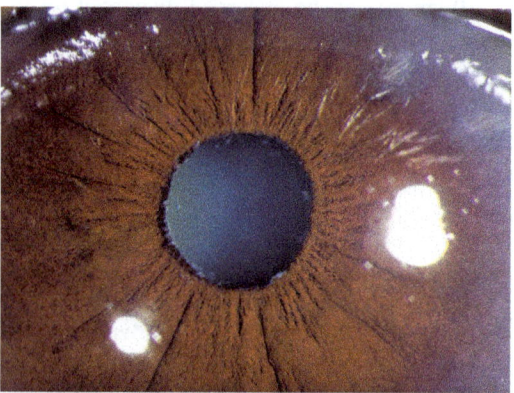

Fig. 1: Whitish powdery ring deposit on anterior lens capsule and pupillary margin.

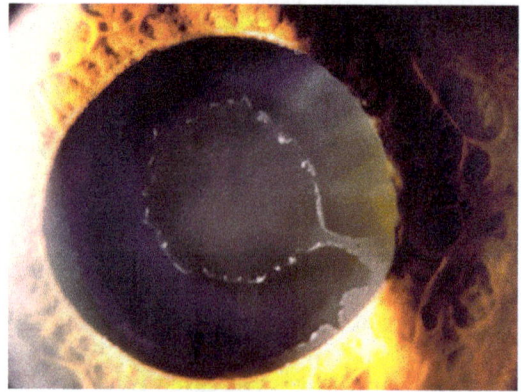

Fig. 2: Peripheral zone of pseudoexfoliative syndrome (PXF) material over lens capsule.

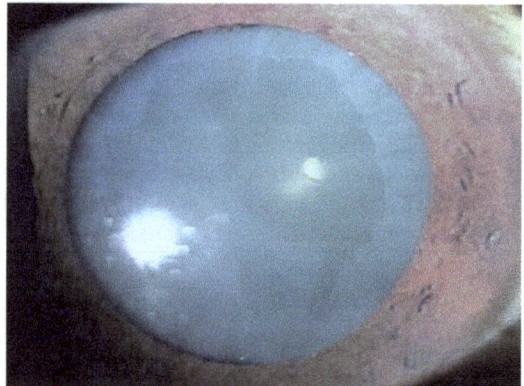

Fig. 3: Peripheral ring of target sign.

along the Schwalbe's line (*Sampaolesi line*) is also seen in PXF. This finding is not exclusive to PXF (also seen in pigment dispersion syndrome and chronic inflammation).[2] In 9–18% angle is occludable in pseudoexfoliation syndrome.[2]

DIFFERENTIAL DIAGNOSIS

A case of PXF has to be differentiated from other forms as discussed here.

Pigmentary Glaucoma

- Common in young age group
- Usually bilateral
- Transpupillary defect is common in midperipheral area of the iris
- Prominent uniform dark pigmentation band of TM is a characteristic feature of pigmentary glaucoma.

True Exfoliation

- Characterized by thin clear membrane like material separating from anterior lens capsule
- Glaucoma is infrequently associated with true exfoliation
- Underlying pathology can be anterior uveitis or exposure to UV rays.

Primary Amyloidosis

- Generalized systemic disorder with numerous ocular manifestations along with glaucoma
- Bilateral ocular involvement is common
- Fine whitish powdery deposits throughout the eye are a characteristic feature.

POAG: Differentiation table in viva questions.

PACG: Can be differentiated by characteristic clinical signs.

Uveitic glaucoma: AC reaction and other signs of uveitis are absent.

INVESTIGATIONS

- Diurnal variation of IOP
- Baseline perimetry
- RNFL imaging
- Specular biomicroscopy shows reduced endothelial cell count
- A-scan biometry for axial length and keratometry
- B-scan ultrasonography in case of hazy media to evaluate retina.

MANAGEMENT

The medical management is similar to that of POAG, including beta-blockers, alpha-adrenergic agonists, carbonic anhydrase inhibitors, or prostaglandin analogs. Monotherapy is usually insufficient to control IOP in PXG so combination therapy is advisable.

Argon/selective laser trabeculectomy is a successful and well-established procedure for reducing IOP in PXG-associated with open angles. Trabeculectomy is indicated when medical or laser therapy has failed to obtain target IOP or when there is progressive of glaucoma.

Combined trabeculectomy and cataract surgery are indicated in PXG with intractable IOP with cataract. Common complications anticipated during combined surgery in PXG are as follows **(Table 1)**:

- Poor dilation of pupil
- Zonular dialysis and vitreous loss
- Dislocation or decentration IOL
- Corneal decompensation
- Postoperative ocular inflammation.

VIVA QUESTIONS

Q.1. What is Sampaolesi line?

Ans. In PXG cases on gonioscopy, a dark, dense, and uneven wavy pigmentation along the Schwalbe's line is known as Sampaolesi line.

Q.2. What are the complications anticipated during cataract surgery in PXG cases?

Ans.
- Poor dilation of pupil
- Zonular dialysis and vitreous loss
- Dislocation or decentration IOL
- Corneal decompensation
- Heightened postoperative inflammation
- Postoperative IOP elevation
- Late intraocular lens implant decentration and prolapse into the posterior segment
- Posterior synechiae and pupillary block.

Table 1: Difficulties and precaution during cataract surgery.

Difficulty	Precaution
Poorly dilating pupil	• Atropine • Stretch the pupil with instruments • Iris hooks • Pupil expansion rings
Endotheliopathy	• Viscoadaptive (Healon 5 or Visco-dispersive viscoelastic (Viscoat) • Ashrinoff's soft-shell technique
Weak zonules	• Chopping techniques or prolapse the lens nucleus out of the capsular bag during phaco • Traditional extracapsular surgery • Capsular tension ring (CTR) • 3-piece intraocular lens implant (IOL)
Postoperative inflammation	Aggressively with postoperative steroids and perhaps for a longer duration
Postoperative pressure spikes	Postoperative Diamox
Capsular phimosis	Nd-YAG laser, placing relaxing incisions in the anterior lens capsule at the four cardinal positions

Table 2: Differentiation between pseudoexfoliative glaucoma (PXG) and primary open angle glaucoma (POAG).

	POAG	PXG
Age of onset	40–50 years	>60 years
Vision loss	Less marked	Marked due to presence of nuclear sclerosis
IOP	>21 mm Hg	High IOP >40 mm Hg
Laterality	Bilateral	Usually, unilateral
Anterior segment	Usually normal	White powdery deposits on pupillary margin, on lens capsule with weak zonules. Subluxated or dislocated lens can be seen
Anterior chamber	Normal	May be normal or shallow Flare may be present
Gonioscopy	Open angle	Marked blotchy pigmentation of trabecular meshwork. Sampaolesi line is characteristic
Disc	Focal or diffuse RNFL defect depending on early or late presentation	Usually, diffuse RNFL defect
Severity of glaucoma	Less	More
Response to therapy	Good	Poor
Surgery	May be required	Often required

(IOP: intraocular pressure; RNFL: retinal nerve fiber layer)

Q.3. How do you differentiate between PXG and POAG?
Ans. *See* Table 2.

Q.4. Cause of zonular weakness in PXF.
Ans. The exact cause is not known; however, the possible mechanisms include following:[2]

- PXF material directly induce zonular damage.
- Accumulation of PXF material at the origin of the zonules on pre-equatorial regions of the lens disrupts zonular architecture.

Table 3: Differential diagnosis.

Parameters	Pigment dispersion	Pseudoexfoliation
Demographics	• 30–50 years • Men • Related to myopia • White race	• 60 years • Men and women • Related to aortic aneurysms (abnormal basement membrane) • Scandinavian countries
Pathomechanism	• Posterior bowing of the iris • Constant rubbing of posterior iris and zonules • *Release of pigments* • Trabecular block	• Systemic disease of *abnormal basement membrane* (skin, viscera, eyes) • Secretion of amyloid like material (oxytalon) in AC • Deposit in trabeculum and zonules • Trabecular block
Clinical features	• Krukenberg's spindle • Deep AC with posterior bowing of iris *(reverse pupillary block)* • Iris atrophy in periphery of iris • Pigment deposit on lens *(Zentmayer's line)*	• White powdery deposits on pupillary margin (pseudoexfoliative material), on lens capsule *(Target sign)* with weak zonules • Subluxated or dislocated lens can be seen • Poorly dilating pupil • Iris atrophy at edge of pupil margin
Gonioscopy	• Heavily pigmented angle • Queer iris pigmentation	• Marked blotchy pigmentation of trabecular meshwork • *Sampaolesi line* is characteristic • Pseudoexfoliative material

(AC: anterior chamber)

- Intrinsic differences between normal and PXF zonules because PXF zonules are composed of modified forms of zonular fibers.

Q.5. How do you differentiate between PXG and pigment dispersion syndrome (PDS)?

Ans. *See* **Table 3**.

Q.6. What are the newer drugs in PXS and PXG?

Ans. Topical latrunculin B is believed to affect the cytoskeleton integrity of TM, acts by increasing aqueous outflow facility by inhibiting cell contractility without any effects on the cornea, and is a new promising agent.

Q.7. Which gene is associated with PXG?

Ans. *LOX1* gene is the most common gene associated with exfoliation syndrome.

■ REFERENCES

1. Stamper R, Lieberman M, Drake M (Eds). Primary open angle glaucoma. Becker-Shaffer's Diagnosis and Therapy of the Glaucomas, 8th edition. New York: Mosby; 2009. pp. 239-65.
2. Desai MA, Lee RK. The medical and surgical management of pseudoexfoliation glaucoma. Int Ophthalmol Clin. 2008;48(4):95-113.

CHAPTER 4

Retina

LONG CASES

VITREOUS HEMORRHAGE

Ritu Nagpal, Ashi Gupta, Shipra Singhi, Brijesh Takkar

■ INTRODUCTION

Vitreous hemorrhage (VH) is defined as the presence of extravasated blood within the space outlined by the internal limiting membrane of the retina posteriorly and laterally, the nonpigmented epithelium of the ciliary body laterally, and the lens zonular fibers and posterior lens capsule anteriorly.[1] The incidence of VH is seven cases per 100,000; which makes it one of the most common causes of acutely or subacutely decreased vision. Such cases are a common reason for surgery and a favorite for long cases. During the work-up, the focus should be on identifying the cause of VH.

■ HISTORY

Chief Complaints

The symptoms of VH are varied but usually include:
- Early or mild hemorrhage cases present with floaters, which the patient describes as cobwebs, ring shadows, multiple insects moving in front of the eye, smoke signals, dark clouds, or even a red hue.
- In severe cases, sudden onset painless unilateral visual loss is the usual complaint (most common presentation). Patients often say vision is worse in the morning as blood has settled to the back of the eye, covering the macula.
- Hemorrhage that is more significant can cause visual field (VF) defects or scotomas.

History of Present Illness

Presentation can be unilateral or bilateral. It may be rapidly progressive. Preceding events such as trauma, Valsalva maneuver, recent surgery or recent retinal laser therapy must be recorded. Many a times the patients would give a history suggestive of the cause of VH, e.g., recurrent pain and redness symptoms of (S/O) uveitis or visual field loss S/O retinal vein occlusion (RVO)/ glaucoma or central scotoma in age-related macular degeneration (ARMD). Scotomas remain fixed in the field whereas generally floaters move with eye movement.[1]

History of Past Illness

History of trauma, diabetes, hypertension, tumor (hemangioma, retinoblastoma, melanoma, and retinal angioma), Valsalva maneuver, shaken baby syndrome, venous occlusion, bleeding disorder, leukemia, ocular surgery (glaucoma surgery, RD surgery, cataract surgery), laser [panretinal photocoagulation (PRP)], vasculitis, chest compression, pseudotumor cerebri must be asked as it may provide a clue to the underlying cause.

Recurrent VH may point toward Eales' disease, PDR, or bleeding diathesis. History from the fellow eye may also be suggestive of ocular predisposition to VH. In cases of trauma, it is necessary to classify as per Birmingham Eye Trauma Terminology System (BETTS), to prognosticate as such cases can often be medicolegal.

Family History

Family history of diabetes, hypertension, bleeding disorder, leukemia, tumor, and vacuities must be recorded.

Past Surgical History

A detailed past ocular surgery must be noted.

Medical History

Medical history of diabetes mellitus (DM), systemic hypertension, drug intake, sickle cell disease, anemia, bleeding diathesis, and cerebral stroke can give a valuable clue even before ocular examination.

■ EXAMINATION

Systemic Examination

Systemic examination is important in the case of VH to rule out the above-mentioned causes. It is especially important in cases of vascular occlusion since there may be some cardiology or associated intracranial events that need immediate attention by a general physician. Similarly, it is not uncommon to discover signs of hematological disorder in patients with unexplained VH. It becomes more important when the disease or causation cannot be localized to the eye.

Ocular Examination

Visual Acuity

Recording of VA of either eye is necessary. The status of the other eye often guides the management plan.

Eyeball

Usually, normal. It may be large in the case of high myopia. Proptosis may be in cases of tumor (axial in cavernous hemangioma).

Lid

Usually, normal.

Conjunctiva

Multiple hemorrhages in the conjunctiva may be there. Conjunctival microvascular abnormality in sickle cell disease *"the comma sign"* is pathognomonic but its pathogenesis remains obscure. In such cases, corkscrew vessels are seen. Similarly, in heart disease conjunctiva may reveal vascular tortuosity or in rare cases bulbar telangiectasia.

Cornea

May be large and corneal thinning may be there in myopes.

Sclera

Scleral thinning may be there (blue sclera in collagen vascular disease).

Anterior Chamber

Keratic precipitates, cells, and flare may be present in inflammatory diseases. The deep anterior chamber (AC) is seen in high myopic eyes. There may be signs of angle closure glaucoma (ACG).

Iris

Iridodialysis, neovascularization of iris (NVI), or neovascularization of angle (NVA) may be there. This is extremely important, as it is prognostic and diagnostic.

Pupil

The presence of relative afferent pupillary defect points unequivocally to an underlying retinal detachment (RD), retinal vascular occlusion, and large macular lesion or optic nerve disease.

Intraocular Pressure

An intraocular pressure (IOP) <9 mm Hg or >22 mm Hg needs to be investigated and explained. A hypotonic globe would suggest RD, a wound leak, or an open globe injury (occult or obvious). Raised increased IOP could be due to neovascular glaucoma (NVG), hemolytic glaucoma, corticosteroid usage, or tumor invasion under conditions of VH.

Gonioscopy

Neovascularization of angle can be seen in cases of PDR, angle recession or cyclodialysis may be there in case of blunt trauma.

Lens

The following points must be noted subluxation, dislocation, zonular dialysis, phacodonesis, and traumatic cataract presence of all these points toward trauma as the underlying cause of VH.

Anterior Vitreous

The presence of vitreous pigments or *Shaffer's sign*, are commonly seen in the presence of an RD but rarely also in the cases of a trauma. The presence of red blood cells (RBCs) or hemosiderin pigments can be typically there. Importantly, retrolental cells may also be seen, their presence however is not specific for uveitis.

Fundus

Posterior vitreous detachment (PVD) can cause VH. If PVD is there scleral, depression is mandatory to rule out a peripheral retinal break. It is important to remember that an acute PVD with VH has up to 70% incidence of retinal tears, compared to a low incidence in acute PVD without VH. Other findings to look for include neovascularization elsewhere (NVE), disc neovascularization (NVD), wet ARMD, DR, familial exudative vitreoretinopathy (FEVR), retinopathy of prematurity (ROP), retinal vasculitis, signs of trauma proliferative sickle cell retinopathy, venous occlusion, retinal macroaneurysm, choroidal melanoma, and angioma. The presence of fresh red hemorrhage mixed with old bleeding is suggestive of recurrent bleeding and indicates retinal neovasculopathy. In old hemorrhage, one should look for the presence of fibrotic clots. The presence of diffuse whitish opacity should indicate the possibility of other causes of media opacity, other than blood. Specific fundus features of individual diseases may be there (see viva section).

Different Forms of Vitreous Hemorrhage

Hemorrhage into Berger's space (retrolental space of Erggelet) and the Canal of Petit (except for the Canal of Hannover) or in a space generated by a PVD (retrohyaloid or subhyaloid hemorrhage) are also considered VH.[1] *Blood within Berger's* space settles down and forms a crescent-shaped pool with the hyaloideocapsular ligament as its inferior border. *Hemorrhage into the Canal of Petit* also has a crescent-shaped superior border, which is also formed by the hyaloideocapsular ligament. *Blood in Cloquet's* canal—outlines its inferior border and, *Blood in the retrohyaloid space*—generated by a vitreous detachment (retro- or subhyaloid hemorrhage) can collect as a meniscus at the inferior vitreoretinal demarcation. A clinically similar appearance is caused by a hemorrhage into the space between the internal limiting membrane and the nerve fiber layer (subinternal limiting membrane hemorrhage). In the latter type of hemorrhage, the blood is under tension and does not shift with changes in the position of the patient's head, as observed in subhyaloid hemorrhage. Subinternal limiting membrane hemorrhage has been described in penetrating ocular injury, Terson's syndrome, anemia, Valsalva maneuver-induced retinopathy, shaken baby syndrome, retinal macroaneurysm, diabetic retinopathy, and branch retinal vein occlusion (BRVO).[1]

In contrast to the abovementioned types of hemorrhage into defined vitreous spaces, bleeding into the vitreous gel (intravitreal hemorrhage) shows no characteristic borders and rapidly clots.

Visual acuity with vitreous VH and retained macular function is primarily determined by the location and density of the hemorrhage. Only small amounts of blood are necessary to cause a substantial reduction in visual acuity. Around 12.5 pL of diffuse blood in a 5 mL aphakic or 10 pL of diffuse blood in a 4 mL phakic vitreous cavity may decrease the visual acuity to hand motions.[1]

Natural Course of Vitreous Hemorrhage

There are certain unique biochemical features of the vitreous in catabolism of blood-like rapid clot formation, slow lysis of fibrin, persistence of intact red blood cells for months and lack of early polymorphonuclear response, extracellular lysis of red blood cells, spontaneous clearance is more common in diseases, which have no recurrent bleeding, syneresis of vitreous gel, and in elderly and aphakic patients. The VH does not clear as spontaneously in patients with diabetic retinopathy, longstanding VH, with an *ochre membrane* (the accumulated red cells and red cell debris suspended in and mixed with vitreous collagen). Complications that can occur must be looked for, such as hemosiderosis bulbi, RD, glial and fibrovascular proliferation, glaucoma (ghost cell, hemolytic, and hemosiderotic), hyphema, and staining of ocular structures.

Fellow Eye

Evaluation of the fellow eye can often help in the diagnosis of VH. The common conditions of the fellow eye that help speculate the cause of VH in the affected eye include diabetic retinopathy, hypertensive retinopathy, ARMD, myopic changes, lattice, vitreous condensation, retinal white without pressure (WWOP) changes, retinal tear, retinal hole, giant retinal tear, peripheral retina breaks/RD, retinal vasculitis (including Eales' disease), ocular ischemic syndrome (OIS), venous occlusions, FEVR, and retinoschisis. We should also look for any RD in the fellow eye.

Fundus Findings in Eales' Disease

Retinal phlebitis—characterized by midperipheral venous dilation, perivascular exudates along the peripheral veins, and superficial retinal hemorrhages. Vascular sheathing ranges from thin white lines limiting the blood column on both sides to segmental heavy exudative sheathing. Peripheral nonperfusion—fine solid white lines retaining configuration of normal retinal vasculature as a remnant of obliterated large vessels, sharply demarcated junction between the anterior peripheral nonperfusion and the posterior perfused retina, vascular abnormalities at the junction between the perfused and nonperfused zones such as microaneurysm, venovenous shunts, venous beading, and occasionally hard exudates, and cotton-wool spots can be seen. Neovascularization: NVE, NVD, recurrent VH, proliferative changes, and TRD. The macula is usually not involved, but when it does, it is termed central Eales' disease. In this variant, all midperipheral lesions appear in the posterior pole and cause loss of vision in the early stage of the disease **(Fig. 1)**. Sea fan new vessels may be there.[1,2]

Differential Diagnosis

These are causes of media opacity and true for old white VH:
- Vitritis
- Amyloidosis
- Lymphoma
- Asteroid hyalosis
- Vitreous degeneration
- Leukemic vitreous infiltration

■ INVESTIGATIONS

Systemic

It is based on the disorder being suspected.

Laboratory Tests

Blood sugar, complete hemogram, coagulation profile, erythrocyte sedimentation rate (ESR), C-reactive protein (CRP), peripheral blood smear,

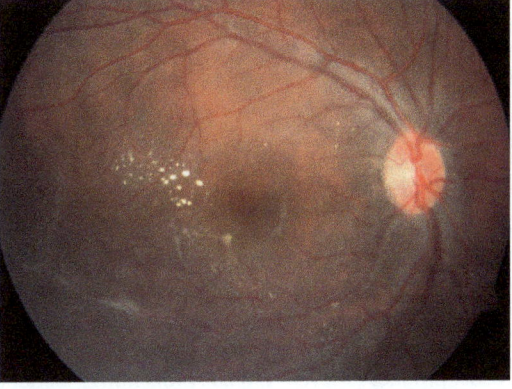

Fig. 1: Central Eales disease.
Note: Sheathing of the major vascular arcade with macular edema.

enzyme-linked immunosorbent assay (ELISA), venereal disease research laboratory (VDRL), Mantoux carotid Doppler scan, electrocardiogram (ECG), chest X-ray, and echocardiography.

Fundus Fluorescein Angiography/ Indocyanine Green

Once media is partially or totally clear angiography can be done for deciding on the management or diagnoses.

Ultrasound

An ultrasound (USG) is extremely important in the management of media haze-related cases. Multiple scans must be taken including transverse and longitudinal just like in a screening USG. If the whole or a part of the underlying retina is obscured due to VH, USG B scans with corresponding A-scan are mandatory to detect any associated RD/mass lesion. During the scan, emphasis should be on three sites: (1) The vitreous cavity, (2) the vitreoretinal interface, and (3) the retinochoroidal layer. With USG, it is possible to differentiate between fresh and clotted hemorrhage. Unclotted hemorrhage with no cellular clumps may not be visible ultrasonically. Asteroid hyalosis is one condition that may appear similar to clotted VH on a B-scan. It allows determination of the location and density of the VH, the location and extent of traction membranes and RD **(Fig. 2)**, and the

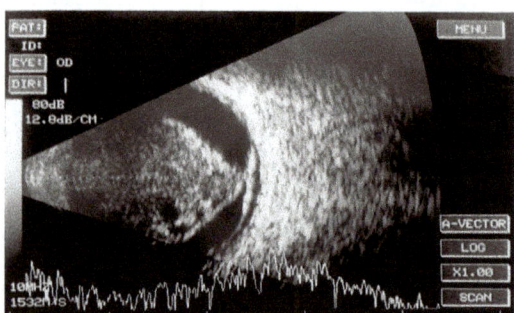

Fig. 2: USG showing VH with TRD in a case of PDR. The membrane persisted on low gain and had poor after-movements. Ruling out RD is necessary as it affects visual prognoses severely. (PDR: proliferative diabetic retinopathy; RD: retinal detachment; TRD: tractional retinal detachment; USG: ultrasound; VH: vitreous hemorrhage)

vitreoretinal relationship, all of which may help to predict the visual outcome after vitreous surgery. The status of PVD and its differentiation from RD is necessary. Rarely retinal breaks may also be picked up.

Some patients may need repeated retinal evaluation and serial ultrasonography in 7–10 days to reaffirm the cause and again rule out any RD/retinal break that would warrant an early surgery. Typically, patients with acute PVD need to repeat USG.

X-ray, Computed Tomography, and Magnetic Resonance Imaging

Occasionally, computed tomography (CT) and magnetic resonance (MR) imaging are performed on patients with VH, for example, in Terson's syndrome to evaluate for intracranial hemorrhage. Computed tomography does not easily differentiate hemorrhage from the surrounding vitreous. They may also be useful in cases of trauma.

Visually Evoked Response (VER)

It may be useful in cases where visual prognoses are doubtful.

■ MANAGEMENT

As discussed earlier, the first part is determining the possible cause of VH, as management involves systemic consultations accordingly. A case of uveitis may need prior treatment with steroids; whereas a case of RD may need urgent surgery.

After establishing etiology, management of VH should be individualized. Management is done in the form of observation, laser photocoagulation, cryotherapy, and pars plana vitrectomy.

The choice depends on several factors. It includes the patient's age, the duration of disease, visual acuity, IOP, presence or absence of neovascularization of the iris, amount of hemorrhage, retinal status, adequacy of photocoagulation if done before the onset of hemorrhage, lens status (phakic or aphakic/pseudophakic), and presence or absence of PVD.[1]

Principles of Management

- *Observation:* Fresh VH often clears in days to weeks to allow evaluation of the retina. Serial

USGs are of paramount importance in such cases.

- *In case of retina attached—in unknown etiology:* In these patients, the patient is asked to rest with the head in an elevated position and we should reevaluate after *3–7 days* to ascertain the possible source of hemorrhage. Oral ascorbic acid (vitamin C) may be given for faster clearance (though not clinically proven), as there is more liquefaction and loss of gel structure in eyes with ascorbic acid. *In known etiology*—in these patients, reevaluation is done *after 3–4 weeks*. This group includes postlaser or postvitrectomy recurrent VHs, VH in Tersons' syndrome, or after acute PVD, and hemorrhage associated with bleeding diathesis.
- *In RD:* Early surgery is recommended in VH associated with RD. In eyes with an attached macula, one may wait for some days for PVD to occur, as this will enhance the technical ease and improve the outcomes of surgery. This includes penetrating trauma without retained intraocular foreign body (and not associated with infection), fresh RD with VH and no PVD, Eales' disease without PVD and rhegmatogenous retinal detachment (RRD), VH in closed globe injury without RD. In macula-off RD with VH, we should do immediate surgery.
- *Laser photocoagulation:* Laser photocoagulation in proliferative vasculopathies should start as soon as any part of the retina is visible. In some cases, one may start laser therapy using an indirect ophthalmoscope delivery system in dense VH, and later on one can shift to slit-lamp delivery. After partial clearing of hemorrhage, one may visualize a retinal break or avulsed vessel that can be treated with a barrage laser. In media haze due to VH, cataract, corneal edema (as in NVG), or poorly dilating pupil, transconjunctival cryopexy mode of laser can be used for panretinal photocoagulation or treatment of retinal breaks. The role of preoperative antivascular endothelial growth factor (anti-VEGF) has been discussed in the chapter on PDR.
- *Anterior retinal cryotherapy (ARC):* Has limited use. Generally, not applied in fresh cases. It may be used for recurrent VH despite adequate PRP or cases of OIS with continued ocular ischemia.
- *Anti-VEGF injections:* These can be delivered as therapeutic in cases where VH is known to be due to ARMD and idiopathic polypoidal choroidal vasculopathy (IPCV). Further, PDR and rebleeds in cases of PDR and OIS may also be treated with anti-VEGF injections in cases where surgery is not possible or is being deferred. More discussion is present in the chapter on PDR.
- *Vitrectomy:* Early vitrectomy is indicated in situations where the underlying pathology is likely to progress fast if left untreated.[1] Surgery can be delayed in eyes with well-lasered proliferative retinopathy with retina attached. Vitrectomy can be deferred till good PVD occurs in eyes with Tersons' syndrome, closed globe injuries, postcataract surgery VH (if not due to peribulbar anesthesia-related globe perforation), VH in bleeding diathesis, etc.

Indications of Vitrectomy

- Severe nonclearing VH over 2–3 months.
- Advanced proliferative retinopathy where the VH does not resolve in 6–8 weeks after adequate laser therapy
- VH with RD
- VH with giant retinal tear
- TRD involving the macula
- Combined TRD and RRDs
- Severe progressive fibrovascular proliferation
- Anterior segment neovascularization with posterior segment opacities
- Dense premacular hemorrhage
- Ghost cell glaucoma
- Macula edema associated with premacular traction
- Anterior hyaloid fibrovascular proliferations
- Fibrinoid syndrome with associated RD
- VH with retained intraocular foreign body
- VH due to AMD and IPCV.

Management of Specific Conditions

Proliferative Diabetic Retinopathy

(See Long Case for PDR)

Eales' disease: Eales' disease usually presents with VH at the time of onset. About 62% of the patients have VH at the time of initial presentation. It can occur due to severe retinal vasculitis or in the proliferative stage due to new vessels and traction. It can be treated with retinal photocoagulation initially. Early vitrectomy has been advocated, with 87% of eyes showing improvement in visual acuity.

Macroaneurysm: VH develops in as many as 30% of the macroaneurysm. It mostly occurs in women over 60 years of age with systemic hypertension. These may resolve spontaneously or may require a laser treatment.

Uveitis: Pars planitis can result in retinal neovascularization and cause VH. Sarcoidosis, Behçets' syndrome, and toxoplasmosis may cause VH due to retinal neovascularization whereas ocular histoplasmosis syndrome causes VH from choroidal neovascularization.

Idiopathic retinal vasculitis, aneurysms, and neuroretinitis (IRVAN) can also present with VH.

Retinal vascular anomalies and tumors: Cavernous hemangioma of the retina and optic disc, capillary hemangiomatosis or juxtapapillary vascular hamartomas of the retina, and congenital arteriovenous anastomoses can lead to VH. Parafoveal telangiectasia and Coats' disease cause VH rarely. A choroidal melanoma does not cause VH until it reaches a considerable size.

Sickle cell disease and leukemia: With peripheral scatter, photocoagulation reduces the risk of VH in Sickle cell hemoglobinopathies. Retinal neovascularization may also develop in chronic cases of chronic myelocytic leukemia and can cause VH.

PVD: Spontaneous VH can occur with PVD. An early diagnosis is crucial because a retinal tear is a common cause of VH. A detailed peripheral retinal evaluation with scleral depression is mandatory to screen for any retinal tears, obscured by VH. B-scan (sometimes dynamic USG) and A-scan may be helpful in detecting the retinal tear and the traction site. Surgery is indicated in the case of RD.

Age-related macular degeneration: VH secondary to ARMD results from subretinal bleeding due to choroidal neovascularization. Ultrasonography shows a highly echogenic subretinal mass temporal to the optic disc typically, without any choroidal shadowing. In these patients, the hemorrhage usually resolves spontaneously.

If surgery is planned, anti-VEGF may be given at the end of surgery.

Miscellaneous: VH may occur in eyes undergoing intracapsular or extracapsular cataract extraction. Most VHs are mild and clear spontaneously; the possibility of needle perforation due to local anesthesia should be excluded. VH in Terson's syndrome occurs due to breakthrough bleeding from the internal limiting membrane of the retina and extends into the vitreous cavity. In a Valsalva maneuver, increased intravascular pressure causes VH due to retinal vein rupture. VH can also occur in warfarin or aspirin users.

VH in children: One of the most common causes of VH in children is trauma. Other causes are shaken-baby syndrome (otherwise unexplained VH in a child), retinoblastoma, and leukemia. In infants, disseminated intravascular coagulopathy or Terson's syndrome are causes of VH. Pediatric retinal diseases that can present with VH include familial exudative vitreoretinopathy retinoschisis, high myopia with retinal tears/detachment, retinopathy of prematurity, and toxocariasis. Early surgery is advocated in these eyes to avoid amblyopia and anisometropia.

VIVA QUESTIONS

Q.1. Describe the causes of VH based on the age of the patient.

Ans. The age of the patient can provide clues about the etiology of VH. For example:
- *Newborn babies*—trauma after spontaneous vaginal delivery (but not after cesarean delivery), shaken baby syndrome, FEVR, and retinopathy of prematurity.
- *Young boys*—X-linked retinoschisis. Children—trauma, FEVR retinoblastoma, leukemia, and other coagulopathies.
- *Young healthy adults*—Eales' disease in the Indian subcontinent is an important cause of VH. Retinals tear with or without associated RD.
- *In the elderly*—choroidal neovascular membrane (CNVM) secondary to age-related macular degeneration (AMD), proliferative retinopathy associated

with diabetes or retinal vein occlusion, and rarely due to retinal tears, PVD, melanoma, IPCV, or systemic anticoagulants.

Q.2. What are the causes of VH?

Ans. *See* **Table 1**. Depending upon the source, the following categories can be seen.
- *Bleeding from abnormal vessels:*
  - Retinal vascular disorders that cause retinal ischemia (due to VEGF, FGF, IGF–NVD, and NVE)
    - PDR
    - Ischemic RVO, more commonly BRVO
    - Eales' vasculitis
    - FEVR
    - Proliferative sickle cell retinopathy
    - Hematological disorders
  - Retinal vascular disorders that are not associated with retinal ischemia
    - Retinal artery macroaneurysm
    - Retinal angioma
    - Severe early vasculitis in the absence of ischemia
- Rupture of a normal retinal vessel:
  - PVD
  - Blunt trauma
  - Terson syndrome
  - Valsalva retinopathy
  - Hematological disorder (anemia, leukemia, and coagulation disorder)
- Breakthrough bleeding:
  - CNVM
  - Choroidal melanoma
  - IPCV
  - Peripheral exudative hemorrhagic chorioretinopathy (PEHCR)

Q.3. What is the role of a fellow eye?

Ans. See chapter.

Q.4. Discuss the USG differentiation of PVR/RD.

Ans. *For RD:* Persistence at low gain, poor after movements, attached to the disc, and quantitative method.

Q.5. What are the reasons for early surgery?

Ans. Unlasered PDR, RD, intraocular foreign body (IOFB), one-eyed patient, other eye lost to VH, zone 3 injuries.

Table 1: Causes of vitreous hemorrhage.	
Ocular causes vascular	Coat's disease, retinal branch artery malformation, retinopathy of prematurity, ocular ischemic syndrome, branch retinal artery occlusion, central retinal artery occlusion, choroidal vascular aneurysm, retinal vein rupture, retinal neovascularization after retinectomy, hypertensive uveitis, persistent hyaloid artery, venous stasis retinopathy, and arteriovenous communications of the retina
Inflammatory	Retinal vasculitis, Behçet's disease, sarcoid posterior uveitis, multiple sclerosis with retinal vasculitis, pars planitis, syphilitic retinitis, and dermatomyositis. Systemic lupus erythematosus and *Toxocara*
Iatrogenic	Retinal laser photocoagulation, after scleral buckling, Molteno implant surgery, trabeculectomy, ocular perforation, during peribulbar injection, secondary IOL, cataract wound neovascularization, and penetrating keratoplasty
Tumor	Retinoblastoma, cavernous hemangioma of the optic disc, combined retinal-retinal pigment epithelial hamartoma, vasoproliferative tumors, retinal angioma, retinal astrocytic hamartoma, and choroidal malignant melanoma
Others	Senile bullous retinoschisis, juvenile retinoschisis, tearing of retinal pigment epithelium, Talc retinopathy, retinitis pigmentosa, extracorporeal membrane oxygenation, and trauma
Indirect causes	Pseudotumor cerebri, valsalva retinopathy, chest compression, and newborn after vaginal delivery
Blood disorders	Thrombocytopenia, idiopathic thrombocytopenic purpura, hemophilia, pernicious anemia, disseminated intravascular coagulation disorder, von Willebrand syndrome, protein C deficiency, and anticoagulant therapy

REFERENCES

1. Spraul CW, Grossniklaus HE. Vitreous hemorrhage. Surv Ophthalmol. 1997;42(1):3-39.
2. Goff MJ, McDonald HR, Johnson RN, Ai E, Jumper JM, Fu AD. Causes and treatment of vitreous hemorrhage. Compr Ophthalmol Update. 2006;7(3):97-111.

CENTRAL RETINAL VEIN OCCLUSION

Ashish Markan, Esha Agarwal, Brijesh Takkar

INTRODUCTION

Retinal vein occlusion is an obstruction of the retinal venous system that may involve the central, hemicentral, or branch retinal vein. The most common etiological factor is compression by adjacent atherosclerotic retinal arteries traveling through the same adventitial sheath. Other possible causes are external compression or inflammation of the vein wall. Central retinal vein occlusion (CRVO) may result from thrombosis of the central retinal vein when the vein passes through the lamina cribrosa. The prevalence of CRVO is reported to be around <0.1–0.4%.[1,2] CRVO is usually a unilateral disease, the risk of developing any type of vascular occlusion in the fellow eye is approximately 1% per year, and about 7% of persons with CRVO may develop CRVO in the fellow eye within 5 years of onset in the first eye.[3,4]

HISTORY

CRVO occurs predominantly in the elderly population (>65 years) and affects males and females equally. These patients may often have ocular or systemic risk factors.

Chief Complaints

- Sudden painless loss of vision
- Rarely pain or redness due to NVG or accompanying high IOP.

History of Present Illness

Patients usually present with sudden painless loss of vision in one eye. Some patients may also present with gradual decline of vision in cases of less severe occlusion. Marked deterioration of visual acuity especially on waking in the morning can be seen in ischemic CRVO. Patients with nonischemic CRVO may have no symptoms and it may be detected as an incidental finding on a routine ophthalmic examination. It is not rare to find some of these patients complaining of episodes of amaurosis fugax before the constant blur.

Patients with partially recovered CRVO may have a history of visual field loss or constriction. Floaters can rarely occur due to accompanying VH.

Decrease in contrast sensitivity, micropsia, macropsia, metamorphopsia, and scotoma can also be there due to associated macular edema. Vision recovery is dependent on the onset and duration of occlusion.

History of Past Illness

Ocular disorders predisposing to crowding/compression at the level of the optic disc, and systemic disorders predisposing to thromboembolic disease or disease of the vascular wall are the most commonly identified risk factors, for example, there may be a history of open-angle glaucoma (OAG) or an angle closure glaucoma, ischemic optic neuropathy, pseudotumor cerebri, tilted optic nerve head, optic nerve head drusen, hypermetropia, hypertension, cardiovascular diseases, carotid insufficiency, diabetes, bleeding/thrombotic disorder, leukemia, multiple myeloma, sickle cell disease, systemic lupus erythematosus (SLE), human immunodeficiency virus (HIV), herpes zoster, syphilis, and sarcoidosis. It may also be presented after retrobulbar block, dehydration, and pregnancy.

There is a small risk of past CRVO in the fellow eye, ~7% in 5 years.

Family History

A family history of risk factors may be there.

Past Surgical History

History of ocular surgery and cardiovascular surgery may be there.

Personal History

There is a history of smoking, alcohol intake, and tobacco use.

Drug History

History of intake of oral contraceptives, diuretics, and the hepatitis-B vaccine must be enquired about.

■ EXAMINATION

General examination/specific systemic examination should be aimed at ruling out the systemic risk factors.

Ocular Examination

- *Visual acuity:* Visual acuity at the time of presentation is variable **(Table 1)**, and is an important prognostic indicator of final visual outcome. Generally, visual acuity better than 20/200 is believed to be a sign of good final prognoses.

Table 1: Types of central retinal vein occlusion (CRVO).

Parameters	Nonischemic CRVO	Ischemic CRVO
Incidence	80%	20%
Age	Young adults and past middle age	Past middle age
Symptoms—vision	The vague blurring of vision Normal/>6/60	Marked deterioration of vision especially on waking in the morning <6/60
Pupil	Normal	RAPD present >0.7 log units (on the neutral density filter)
Site of occlusion	Further back in the retrolaminar region	At or near the retrolaminar region
Early stages	Mild to moderate dilatation of all branches of the central retinal vein	Marked tortuosity and engorgement of retinal vein
Retinal hemorrhages	Mild to moderate, more in the periphery	Extensive hemorrhages involving the periphery and posterior pole
Cotton-wool spots	Rare	Common
Optic disc	Hyperemic and may be edematous	Marked optic disc edema
Macula	Normal or may show edema	Gross hemorrhages and edema
Late ophthalmoscopic finding	• Veins—mild to moderately engorged • Sheathing +/− • No neovascularization • Macula—normal/CME	• Veins—mild to moderately engorged • Sheathing—frequently seen • Hemorrhages—none or few • Retina has—aneurysms, neovascularization, preretinal/vitreous hemorrhages • Optic disc—pale • Macula—degenerative/pigmentary disturbances
FFA	<10-disc area of capillary nonperfusion	>10-disc areas of capillary nonperfusion
ERG	Minimal or no change	Marked reduction of b-wave amplitude <60%

Contd...

Contd...

Parameters	Nonischemic CRVO	Ischemic CRVO
Goldmann perimetry	No or minimal defects	Marked peripheral visual field defects
Complications	Macular edema, macular degeneration	Macular edema, macular degeneration, preretinal hemorrhages, vitreous hemorrhage, NVE, NVD, NVG
Prognosis	Good	Poor
(ERG: electroretinogram; FFA: fundus fluorescein angiography; NVE: neovascularization elsewhere; NVD: neovascularization of the disc; NVG: neovascular glaucoma; RAPD: relative afferent pupil defect)		

- External and anterior segment evaluation can reveal signs of systemic risk factors.
- *Eyeball:* Proptosis in case of tumor (abaxial in sarcoid)
- *Lid:* Signs of other systemic risk factors may be present.
- *Conjunctiva:* Multiple hemorrhages in conjunctiva may be seen (bleeding disorders)
- *Cornea:* Peripheral ulcerative keratitis (PUK) in case of SLE and PAN
- *Sclera:* Nodular scleritis
- *Anterior chamber:* It may be shallow in patients with angle closure glaucoma or short axial length. Keratic precipitates, cells, and flare may be present in inflammatory diseases (vasculitis, sarcoidosis, and HIV). Flair may be noted in patients with NVI and the presence of hyphema is uncommon.
- *Gonioscopy:* Undilated gonioscopy is essential to determine the presence of NVA or evidence of angle closure. NVA may be present without neovascularization of the iris (NVI) in 12% of eyes.[5]
- *Iris:* NVI or NVA may be there. The pupillary margin should be carefully examined for the presence of NVI. As later discussed, it is an important sign in deciding on management.
- *Pupil:* The presence of a relative afferent pupillary defect is an ominous sign. It is important to look for relative afferent pupil defect (RAPD) before pupil dilation whenever one is suspecting vascular occlusion.
- *Lens:* Generally normal or age-related nuclear sclerosis. Complicated cataracts can be seen in inflammatory conditions.
- *IOP:* An IOP >22 mm Hg needs to be investigated and explained. Raised IOP could be due to NVG, underlying open-angle

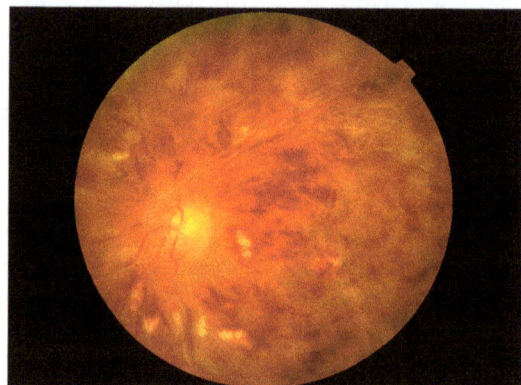

Fig. 1: Fundus picture of ischemic central retinal vein occlusion (CRVO) with macular edema. Four quadrant retinal hemorrhages can be seen along with soft exudates and retinal edema.

glaucoma. Angle-closure glaucoma attacks around the time of CRVO are not uncommon. It may be both causative as well as the effect of CRVO.
- *Posterior segment* **(Figs. 1 to 3)***:* The typical clinical constellation in CRVO includes retinal hemorrhages (both superficial flame-shaped and deep blot type) in all four quadrants with dilated, tortuous retinal veins (classic "blood and thunder appearance"). Optic nerve head swelling, cotton-wool spots, splinter hemorrhages, and macular edema are present to varying degrees. Macular edema may be accompanied by accumulation of subretinal fluid. In severe cases, the retinal thickening maybe 4–5 times normal. With time, retinal hemorrhages may decrease or resolve completely with secondary retinal pigment epithelium alteration. An epiretinal membrane may form.

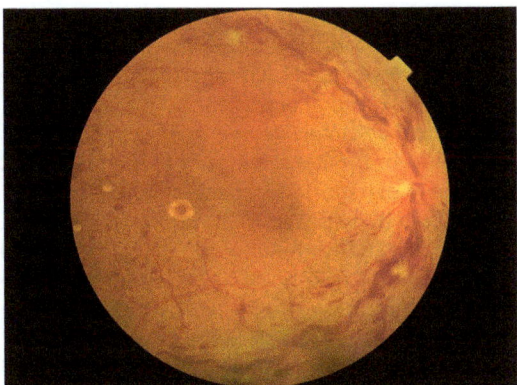

Fig. 2: Fundus picture of central retinal vein occlusion (CRVO) showing venous tortuosity.

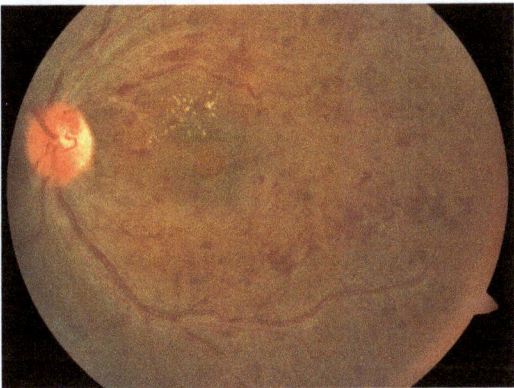

Fig. 3: Fundus picture of old central retinal vein occlusion (CRVO) with macular edema. Collaterals have developed over the optic disc.

Optociliary shunt vessels (disc collaterals) can develop on the optic nerve head and are very important clues to an old RVO. With time disc pallor ensues. NVD or NVE may develop. A careful 90D examination should be done to differentiate disc collaterals from NVD. The vessels that comprise NVD are typically of smaller caliber than optociliary shunt vessels and branch into a vascular network. Fibrovascular proliferation from NVD or NVE may result in VH or traction RD.

Gross signs of vascular sclerosis may be present and clues to systemic disorders may be discussed before. One should always look for the presence of atherosclerosis in the retinal arteries.

Fellow eyes should be examined carefully to look for signs of hypertensive retinopathy, diabetic retinopathy, vasculitis, or signs of vascular occlusion. Gonioscopy should be performed to rule out occludable angle (vascular occlusion may be secondary to angle closure glaucoma).

- *Complications associated with CRVO:* A careful examination must be done to rule out any of these complications of CRVO.
- Macular edema
- Macular ischemia
- NVG
- VH
- TRD
- Optic atrophy.

■ DIFFERENTIAL DIAGNOSIS

A case of CRVO may have to be differentiated from the following:
- OIS
- Diabetic retinopathy
- Papilledema
- Radiation retinopathy
- Retinopathy due to anemia
- CRAO with CRVO
- Venous stasis retinopathy.

■ INVESTIGATIONS

One important part of the work-up includes identifying appropriate risk factors, ocular or systemic. Ocular risk factors enlisted before should be ruled out as appropriate.

Systemic Work-up

It is generally not indicated in elderly patients with known systemic vascular risk factors for CRVO. However, routine blood pressure, fasting blood glucose, and lipid profile should be checked. A cardiac consultation should be done when possible.

Younger patients, patients with bilateral simultaneous vascular occlusion, prior occlusion in the fellow eye, prior systemic thrombotic disease, and family history of thrombosis require detailed evaluation for hypercoagulable conditions as these persons may be at risk for future, nonocular thrombotic events. These investigations include:
- Complete hemogram with peripheral smear
- ESR
- Plasma homocysteine level

- Chest X-ray—to rule out tuberculosis (TB), sarcoidosis, and left ventricular hypertrophy.
- CRP
- Thrombophilia screen—PT, TT, activated partial thromboplastin time (aPTT), protein C, protein S, activated protein C resistance, factor V Leiden mutation, lupus anticoagulant, and anticardiolipin antibody.
- Autoantibodies—ANA, ANCA, anti-DNA antibody, rheumatoid factor.
- Serum angiotensin-converting enzyme
- Treponemal serology
- Carotid Doppler scan

Ocular Investigation

- *Fundus fluorescein angiography (FFA):* Fluorescein angiography in CRVO **(Fig. 4)** shows marked delay in arteriovenous transit time, blocked fluorescence due to retinal hemorrhages, vessel wall staining, areas of nonperfusion, collaterals, NVD, NVE, and macular edema. Blocked fluorescence of the underlying retinal circulation occurs if extensive intraretinal hemorrhages are present, especially in the early part of the disease and therefore FFA may not reveal useful information. So, best to wait for the resolution of hemorrhages.

  FFA is indicated to rule out macular ischemia, to determine the type of CRVO (ischemic vs. nonischemic), and to detect NVD and NVE. CRVO is said to be nonischemic if capillary nonperfusion is <10 disc areas and ischemic if capillary nonperfusion is >10 disc areas (definition of CVOS).
- *Optical coherence tomography (OCT):* OCT is useful in the assessment of macular edema, and particularly in monitoring its course, especially with the treatment of the edema. It can readily detect cystic spaces, retinal thickening, and serous RDs, all of which are rather frequent in CRVO. In long-standing cases, it helps to detect ERM and VMA. OCT B scans (DRIL, thinning, and hyperreflective dots) and OCT—angiography can also help in detecting features of retinal ischemia.
- *Ultrasonography:* If the whole or a part of the underlying retina is obscured due to VH, a USG B-scan with a corresponding A-scan is mandatory to detect any associated RD/mass lesion. Also useful in detecting hypermetropia and disc drusen.
- *Electroretinogram (ERG):* This is an objective functional test, very useful in the differentiation of ischemic from nonischemic CRVO. In ischemic CRVO, there is reduced b-wave amplitude (<60% of normal), reduced b:a ratio, and prolonged b-wave implicit time on the ERG.
- *Perimetry:* VF plotting with a Goldmann perimeter helps in the differentiation of ischemic (defective V4e target) from nonischemic CRVO.

■ MANAGEMENT

The goals of treatment in CRVO are to identify and treat predisposing medical conditions, to maintain central visual acuity by minimizing macular edema, to reduce the risk of bleeding into the vitreous cavity by producing regression of retinal neovascularization, and to prevent NVG. Previously there has been a lot of interest in relieving the obstruction or bypassing it, but none of the therapies have proven to be of benefit (discussed later).

Macular Edema

Before the advent of intravitreal pharmacotherapy, observation was the standard of treatment for macular edema associated with CRVO as

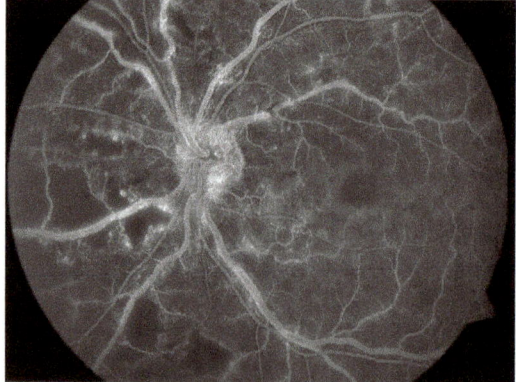

Fig. 4: Fluorescein angiography picture of central retinal vein occlusion (CRVO) showing collateral vessels, severe retinal ischemia, and microaneurysms.

recommended by CVOS. In CVOS group M, no significant improvement in visual acuity was seen with grid laser as compared to the untreated group, though macular edema was decreased angiographically. Hence, macular grid is not routinely recommended.

Intravitreal steroids by reducing vascular permeability and inhibiting the expression of the VEGF gene and the metabolic pathway of VEGF play an important role in the treatment of macular edema due to CRVO (SCORE trial, GENEVA trial). Ozurdex (sustained release intravitreal dexamethasone delivery system) is also now FDA-approved for the treatment of macular edema secondary to CRVO, but it has complications, such as cataracts and increased IOP. Intravitreal anti-VEGF agents are currently the first-line therapy for macular edema. Various trials have shown their efficacy ranibizumab in the CRUISE trial, VEGF trap (aflibercept) in Galileo and Copernicus, and they have now replaced observation established by CVOS as the standard of care for the treatment of macular edema associated with CRVO. Anti-VEGF drugs are also FDA-approved for the treatment of macular edema due to CRVO. A common dosing would be 3 or 6 monthly injections of ranibizumab followed by a required dosage as the shunt vessels develop and the RVO relieves itself with time, the need for injections decreases. It is less needed in nonischemic CRVO. Targeted peripheral scatter laser has also been tried but with minimal gain.

Ocular Neovascularization

Panretinal photocoagulation should be promptly delivered after the development of NVI/NVA to prevent secondary complications. CVOS did not recommend prophylactic PRP in ischemic CRVO. PRP in patients without NVI has the risk of making future NVI refractory and is not indicated. The laser should be delivered as anterior as possible and supplementary cryotherapy may be added as needed.

Prophylactic PRP can how however be considered in cases of ischemic CRVO where follow-up is not possible in high-risk cases.

Anti-VEGF agents result in rapid regression of neovascularization, but these should be used as temporizing adjunctive measures with subsequent PRP as definitive treatment.

Role of Vitrectomy

It is indicated in cases of nonresolving VH or TRD secondary to retinal neovascularization.

Pars plana vitrectomy with internal limiting membrane (ILM) peeling has also been investigated for macular edema secondary to CRVO and has shown variable results.

Other Modalities

- The role of *systemic anticoagulants* in the management of CRVO is unclear; though it does not alter the natural course of CRVO they may help to prevent nonocular thrombotic events.
- Role of *oral pentoxifylline (vasodilator)/ hemodilution* in the management of CRVO is still controversial.
- *Recombinant tissue plasminogen activator (r-tPA)* has been administered by several routes of systemic, intravitreal and endovascular cannulation of retinal vessels for the treatment of CRVO and has shown variable results.
- *Chorioretinal venous anastomosis* between the nasal branch retinal vein and the choroidal circulation has been created using Nd:YAG laser in nonischemic CRVO. It may allow transretinal retrograde flow of the venous blood from the eye and may prevent retinal ischemia. Studies have shown limited visual recovery even after successful anastomosis due to thrombosis of the treated retinal vein.
- *Radial optic neurotomy* involves a transvitreal incision of the nasal scleral ring to release pressure on the central retinal vein at the level of the scleral outlet. Some studies have shown improvement in visual acuity, but its use has been abandoned owing to significant risks.

VIVA QUESTIONS

Q.1. What are the various risk factors for CRVO?
Ans. Refer text.

Q.2. What is the pathogenesis of CRVO?
Ans.
- The site of occlusion in CRVO is at or just proximal to the lamina cribrosa.
- The central retinal artery and vein are aligned parallel to each other in

a common tissue sheath within the retrolaminar portion of the optic nerve and they are naturally compressed as they pass through rigid sieve-like openings in the lamina cribrosa but they typically give off branching collateral vessels just before piercing the lamina. These vessels may be subject to compression from an increase in IOP which causes posterior bowing of lamina cribrosa due to mechanical stretch or occlusion of the central retinal vein can be due to compression by an atherosclerotic central retinal artery or it can be primarily due to inflammation of the central retinal vein. Hemodynamic alterations may lead to thrombus formation in the central retinal vein by Virchow's triad (diminished blood flow, increased blood viscosity, and altered lumen wall).

- Occlusion of both the retrolaminar central retinal artery and central retinal vein posterior to lamina cribrosa and before the branching of collateral channels from the main trunk is required to produce ischemic CRVO while nonischemic CRVO is due to occlusion of the central retinal vein at a site further posterior, allowing normal collateral channels to provide alternative routes of venous drainage.
- Resistance to venous flow, blood stagnation, and ischemia stimulates the production of VEGF resulting in neovascularization and macular edema.

Q.3. What are the types of CRVO and how to differentiate between them?

Ans. Refer to **Table 1**.

Q.4. What is the risk of nonischemic CRVO converting to ischemic CRVO?

Ans. About one-third of cases of nonischemic CRVO convert to ischemic CRVO over a period of 1 year.

Q.5. What is the common site of neovascularization in CRVO?

Ans. The following are the sites:
- Iris
- NVI develops in about 50% of eyes, usually in 2–4 months (100 days glaucoma).
- NVG develops in one-third of cases with NVI.
- Retinal neovascularization is seen in 5% of the cases.

Q.6. What is an ischemic index and what is its importance?

Ans. Ischemic index[6] = $\dfrac{\text{Nonperfusion area}}{\text{Total area of retina}}$

An ischemic index of 50% corresponding to about 10-disc areas of retinal capillary nonperfusion was considered the threshold for a significant risk of neovascular complications.

Q.7. When will you call anterior segment neovascularization significant?

Ans. When there is NVI of >2 clock hours or there is the presence of NVA.

Q.8. What are the objectives and conclusion of CVOS?

Ans. The main objectives of the CVOS study are:
- To assess whether grid-pattern photocoagulation therapy will reduce loss of central visual acuity due to macular edema secondary to central vein occlusion (CVO).
- To determine whether photocoagulation therapy can help prevent iris neovascularization in eyes with CVO and evidence of ischemic retina.

Its conclusion is:
- There is no visual benefit to treating macular edema from a CRVO with grid laser photocoagulation.
- There is no benefit to treating ischemic CRVO with early (prophylactic) PRP.

Interpretations: Delaying treatment with PRP until the development of NV resulted in significant regression of neovascularization and no additional risk of NVG compared to patients treated with prophylactic PRP.

The study also suggested a follow-up schedule, which basically advised regular monthly follow-up for the first 6 months and then tapered follow-up. However, on the day of anti-VEGF treatment, the discussion is rather arbitrary.

Q.9. What are the indications for FFA in CRVO?
Ans. Refer text.

Q.10. When is PRP indicated in CRVO?
Ans. Refer text.

Q.11. What is the treatment of choice for macular edema in CRVO?
Ans. Refer text.

Q.12. What are the causes of CRVO in the young?
Ans. Refer to risk factors and work-up.

Q.13. What are the risk factors for the development of NVI in CRVO cases?
Ans. Risk factors of NVI include:
- >10 DD of nonperfusion in the posterior pole (greater risk with greater nonperfusion)
- RAPD
- Decreased visual acuity
- *ERG:* Decreased b:a ratio if <1 (normal 2:1)
- Elevated central retinal venous pressure
- Duration <1 month

Q.14. What is CRAO with CRVO?
Ans. In this case, the retinal hemorrhages are scattered and less due to the accompanying RAO. These cases are at very high risk of developing NVI, with some figures as high as 80%.

Q.15. Why does CRVO cause more of NVI and BRVO cause more of retinal new vessels?
Ans. In CRVO, particularly, the ischemic variant, the ischemia is so severe that the retinal tissue may not be able to respond to VEGF load to develop new vessels. Hence, retinal new vessels are much less frequent than in BRVO.

Q.16. What is the current role of laser in CRVO macular edema?
Ans. As discussed above macular laser has no or poor role in treating macular edema. Recent studies, RELATE study for CRVO, are indicating the role of peripheral laser for treating edema refractory to injections. The earlier the laser is done the more the chance of it being effective. With the availability of widefield FA, the targeted laser may be attempted to knock off the VEGF-producing CNP areas.

■ REFERENCES

1. Mitchell P, Smith W, Chang A. Prevalence and associations of retinal vein occlusion in Australia. The Blue Mountains Eye Study. Arch Ophthalmol. 1996;114(10):1243-7.
2. Klein R, Klein BE, Moss SE, Meuer SM. The epidemiology of retinal vein occlusion: the Beaver Dam Eye Study. Trans Am Ophthalmol Soc. 2000;98:133-41.
3. Hayreh SS, Zimmerman MB, Podhajsky P. Incidence of various types of retinal vein occlusion and their recurrence and demographic characteristics. Am J Ophthalmol. 1994;117(4):429-41.
4. The Central Vein Occlusion Study Group. Natural history and clinical management of central retinal vein occlusion. Arch Ophthalmol. 1997;115(4):486-91.
5. Browning DJ, Scott AQ, Peterson CB, Warnock J, Zhang Z. The risk of missing angle neovascularization by omitting screening gonioscopy in acute central retinal vein occlusion. Ophthalmology. 1998;105(5):776-84.
6. Magargal LE, Donoso LA, Sanborn GE. Retinal ischemia and risk of neovascularization following central retinal vein obstruction. Ophthalmology. 1982;89(11):1241-5.

BRANCH RETINAL VEIN OCCLUSION

Pulak Agarwal, Shorya Vardhan Azad

■ INTRODUCTION

Retinal vein occlusion is the second most common retinal vascular disease. Amongst vascular occlusions, branch retinal vein occlusion (BRVO) is commoner (78%). Most patients are in the sixth decade of life; however, it can occur in younger populations. In such cases, systemic investigation becomes imperative for finding the underlying cause. Risk factors for BRVO are summarized in **(Table 1)**. BRVO patient is usually given a long case or spotter.

Table 1: Risk factors for BRVO.

Risk factors	What to look
Systemic:	
Age	>60 years
Hypertension	Blood pressure
Diabetes mellitus	RBS, PPBS, and HbA1C
Coagulopathies: • Hyperhomocysteinemia • Factor V Leiden mutation • Antiphospholipid antibody syndrome • Protein C/S deficiency	• Serum homocysteine • *Screening blood test:* Activated protein C resistance • *Antiphospholipid antibodies (aPL):* Anticardiolipin antibodies (aCL) Lupus anticoagulant (LA) anti-β2-glycoprotein-1 (anti-B2GP1) • Free protein C/S antigen
Inflammatory: • Behçets • Sarcoidosis • Wegener's	• HLA B51, and pathergy test • Serum ACE, chest X-ray, and chest CT • C-ANCA, chest X-ray
Infections: • TB • Syphilis • Lyme's • HIV	• Mantoux test and chest X-ray • VDRL • ELISA and Western Blot • ELISA
Chronic renal failure	RFT
Others: • Smoking • Oral Contraceptive • Dehydration	History
Ocular:	
Glaucoma	Intraocular pressure
Short-axial length	Axial length
(ELISA: enzyme-linked-immunosorbent assay; PPBS: postprandial blood sugar; RBS: random blood sugar; RFT: renal function test; VDRL: venereal disease research laboratory)	

■ HISTORY

Chief Complaints

Branch retinal vein occlusion is most commonly present in an elderly patient with complaints of:
- Sudden, painless diminution of vision/blurred vision/onset of field defect.
- The patient may also have metamorphopsia, which will indicate toward macular edema.
- Occasionally, patients with old occult RVO may present with sudden onset of floaters, leading to complete loss of vision. In such cases, the patient may have VH.
- Lastly, in certain cases the patient may entirely be asymptomatic and a peripheral BRVO may be detected on routine clinical examination.

History of Present Illness

It includes complete documentation of onset duration and progress of visual complaints. Associated ocular and systemic symptoms (discussed above) should also be enquired. There may be a history of similar episodes in the same or the other eye, for which the patient might have sought medical attention.

Medical/Treatment History and Past History

It should include the following:
- Detailed history of the patient's systemic status, such as hypertension, diabetes, hyperlipidemia, hypercholesterolemia, cardiovascular disease, and any other drug intake.
- Young people should be specifically asked about their previous history of hypercoagulability (bruises elsewhere in the body, blood transfusions, etc.), HIV or other infectious diseases, and use of OCPs.
- Personal history should include smoking, chewing tobacco, and alcohol consumption.
- The patient may have received some form of laser or intravitreal therapy, which needs careful documentation.
- Careful documentation of past ocular disorders and therapies, e.g., for glaucoma and retinal vasculitis must be obtained.

■ EXAMINATION

Systemic Examination

Detailed systemic examination should be carried out **(Table 1)**. In patients with VH, another eye may reveal the predisposition to BRVO.

Ocular Examination

Visual Acuity

It is paramount to note the best-corrected vision with correction, as it would decide the need to treat. In treated cases, it is important, as it would help in monitoring the response to therapy. In addition, initial visual acuity could be a prognostic factor for postintervention success.

Ocular Adnexa and Globe

Ocular adnexal skin can be examined for signs of coagulopathy, collagen vascular disorders, and infections. There is no significant examination regarding ocular alignment or movements. Lids, eyebrows, and eyelashes are within their limits for the age.

Conjunctiva

Patients with glaucoma may have conjunctival blebs. Conjunctival hemorrhages may be present in coagulopathies.

Cornea

Involvement is rare, except in collagen vascular disorders.

Anterior Chamber

It may be shallow if the patient has a preexisting glaucoma or short axial length. AC should be inspected for signs of uveitis. Similarly, gonioscopy may reveal NVA in selected cases.

Pupil

Rarely neovascularization may be present at the pupillary border. The presence of RAPD may indicate CRVO or HRVO or anterior ischemic optic neuropathy (AION) rather than BRVO. Even major BRVOs will not have RAPD.

Lens

As patients are elderly, there may be cataractous changes present in the lens.

Posterior Segment

It requires +90D/78D and +20D examination after pupillary dilatation.
- Vitreous is mostly clear except when there may be vitreous haze present posthemorrhage with red blood cells floating in the vitreous.
- The next important structure for assessment is the optic disc and the peripapillary area to rule out signs of glaucoma and NVD and AION.
- As most of the patients are hypertensive, signs of hypertensive retinopathy should be noted. Splashed tomato and blood and thunder appearance must be kept in mind in cases of RVO.
- Macular assessment on slit-lamp biomicroscopy with a +90D lens may reveal macular

edema seen as an elevation of the retina with loss of foveal reflex. Long-standing cases may have intraretinal hard exudates and cystic type of edema.
- Meticulous inspection of the vitreoretinal interface may show the area of vitreomacular adhesion or an epiretinal membrane in recalcitrant cases.
- Mostly BRVO occurs in the superotemporal quadrant **(Fig. 1)**, as more arteriovenous (AV) crossings are present in this area. AV crossing should be carefully evaluated as it may reveal the site of occlusion.
- In contrast, a nasal BRVO or a peripheral BRVO may even go unnoticed. There will be dilated, tortuous vessels proximal to the occlusion. Intraretinal flame-shaped hemorrhages; microaneurysms can be present along the occluded vessel. Cotton-wool spots are also seen.
- Old cases may have collaterals, telangiectatic vessels, and neovascularization.
- Neovascularization can be present on the disc or at the junction of perfused and nonperfused retina. After 6–12 months, the acute findings will resolve and there will be venous sheathing and sclerosis. Macular edema can also be seen with +90D or +78D.

Amsler grid testing: It is important to monitor the response of the patient. Patients at their homes can do it. It can provide objective evidence to the patient if there is a sudden increase in metamorphopsia or blurring of vision so that the patient can seek medical attention in time. This is more important for patients who present with vision of >6/12 and hence a follow-up is recommended for monitoring any deterioration in vision.

Major Complications Associated with Branch Retinal Vein Occlusion

- Macular edema—the main cause of low vision
- Macular ischemia
- Neovascularization leading to VH. NVE develops in 40% of the cases
- NVI develops rarely (1%)

◾ DIFFERENTIAL DIAGNOSIS

In patients with NVs or VH or macular edema, differentials are essentially the same (*See* relevant chapters). For intraretinal hemorrhages, differentials include DR, CRVO, AION, CNVM, PEHCR, coats, homocysteine disorders, retinitis, vasculitis, etc. Usually, the typical sectoral or quadrantic appearance in a predisposed patient is the clincher for BRVO.

◾ INVESTIGATIONS

Systemic Investigation

In a person aged >60 years, BRVO may occur as an age-related vasculopathy even in the absence of hypertension. However, routine blood pressure, fasting blood glucose, and lipid profile should be checked.

In a young person, the investigations that should be done are:
- Plasma homocysteine level
- Chest X-ray to rule out TB, sarcoidosis, and left ventricular hypertrophy.
- CRP
- Thrombophilia screen—PT, TT, aPTT, protein C, protein S, activated protein C resistance, factor V Leiden mutation, lupus anticoagulant, and anticardiolipin antibody.
- Autoantibodies—antinuclear antibodies (ANA), antineutrophil cytoplasmic autoantibodies (ANCA), anti-deoxyribonucleic acid (anti-DNA) antibodies, and rheumatoid factor.
- Serum angiotensin-converting enzyme
- Treponemal serology
- Carotid duplex imaging
- Full blood count

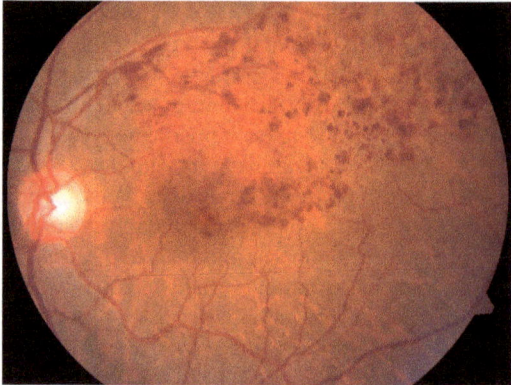

Fig. 1: Clinical photograph of fresh superior temporal BRVO depicting scattered hemorrhages in the area of drainage of the major vein and macular hemorrhages.

Ocular Investigation

It includes the following:
- *Fluorescein angiography (FA):* Although the diagnosis of BRVO is purely clinical, FA does reveal additional findings that help in treatment and prognostication. FA may not be useful in acute onset BRVO due to extensive areas of hemorrhage resulting in blocked fluorescence and masking of underlying features. Therefore, the best time to do FA would be when substantial clearing of hemorrhage is seen. The characteristic findings of FA are delayed filling of the occluded retinal vein, blocked fluorescence due to intraretinal hemorrhages, microaneurysms, dye extravasation secondary to macular edema, telangiectatic collateral vessels, capillary nonperfusion, and retinal neovascularization **(Fig. 2)**.
- The two most important features to note on FA are the type of macular edema and BRVO. Macular edema may be perfused or nonperfused (ischemic). In perfused, FA would reveal areas of macular leakage with a normal foveal avascular zone (FAZ), whereas ischemic edema may have a distorted and enlarged FAZ apart from leakage. Type of edema will help guide our treatment, as ischemic cases have shown not to benefit from any intervention. Secondly, it helps us assess whether BRVO is Ischemic, marked by the presence of >5-disc area of capillary nonperfusion. These cases have more chances of developing neovascularization and may need to be lasered. Another recent concept is to map peripheral ischemic areas, which may be responsible for the constant production of VEGF leading to chronic macular edema. These areas may need targeted laser ablation to decrease VEGF load. FA is also essential for follow-up.

Wide-field Angiography

UWA gives a 200° field of vision. A single image helps in delineating the extent of peripheral capillary nonperfusion and can help in targeted laser. In addition, it can pick up any neovascularization, as dynamic FA may lead to skipping areas.

Optical Coherence Tomography

It is a noninvasive and highly informative investigation. Even in acute BRVO where FA might not be helpful, OCT is minimally affected by extensive intraretinal hemorrhages. Characteristic findings may include intraretinal edema, cystoid macular edema, intraretinal hyperreflectivity from hemorrhages, shadowing from edema, and occasional neurosensory detachment. Some studies have also assessed IS-OS junction abnormalities in chronic cases. Chronic cases may also show ERM or VMA.

It is the most preferred investigation for following up on cases of macular edema and response to therapy.

■ MANAGEMENT

Systemic conditions should be taken care of properly. Anticoagulants are not of much benefit. Oral contraceptives (OCPs) and hormone replacement therapies (HRTs) may be avoided if possible. Treatment for BRVO is usually done for its complications.

The treatment of BRVO macular edema (See Table, also See Chapter on CRVO) until recently was guided by the Branch Vein Occlusion Study (BVOS), which recommended grid laser for perfused macular edema of >3 months duration with best-corrected vision <6/12. They showed 63% of these patients recovered more than two Snellen's lines at 3 years follow-up following laser treatment

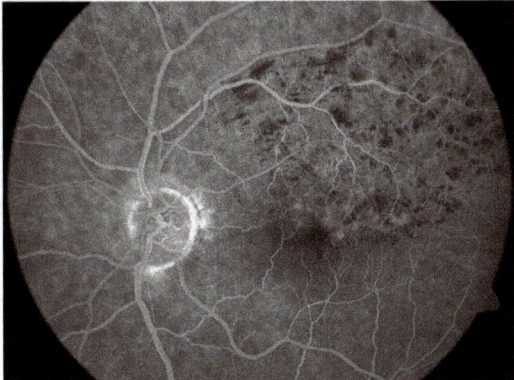

Fig. 2: Late fluorescein angiography (FA) picture showing blocked fluorescence in the area of the hemorrhages along with minimal leakage of the capillary bed.

in comparison to shams 36%. However, the visual gain was delayed and somewhat incomplete, and hence treatment options hastening recovery were explored. Although various forms of steroids (SCORE trial and GENEVA trial) have been used, their efficacy is less than anti-VEGF agents, along with an increased risk of glaucoma and cataract. The second most important trial was the BRAVO study, which evaluated the efficacy of intravitreal ranibizumab in macular edema. They concluded that ranibizumab-treated patients gained more than three-line improvement in nearly 60% of the patients and maintained it at a 2-year follow-up (HORIZON trial, not to be confused with the ARMD Horizon trial). Thus, the first line of treatment is anti-VEGF. Single monthly injection for the first 3 months followed by PRN dosing is preferred, though the trials gave continuous monthly injections for 6 months. Laser can be used as a second line of treatment. Recalcitrant cases should be assessed for cause—chronic breakdown of the blood-retinal barrier, peripheral ischemia, or epiretinal membrane (ERM). Most cases respond well to steroids, others may need a targeted laser to peripheral ischemic areas or vitrectomy for significant ERM. Later, neovascularization may occur and complicate further by VH, which may require vitrectomy in nonresolving cases. Recently another anti-VEGF aflibercept has also shown equal efficacy with a longer duration of action (VIBRANT trial). Combination treatment of anti-VEGF with laser is ongoing and has shown no additional benefit of laser with anti-VEGF (RELATE and BRIGHTER trial).

These case scenarios may be encountered:
- *Condition 1:* Patient having BRVO with no macular edema or neovascularization. FFA shows <5DD of capillary nonperfusion.
  Rx: Follow up.
- *Condition 2:* Patient having macular edema but no neovascularization. FFA shows <5DD of capillary nonperfusion.
  Rx: Determine the cause of macular edema by fluorescein angiography. If the cause is leaking capillaries, but the vision is 6/9 or better, observation can be employed with serial follow-up. If the vision is worse than 6/12 or hampers the patient's activities, an anti-VEGF injection can be given. In chronic cases or recalcitrant edema steroids in the form of triamcinolone (SCORE trial) or dexamethasone (GENEVA trial) can be given with the risk of side effects, such as IOP elevation and cataract. In cases of macular ischemia, only observation can be done, and the macular edema usually resolves within 1 year with a gain of visual acuity. BVOS had suggested a wait period of 3 months, though current studies do not suggest the same.
- *Condition 3:* Patient having BRVO with no macular edema or neovascularization. FFA shows > 5DD of capillary nonperfusion.
  Rx: More stringent follow-up, as the chances of developing neovascularization are higher in these cases.
- *Condition 4:* Patient having BRVO with no macular edema but with neovascularization present, either NVE or NVD.
  Rx: According to a branch retinal vein occlusion study, sectoral retinal photocoagulation. Now with wide-field angiography available trend has shifted toward targeted laser photocoagulation with repeat fluorescein angiography after 6 months to look for any new areas of capillary nonperfusion or neovascularization and repeat laser.
- *Condition 5:* Patient having BRVO with macular edema and neovascularization.
  Rx: Determine the cause of macular edema as to ischemia or leakage. Laser of peripheral capillary nonperfusion areas has to be done. However, before that, an anti-VEGF intravitreal injection may be considered to reduce macular edema in cases of leaking capillaries as laser photocoagulation increases macular edema. OCT should be done to document macular edema. This is the current gray zone. In patients with NVs, though BRVO is likely to be long-standing and so the chronic edema, it may be prudent to treat the NVs first followed by sequential/simultaneous and rapid management of edema.

VIVA QUESTIONS

Q.1. What are the common causes of BRVO? What are risk factors in young patients and how will you work with such a patient?
Ans. Refer text.

Q.2. What is the pathogenesis of BRVO?

Ans. The obstruction occurs at the A/V crossing. Most of the time the artery is above the vein and can lead to compression of the other as they share the common adventitial sheath. Vitreous has also been implicated, with greater vitreomacular attachments at greater risk for developing BRVO. Thus turbulent flow may lead to endothelial swelling, an increase in vessel wall size, and obstruction. The resulting venous obstruction leads to elevation of venous pressure that may overload the collateral drainage capacity and lead to macular edema and ischemia. An increase in venous pressure can also result in rupture of the vessel wall with intraretinal hemorrhage. Recently increased VEGF load has been shown to lead to a lessening of endothelial cells and an increase in permeability of capillaries, thereby validating the use of anti-VEGF.

Q.3. What is the classification of BRVO?

Ans. It is classified based on anatomical location—Major and macular. Major is when the vessel supplying the entire quadrant gets affected. Macular is when a macular branch gets affected.

It can also be classified based on the area of capillary nonperfusion—Ischemic or nonischemic. Ischemic had more than five-disc diameter areas of CNP. These cases are more likely to develop neovascularization.

Q.4. Which is the most common quadrant for BRVO and why?

Ans. The superotemporal quadrant is the most commonly involved quadrant as the superior hemi retina has the greatest number of A/V crossing changes and superonasal BRVO is not present due to lack of symptoms.

Q.5. What is the most common cause of defective vision due to BRVO?

Ans. The most common cause is macular edema. However, it is imperative to rule out FA whether it is perfused or nonperfused as it guides the further course of treatment.

Q.6. What are the common complications of BRVO? What are the chances of a nonischemic BRVO converting into an ischemic BRVO?

Ans. The most important complications are macular edema, macular ischemia, and neovascularization sequelae. Neovascularization may progress to VH, TRD, and NVG. Patients with macular edema with vision <6/12 are treated with above mentioned therapeutic options. Macular ischemia has not been shown to benefit from treatment. Neovascularization sequelae are expected in 11% of nonischemic and 40% of ischemic BRVO. It can occur up to 3 years of BRVO, although in most cases it occurs between 6 and 12 months. Laser is recommended only after the development of new vessels. There is no additional benefit of prophylactic laser in ischemic cases without new vessel formation.

Q.7. What investigations would you do in the case of BRVO and what would they reveal?

Ans. Refer text.

Q.8. When do you treat a patient of BRVO and what are the treatment options?

Ans. Refer text.

Q.9. Name two landmark clinical trials.

Ans. BVOS and BRAVO. Refer text.

Q.10. What is the first line of treatment for macular edema?

Ans. Refer text.

Q.11. What are the treatment options for recalcitrant macular edema?

Ans. Refer text.

Q.12. What is the role of laser in the management of macular edema?

Ans. Refer text. RELATE and BRIGHTER (ongoing).

Q.13. Compare modalities for managing macular edema in BRVO.

Ans. *See* Discussion.

BIBLIOGRAPHY

1. Hayreh SS, Zimmerman MB. Fundus changes in Branch Retinal Vein Occlusion. Retina. 2015; 35(5):1016-27.
2. Jaulim A, Ahmed B, Khanam T, Chatziralli IP. Branch retinal vein occlusion: epidemiology, pathogenesis, risk factors, clinical features, diagnosis, and complications. An update of the literature. Retina. 2013;33(5):901-10.
3. Rogers SL, McIntosh RL, Lim L, Mitchell P, Cheung N, Kowalski JW, et al. Natural history of branch retinal vein occlusion: an evidence-based systematic review. Ophthalmology. 2010;117(6):1094-101.

PROLIFERATIVE DIABETIC RETINOPATHY

Brijesh Takkar, Dhaval Patel, Rajesh Pattebahadur

INTRODUCTION

Diabetic retinopathy (DR) is the leading cause of vision loss in the middle-aged population. The worldwide prevalence of DR is 34.6% and that of vision-threatening DR is 10.2%.[1] Broadly, diabetic retinopathy is classified into NPDR, PDR, and diabetic maculopathy. It is important that students undergoing examination should be able to examine and identify the changes in DR and PDR, which are harbingers of severe visual loss.

HISTORY

Chief Complaints

Proliferative diabetic retinopathy generally presents in a known case of DM along with an established diagnosis of DR under the follow-up. Nevertheless, it is not uncommon to see a patient with the presentation of PDR on a first ophthalmic visit. The different presenting symptoms depend on the stage and complications of PDR and are as follows:
- *Gradual loss of vision:* Due to deterioration of DR, macular edema, or associated progression of cataract or tractional papillopathy/retinopathy
- *Acute loss of vision:* When associated with VH or TRD involving macula or diabetic macular edema (DME)
- *History of floaters:* Due to VH (mild) or vitreous degeneration associated with PDR
- *Acute pain, redness, and loss of vision:* Due to associated NVG

History of Present Illness

While taking a history of such cases, the onset and progression of decrease of vision (DOV) is important, because the sudden onset implies causes, such as VH and RD (secondary RRD). Whereas, the slow onset DOV can be caused by complications, such as diabetic macular edema and clinically significant macular edema.

History of Past Illness

See chapters on NPDR and DME for history.

Past Surgical History

See the chapter on NPDR/DME.

Family History

Family history of DM, hypertension, and other risk factors for DR.

Personal History

History of smoking, alcohol intake, and tobacco chewing.

EXAMINATION

General Examination/Specific Systemic Examination

Diabetes is a multisystem disorder involving causes vasculopathy and neuropathy. So, a detailed systemic evaluation of the cardiovascular system, respiratory system, central and peripheral nervous system, and renal system should be done to rule out the comorbidity associated with DM.

Ocular Examination

The examination findings are similar to a case of NPDR. A few important points for PDR are summarized further.

Visual Acuity

Uncorrected visual acuity (UCVA) and best corrected visual acuity (BCVA) must be noted. This is important for decision-making.

Eyeball

Usually, it is normal in such a case. In a few cases, squint can be seen due to associated ischemic mononeuropathy involving the cranial nerve (CN) third, fourth, or sixth (classically pupil sparing III CN palsy or seventh CN palsy).

Cornea

The following points must be noted:
- Corneal hypoesthesia (risk of neurotrophic keratitis)
- Decrease corneal healing (risk of recurrent corneal erosion and persistent epithelial defect)
- Tear film abnormalities (Dry eye due to autonomic neuropathy affecting sensory nerves associated with tear secretion)
- The corneal endothelium is usually normal in clinical examination. However, specular microscopy significantly higher coefficient of variation, a decrease in the percentage of hexagonal cells, and a low figure coefficient.

Iris

Check for NVI. The pupillary margins are the earliest site where neovascularization of the NVI. (See chapter on NPDR and DME)

Pupil

The following points must be noted:
- Ectropion uvea (the fibrous tissue accompanying neovascularization contracts which caused eversion of the posterior pigmented layer at the pupillary margin).
- Increase pigment at angles.
- Difficulty in dilating pupils (manifestation of diabetic neuropathy resulting in reduced functional innervation of the dilator muscle). The maximum pupillary dilatation should always be noted. In DM the pupils dilate poorly. This is important because every surgery including cataract and retinal surgery will need the maximum papillary dilatation. Diabetic pupil dilates poorly in response to standard anticholinergic eye drops (tropicamide, homatropine, and cyclopentolate that act by paralyzing the iris sphincter muscle). This failure of dilatation is due, at least in part, to a sympathetic dysfunction related to the autonomic neuropathy of these patients. The addition of phenylephrine (which acts directly by stimulating α-adrenergic receptors on the iris dilator muscle, producing contraction of the dilator muscle of the pupil), which utilizes the denervation super sensitivity (a sharp increase of sensitivity of postsynaptic membranes to a chemical transmitter after denervation) of the small diabetic pupil, greatly improving the mydriatic drug response in diabetic patients.
- Argyll Robertson pupils (bilateral small pupils that reduce in size on a near object (they "accommodate"), but do *not* constrict when exposed to bright light (they do not "react" to light) and useful mnemonic **A**ccommodation **R**eflex **P**resent).

Intraocular Pressure

Raised IOP can be there due to POAG (6 to 11%), NVG, or ghost cell glaucoma (in long-standing cases of VH) can be seen in DM.

Lens

See the chapter on NPDR.

Vitreous following findings can be there:
- The vitreous in diabetic patients undergo abnormal collagen crosslinking and nonenzymatic glycation, which lead to precocious liquefaction and PVD.

- Asteroid hyalosis
- In cases with secondary RRD along with TRD, tobacco dust (Schaffer's sign) is seen.

Fundus

The following signs must be noted:
- *Early PDR:* New vessels at the disc or within 1 DD of the disc (NVD) or new vessels elsewhere (NVE).
- *High-risk PDR:* The presence of any three of the following four features characterizes DRS.
  1. Neovascularization (at any location)
  2. Neovascularization at the optic disc (NVD)
  3. *Severe neovascularization:*
     - New vessels within one disc diameter of the optic nerve head (NVD) that are >1/4–1/3-disc area in size
     - NVE at least ½-disc area in size
  4. *Vitreous or preretinal hemorrhage*: To simplify presence of the following indicates the need for treatment
     - NVD > 1/3–1/4 of disc area
     - Any NVD with associated VH
     - NVE greater than 1/2 with vitreous or preretinal hemorrhage

TRD: It is important to note if TRD is involving the macula and TRD is threatening the macula **(Figs. 1 and 2)**.

TRD threatening macula: Retinal elevation of at least 4 DD area whose at least some part is within 30° of the center of the macula or retinal elevation of <4DD, along with one or more vitreoretinal adhesion causing elevation of the retina within 30° of the center of macula in presence of new vessel or fresh bleed VH.

TRD involving macula: Vitreoretinal traction along the arcade or disc or retinal traction lines extending through the fovea and causing progressive vision loss.

The presence of TTPH, vitreomacular traction (VMT), and CSME should always be noted as they affect treatment management. Very commonly these attachments are around the arcades.

Advanced DR: Also known as end-stage DR or burnt-out DR. The retina becomes featureless with sclerosed vessels and loss of sheen. There may be massive TRD and accompanying absolute NVG.

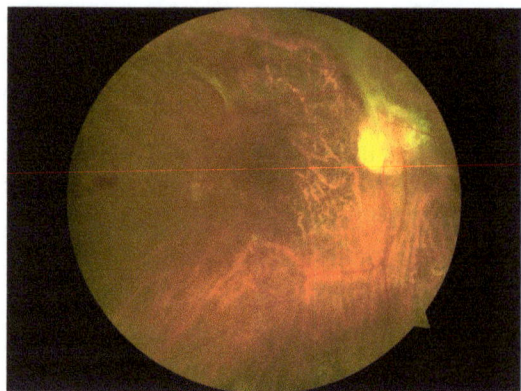

Fig. 1: Fibrovascular proliferation on disc and along arcades can be seen in the fundus photograph.

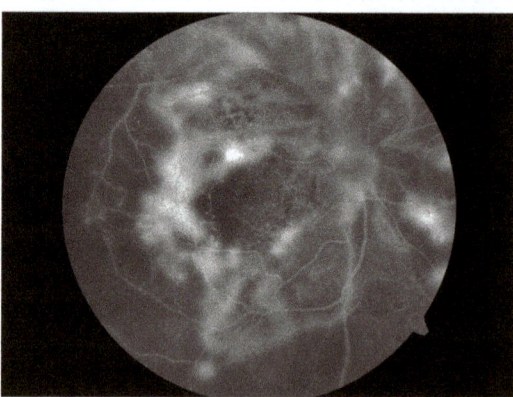

Fig. 2: FA picture is suggestive of NVD and NVEs. Severe peripheral ischemia and macular ischemia are also visible. (FA: fluorescein angiography; NVD: neovascularization at the disc; NVEs: neovascularization elsewhere)

■ DIFFERENTIAL DIAGNOSIS

See the chapter on DME and NPDR.

■ INVESTIGATION

(*See* chapter on DME and NPDR)
- UWFA may be very helpful in picking up peripheral anterior ischemia with peripheral new vessels. Predominant peripheral DR can also be differentiated. General FFA is helpful in differentiating between OIS and early PDR.
- *OCT-A:* This modality can detect and measure changes in differences and types of NVD.

- UWF OCT angiography is a noninvasive method of differentiating between advanced NPDR and PDR. The test, however, is not well validated against FFA yet.
- USG should be done in VH. It also helps in prognostication. It can also guide to severity and location of TRD.

■ MANAGEMENT

[Also *See* Chapter on VH, NPDR and DME **(Table 1)**].

Non High-risk PDR

Conventionally, these cases are treated with careful follow-up (at 2–4-month intervals) and prompt panretinal photocoagulation (PRP) if progression to high-risk PDR occurs. However, PRP was suggested under the following circumstances:
- The patient has poor DM control with associated DM complications (nephropathy).
- The patient will not or cannot be followed closely
- Access to health care is difficult
- Fellow eye is blind from DR
- Poor patient compliance with follow-up
- Before cataract operation or pregnancy (controversial)
- Whenever iris or angle neovascularization is seen, early PRP should be done irrespective of the presence or absence of retinal HRC.

As of now recommendations by the International Council of Ophthalmology are to treat any PDR.

Table 1: Comparison of anti-VEGF.

	Pegaptanib	*Bevacizumab*	*Ranibizumab*	*Aflibercept*
Composition	Aptamer (single strand of RNA or DNA	Full-length antibody	Antibody fragment	Recombinant protein combined with Fc portion of IgG
Molecular weight	50 kD	149 kD	48 kD	115 kD
	VEGF-165 isoform	All isoforms of VEGF-A	All isoforms of VEGF-A	All isoforms of VEGF-A, VEGF-B, PLGF-1 and 2
Half-life	2 days	5 days	3 days	7 days
Doses	0.3 µg/0.9 mL	1.25 mg/0.05 mL	0.5 mg or 0.3 mg/0.05 mL	2 mg/0.05 mg
Systemic side effect	• Bronchitis • Plural effusion • Diarrhea • Nausea • Vomiting • Carotid artery occlusion • CVA • TIA • Contact dermatitis • HS reaction/anaphylactic reaction	• Arterial thromboembolic events • CHF • Dizziness • Confusion • CVA	• Acute HTN • CVA • MI • Facial skin redness • Itchy skin rash	• CVA • HT

(CHF: congestive heart failure; CVA: cerebrovascular accident; DNA: deoxyribonucleic acid; RNA: ribonucleic acid; HS: hypersensitivity; MI: myocardial infarction; PLGF: placental growth factor; TIA: transient ischemic attacks; VEGF: vascular endothelial growth factor)

High-risk PDR

- High-risk PDR requires immediate *panretinal photocoagulation* (PRP) or scatter photocoagulation
- Patients with HRC treated with PRP have a 50% reduction in risk of severe visual loss. The rate of severe visual loss (visual acuity <5/200) was reduced by treatment from 16% in nontreated eyes over 2 years to 6% in treated eyes, a reduction of 57% in DRS.[1,2]
- The following points must be remembered, PRP:
  - Does not improve visual acuity
  - May cause worsening macular edema and loss of peripheral vision and night vision
  - Indications for supplementation are uncertain
  - Does not always cause regression of NVD/NVE: Regression of neovascularization occurs in 30–55% of eyes after laser photocoagulation. Complete regression of NVD was found in 29.8% and partial regression in 24.5% of eyes at 12 months after treatment in DRS.[1,2] Regression is marked by fibrotic changes.
  - Is also indicated in patients with NVI from PDR even in the absence of NVD/NVE or in the presence of widespread retinal ischemia and capillary drop-out on fluorescein angiography
  - Protocols of Diabetic Retinopathy Clinical Research Network (DRCR.Net) have attempted management of NVs with monthly intravitreal ranibizumab alone, though there is no benefit in terms of vision in comparison to laser PRP, which is an economically easier therapy (Protocol S).
  - Injections are generally avoided in the presence of traction and TRD.
- If CSME is also present in addition to high-risk PDR, combined anti-VEGF therapy and PRP at the first treatment session should be considered. In the days of LASER and early treatment diabetic retinopathy study (ETDRS), it was suggested that diabetic macular edema (DME) should be managed before PDR to prevent its worsening. However, now intravitreals are preferred which act on NVs also, making decisions easier.
- Complications of PRP
- *Transient side effects:* Blurring of vision, Macular edema, CD, Headache, iritis
- *Medium-term side effects:* Macular edema may persist for >3 months
- *Long-term:* Foveal burn, macular edema, choroidal neovascularization, PVD, retinal, subretinal, or choroidal hemorrhage due to excessive power of the laser, exudative RD, VH, increased IOP, mydriasis, and paresis of accommodation, loss of visual field, loss of dark adaptation/nyctalopia, lens opacities, increase in traction detachments.

High-risk PDR—not Amenable to Photocoagulation

In the presence of severe vitreous or pre-retinal hemorrhage, it may not be possible to deliver laser photocoagulation adequately. In such cases, retinal cryopexy or vitrectomy has to be considered.[3] Reported benefits of peripheral retinal cryotherapy include resorption of VHs and regression of NVD, NVE, and NVI. The main complication is the development or acceleration of traction RD in 25–38% of eyes.[1] Therefore, this treatment should be avoided in patients with known traction RD, and all patients must be monitored carefully. Nowadays, generally, surgery is preferred.

Vitrectomy in diabetic patients: The following are the indications of vitrectomy in PDR:
- Nonclearing hemorrhage-vitreous/subhyaloid/premacular
  - The Diabetic Retinopathy Vitrectomy Study (DRVS) was the landmark randomized controlled trial to evaluate indications and timing of pars plana vitrectomy for the management of advanced DR.
  - Early vitrectomy (within 3 months) for treatment of VH secondary to DR was highly cost-effective in a cost-utility analysis using DRVS results.
    - The benefits of early vitrectomy for nonresolving severe VH are greater for patients with T1DM and lower for T2DM.
    - With diffuse or chronic DME, or a thickened or taut posterior hyaloid, early vitrectomy reduces DME.

- If RD is present, an early vitrectomy is usually suggested.
- Patients with bilateral severe VH generally should undergo vitrectomy in one eye when they are medically stable.
• TRD not involving the macula may remain stable for many years. When the macula becomes involved, immediate vitrectomy is generally recommended.
• Combined tractional and RRD may progress rapidly, and early surgery should be considered in these patients.
• Anterior segment neovascularization with postsegment opacity
• TRD threatening/involving the macula
• Ghost cell/hemolytic glaucoma
• Anterior hyaloid fibrovascular proliferation
• Epiretinal membrane
• Concurrent internal limiting membrane (ILM) peeling may be done for cases with DME.
• Anterior retinal cryopexy has a limited role.

VIVA QUESTIONS

Q.1. Define NVD and NVE.
Ans. When neovascularization arises on or within 1 disc diameter of the optic disc they are referred to as neovascularization of the disc (NVD). When they arise further than 1 disc diameter away, they are called NVE.

Q.2. What is the prevalence of retinopathy in diabetes?
Ans. The overall prevalence is about 25%. It is 40% in insulin-dependent diabetes mellitus (IDDM) and 20% in noninsulin-dependent diabetes mellitus (NIDDM).

Q.3. What associated systemic conditions worsen diabetic retinopathy?
Ans. These are—pregnancy, hypertension, anemia, and renal failure.

Q.4. What do you know about the pathogenesis of retinal new vessel formation?
Ans. It is not completely understood, and current theories emphasize the production of angiogenic factors by areas of ischemic and hypoxic retina. More recently, VEGF has been isolated from ocular fluid and is an endothelial cell-specific angiogenic factor whose production is increased by hypoxia: it has been implicated in the neovascularization seen in diabetic retinopathy and retinal vein occlusion.[2,4]

Q.5. Enlist non-DR causes of visual loss in diabetic subjects.
Ans. These are as follows:
- Trauma and injury
- Amblyopia
- ARMD
- Retinal vein and artery occlusion, ischemic optic neuropathy
- Cataract
- Glaucoma
- Hypertension (and macroaneurysms)
- RD
- Optic atrophy
- Retinal dystrophies and myopic degeneration.

Q.6. Write a note on PASCAL (Pattern-scanning retinal laser).
Ans. PASCAL technology is a semi-automated pattern generation method using short laser pulse durations of typically 20 milliseconds (five times shorter than conventional systems). These laser pulses are delivered in a rapid pre-determined sequence resulting in precise even burn patterns as well as improved safety, patient comfort, and a significant reduction in treatment time when compared to single-shot photocoagulation. Multiple spot lasers are similar technology.

Q.7. What is the role of anti-VEGF injections in the surgical management of PDR?
Ans. It is helpful in managing unlasered cases posted for surgery to prevent bleeding. It should be given 1–3 days before surgery. In patients with TRS, however, caution should be executed for risks of conversion to secondary RRD. Some surgeons also leave it at the end of surgery as it may help in managing concurrent DME and prevent rebleed to some extent.

Q.8. What is rebleed?
Ans. Up to 20% of patients may have recurrent VH following PPV. Early causes include dispersed hemorrhage, hypotony, and port

site bleeds. Late causes include inadequate laser, poor hyaloidal dissection with retinal breaks poor systemic status, and port site new vessels.

Q.9. How is diabetic PPV different from other surgeries?

Ans. After core vitrectomy, the surgeon should cauterize all possible bleeders first and then identify VR adhesions. Vitreoschisis is frequent in such cases. PVD should not be induced before clearing all adhesions to the retina or new vessels. Intraoperative bleeding is very common, and the surgeon should be prepared for it. Keep suction and other parameters low. An old protocol would involve segmentation, delamination, and en bloc methods of dissection. These days the role of MIVS cutter as a multipurpose instrument has made surgery much easier. Meticulous PRP should be done and ILM peeling as needed. At the end of surgery, again all bleeders must be cauterized.

Q.10. Discuss the management of NVG.
Ans. See glaucoma chapters.

Q.11. What are the specifications for PRP?
Ans.
- 300–500 μm laser spot size depending on the type of lens used (for magnification adjustment)
- Laser power starts at 100 mW and increase
- Spot distance half-one spot size apart
- Total spots around 2,000–2,500
- To be done in 2-3 sittings to avoid exudative RD, angle closure, and CD
- Mark the boundary and start inferiorly first
- Stay 500 μm far nasal to disc, just outside/within arcades, and always at least 2DD away from the fovea
- Augmentation may be done as needed.

REFERENCES

1. American Academy of Ophthalmology. Preferred Practice Pattern® Guidelines. [online] Available from https://www.aao.org/education/about-preferred-practice-patterns [Last accessed February, 2024].
2. Nentwich MM, Ulbig MW. Diabetic retinopathy—ocular complications of diabetes mellitus. World J Diabetes. 2015;6(3):489-99.
3. Eliott D, Lee MS, Abrams GW. Proliferative diabetic retinopathy: principles and techniques of surgical treatment. In: Ryan SJ (Ed). Retina, 4th edition. Philadelphia: Elsevier Mosby; 2006:2413-49.
4. Heng LZ, Comyn O, Peto T, Tadros C, Ng E, Sivaprasad S, et al. Diabet Med. Diabetic retinopathy: pathogenesis, clinical grading, management, and future developments. 2013;30(6):640-50.

NONPROLIFERATIVE DIABETIC RETINOPATHY

Dhaval Patel, Brijesh Takkar, Rajesh Pattebahadur

INTRODUCTION

Broadly, diabetic retinopathy (DR) is classified into NPDR, PDR, and diabetic maculopathy. The previous concept of background retinopathy generally falls under NPDR. DR is a very common disorder inwards and retina clinics. Hence, the chances of getting DR as short or long cases are very high. Particularly the viva revolves around the landmark studies done for DR. In India, most of the results seen in western trials have been echoed by the Sankara Nethralaya Diabetic Retinopathy Epidemiology and Molecular Genetic (SN-DREAMS) study conducted in southern India.

HISTORY

Chief Complaints

It primarily depends upon whether associated maculopathy is present or not. The various modes of presentation can be
- Gradual or acute loss of vision (macular edema)
- History of floaters
- Paracentral scotomata
- Some patients may be asymptomatic if the macula is spared
- Detection during DR screening.

History of Present Illness

Typically, the patient has a known case of DM often referred by a general physician for screening. In India, it is not uncommon for ophthalmologists to see a case of DR without a previous diagnosis of DM.

History of Past Illness

Unlike many ocular disorders, this is very important in the case of diabetic retinopathy.

The following points must be noted in history:
- *History of DM:* It is very important to note down the following:
  - *Type of DM:* Screening of DR is done immediately after diagnosis in type 2 and within 5 years of diagnosis in cases of type 1 DM. Typically diabetic macular edema (DME) is a more common presentation of type 2 DM and PDR is more common in type 1.[1]
  - *Duration of DM:* Duration of DM is directly proportional to the risk of DR. After 5 years, approximately 25% of *type 1* patients will have retinopathy.[1] After 10 years, almost 60% have retinopathy, and after 15 years, 80% have retinopathy. In the Wisconsin Epidemiologic Study of Diabetic Retinopathy (WESDR), most vision-threatening complications were present in approximately 50% of *type 1* patients who had the disease for 20 years.[1] In the Los Angeles Latino Eye Study (LALES) and Proyecto VER (Vision, Evaluation, and Research), 18% of participants with diabetes of >15 years' duration had PDR, with no difference in the percentage with PDR between those with type 1 versus type 2 diabetes.[1,2] *Type 2* patients with a duration of diabetes of <5 years, 40% of those patients taking insulin, and 24% of those not taking insulin have DR.[1] These rates increased to 84 and 53%, respectively, when the duration of diabetes was 19 years.[1,2] It is generally believed that almost all diabetics develop some form of DR over time, whether treatable or not.
  - *DM control:* Poorly controlled DM is highly likely to be associated with DR. *Duration of diabetes and severity of hyperglycemia* is the major risk factor for developing retinopathy. Remember HbA1c is the most important parameter to evaluate control of (DM) over a period of 3 months. As per guidelines, HbA1c of 7% or lower is the target for glycemic control in most patients with DM. As per the Diabetes Control and Complications Trial (DCCT) for each 10%, decrease in the HbA1c, the risk of progression of retinopathy decreases by 39%.[1,2]
  - *Insulin use:* Recent change from oral hypoglycemic agents (OHAs) to insulin can be associated with a high-risk of having DR. Among the *type 2* patients a higher proportion of cases of insulin develops DR compared to those not taking insulin (40% vs. 24% at 5 years and 84% vs. 53% at 19 years.[1] Certain oral hypoglycemic agents (OHAs) may in fact precipitate DME.
  - *Associated nephropathy:* The development of PDR parallels an increased risk of nephropathy, myocardial infarction, and/or cerebral vascular accidents;[1] however, the same cannot be said for DME as nearly all the studies on the topic have failed to find an association between nephropathy and DME.
  - *The history of retinal laser* for DR may be present, type, and number of settings must be noted.
  - *History of* prior treatment with *intravitreal injections* should always be asked as leading questions.
- *Hypertension:* Intensive management of hypertension may slow retinopathy progression.
- *Hyperlipidemia:* Management of serum lipids may reduce retinopathy progression and the need for treatment. This has been noted both in Action to Control Cardiovascular Risk in Diabetes (ACCORD) and Fenofibrate Intervention and Event Lowering in Diabetes (FIELD) Trials.[1]
- *Anemia/use of angiotensin-converting enzyme inhibitor/clotting factors* has been described to influence the onset of DR, although the evidence is inconclusive. Overall,

ACE inhibitors were not found to have any conclusive effect on DR progression.[1,2]
- *Pregnancy:* DR can worsen during pregnancy. This is due to the physiologic changes of pregnancy and the changes in overall metabolic control. During the first trimester, an eye examination should be performed, and subsequent follow-up visits must be scheduled depending on the severity of retinopathy.

  If there is no DR, then at least one examination should be done in every trimester. FA, intravitreal injections, and lasers should be avoided if possible. The retinopathy can eventually subside on its following delivery.
- Cardiac disease and neurological disease.

Past Surgical History

The previous history of any cataract surgery must be enquired about. The effects of cataract surgery on the acceleration of the progression of DR are controversial. Some reports suggest that eyes that had phacoemulsification had a two-fold increased risk of developing retinopathy compared with eyes that were not subjected to cataract surgery and cataract surgery may deteriorate the progression of diabetic macular edema.[1,2] However the Early Treatment Diabetic Retinopathy Study (ETDRS) did not find an association between clinically significant macular edema and cataract extraction.

■ EXAMINATION

General Examination/Specific Systemic Examination

- A detailed general examination must be done to rule out other complications of DM such as neuropathy, nephropathy, and diabetic foot.
- Other medical problems (often coexisting with DM) must be looked for such as:
  - Hypertension
  - Smoking
  - Obesity
  - Hyperlipidemia
  - Anemia

Ocular Examination

- *Visual acuity:* Reversible refractive errors with changes in glycemic levels even during a day should be kept in mind while performing vision testing. Best-corrected visual acuity is often helpful in deciding the treatment modality in the presence of macular edema.
- *Eyeball:* CN palsies (classically pupil sparing third CN palsy or sixth CN palsy as a sign of reversible ischemic mononeuropathy).
- *Lid:* Xanthelasma (suggestive of hyperlipidemia), recurrent hordeola, and blepharitis in uncontrolled diabetes can be seen.
- *Conjunctiva:* There is an increased risk of developing conjunctival bacterial infections. In addition, microaneurysms can be seen in the bulbar conjunctiva.
- *Cornea:* Look for the following:
  - Corneal hypoesthesia (due to associated neuropathy; risk of neurotrophic keratitis)
  - Decrease corneal healing (risk of recurrent corneal erosion)
  - Tear film abnormalities (a manifestation of autonomic neuropathy).
- *Iris:* Check for NVI that indicates the presence of PDR.
- *Pupil:* Look for the following:
  - Ectropion uvea (the fibrous tissue accompanying neovascularization contracts which caused eversion of the posterior pigmented layer at the pupillary margin)
  - Increase pigment at angles
  - Difficulty in dilating pupils (manifestation of diabetic neuropathy resulting in reduced functional innervation of the dilator muscle)
  - Argyll Robertson pupils (bilateral small pupils that reduce in size on a near object (they "accommodate"), but do *not* constrict when exposed to bright light (they do not "react" to light)—a useful mnemonic **A**ccommodation **R**eflex **P**resent).
- *IOP:* DR can be associated with primary open-angle glaucoma (POAG) and NVG.
- *Lens:* Look for the following:
  - Reduction in accommodative ability.
  - DM can produce the following forms of cataract:
    - Typically, nuclear and cortical cataract formation is chronic and progressive cases

- Acute cortical cataract formation with profound elevations in blood glucose
- Snowflake cataracts, which are white subcapsular opacifications, have been described in young type 1 diabetic patients. This type of cataract is less commonly seen today because it is usually associated with long-term untreated hyperglycemia.
- Rapid progression of senile cataract occurs in DR.
- *Vitreous:* The vitreous in diabetic patients undergo abnormal collagen cross-linking and nonenzymatic glycation, which lead to precocious liquefaction and PVD. Asteroid hyalosis can also occur.
- *Fundus:* The different changes that can be seen in DR are summarized in **Tables 1 and 2**.

Stages of NPDR

- *Mild NPDR:* Microaneurysm (one or more) **(Fig. 1)**
- *Moderate NPDR:* Microaneurysm, retinal hemorrhages (dot and blot), hard exudates, cotton-wool spots (CWS), venous beading, arteriolar narrowing, intraretinal microvascular abnormalities (IRMA) **(Figs. 2 and 3)**.
- *Severe NPDR:* All of the above plus any of the following three (the famous 4:2:1 rule in ETDRS) **(Fig. 4)**:
  1. Blot hemorrhages in four quadrants
  2. Venous beading in two quadrants
  3. IRMA in one quadrant
- *Very severe NPDR:* More than one of the aforementioned rules.

Clinically Significant Macular Edema

- Retinal thickening or edema at or within 500 μm of the center of the macula
- Hard exudates at or within 500 μm of the center of the macula associated with retinal thickening of the adjacent retina
- An area or areas of retinal thickening at least one disc area in size at least part of which is within one disc diameter of the center of the macula.

Retinovascular Disease

- Retinal vein and artery occlusion
- Ischemic optic neuropathy

Diabetic Papillopathy

- It is a rare cause of bilateral (or sometimes unilateral) disc swelling in patients with type-1 DM.
- Disc edema is often associated with capillary telangiectasias overlying the disc surface.
- It differs from AION in that there is often bilateral and simultaneous optic nerve involvement.

Table 1: Fundus changes in diabetic retinopathy.

Clinical sign	Pathogenesis	A layer of the retina affected	Effect of treatment
Cotton-wool spot	Nerve fiber layer ischemic necrosis	Nerve fiber layer	Persists
Microaneurysms	Secondary to capillary wall outpouching due to pericyte loss	Superficial retinal layers	Resolves if controlled
Dot and blot hemorrhages	Microaneurysms rupture in the deeper layers of the retina	Inner nuclear and outer plexiform layers	Resolves gradually
Flame-shaped hemorrhage	Splinter hemorrhages that occur in the more superficial nerve fiber layer	Superficial layers	Resolves gradually
Retinal edema and hard exudates	Breakdown of the blood–retina barrier, allowing leakage of serum proteins and lipids from the vessels	Deeper layers	Resolves but complete resolution unlikely

Table 2: International diabetic retinopathy severity scale.

Disease severity level	Dilated ophthalmoscopy findings
No apparent DR	No abnormalities
Mild nonproliferative DR	Microaneurysms only
Moderate nonproliferative DR	More than "mild" but less than "severe"
Severe nonproliferative DR	Any of the following: • 20 or more intraretinal hemorrhages in four quadrants • Definite venous beading in two or more quadrants • Prominent IRMA in 1 or more quadrants and no neovascularization
Proliferative DR	One or more of the following: • Definite neovascularization • Preretinal or vitreous hemorrhage

(DR: diabetic retinopathy; IRMA: intraretinal microvascular abnormalities)

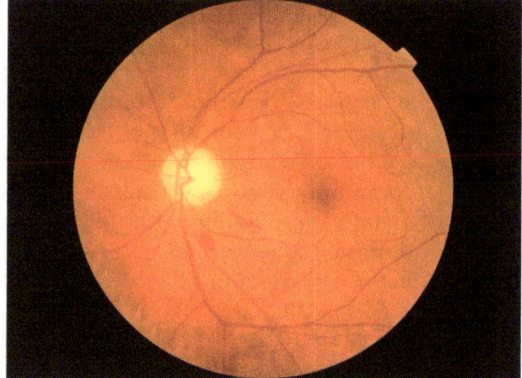

Fig. 1: Mild NPDR with microaneurysm and hemorrhage.

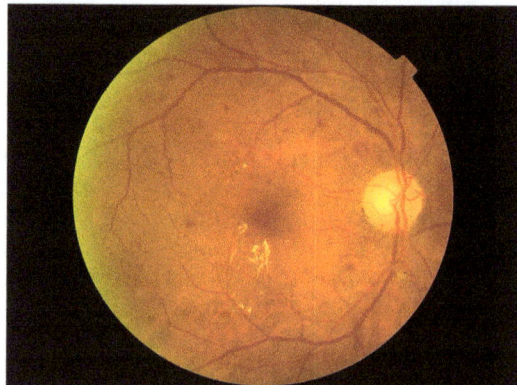

Fig. 2: Moderate NPDR with retinal hemorrhages and venous bleeding.

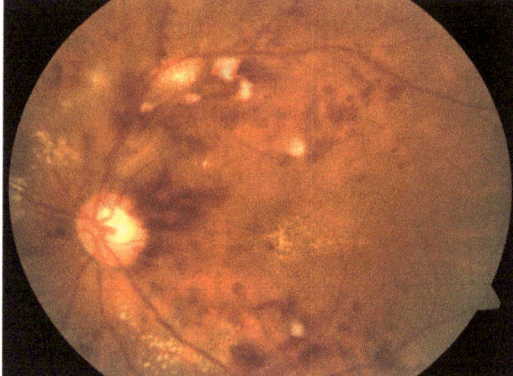

Fig. 3: Very severe NPDR with retinal hemorrhages, hard exudates, CWS, and venous beading. (CWS: cotton-wool spots; NPDR: nonproliferative diabetic retinopathy)

- Visual acuity is often normal
- The pathogenesis is impaired blood flow causing disc swelling, but not have sufficient to significantly affect optic nerve function.
- In most cases, the optic disc edema resolves without residual visual deficit.

■ DIFFERENTIAL DIAGNOSIS

The characteristic clinical findings and history of DM often differentiate DR from other disorders. However, the following disorders must be kept in mind that can mimic NPDR, especially in unilateral cases:
- Hypertensive retinopathy
- RVO (branch or central)
- Hemoglobinopathies
- Anemia or leukemia
- Ocular ischemic syndrome
- Radiation retinopathy
- Idiopathic juxtafoveal telangiectasis
- Coats' disease
- Vasculitis (e.g., sarcoidosis and lupus)

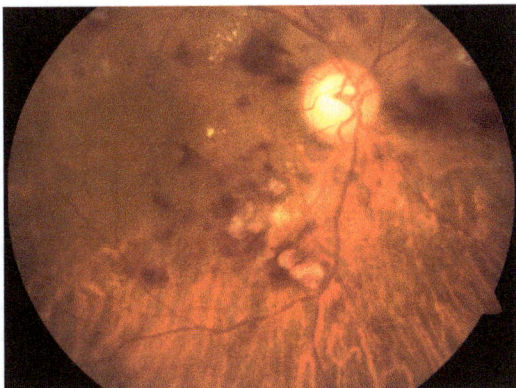

Fig. 4: Severe CWS and arterial attenuation along with features of NPDR in a case of combined retinopathy. (CWS: cotton-wool spots; NPDR: nonproliferative diabetic retinopathy)

■ INVESTIGATION

- *Systemic investigations:* The following points are specific for DR:
    – Fasting and postprandial blood sugar test
    – Glucose tolerance test
    – Hemoglobin A1c
    – Renal function test
    – Others for the systemic entities listed before
- *Fundus photography:* Color fundus photography is commonly used to document retinal disease and its evolution in diabetic patients. It is used for tracking disease progression and is accepted as the best screening method for DR especially in teleophthalmology. It also aids in teleophthalmology-based and artificial intelligence-based screening. By virtue of UWF imaging, peripheral predominant DR can be identified, which has a linkage to cardiac disorders.

Optical Coherence Tomography

- Noninvasive imaging technique
- It is important in managing diabetic macular edema (see the short case on DME).

Following are the uses of OCT in DR:
- To investigate cases with unexplained visual acuity loss
- To detect areas of VMT
- To evaluate patients with difficult and/or questionable examinations for DME
- To rule out other causes of macular edema
- To screen a patient with no or minimal diabetic retinopathy.

FFA

Following are uses of FFA in DR.
- *Diagnosis:*
    – Ischemic maculopathy
    – Areas of capillary nonperfusion
    – To rule out other causes of macular swelling
    – Differentiate between new vessels from IRMA
        ♦ To identify suspected but clinically obscure retinal neovascularization
        ♦ To evaluate unexplained visual loss.
- *Aid in treatment:*
    – To guide laser treatment of CSME
    – Delineate fovea and fovea avascular zone
    – Delineate the area of leakage
    – To detect areas of untreated retinal capillary nonperfusion that may be the cause for persistent retinal or NVD after previous scatter laser photocoagulation.

Ultrawide imaging: Instead of the previously used seven-field fundus imaging, now the focus is shifting toward ultrawide-field imaging for monitoring NPDR.

Red-free imaging: This is helpful in identifying new vessels, which may not be visible to the clinician.

ERG: Full field and multifocal ERG are helpful in diagnosing what has been called diabetic neuroretinopathy. This entity particularly can cause mild/minimal/functional/qualitative visual loss in patients without maculopathy. Together with FFA, it will also help in identifying OIS.

OCT angiography: The role is under evaluation, and the current concept involves imaging microaneurysms and FAZ changes.

■ MANAGEMENT

The following points are important in the management of NPDR:
- Joint management with family physicians or endocrinologists

- Stress should always be on systemic control first, and ocular management later
- Ensure good DM control (good glycosylated hemoglobin levels)
- Treat associated systemic diseases most important among them is maintaining, serum lipids, and blood pressure.
- Worsening DR is an indicator of poor systemic control.

Normal or minimal NPDR (with rare microaneurysms): Follow-up patient and watch for progression and macular edema. Remember within 1 year 5–10% of such patients can progress to advanced stages of DR.[1]

Mild to moderate NPDR without macular edema: Reexamine within 6–12 months. Approximately 16% of cases of mild and 23% of cases of moderate NPDR patients may progress to proliferative stages within 4 years.

Mild to moderate NPDR with CSME: If it is center-involving (ci-CSME) anti-VEGF is the treatment of choice. If it is noncenter-involving (nci-CSME) then focal/grid laser surgery guided by the ETDRS is the treatment of choice. (Refer to the chapter short case diabetic macular edema for details on the management of macular edema).

Severe and very severe NPDR: Follow-up patient very closely (2–4 months). In half of patients with in case of severe NPDR 50% of the cases progress PDR within 1 year, and 15% will develop high-risk PDR. Similarly, in cases with very severe NPDR 75% of the cases develop PDR within 1 year while 45% will develop high-risk PDR. Therefore, a close follow-up of such cases is required.

Screening for NPDR and advancing DR has seen a paradigm shift, with the inclusion of teleophthalmology and artificial intelligence. While commercial tools are also available, it has not gone to a level of inclusion in daily practice yet. Nonophthalmologists may also be employed in such screening protocols.

Classic indication of PRP is high-risk PDR; however, it may be done even without CSME in special situations such as:
- The patient is a young insulin-dependent diabetic (IDDM)
- Patient has poor DM control with associated DM complications (nephropathy)
- Fellow eye is blind from DR
- Family history of blindness from DR
- Poor patient compliance with follow-up
- Before cataract operation or pregnancy.

VIVA QUESTIONS

Q.1. Describe the pathophysiology of micro aneurysm development.

Ans. Normally there is one pericyte per endothelial cell. Pericytes are contractile cells that play an important role in microvascular autoregulation and maintaining the blood-retinal barrier. In people with diabetes, the pericytes die off and are decreased in number (SORBITOL accumulation). Their absence weakens the capillaries and permits thin-walled dilatations, which are known as microaneurysms. Naturally, these microaneurysms tend to collapse upon themselves but may leak causing disease.[3]

Q.2. Describe the pathophysiology of macular edema development.

Ans. The breakdown of the blood-retina barrier is an important pathophysiologic feature of diabetic retinopathy that leads to the development of macular edema.

Q.3. How would you differentiate between microaneurysm and small dot hemorrhage?

Ans. It is often difficult to distinguish a small dot hemorrhage from a microaneurysm by ophthalmoscopy alone. On fluorescein, angiography patent microaneurysms will fill with dye quickly and then leak, unlike a small dot hemorrhage that will block fluorescence.

Q.4. Describe the pathophysiology of dot-blot and flame-shaped hemorrhage.

Ans. If the hemorrhage is deep (i.e., in the inner nuclear layer or outer plexiform layer), it usually has a round or oval shape (dot or blot hemorrhage). Superficial (nerve fiber layer) hemorrhages, on the other hand, become flame or splinter shaped. This is due to the peculiar arrangement of nerve fibers in respective layers. Superficial hemorrhages may be associated with CWS, which represents blocked axoplasmic flow in the RNFL following focal ischemia.[3]

Q.5. Discuss about IRMAs.

Ans. These are shunt vessels and appear as abnormal branching or dilation of existing blood vessels (capillaries) within the retina that appear to supply the areas of nonperfusion. These vessels represent either new vessel growth within the retina or remodeling of pre-existing vessels through endothelial cell proliferation stimulated by hypoxia bordering areas of capillary nonperfusion. When compared to neovascularization (NV) in PDR, IRMAs are slightly larger in caliber with a broader arrangement and are always contained to the intraretinal layers. Conversely, NV tends to be much finer and delicate in caliber and is sometimes more focal in location depending on its severity. In severe cases, NV tends to grow along the posterior hyaloid interface, especially around the optic nerve (NVD) and periphery (NVE). On fluorescein angiography, NV will often show late leakage whereas IRMAs traditionally do not leak.[3]

Q.6. How often would you screen diabetic patients for retinopathy?

Ans. *Type-1 (Insulin-dependent diabetics):*
- 5 years after diagnosis then annually. In type 1 diabetes, substantial retinopathy becomes apparent as early as 6–7 years after the onset of the disease. In addition, the disease is diagnosed early because of its severity; hence screening is recommended beginning 5 years after the diagnosis of Type 1 diabetes.
- *Type-2 (Noninsulin-dependent diabetics):* Screening is done at diagnosis and then annually. The diagnosis of DM may be delayed in these cases and when the diagnosis is made, it is assumed that the disease might have already been present for the last 4–5 years. About 30% of patients will have some manifestations of DR at diagnosis hence screening has to be done immediately after diagnosis.

Pregnancy (Type 1 or Type 2):
- First examination—soon after conception and early in the first trimester.
- Follow-up—no retinopathy to mild or moderate NPDR: every 3–12 months. If severe NPDR or worse is present, then follow-up: every 1–3 months.

Q.7. What is the earliest sign of retinal change in diabetes?

Ans. Microaneurysms at the posterior pole are the first clinical signs. An increase in capillary permeability, evidenced by the leakage of dye into the vitreous humor after fluorescein injection, is the earliest sign of retinal change in DM.

Q.8. What are the three questions that ETDRS addressed and what are the inferences?

Ans. 1. What is the role of aspirin in diabetic retinopathy?
   Ans: It neither improves nor worsens retinopathy.
2. What is the role of initiating early laser (as compared to DRS high-risk criteria) in the management of severe nonproliferative and early proliferative retinopathy?
   Ans: Inconclusive. No strong benefit to early scatter PRP was found. Certain clinical circumstances (e.g., poor compliance with follow-up examinations, rapid progression in the fellow eye, and very poor cardiorenal status) may justify early initiation of PRP.
3. What is the role of laser (PRP or focal macular laser, or both) in the management of macular edema?
   Ans: Traditionally, there is no role for PRP in the treatment of macular edema. Macular laser is of benefit, reducing the risk of moderate visual loss by 50%. Patients with CSME should be treated. However, now research focus is toward targeted laser for peripheral ischemic areas detected upon wide FA.

Q.9. What is the international DR severity scale?

Ans. A workshop was held in April 2002 in conjunction with the International

Congress of Ophthalmology to develop and build broad-based consensus around a *clinically relevant* and *simplified DR disease severity scale* that is summarized in **Table 2**.

Q.10. What is subthreshold micropulse diode laser photocoagulation?
- *Subthreshold:* The intent of treatment is to lightly affect the retinal pigment epithelium alone, restricting the lateral spread of heat and thus, sparing damage to the overlying photoreceptors and midretinal interneurons
- *Micropulse:* Employs repetitive trains (50–500) of laser pulses of short duration (0.8–5.0 milliseconds) and extending the "off-time" between micropulses.
- *Diode laser:* Using a longer wavelength near-infrared 810 nm diode laser.

Q.11. How does laser act in macular edema?
Ans. It acts by the following mechanism:
- Reduces metabolic need.
- Direct diffusion of oxygen from the choriocapillaris through the scar to the inner retina.
- Stimulates endothelial repair process.

Q.12. How will you differentiate between diabetic papillopathy and AION?
Ans. See fundus changes above in the chapter.

Q.13. Discuss the preoperative/intraoperative/postoperative precautions for cataract surgery in the presence of NPDR with CSME.
Ans. The following are the precautions:
Preoperative care:
- In patients with existing rubeosis, this should be treated preoperatively with panretinal photocoagulation.
- Laser of macular edema or anti-VEGF injection should be given.
- Topical nonsteroidal anti-inflammatory drugs (NSAIDs) can prevent intraoperative miosis.

Intraoperative care:
- It is advisable to perform a large capsulorrhexis with a 6 mm optic lens, thus allowing better visualization of the fundus for PRP if required.
- Multifocals are contraindicated as they reduce the contrast and fundus evaluation is difficult.

Postoperative care:
- Patients with diabetes are at slightly greater risk of cystoid macular edema which may be difficult to differentiate from true diabetic maculopathy (see DME chapter).
- Incidence of capsular opacification is greater in diabetics than in nondiabetics. Therefore, a large yttrium aluminum garnet (YAG) capsulotomy to improve vision or improve visualization of the retina may become necessary.

Q.14. What is the role of NSAIDs?
Ans. DM induces inflammatory reactions by many mechanisms including, oxidative stress NF-κB activation, NOS dysregulation, AGEs formation, hypertension, dyslipidemia, and impaired anti-inflammatory pathways. Topical nonsteroidal anti-inflammatory medications are common treatments for DME. These agents are directed at decreasing intraocular prostaglandin levels, which have been implicated in the pathogenesis of DME. Bromfenac perhaps has the highest vitreal penetration.

REFERENCES

1. American Academy of Ophthalmology. Preferred Practice Pattern® Guidelines. [online] Available from https://www.aao.org/education/about-preferred-practice-patterns [Last accessed February, 2024].
2. Nentwich MM, Ulbig MW. Diabetic retinopathy—ocular complications of diabetes mellitus. World J Diabetes. 2015;6(3):489-99.
3. Heng LZ, Comyn O, Peto T, Tadros C, Ng E, Sivaprasad S, et al. Diabet Med. Diabetic retinopathy: pathogenesis, clinical grading, management and future developments. 2013;30(6):640-50.

RETINITIS PIGMENTOSA

Jyotiranjan Mallick, Prafulla Kumar Maharana

INTRODUCTION

Retinitis pigmentosa (RP) is a retinal dystrophy affecting the rod photoreceptors, to begin with, and subsequently cones resulting in severe visual loss. The prevalence is 1:3500 to 1:4000. The inheritance pattern is complex. It is usually presenting clinically in the second or third decade. Central vision is preserved late in the course of the disease. However, earlier loss of central vision may be attributed to cystoid macular edema occurring in 10–50% of individuals.[1-3] Typically X-linked variants present very early in childhood whereas autosomal recessive (AR) variants present around 10–12 years of age. Autosomal dominant (AD) linked and spontaneous variants present later. In exams, it is usually given as a long case.

HISTORY

Chief Complaints

The usual presenting complaints are the following:
- Dark adaptation difficulty (earliest, but patient often fails to recognize)
- Night blindness (most common presentation)
- Progressive loss of peripheral visual field—rarely the patient can present with tunnel vision when the central field is the only vision left.
- The gradual decrease in visual acuity—central visual acuity is usually preserved until the end stages of RP. Early central acuity loss can occur from cystoid macular edema (CME), complicated cataract, or an atypical form of RP.
- Acquired tritan color vision defect
- Noted during sibling screening
- Noted during fundus evaluation after medical advice.

History of Present Illness

- The disease usually begins in childhood or adolescence. The initial symptom is difficulty in dark adaptation. The earlier the onset of defective dark adaptation, the more severe the course of RP.
- The loss of red cell functioning in the retina of RP patients leads to many glare-related problems. In low light, these patients have night blindness. However, in bright light, they can experience "white out" glare. Parents may note an affected child bumps into objects at night.
- Subsequently, there occurs constriction of the visual field with preserved central vision until late in the disease. A careful history can often reveal frequent bumping or frequent accidents while driving a vehicle in cases unaware of their constricted field of vision.

History of Past Illness

Past medical and surgical history must include careful history to rule out the systemic associations of RP. This is more important in X-linked and AR variants. There may be a past history of associations of RP as well.

Family History

Meticulous family history should be taken and a pedigree should be prepared. A three-generation pedigree chart must be prepared in all such cases. Efforts should be made to identify the inheritance pattern if present.

EXAMINATION

General Examination

A detailed systemic examination is done to know any associated sensory neural hearing loss, vestibular nerve function, ataxia, and speech disorder. RP can be associated with multiple syndromes; some of them and their systemic features are summarized in **Table 1**. Associated sleep disturbance and headache are common in RP patients.[1-3]

Ocular Examination

- *Visual acuity:* The visual acuity is normal in early cases. Early central acuity loss can occur from cystoid macular edema (CME), epiretinal membrane (ERM), and complicated cataract or in an atypical form of RP.

Table 1: Common forms of syndromic retinitis pigmentosa.

Syndrome/disease	Characteristic features	Etiology
Usher syndrome	• Bilateral sensory neural hearing loss • Lack of development of speech • Vestibular nerve dysfunction • Ataxia	Most commonly due to mutations in the *MYO7A* gene on chromosome 11q
Laurence–Moon–Bardet–Biedl syndrome (BBS)	• Obesity • Mental retardation or mild psychomotor delay • Postaxial polydactyly • Hypogenitalism • Renal abnormalities/renal failure	Mutation involving at least six distinct loci
Refsum disease	• Neuropathy • Ataxia • Deafness • Arrhythmia	Recessively inherited condition in which the patient accumulates exogenous phytanic acid
Bassen–Kornzweig syndrome (abetalipoproteinemia)	• Acanthocytosis • Malabsorption • Ataxia	A malabsorption syndrome associated with the absence of low-density plasma lipoproteins or so-called β-lipoproteins
Freidreich-like ataxia with retinitis pigmentosa	Friedreich-like ataxia, dysarthria, hyporeflexia, and decreased proprioceptive and vibratory sensation, as well as markedly decreased serum vitamin E levels	Recessively inherited, mutation in the α-tocopherol-transfer protein (α-TTP) gene
Kearns–Sayre syndrome	Conduction defects of heart External ophthalmoplegia RP	Mitochondrial DNA disorder

- *Eyeball:* Myopia is a common association with RP (22–75% of people with RP have myopia of about –2D).
- *Lid/conjunctiva/cornea/sclera:* These are usually within normal limits (WNL). There may be fat atrophy of the orbits due to frequent rubbing, typically seen in LCA. Keratoconus may be noted as an association of RP.
- *Iris:* Forward shifting of iris lens diaphragm may occur due to zonular weakness.
- *Pupil:* As per traditional teaching, afferent papillary defect (APD) does not occur in normal room luminance, as the light reflex pathway dependent on melanopsin RPE cells is still functional. Relative afferent pupillary defect (RAPD) suggests underlying optic atrophy. However, RAPD can be absent despite optic atrophy as RP is a bilateral disorder.
- *IOP:* An increase in IOP may occur in cases with RP with glaucoma, open-angle glaucoma is an association.
- *Lens:* Posterior subcapsular cataract (PSC) may occur in some cases (41–53%). Zonular weakness, although rare, can also occur in RP.
- *Vitreous:* Vitreous degeneration and early PVD can occur. Dust-like particles can be seen in the vitreous. These particles are fine, colorless, consisting of free melanin pigment granules, pigment epithelium, uveal melanocytes, and macrophage-like cells. They are found evenly distributed throughout the vitreous cavity. Observation of these particles can be helpful in the diagnosis of early RP before fundus changes are apparent. Retrolental cells may also be noted, as pars planitis is known to be associated with RP.
- *Fundus:* The following signs can be seen in a case of typical RP:
  - Arteriolar narrowing (most common but not earliest, seen in 90–95% of cases)

- *Pigmentary changes:* (Some authors list this as the first and most prevalent sign)
    - Earliest changes include fine dust-like intraretinal pigmentation and loss of pigment from the pigment epithelium.
    - The pathognomonic pigment clumps in a characteristic *"bone spicule"* configuration appear subsequently as the photoreceptor deterioration progresses, and there is increasing loss of pigment from the pigment epithelium with intraretinal clumping of melanin **(Fig. 1)**.
    - The term bone spicules is used to refer to the type of small cells that are laid down in the formation of a new bone matrix. These spicules in bone have a similar shape to the classic pigment finding in RP, thus the name.
    - The bony spicules are characteristically perivascular. Remember the spicules are initially more around the venules. They appear first in the midperiphery.
- In advanced cases waxy pallor of the optic disc is seen (50–55%) **(Fig. 2)**.[4]
- Associated cystoid macular edema (CME) is seen in 19–70% of cases **(Fig. 3)**.[1,4]
- The macula may show atrophy or epiretinal membrane (ERM) formation.
- Optic disc drusen can be seen in cases of RP.
- There may be a golden ring around the optic disc sign.

Atypical Retinitis Pigmentosa

In 20–30% of cases of RP the classical triad of attenuated vessels, bone spicules, and waxy pallor may not be seen. These forms of RP are known as atypical forms.

- *Retinitis pigmentosa sine pigmento:* Fundus appears normal but there is evidence of photoreceptor dysfunction in ERG.
- *Retinitis punctata albescens:* Retinal pigment epithelial degeneration appears as the presence of deep white dots at the level of RPE.
- *Sectoral RP:* Only one quadrant or one-half of the fundus has degenerative changes of retinitis pigmentosa. Most commonly, the inferior and nasal quadrants are involved, and the involvement is often symmetrical.

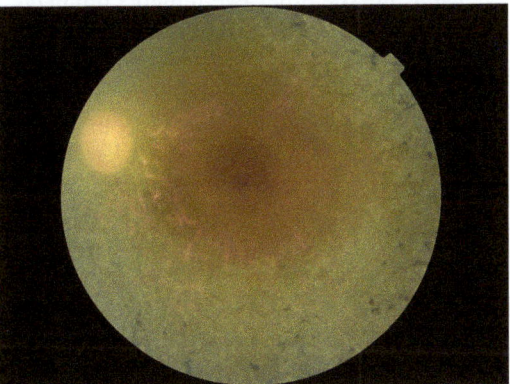

Fig. 2: Fundus photograph in case of RP showing severe vascular attenuation.

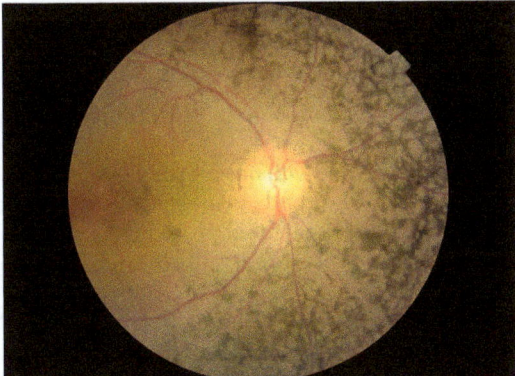

Fig. 1: Fundus photograph showing bony spicules with waxy disc pallor.

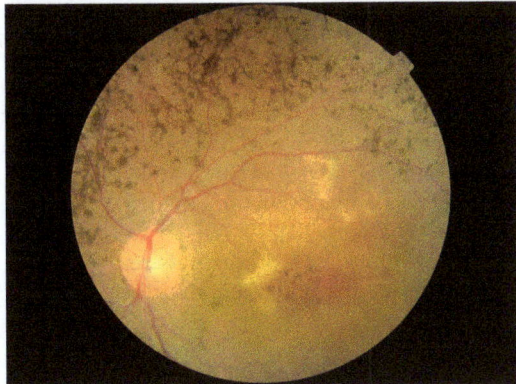

Fig. 3: Macular scarring in a case of RP with CME.

- *Retinitis pigmentosa inversus or pericentric RP:* Changes in RP primarily affect the macula and posterior pole. Thus, it can mimic hereditary fundus dystrophies. Visual acuity and color vision are affected early in the course of the disease. It progresses at a slower rate than typical RP and in advanced cases, the central vision is severely affected but the peripheral vision is retained. The visual field defect is near the midperipheral scotoma extending from the 5 to 30° isopter in contrast to the 20–40° isopter seen in cases of typical RP.
- *Unilateral RP:* It is characterized by fundus changes of RP in one eye and no evidence of RP in the fellow eye. ERG findings are substantially reduced in the affected eye but normal in the fellow eye. The RP progresses in the affected eye while the other eye remains unaffected. DDs of pseudo-RP must be evaluated.
- *Paravenous RP:* In this form, the ERG changes, and intraretinal pigment and atrophy of the pigment epithelium remain confined to the distribution of the retinal veins in each eye. Patients may lose central vision but, like pericentral RP, they retain peripheral vision into later life.

Syndromic RP
- RP associated with systemic disorder
- Usually, AR or mitochondrial inheritance
- Usher syndrome, Kearns–Sayre syndrome, Bassen–Kornzweig syndrome, refsum disease, and Bardet–Biedl syndrome (**Table 1**).

■ DIFFERENTIAL DIAGNOSIS

Pseudoretinitis Pigmentosa

This term refers to the conditions that mimic the fundal appearances of retinitis pigmentosa.[1-3] This can occur in the following conditions:
- Syphilis (leopard skin retinopathy)
- Congenital rubella
- *Drug-induced:* Thioridazine streaks, chloroquine, quinine, and phenothiazine
- Laser scars
- Old RD
- Trauma
- Chronic uveitis
- Cancer-associated retinopathy.

Choroideremia

- X-linked disease
- *Early stage:* Fine pigmentary stippling and atrophy of fundus
- *Later stage:* Patchy RPE and choroidal atrophy which gradually coalesce.

Gyrate Atrophy of Retina and Choroid

An AR disorder. Discrete round patches of choroidal and retinal atrophy occur in the midperipheral fundus. Gradual coalescence of the lesions occurs leading to sharply defined scalloped defects. There are 10–20-fold increases in plasma ornithine levels due to ornithine ketoacid aminotransferase deficiency.[1]

Cone and Rod Dystrophy

In contrast to typical retinitis pigmentosa (known as rod-cone dystrophies), cone-rod dystrophies reflect the opposite sequence of events, where cone cells are primarily first affected by later loss of rods. Thus, the presenting features are difficult with the clarity of vision, color vision problems, and light sensitivity. It can occur in association with Alstrom syndrome, Bardet–Biedl syndrome, neuronal ceroid lipofuscinosis, Joubert syndrome, and related disorders. Remember few clinicians term this as inverse RP, but this is better termed as inverse retinal pigmentary dystrophy; in inverse RP although the lesion starts around the macula or posterior pole the pathogenesis is the same, unlike cone-rod dystrophy where cones are primarily affected.[1]

Leber's Congenital Amaurosis

The following points help in differentiating from RP.[1-3]
- AR inheritance with onset in first year of life.
- Severely reduced visual function with nystagmus/nystagmoid movements, sluggish pupillary response, photophobia, and hyperopia.
- *Oculodigital sign:* Characterized by orbital fat atrophy (apparent by the deep sockets with a prominent eyeball), and development of keratoconus if the child survives into later decades. This is because the child repeatedly

rubs, pokes, and presses the eyes to elicit retinal stimulation.
- Initially, the fundus appears normal but later in childhood, pigmentary retinopathy changes develop. *Toxoplasma*-like scars can occur.
- ERG is nondetectable and severely abnormal quite in the early stage of the disease.
- SECORD (Severe childhood-onset retinal dystrophy): Similar to LCA but with better visual acuity than LCA later in life.

■ INVESTIGATION

- *ERG:* It shows early and severe reduced rod response, decreased a- and b-wave amplitude, prolonged implicit time, and reduction in cone response in advanced cases.
- *Visual field:* In early RP, there is the presence of ring scotoma in midperiphery (20–25° from fixation). It usually starts as a group of isolated scotomas around 20–25° from fixation and gradually coalesces to form a partial followed by a complete ring. The outer edge of the scotoma expands relatively rapidly, while the inner edge constricts slowly toward fixation. In advanced cases, the inner edge progresses to the center giving rise to tunnel vision. (It must be remembered that when visual acuity is low only Goldman's visual field is possible and this is the preferred modality in RP).
- *OCT:* It is done to rule out any macular pathology. This must be done in any case presenting with early loss of central vision or acute loss of vision during the course of RP. Choroidal changes have also been studied in RP but have been found to not relate to visual acuity in these patients.
- *Fluorescein angiogram:* It shows diffuse hyperfluorescence due to RPE window defects.
- *Ultrawide imaging* helps in documenting peripheral changes.
- *Color vision and contrast sensitivity* may also be done for evaluation.

■ CLASSIFICATION

- *Nonsyndromic or simple:* It does not affect other systems of the body. It may occur in AD, AR, X-linked, and digenic forms.
- *Syndromic:* Affects other neurosensory systems of the body such as hearing **(Table 1)**
- *Systemic:* Affects multiple organs of the body.

■ STAGING

The typical form of RP has been divided into the following three stages:[1-3]

Early Stage
- Involvement occurs in the first years of life
- Night blindness
- Very early minimal visual field defect
- Normal fundus appearance
- ERG shows decreased b wave amplitude, particularly in scotopic conditions.

Mid Stage
- Peripheral visual field defect in daylight
- Fundus changes, such as bony spicule-like pigmentary changes, attenuated vessels, and optic disc pallor.
- ERG: Unrecordable in scotopic conditions and hypovolted cone response.

End Stage
- Tunnel vision
- Decreased visual acuity due to cone involvement
- Unmasking of choroidal vessels giving the fundus tessellated appearance
- Unrecordable ERG.

■ COMPLICATIONS

- Keratoconus
- Posterior subcapsular cataract
- Open-angle glaucoma (3%)
- Occasional intermediate uveitis
- Exudative vasculopathy is often called coat-like disease.

■ MANAGEMENT

Currently, there is no definitive treatment for retinitis pigmentosa. The visual prognosis in advanced cases is usually poor. Various treatment modalities are under trial to slow down the disease progression, treatment of complications, and improve the visual rehabilitation of RP patients.[1-4]
- Smoking should be avoided
- *Optical aids and light protection:*
  - *UV A and UV B blocking sunglasses*: They reduce retinal degeneration by reducing

short wavelength light exposure. The use of CPF 550 lenses filters out 97–99% of spectral and UV rays.
  - Low vision aids, e.g., magnifiers, and closed circuit television are given to people with decreased central vision.
  - Wide-field bright intensity flashlight improves night vision by producing a bright wide beam of light.
- *Vitamin A palmitate:* It is prescribed at a dose of 15,000 IU/day. However, the use is highly controversial. Pregnancy is a contraindication as there is a risk of teratogenicity. It should not be given to children <18 years and persons with ABCA4 deficiency due to the risk of accumulation of toxic product A2E. Vitamin E in high doses has been shown to adversely affect the course of RP and should therefore be avoided.
- Increased intake of docosahexaenoic acid and lutein-zeaxanthin has shown promising results in decreasing progression.
- Systemic carbonic anhydrase inhibitors in a dose of 500 mg daily have been shown to reduce the cystoid macular edema associated with RP. However, the CME is chronic and often difficult to treat. Topical carbonic anhydrase inhibitors are not very effective in treating CME.
- Intravitreal triamcinolone and anti-VEGF injections have been shown to reduce CME.
- Cataract extraction is often indicated for decreased vision due to posterior subcapsular cataract, especially in cases with <10° of the visual field.
- Hyperbaric oxygen therapy to promote photoreceptor survival, retinal cell transplantation, calcium channel blockers, and neurotrophic growth factors (CTNF, GDNF, cardiotrophin 1, b FGF, BDNF, topical brimonidine tartrate 0.2%) are various treatment modalities which are under trial.
- Gene therapy with surgical administration of AAV vectors having RPE65C DNA to subretinal space were found to save vision in LCA in an animal model. This is an upcoming treatment under advanced phases of studies in humans. This is likely to benefit LCA/SECORD.
- Retinal prosthesis like microphotodiode that capture light and stimulate the retina, optic nerve, and visual cortex are being developed.

- Psychological and visual rehabilitation is often necessary, and patients should be trained to develop new professional skills.
- *Follow-up:* Goldmann visual perimetry and dilated fundus examination by ophthalmoscopy should be done annually and biannually. In cases with RP associated with CME, more frequent follow-ups are necessary.
- Examination of other family members of the affected person is recommended. People who are undergoing family planning should have proper genetic counseling regarding the mode of inheritance and possible affection of the offspring and manifestations of RP to help them make proper decisions.

VIVA QUESTIONS

Q.1. Discuss the mechanism of glaucoma in RP.

Ans. RP can be associated with both angle closure and open-angle glaucoma.
- *Angle closure glaucoma:* There is increased zonular instability with anterior shifting of the iris lens diaphragm resulting in angle narrowing and angle closure glaucoma.
- *POAG, NTG, and JOAG:* Attributed to the mutation of the gene for retinitis pigmentosa GTPase regulator-interacting protein 1 (RPGRIP1) on chromosome 14q11.

Q.2. Discuss the differential diagnosis of tunnel vision.

Ans. The loss of peripheral vision with retention of central vision gives rise to tunnel vision. Tunnel vision can be caused by:
- *Common:* Glaucoma, retinitis pigmentosa
- *Rare:*[1-4]
  - Blood loss (hypovolemia)
  - Alcohol consumption
  - Sustained, i.e., 1-second or more high accelerations, (typically, flying an airplane with a centripetal acceleration of up to or over 39 m/s² with the head toward the center of curvature, common in aerobatic or fighter pilots)

- Hallucinogenic drugs (dissociative)/extreme fear or distress/intense physical fight/excitement or extreme pleasure (causing a surge of adrenaline in the body)
- Altitude sickness/hypoxia in passenger aircraft/exposure to oxygen at a partial pressure above 1.5–2 atmospheres (producing central nervous system oxygen toxicity, called narcosis)
- Pituitary tumors (or other brain tumors that compress the optic chiasm)
- Advanced cataract, during the aura phase of a migraine, intense anger (due to the body being rapidly flooded with adrenaline and oxygen)
- A bite from a Black Mamba and other snakes
- Mercury poisoning (especially Methyl mercury).

Q.3. Why do bony spicules occur in the perivascular region? Why is there thinning of blood vessels in RP?

Ans.
- *Bony spicules:* It is referred to the type of small cells that are formed during the formation of a new bone matrix. In RP, the appearance of pigment has a similar shape to spicules in bone.
- *Attenuation of vessels:* Due to progressive damage of the outer retina the vascular demand of the retina on the choriocapillaris and inner retinal arteries decreases.
- *Perivascular distribution:* In RP due to progressive outer photoreceptor and outer retinal damage the inner retina and the inner retinal blood vessels lie in contact with RPE. This blood vessel-RPE contact sends a trigger signal for bony spicule-like pigment formation. Progressive attenuation of inner retinal arteries leads to gradual hypoxia and subsequent damage to the cells forming the inner blood-retinal barrier. The bony spicule-like pigment (along with RPE cells) migrates along the vessels in order to reform the inner blood-retinal barrier. The RPE cells seal the vessels with tight junction linkage, deposit perivascular extracellular matrix, and induce fenestrations in the vascular endothelium of the cuffed vessels that lead to the characteristic "spicule" pattern.[1-4]

Q.4. What is the significance of bionic eye in RP?

Ans. In RP patients who are blind several prosthesis prototypes have been tested that electrically stimulate the inner retina. These devices can induce phosphenes and can improve performance on some tests of visual function. However, it needs a functional optic nerve and its role in RP with optic atrophy is unclear.

Q.5. What is stem cell transplant?

Ans. Several studies have demonstrated *in vitro* differentiation of embryonic and adult stem cells into retinal cell types. The *in vivo* transplantation of these cells as well as fetal retinal cells to animal models has given promising results. Some studies of stem cell transplantation on individuals with RP have shown improvement in visual function.

Q.6. Can an RP patient be legally blind despite having good central vision?

Ans. Yes, the visual field of <10° is considered blind even when the visual acuity is 6/6.

Q.7. What is the role of multifocal ERG? Discuss.

Ans. Records local response from the macula and can detect residual macular functions in advanced cases. Thus, in cases with advanced RP, long-term follow-up and monitoring of visual function can be done with multifocal ERG.

Q.8. Write a note on full-field ERG.

Ans. It stimulates the full visual field and records responses from the entire retina. It is used traditionally to follow the disease progression in RP.

Q.9. Discuss about genetics and RP.

Ans. The different genes associated with RP are described below.[1-4]
- *AD RP:* These are the mildest forms with some cases occurring after age 50. RHO (most common), PRPF 31, PRPH2, RP1, IMPDH1, PRPF8, KLHL7, NR2E3, CRX,

PRPF3, TOPORS, CA4, NRL, ROM1, RP9, RDH12, SNRNP200, AIPL1, BEST1, PRPF6, RPE 65, GUCA1B, FSCN2, SEMA4A.
- *Sporadic:* May have a favorable prognosis. Retention of central vision until 6th decade or later.
- *AR RP:* Usually starts in the first decade. USHA2A (most common), ABCA4, PDE6A, PDE6B, RPE65, CNGA1, BEST1, C20RF71, C80RF37, CLRN1, CNGB1, DHDDS, FAM161A, IDH3B, IMPG2, LRAT, MAK, MERTK, NRL, PDE6G, PRCD, PROM1, RBP3, RGR, RHO, RLBP1, RP1, SPATA7, TTC8, TULP1, ZNF513, ARL6, NR2E3, EYS, CRB1, CERKL, SAG.
- *X-linked:* Early onset and frequently associated with myopia. The least common, but most severe, is usually complete blindness by third or fourth decade. In most of the cases, transmission is recessive. RPGR, RP2.
- *Digenic (very rare):* Inherited in pseudodominant pattern. Simultaneous presence of PRPH2 and ROM1.
- *Prognosis:*
  - Best prognosis: AD.
  - Worst prognosis: XR.
  - AD>Sporadic>AR>XR
- *MC mode of inheritance:*
  - Sporadic/simplex (40-50%)
  - AD (15-25%)
  - AR (5-20%)
  - X-linked (5-15%)
  - Digenic (very rare)

Q.10. What are the types of sunglasses preferred in RP?

Ans. Some clinicians prefer orange photochromic sunglasses with tinted side shields or dark amber sunglasses with tinted side shields. However, no particular type of sunglasses has been shown to delay the progression of the disease. Sunglasses should be selected for outdoor use that provides maximal comfort to the vision without compromising vision.

Q.11. Discuss the causes of completely extinguished ERG.

Ans.
- Leber's congenital amaurosis
- Severe retinitis pigmentosa
- Retinal aplasia
- Total detachment of retina
- Ophthalmic artery occlusion
- Advanced siderosis.

■ REFERENCES

1. Fahim AT, Daiger SP, Weleber RG. Retinitis pigmentosa overview. In: Pagon RA, Adam MP, Ardinger HH, Wallace SE, Amemiya A, Bean LJH, et al. (Eds). Nonsyndromic Retinitis Pigmentosa Overview. Seattle (WA): GeneReviews(R), University of Washington; 1993.
2. Bowling B, Kansi JJ. Kanski's clinical ophthalmology: a systematic approach, 8th edition. Edinburgh: Elsevier; 2015.
3. In: Albert DM, Miller JW, Azar DT (Eds). Albert and Jakobiec's Principles and practice of ophthalmology, 4th edition. Switzerland AG: Springer Nature; 2008.
4. Hartong DT, Berson EL, Dryja TP. Retinitis pigmentosa. Lancet. 2006;368(9549):1795-809.

MACULAR HOLE

Vaishali Ghanshyam Rai, Brijesh Takkar

■ INTRODUCTION

A macular hole (MH) is an anatomic discontinuity of the neurosensory retina that develops in the center of the macula or fovea. Idiopathic macular hole is the most common type seen in clinical practice. Typically, the patient presents with metamorphopsia and decreased visual acuity. In examinations, MH can be given as a long case and needs an elaborate workup. Most discussion is around full-thickness idiopathic MH.

■ HISTORY

Epidemiology/Demography

The incidence of MH ranges between 7 and 9 eyes per 100,000 people per year.[1-4] Females are affected more than males (approximately 2:1). Most cases occur in the sixth to seventh decade. However, young myopes can be present in the third decades of life, as do patients with traumatic MH. The 5-year risk of a patient with a full-thickness macular hole (FTMH) of developing an FTMH in the fellow eye is approximately 10–15%.[1-4] Rarely, they are with simultaneous presentations.

Chief Complaints

A case of MH can be presented in the following manners:
- Asymptomatic-early stages of MH are asymptomatic, especially if the other eye is normal. Such cases may be detected during fundus examination for other causes, most commonly cataract due to the age group affected.
- Late stages of MH can present with significantly reduced visual acuity (VA), metamorphopsia, and loss of central vision with a central scotoma. VA is inversely correlated with the size of the MH.
- Symptoms of VMT and vitreous traction—may precede or be the only presentation in early cases of MH. These symptoms include metamorphopsia (distorted VA), micropsia (a diminution of objects within the visual field), and photopsia (flashes of light).

History of Present Illness

The formation of an MH typically evolves over a period of weeks to months. However, it is frequently detected when the patient's symptoms change relatively abruptly. Thus, the onset can be subacute or acute and the visual acuity progressively deteriorates. Typically, metamorphopsia would precede significant visual loss.

History of Past Illness

Any preceding history of trauma, ocular surgery, sun or eclipse gazing, or use of myopic glasses must be recorded. This will help in identifying the cause of MH. Other eye history may be pertinent in indicating interface anomalies. There may be a history of diabetic retinopathy (DR), RVO, or radiation exposure in secondary cases. The history of similar complaints in the fellow eye must be enquired, as MH is bilateral in 10–15% of the cases. Medication use that may be related to macular cystoid edema (e.g., systemic niacin and topical prostaglandin analogs) should be asked. Lastly, a history of glaucoma, cataract, or ARMD must be ruled out as these may coexist with MH and may account for poor visual acuity.

Systemic History

Since most of the cases occur in 60–70 years of life-coexisting systemic diseases such as DM, hypertension, bronchial asthma, and any posture-related issues (cervical spondylitis and kyphoscoliosis) must be checked. Following MH surgery, the patient may be advised certain postures for a few days, hence posture-related problems must be enquired about carefully.

■ EXAMINATION

Systemic Examination

As discussed earlier coexisting systemic diseases, due to the age factor, must be ruled out. In addition, any posture-related issues must be looked for.

Ocular Examination

- *Visual acuity (VA):* VA measurement, especially best corrected (BCVA) is extremely important in cases of MH. A BCVA <6/60 or 20/200 is rare in MH and in the presence of such low acuity, other causes of loss of VA (such as ARMD, cataract, or glaucoma) must be ruled out. Poor BCVA is also an indicator of poor prognoses.
- Examination should cover all the aspects of the external eye and intraocular structures should be done to look for secondary causes of MH. Pupil dilation is of the essence for further management.
- *Lens:* MH surgery invariably leads to cataract formation (almost 100%) hence many surgeons prefer to perform the cataract surgery during vitrectomy itself. The presence of PSC is especially hampering during macular surgery. In addition, cataract and MH may coexist and few cases may benefit from only cataract surgery and observation.
- *Posterior segment:* Slit-lamp biomicroscopy is the best technique to evaluate the MH **(Fig. 1)**. The MH progresses characteristically through four stages (Gass classification).[1-4] The clinical findings of these stages are described below:

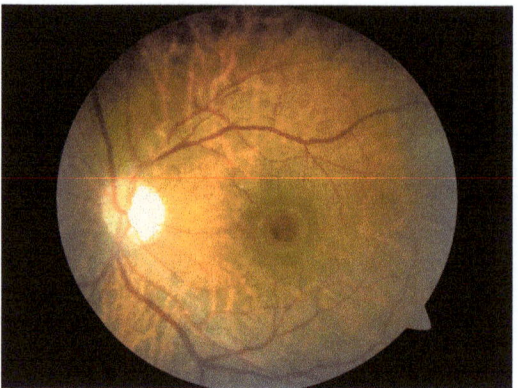

Fig. 1: Fundus photograph showing an old macular hole of the left eye. Large diameter along with pigment changes the base and disc pallor are noticeable.

- *Stage 1:* Impending macular holes
  - *Stage 1A:* Loss of the foveal depression associated with a small yellow spot (foveal pseudocyst)
  - *Stage 1B:* Loss of the foveal depression associated with a small yellow ring
  - Typically includes central vision loss (with visual acuity typically measuring 20/25 to 20/60) and metamorphopsia.
- *Stage 2:*
  - Macular hole represents the progression of a foveal pseudocyst to a full-thickness dehiscence
  - Small opening in the inner layer (<400 μm diameter) may be either centrally or eccentrically located
  - Visual acuity 20/25 to 20/80
  - May have a partially detached operculum.
- *Stage 3:*
  - Macular hole is a fully developed hole (>400 μm diameter), typically accompanied by a rim of thickened and slightly elevated retina.
  - Visual acuity may range from 20/100 to 20/400.
  - The posterior hyaloid is detached from the macula but remains attached to the optic disc.
  - A detached operculum is present on the posterior hyaloid over the hole and is visible clinically or by means of OCT.
  - A cuff of subretinal fluid may be detected along with intraretinal edema and cysts.
  - Drusen-like or yellow deposits may be occasionally seen in the base of the hole. These deposits represent macrophage activity at the level of the retinal pigment epithelium, suggesting chronicity of disease. These typically have poor outcomes.
  - A rim of retinal pigment epithelium hyper/hypopigmentation is often present at the junction between edematous or detached retina and normal-appearing attached retina in long-standing cases.
  - Epiretinal membranes may be present.
- *Stage 4:*
  - A full-thickness hole with a diameter usually larger than stage 3 (>400 μm in diameter).
  - A complete PVD with a Weiss ring.
  - A cuff of subretinal fluid, intraretinal edema, and cystoid changes are usually present.
  - Drusen-like deposits may be occasionally seen in the base of the hole.
  - Epiretinal membranes are more frequent.
  - Visual acuity is more profoundly decreased from 20/100 to 20/400.

Following macular examination, the periphery must be examined for the presence or squeal of anomalous PVD. These patients commonly have VR problems as pathogenesis revolves around anomalous vitreous traction. In addition, peripheral lesions would need attention during the surgery, as these patients are especially prone to peripheral iatrogenic breaks as well. Signs of trauma or other secondary causes may also be picked up.

Traumatic hole: Apart from other history and signs of trauma, these holes typically have irregular/ragged borders secondary to contusion necroses, irregular margins, and shape, larger (usually >1,000 μm) with underlying pigmentary changes, and PVD may be absent. The surrounding retina may appear atrophic.

Diagnostic Tests (Help in Differentiating Lamellar Holes)

Watzke–Allen Test

This test is performed at the slit-lamp biomicroscope by using a fundus/macular lens and placing a narrow vertical slit beam through the center of the macula. In a FTMH a positive test is noted, that is the patient detects a break in the bar of light.

The Laser Aiming-beam Test

This is similar to the Watzke–Allen test. It is performed similarly using a macular/fundal lens and placing a 50-μm laser (Helium Neon) aiming beam through the center of the macula. In the presence of FTMH, a positive test is observed when the patient cannot detect the aiming beam within the hole area but is able to detect it in surrounding intact tissue. This test is possibly *more sensitive* and *more specific* for FTMH.

Amsler Charting

It is useful in the early stages of holes to document clinical progression and also to document metamorphopsia.

■ DIFFERENTIAL DIAGNOSIS

Pseudomacular Holes

Pseudomacular holes associated with epiretinal membranes can be differentiated by the presence of retinal vascular tortuosity and compression and the absence of the rim of subretinal fluid. Watzke–Allen test and red beam tests are negative in the pseudomacular hole.

Lamellar Macular Holes

These are sharply circumscribed, partial-thickness defects of the macula usually seen following chronic cystoid macular edema or an aborted FTMH. In contrast, in FTMH a "well" is noted depicting the boundaries of the hole. A flat, reddish hue-type lesion with intact outer retinal tissue characterizes a lamellar macular hole (LMH). Unlike true FTMH, they do not have subretinal fluid, drusen-like yellowish deposits in the base of the hole or operculum. Watzke–Allen and laser aiming beam tests are negative. LMH does not progress to full-thickness lesions.

Other lesions that may be confused with MH include the following:
- Vitreomacular traction syndrome
- Foveal drusen
- CVNM
- Solar retinopathy
- Central serous chorioretinopathy
- Macular atrophy
- Macular hemorrhage.

All these lesions can be easily differentiated, as the characteristic findings of FTMH are absent. In doubtful cases, OCT often confirms the diagnosis.

■ INVESTIGATION

Optical Coherence Tomography

The gold standard tool for diagnosing, staging, prognosticating, planning for macular hole surgery, and following up later **(Fig. 2)**. Several indices have been described based on OCT that often help in predicting the prognosis of surgery. These are described here.[1-5]

- *MH minimum diameter* also known as the minimum linear dimension of MH—a smaller minimum diameter is associated with better postoperative visual acuity, irrespective of the presence/absence of a statistical significance, eyes with MHs smaller than 400 μm tended to have greater visual acuity improvement.
- The *basal hole diameter* is a linear dimension of MH at the level of the retinal pigment epithelium layer. The smaller the basal hole diameter becomes, the better the postoperative visual acuity.
- *The hole form factor (HFF)* is the first calculated OCT index used as a prognostic factor. The HFF is the quotient of the summation of the left and right arm lengths divided by the basal hole diameter. The HFF is reported to be positively

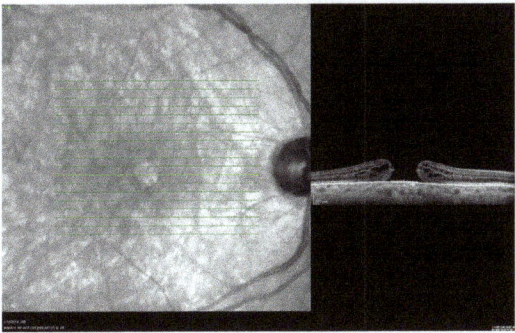

Fig. 2: EDI OCT of a right eye macular hole showing a large full-thickness hole with cystoid spaces.

correlated with the postoperative visual acuity. HFF >0.9 indicates better prognoses.
- *MH height:* The hole height is another preoperative OCT parameter, defined as the greatest distance between the retinal pigment epithelium layer and the vitreoretinal interface. Previous studies concluded that there is no significant relationship between the hole height and postoperative visual outcomes, with the exception of one retrospective study showing a negative correlation between the hole height and visual acuity >5 years after MH surgery.
- The photoreceptor *inner segment/outer segment (IS/OS) junction* line (now termed the EZ): It is recognized as a hyper-reflective band by spectral domain OCT imaging. There are studies reporting that the preoperative IS/OS junction defect length is associated with postoperative macular sensitivity and visual acuity.
- Similarly, ELM and COST have also been used as markers for visual prognostication in MH.
- *Macular Hole Index (MHI):* The MHI is defined as the ratio of the hole height to the basal hole diameter and is reported to be positively correlated to postoperative visual acuity in several studies. The visual outcomes are better in patients with an MHI value ≥0.5 compared to a value of <0.5.
- *Diameter Hole Index (DHI):* It is calculated by the ratio of minimum hole diameter and basal hole diameter. It indicates *tangential traction strength*.
- *Enface OCT:* This modality has linked the shape and orientation of macular holes to outcomes. It is still under investigation.
- *Tractional Hole Index (THI):* It is defined as the ratio of the hole height to the minimum diameter. It is another OCT index useful as a predictor for visual outcomes. It indicates anteroposterior VMT. A larger THI indicates stronger AP VMT and weaker tangential traction and hence a better outcome.

Remember Min hole Diam of <310 μ and THI >1.4 are associated with good visual outcome following MH surgery.[1,5]

Fluorescein Angiography

Fluorescein angiography (FFA) may be a useful test in differentiating macular holes from masquerading lesions, such as CME and choroidal neovascularization (CNV). Full-thickness stage 3 holes typically produce a window defect early in the angiogram and do not expand with time. No leakage or accumulation of dye is observed as opposed to other lesions.

■ TREATMENT

The treatment depends upon the stage of the disease **(Table 1)**.[1-5]
- Stage 1 can be followed up regularly. Only about 50% of the early stages progress to an FTMH. In a small number of cases, VMT resolves spontaneously without intervention (reported incidences are 10–11%).
- Stages 2, 3, and 4 require surgical intervention.
- Patients with very good visual acuity may be followed up.
- *MIVI-TRUST trials:* These have found up to 40% success with ocriplasmin for MH closure. However, the results are still in the initial phase of the study.

Surgery for Macular Hole

Indication

Lifestyle hampering metamorphopsia or significant visual acuity loss, usually taken as <6/12

Table 1: Management of macular hole.

Stage	Management	Follow-up
1-A and 1-B	Observation	2–4 months with prompt return if new symptoms develop Monitoring with Amsler grid
2	Vitreoretinal surgery	Depending on the outcome of surgery and the patient's clinical course
	Vitreopharma-colysis	Follow-up at 1 week and 4 weeks, or with new symptoms (i.e., retinal detachment symptoms)
3 and 4	Vitreoretinal surgery	Depending on the outcome of surgery and the patient's clinical course

is considered to be the criteria for surgery by most clinicians. Cautious decisions have to be taken in one-eyed patients measuring the risk-benefit ratio. Stage 1 holes are usually kept under observation.

Aim

Surgical repair of macular holes includes relief of all tangential traction and AP traction, to use of vitreous substitute or reverse ILM flap to allow the repair process to heal the hole.

Technique

A standard pars plana vitrectomy (PPV) with ILM peeling with gas injection is the most common procedure done. Three sclerotomies are created 3.5 mm from the limbus for the infusion cannula, illumination pipe, and vitreous cutter. Using active aspiration (150–250 mm Hg), a silicone-tipped suction cannula/vitreous cutter, using suction only is used very effectively for PVD induction— *"fish strike sign"* or *"diving rod sign".* Once the vitreous is completely detached, vitrectomy is completed.

Internal Limiting Membrane Peeling

Several studies have reported excellent macular hole closure rates (87–96%) using internal limiting membrane (ILM) peeling techniques.[1] The ILM acts as a scaffold for cellular proliferation or attachment of contractile tissue elements that may cause persistent traction. Thus, failure of the original surgery or late reopening of initially successfully closed holes may occur without removal of the ILM. However, the limitation of ILM peeling is the loss of its structural role or secondary collateral nerve fiber layer loss during removal. ILM peeling can be done using indocyanine green (ICG), trypan blue (TP), brilliant blue (BB), and triamcinolone acetonide (TA), to optimize visualization of the ILM during surgery. ICG was used initially but reports of visual field defects and retinal pigment epithelium abnormalities in the foveal center raised concerns for possible toxicity. Importantly, when the surgeon prefers ICG to stain the ILM, the lowest possible concentration with the correct osmolarity of ICG should be used. Currently ICG and infracyanine green have fallen out of favor due to toxicity and stringent use conditions. Trypan blue was commonly advocated, it is a "real vital dye" staining the ERM more than an ILM. However, it required injection under air and a wait period of 5–8 minutes for proper staining. Next BBG was introduced which is more active in staining ILM, though it may also stain ERMs. Steroid crystals typically attach to hyaloids/ERM, rather than actual staining. A combination of trypan blue and BBG has been used, and pegylated BBG is heavier than BBG and may offer better staining. Blood has also been used in combination with another dye or as the sole agent for this purpose. "Negative staining" is useful in cases where both ERM and ILM are planned to be removed.

Peeling is carried out using the ILM forceps. *The pinch and peel technique* is commonly applied. Peel the ILM across the hole to relieve all traction at the edge of the hole. Few surgeons prefer peeling from arcade to arcade. Adequately sized peel is debated, for usual stage 2–3 holes, 1 disc diameter (DD) peel usually suffices. For larger holes, up to 2 DD peels may be done. Total fluid-air exchange is performed; nonexpansile concentration of gas is exchanged for air.

Postoperatively, a prone position is advised for 3–5 days. There is no clear consensus regarding the duration of facedown positioning to seal macular holes following vitrectomy surgery, but longer positioning may be required for holes larger than 400 μm or those with inadequate tamponade.

ILM flaps: Inverted ILM flaps, free flaps, pedunculated flaps, stuffed flaps, and other techniques have shown higher hole closure in larger holes. However, improvement in visual acuity remains limited.

Post-ILM peeling OCT features: These may be early or late. Early features include dimpling of the inner retina, and double or split in the nerve fiber layer. Late changes include thinning of the retina, ganglion cell layer, and nasalization of the fovea.

Common Complications

- *Nuclear sclerotic cataracts:* Almost all cases (80–98%) develop cataract within a few years of surgery.[1-5] In addition, a closed macular holes may reopen after cataract surgery, and cystoid macular edema after surgery further increases the risk by seven-fold. Thus, some surgeons advocate combining macular hole surgery with phacoemulsification and placement of an intraocular lens.

- *Peripheral retinal breaks:* Occur in 3-17% of macular hole surgeries and most occur inferiorly.[1-4]
- *RRD:* Most series report an incidence of 1-5%. The detachment is typically located inferiorly and caused by tears at the posterior vitreous base.[1-5]
- *Visual field defects:* The reported incidence is 10-20% of patients. Most believe that this field loss is caused by either mechanical injury (such as trauma to the peripapillary retinal vasculature or nerve fiber layer) or dehydration damage to the retina as a result of air streaming from the temporally placed infusion cannula during the air-fluid exchange.
- Enlargement of the hole and late reopening of the hole occurs in 2-10% of the cases.[1,2,5]
- *Endophthalmitis:* Endophthalmitis has been reported rarely.

Success rate: Recent reports on acute (<6 months) idiopathic macular holes are showing anatomic success rates from 89 to 100% and improvement in visual acuity of two or more lines in 72-95% of patients.[1,3,5]

VIVA QUESTIONS

Q.1. What is a stage 0 macular hole?

Ans. An abnormal vitreofoveal traction observed on OCT in the contralateral eye of a patient with a macular hole is associated with an elevated risk of macular hole formation in the contralateral eye. May be present in an extremely high number of contralateral eyes.

Q.2. What is an LMH?

Ans. A hole in the macular region that is not full thickness. It may be outer or inner. It may also be an early stage toward a full-thickness hole or an aborted full-thickness hole that may spontaneously close. Inner holes usually occur secondary to rupture following CME, such as in uveitis and DR. Outer holes are seen typically after solar retinopathy, macular dystrophy, PFT, etc. ERMs typically accompany inner holes; surgery is controversial and usually reserved for a few cases.

Q.3. Discuss the prognosis factor for macular hole.

Ans. The following are prognostic factors for macular hole surgery:
- Better closure rates and better final visual acuities have been reported when the duration of symptoms is <6 months.
- Patients whose macular holes fail to seal after the first surgery usually have a less favorable visual acuity outcome when compared with primary closure.
- Hole size >400 μm is associated with poor prognosis.
- *Presenting visual acuity:* <6/60 is associated with poor prognosis.
- *OCT indices:* Smaller base diameter, smaller inner opening size, shorter minimum linear dimension, and larger THI are associated with good visual outcomes and hole closure.
- Traumatic holes and those related to secondary pathologies have usually poor outcomes.

Q.4. Discuss the controversies of macular hole.

Ans.
- *ILM peeling:* The role of the internal limiting membrane (ILM) peeling its necessity, preferred technique, and potential complications, including the toxicity of adjuvant agents are far from definitively established. Removal of the ILM increases the rate of macular hole closure and perhaps improves the final visual acuity. Closure rates as high as 88-100% have been reported.[1-3] There is controversy, however, as to whether all sizes of macular holes require ILM peeling. IMH of <400 μm in diameter may close equally with and without ILM peeling. In addition, ILM peeling can lead to reduced retinal sensitivity and microscotomas. Lastly, various dyes used to facilitate ILM peeling (especially ICG) can lead to retinal toxicity.
    - *Duration of face-down positioning:* The ideal duration of positioning (short vs. prolonged) is not well defined. Most vitreoretinal surgeons

recommend strict face-down positioning for at least 1 week postoperatively. However prolonged positioning may be required especially in large-diameter holes. Most holes close by 1 day, up to 80% by 3 days, as proved with face-down positioned OCT.
- *Surgical adjuvants:* The effect of adjuvants on the MH closure rate is controversial. Most surgeons do not currently use adjuvant agents in the surgical repair of macular holes.
- *Role of silicone oil:* Few surgeons advocate silicone oil tamponade instead of gas tamponade for a prolonged effect. However, the visual acuity and closure rates are better among eyes undergoing surgery with gas tamponade compared with silicone oil. The use of silicone oil for postoperative tamponade can be considered for patients unable to position or when prolonged positioning is required.
- *Combined phacovitrectomy or sequential vitrectomy and phacoemulsification (during the first year following vitrectomy):* Since almost all the patients develop cataract following VR surgery in MH few surgeons advocate phacovitrectomy. However, there is no clear evidence that combined phacovitrectomy affects the long-term results of PPV for IMH but visual recovery is quicker.
- *Role of vitreous substitute:* The major function of vitreous substitutes (air/SF6/C3F8/silicone oil) is to segregate the hole from the fluid-filled vitreous cavity, allowing the healing process to occur. Typically, a short-acting substitute like SF6 is preferred.
- *Other techniques (adjunctive or sole):* These include ILM flap techniques (pedunculated/detached/multilayered, etc.), MH tapping, temporal arcuate retinectomy, fluid injection at MH base, blood in MH well, and others. Fibrin glue has also been attempted. Such techniques are usually reserved for holes with poor chances of postoperative closure or those undergoing second surgeries.

Q.5. What are the types of hole closure?

Ans. As per postoperative OCT, U, V, and W types of closures have been seen. U closure has the best outcomes. Closure, as proved on OCT, would typically occur in 3 days, though visual acuity increases slowly. Type 1 closure includes U and V. Type 2 closure (W types) indicates poor visual outcome, seen in advanced stages and traumatic holes.

Q.6. Write a note on ILM peeling.

Ans.
- Techniques for removal of the ILM involve establishing an elevated edge of the ILM and then peeling the ILM from around the macular hole. Establishing an initial edge may be accomplished with the use of a barbed microvitreoretinal blade with a Tano Diamond-Dusted scraper or with the use of fine intraocular end-grasping forceps to 'pinch' and elevate the ILM. Peeling is generally carried out using a pinch-peel technique with fine-tipped forceps.
- The ILM peel is most often performed in a circular motion around the hole (Maculorhexis). The ILM is usually peeled to a radius of approximately one disc diameter around the hole.
- *It works by:* Removing residual adherent vitreous cortex remnants on the ILM surface; removing associated fibrocellular collections; removing the rigid and less compliant ILM (relative to the retina itself); and causing a retinal glial cell proliferation that may help macular hole contraction and repair.

Q.7. Discuss about macular hole formation, pathogenesis, and tangential traction.

Ans. Gass hypothesized that IMHs begin with tangential traction of the prefoveal vitreous cortex, which results in a foveal dehiscence that progresses from foveolar detachment to a full-thickness IMH. However, more recent research (using USG and OCT) has elucidated that IMHs are initiated during perifoveal PVD as a consequence of anteroposterior and dynamic VMT.[1,2]

The anterior tractional forces acting at the foveola first produce an intrafoveal split, which evolves into a foveal pseudocyst. Dehiscence of the foveal cyst creates a full-thickness defect. Complete detachment of the cyst roof is observed by the appearance of an operculum within the vitreous gel.[1,2]

Q.8. Discuss about adjunctive therapy in macular hole repair.

Ans. The role of adjunctive therapy in macular hole repair is controversial. The adjuvants are applied to the site of the macular hole in hopes of stimulating a cellular reparative response and hole closure. Examples include autologous serum, autologous platelet concentrate, thrombin-activated fibrinogen, thrombin, transforming growth factor beta-2 (TGF β-2), and tissue glue.

Q.9. Discuss the IVMTS classification.

Ans. *See* **Table 2**.

Table 2: International Vitreomacular Traction Study Group optical coherence tomography (OCT)-based anatomic classification system for diseases of the vitreomacular interface (VMI).

Anatomic state	Definition	Classification		
VMA	• Evidence of perifoveal vitreous cortex detachment from the retinal surface • Macular attachment of the vitreous cortex within a 3-mm radius of the fovea • No detectable change in foveal contour or underlying retinal tissues	By size of attachment area • Focal (≤1,500 µm) • Broad (>1,500 µm, parallel to RPE and may include areas of dehiscence)	By the presence of concurrent retinal conditions (other associated macular abnormalities, including ARMD, RVO, and DME) • Isolated • Concurrent	
VMT	• Evidence of perifoveal vitreous cortex detachment from the retinal surface • Macular attachment of the vitreous cortex within a 3-mm radius of the fovea • Association of attachment with distortion of the foveal surface, intraretinal structural changes, and/or elevation of the fovea above the RPE, but no full-thickness interruption of all retinal layers	By size of attachment area • Focal (≤1,500 µm) • Broad (>1,500 µm, parallel to RPE and may include areas of dehiscence)	By presence of concurrent retinal conditions • Isolated • Concurrent	

Contd...

Contd...

Anatomic state	Definition	Classification		
FTMH	Full-thickness foveal lesion that interrupts all macular layers from the ILM to the RPE	By size (horizontally measured linear width across the hole at the narrowest point, not ILM) • Small (250 μm) • Medium (>250 and 400 μm) • Large (>400 μm)	By presence or absence of VMT	By cause • Primary (initiated by VMT) • Secondary (directly due to associated disease or trauma known to cause a macular hole in the absence of prior VMT)
LMH	• Irregular foveal contour • Defect in the inner fovea (may not have an actual loss of tissue) • Intraretinal splitting (schisis), typically between the outer plexiform and outer nuclear layers • Maintenance of an intact photoreceptor layer			
Macular pseudohole	• Invaginated or heaped foveal edges • Concomitant ERM with a central opening • Steep macular contour to the central fovea with near-normal central foveal thickness • No loss of retinal tissue			

(ARMD: age-related macular degeneration; DME: diabetic macular edema; ERM: epiretinal membrane; FTMH: full-thickness macular hole; ILM: internal limiting membrane; IVTS: International Vitreomacular Traction Study; LMH: lamellar macular hole; RPE: retinal pigment epithelium; RVO: retinal vein occlusion; VMA: vitreomacular adhesion; VMT: vitreomacular traction)

REFERENCES

1. Ryan SJ, Schachat AP, Wilkinson CP, Hinton DR, Sadda SR, Wiedemann P. Retina, 5th edition. Philadelphia: Saunders; 2012.
2. Duker JS, Yanoff M. Ophthalmology, 4th edition. London: Elsevier/Saunders; 2013.
3. In: Albert DM, Miller JW, Azar DT (Eds). Albert and Jakobiec's Principles and Practice of Ophthalmology, 4th edition. Switzerland AG: Springer Nature; 2008.
4. Steel DHW, Lotery AJ. Idiopathic vitreomacular traction and macular hole: a comprehensive review of pathophysiology, diagnosis, and treatment. Eye (Lond). 2013;27(Suppl 1):S1-21.
5. Bowling B, Kansi JJ. Kanski's Clinical Ophthalmology: A Systematic Approach, 8th edition. Edinburgh: Elsevier; 2015.

RETINAL DETACHMENT

Pranayee Behera, Rajesh Pattebahadur, Raghav Ravani

INTRODUCTION

Retinal detachment refers to the separation of the neurosensory layers of the retina from the underlying retinal pigment epithelium (RPE).

Retinal detachment occurs by 3 basic mechanisms and thus is classified into the following three main types **(Table 1)**:

1. *RRD (the most common type):* This results when a hole, tear, or break in the neuronal layer allows fluid from the vitreous to seep between and separate sensory and RPE layers **(Fig. 1)**.
2. *Traction retinal detachment:* This results from adhesions between the vitreous gel/fibrovascular proliferation and the retina **(Fig. 2)**.
3. *Exudative (serous) RD:* This results from the exudation of material into the subretinal space

Table 1: Types of retinal detachment.

	Rhegmatogenous	Tractional	Exudative
History	Photopsia, visual field defects	Diabetes, penetrating trauma, sickle cell disease	Malignant hypertension, eclampsia, renal failure, uveitis, tumor
Retinal break	Present	No primary break. May develop a secondary break	No break or coincidental
Extent of detachment	Extends to Ora early	Does not extend to ora	Gravity dependent
Retinal shape	Convex	Elevated to a level of traction, concave	Extremely high convex
Motility	Undulating	Taut. Peaks to traction point	Smoothly elevated bullae
Subretinal fluid	Clear	Clear. No shift	May be turbid. Shift rapidly to a dependent location
Choroidal mass	None	None	May be present
Proliferative vitreoretinopathy (PVR)	+	–	–

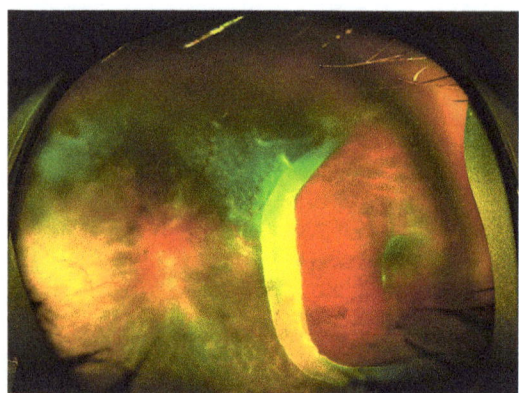

Fig. 1: Ultrawide-field pseudocolor image of rhegmatogenous retinal detachment with a large tear.

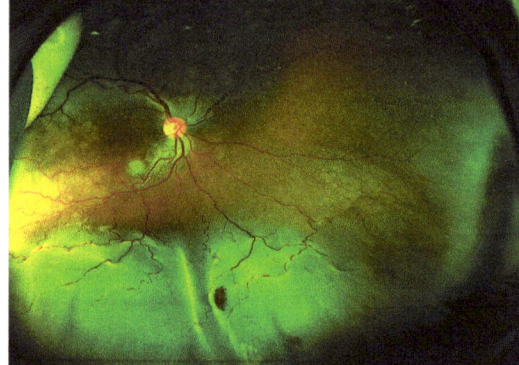

Fig. 2: Ultrawide-field pseudocolor image of choroiditis with inferior exudative retinal detachment.

(**Fig. 3**) from retinal vessels (as in hypertension, central retinal venous occlusion, vasculitis, or uveitis, tumors, infective disorders, chronic rhinosinusitis, etc.).

The RRDs are usually kept as long cases and the subsequent discussion particularly revolves around it.

■ HISTORY

Chief Complaints

A case of RRD may present with the following:
- Flashing lights
- Floaters
- Visual field defect
- Visual loss.

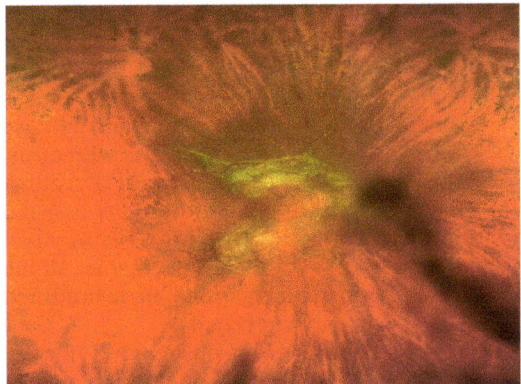

Fig. 3: Ultrawide-field pseudocolor image of tractional retinal detachment.

History of Present Illness

- *Photopsia:* It includes the sensation of a flashing light related to retinal traction. Typically described as a sensation of falling stars, even when the eyes are closed or in a dark room. A shower of floaters and vision loss often accompanies it.
- *Floaters:* Floaters are a very common visual symptom in the population; thus, distinguishing their etiology requires eliciting a detailed history.

  The sudden onset of large floaters in the center of the visual axis may indicate PVD. The patient observes a circular floater when the vitreous detaches from its annular ring surrounding the optic nerve (Weiss ring). More serious is the description of hundreds of tiny black specks or multiple small insects floating in front of the eye, as this is suggestive of a VH, resulting from a tear of a retinal blood vessel caused by a retinal tear or mechanical traction of a vitreoretinal adhesion. A few hours after the initial shower of black spots, the patient can note cobwebs that result from blood-forming irregular clots. Generally, the new onset of floaters associated with flashing lights is highly suggestive of a retinal tear, full thickness, or otherwise.
- *Field defect:* The patient may report a black curtain or shadow in the peripheral visual field, which, over a period of a few days, may spread to involve the entire visual field. Bullous (i.e., large ballooning) detachments produce dense visual field defects (i.e., blackness), and flat detachments produce relative field defects (i.e., grayness). The visual field defect can be helpful in guessing the probable quadrant of detachment.
- *Visual loss:* If the RD involves the central visual area or the macula, the complaint is sudden onset painless visual loss. The patient may describe this as cloudy vision. The intensity of the same depends on the height and duration of the macular detachment.

History of Past Illness

For RRD, one should inquire regarding a family history of retinal disorders or degenerations, myopia, or prior retinal therapies. History of past intraocular surgeries should always be identified in detail (see further), and history of trauma should be asked leading questions, especially if suggestive by signs.

Systemic history is very essential for TRD and exudative RD. One may find the history of DM, hypertension, TB, tumors, and other syndromes **(Box 1)** as applicable in the case.

Past Surgical History

The following points should be noted:
- History of vitreous loss during cataract surgery.
- Previous laser capsulotomy.
- Intraocular foreign body removal.

Family History

It may be helpful in certain cases of familial RD, where retinal degenerations are hereditary. Such cases may also be syndromic, e.g., Stickler's, Marfan's, and Wagner's, etc. **(Box 1)**.

■ CLINICAL EXAMINATION

- *Visual acuity:* Check visual acuity at near and distance, correcting for refractive error should be noted. Always look for myopia in the fellow eye.
- *External examination:* For signs of trauma (*See* chapter on traumatic RD).
- *Anterior segment:* Look for signs of trauma, stability of lens barrier/status, media clarity, etc. Uveitis and neovascularization of the iris (NVI) may be seen in TRD/exudative RD.

Box 1: Disorders associated with retinal detachment.

Familial vitreoretinal disorders:
- Familial exudative vitreoretinopathy
- Goldmann-Favre vitreoretinal degeneration
- Familial retinal dialysis
- Stickler syndrome (types I and II)
- Knobloch syndrome
- Enhanced S-cone syndrome
- Autosomal dominant vitreoretinochoroidopathy
- Wagner disease
- Snowflake vitreoretinal degeneration

Hereditary systemic disorders:
- Marfan syndrome
- Homocystinuria
- Ehlers–Danlos syndrome
- Sickling hemoglobinopathies

Other causes of RD:
- Infections
- Inflammatory conditions
- *Toxoplasma*
- *Toxocara*
- Pars planitis
- ROP

(RD: retinal detachment; ROP: retinopathy of prematurity)

- *Pupil Reaction:* A fixed dilated pupil may indicate previous trauma; a positive Marcus-Gunn pupil can occur with any disturbance of the afferent pupillomotor pathway, including RD. Relative afferent pupillary defect (RAPD) is more likely to be seen clinically if the RD is bullous, >2 quadrants, and especially if the macula is off.
- *IOP:* A relative hypotony of >4–5 mm Hg less than the fellow eye is common. If IOP is extremely low, choroidal detachment may be present. It may be raised in Schwartz-Matsuo syndrome in which RRD is associated with mild anterior uveitis due to blockage of the angles by parts of photoreceptors. This is also seen due to retinal dialysis due to prior blunt trauma in a young man.
- *Vitreous:* Look for signs of pigment or tobacco dust (i.e., Shaffer sign), which is suggestive of retinal tears in 70% of cases with no previous eye disease or surgery, hence a sign of RRD. Other findings that must be looked for include VH in TRD, RL cells in exudative RD, and vitreous degeneration in RRD.
- *Fundus examination:* Indirect ophthalmoscopy is the definitive means of diagnosing RD. Direct fundoscopy may detect VH and large detachment of the posterior pole, but it is inadequate for complete examination because of the lower illumination, lack of stereopsis, and limited view of the peripheral retina. However, following IO, either 90D-assisted biomicroscopy or direct fundoscopy must be done to assess the macular status. All the findings must be recorded in a modified Amsler–Dubois chart **(Fig. 4)**.
- Obvious detachment is observed as marked elevation of the retina, which appears gray due to loss of transparency with dark blood vessels that may lie in folds. The detached retina may undulate and appear out of focus. Shallow detachments are much more difficult to detect; thus, comparing the suspected area with an adjacent normal quadrant is helpful in detecting any change in retinal transparency. A pigmented or nonpigmented line may demarcate the limit of a detachment.
- *Specifically, for RRD:*
  - Identify the extent of RD, identify fresh or old, and identify the location, types-numbers of retinal breaks, grade of PVR, macular status, and presence of risk factors. See viva questions for a detailed discussion.
  - For exudative RD and TRD, *See* the differentiating features in **Table 1**.
  - *Remember the triad of cardinal signs:* RAPD, gray reflex, and hypotony for presumptive diagnosis of RRD.
  - A thorough fellow eye examination must be done for risk factors of RD, or signs of causative etiology of TRD and exudative RD.

DIFFERENTIAL DIAGNOSIS

- Posterior uveitis/scleritis
- PVD
- VH
- Vitreous syneresis
- Thick hyaloid
- Vitreous membranes
- Retinoschisis
- Retinal cyst
- Subretinal exudates
- Other differentials of TRD/exudation
- Retinal mass
- CD.

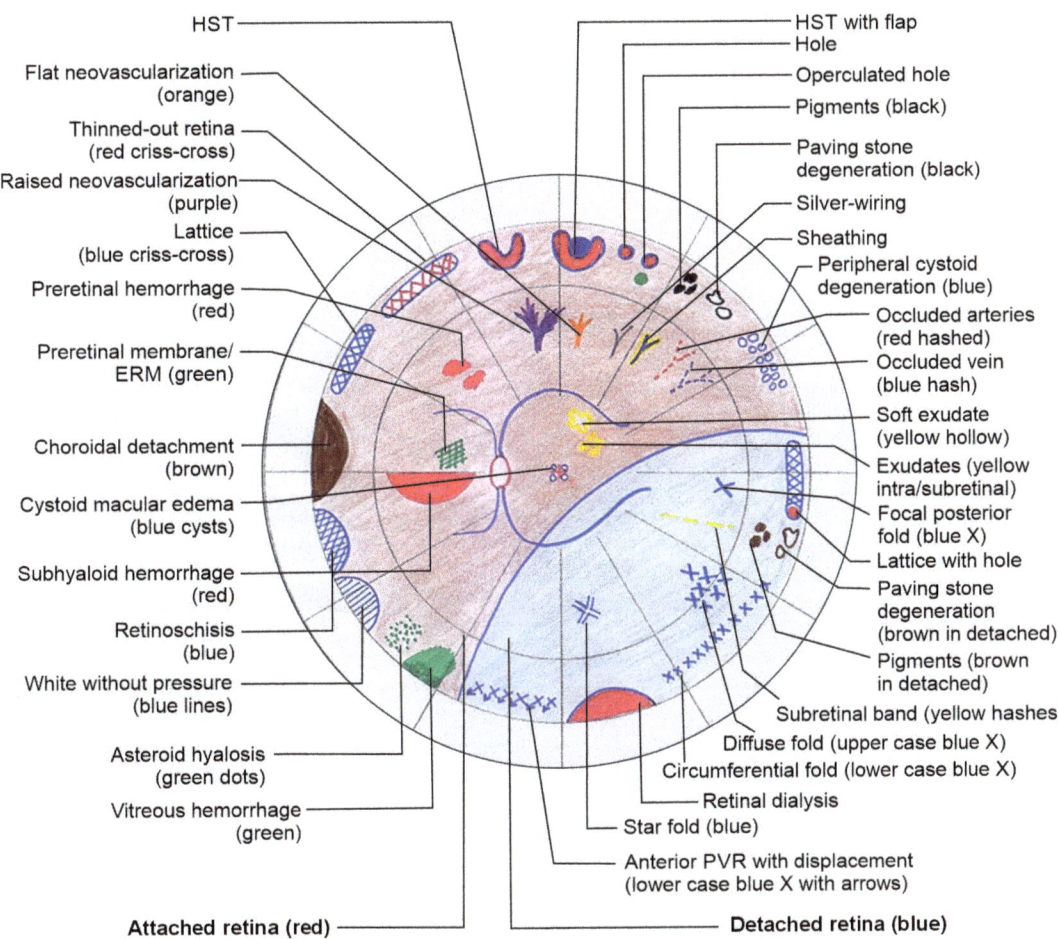

Fig. 4: Modified Amsler–Dubois retinal detachment chart with color coding.

■ INVESTIGATION

- *USG B-SCAN:* In the presence of media haze USG helps in differentiating the type of membrane, ruling out IOFB, subretinal mass, CD, etc.
- Systemic investigations as needed
- Other eye investigations may depend on complete diagnoses.

■ MANAGEMENT

The management of RRD is usually surgical. In certain poor prognoses cases, surgery may be deferred, while in certain others like subclinical RD medical management may be opted for. Broadly for RRD, the surgical options include vitrectomy, scleral buckling, and pneumatic retinopexy **(Table 2)**. *See* viva questions as to how to choose for best plan. In all cases, fellow eye treatment must be considered as optimum.

The management for TRD may be observation or vitrectomy depending on macular status. In all cases, efforts should be made to identify the cause of TRD. For exudative RD, either observation or management with steroids is done. Like TRD, efforts should be made to discern the cause and initiate treatment accordingly. *See* relevant chapters for further discussion.

Table 2: Surgery for retinal detachment.

	Scleral buckling	VR surgery	Pneumatic retinopexy
Indications	• RRD (PVR < C1) • Inferior retinal breaks • Retinal dialysis • Pediatric RD	• RD with PVR changes • RD with GRT • RD with vitreous hemorrhage • RD with intraocular FB	• A detachment caused by a single break, in superior 8 clock hours • The break should not be >1 clock hour • Multiple breaks but within 1–2 clock hours of each other
Contraindications	• Posterior breaks • Opaque media • Vaso-occlusive diseases like sickle cell anemia • PVR > C2	• Bleeding disorders • Suspected tumors, such as RB and melanoma	• Break larger than 1 clock hour or multiple breaks in >1 clock hour • Break in inferior 4 clock hours • PVR grade C or D • Patient not able to maintain the head position • Severely uncontrolled glaucoma or recent cataract surgery • Hazy media preventing adequate visualization of the retina
Complications	• Perforation • Rise in IOP • Extrusion • Infection • Diplopia • Anterior segment ischemia • Extrusion of explants • Epiretinal membrane (ERM) • Recurrent retinal detachment	• Iatrogenic breaks • Lens trauma • Re-detachment • Secondary glaucoma • PVR • Cataract progression	• Incarceration of vitreous • Subconjunctival gas • New or missed breaks • PVR • Re-detachment • Persistent subretinal fluid • Re-opening of original break • Vitreous haze • Sudden rise in IOP
Benefits	Excellent anatomic results, longevity, and good visual outcomes	Visualization of all tears/breaks, removal of opacities/synechiae, anatomic success in complicated detachments	In-office procedure, minimally invasive, reduced recovery time, better postoperative visual acuity

(RD: retinal detachment; RRD: rhegmatogenous retinal detachment; PVR: proliferative vitreoretinopathy; IOP: intraocular pressure; GRT: giant retinal tear; RB: retinoblastoma)

VIVA QUESTIONS

Q.1. What keeps the retina attached?
Ans. Embryologically, RPE and the neurosensory retina arise from different neuroectodermal layers, hence the potential space. Normally, the hydrostatic pressure of the fluid dynamics, mechanical vitreous pressure, and glycoprotein matrix between these layers keeps the retina in position.

Q.2. How to identify ora serrata on examination?
Ans. The ora is the anterior-most limit of the retina. The dentate process, oral bays, meridional folds, and oral bays are present. The choroid also ends there with the beginning of the pars plana.

Q.3. Define vitreous base.
Ans. This is a 3–4 mm wide zone of condensed and firmly adherent vitreous cortex straddling either side of the ora. It starts around 5 mm from the limbus.

Q.4. Enumerate some retinal degenerations not leading to RD.
Ans. Microcystoid (most common), paving stone, reticular, WWOP. WWOP is considered by some as an optic illusion.

Q.5. What are the normally strong adhesions of vitreous?
Ans. Fovea, vascular arcades, optic disc, and vitreous base (strongest).

Q.6. What is the retinal break?
Ans. Retinal break is a full-thickness deficiency in the neural retina. Holes, Horseshoe tears, and retinal dialysis are the types. Scleral depression may be needed to identify peripheral breaks.

Q.7. Which retinal degenerations are associated with RD?
Ans.
- *Lattice:* It is the most important degeneration. Though it may be seen in up to 8% of the normal population, it is present in up to 50% of RD and causes up to 20%. It is bilateral in 50%. It can develop HSTs at the posterior border or atrophic holes. Clinically it is seen as a cigar-shaped, pigmented or nonpigmented peripheral circumferential lesion, though it may be radial also like in Stickler syndrome. It has hyalinized criss-cross vessels, a thin retina with overlying liquefied vitreous, strongly adherent on its posterior border.
- *Retinoschisis:* This is split into retinal layers. It may be typical (split in OPL) and reticular (split in NFL layer). Reticular is seen in congenital schisis as the X-linked retinoschisis syndrome. It is characterized by bicycle maculopathy, vitreous veils, pockmarks, and snowflakes and is seen as hypermetropes. Some children may develop RD or VH rarely. In contrast, degenerative schisis is seen elderly, in the inferior temporal region, and may or may not be bilateral. This develops due to the coalescence of cystoid degeneration. The retinal breaks may develop in the inner layer or outer layer of schisis. While inner breaks do not lead to RD, outer layer breaks singularly, or in combination can lead to RD and should be treated. Retinoschisis has an absolute scotoma in contrast to RD, and diagnostic differentiation is the laser uptake test in schisis.
- *Snail-track degeneration:* White frost-like peripheral degeneration, HSTs are uncommon due to less traction. Some believe it to be a lesser form of lattice.

Q.8. What are flashes due to?
Ans. The perception of flashes or photopsia is due to the production of phosphenes by pathophysiologic stimulation of the retina. During PVD, as the vitreous separates from the retinal surface, the retina is disturbed mechanically stimulating a sensation of light. Ocular migraine is a differential diagnosis.

Q.9. What is the significance of floaters?
Ans.
- Sudden appearance of one large floater near the visual axis is mostly due to PVD (Weiss ring)
- Appearance of numerous curvilinear opacities within the visual field indicates vitreous degeneration
- Floaters due to VH are characterized by numerous tiny black dots, followed by cobwebs as the blood forms clots. While a single floater has a low (~15%) risk of having a retinal tear, multiple floaters have a higher risk (70%). PVD with VH is particularly ominous.

Q.10. Why is the IOP decreased in RRDs?
Ans. An eye with RRD typically has decreased IOP and it is due to the following factors:

- *Early transient pressure drop* may result from inflammation and reduced aqueous production. A vicious cycle sets up between CD and inflammation.
- *Prolonged hypotony* may be caused by posterior flow, presumably through a break in the RPE and even anterior PVR and CD.

Q.11. What is Schwartz–Matsuo syndrome?

Ans. RRD is typically associated with decreased IOP. Schwartz described a condition in which the patient presents with unilateral IOP elevation, RD, and open anterior chamber angle with 'cells' in the anterior chamber. Elevated IOP is often seen in the evening. The detachment is typically caused by dialysis at the ora serrata or a break in the nonpigmented epithelium of the pars plana or pars plicata of the ciliary body. The elevated IOP is usually discovered incidentally at the time of diagnosis of the RD, and resolves without specific treatment when the retina is reattached.

The proposed hypothesis for raised IOP: The cells in the aqueous were photoreceptor outer segments rather than inflammatory cells. These fragments are derived from the rods. The peripheral retinal break allows free communication between the subretinal space and aqueous humor. Outer segments then flow into the aqueous and obstruct the trabecular meshwork.

Q.12. Why is IOP raised in certain RDs?

Ans.
- Chronic low-grade uveitis in RDs damage the trabecular meshwork
- In long-standing RDs, rubeosis iridis (NVI) is followed by increased IOP due to NVG.

Q.13. What is "tobacco dusting"?

Ans.
- Pathognomonic of RRD
- Present in the anterior vitreous phase
- The cells represent macrophages containing shed RPE.

Q.14. What is the incidence of RD in myopes?

Ans. 40% of all RDs occur in myopes. The reasons for high myopes to have RRD include the following:
- Increased stretch of the retina over the bigger eyeball
- Incidence of lattice generation is higher
- Incidence of PVD is higher
- Macular hole
- Vitreous loss during cataract surgery
- Diffuse chorioretinal atrophy

Q.15. What is high myopia, or pathological myopia? What are the signs of myopia?

Ans. A refractive error greater than 6D, or axial length >26 mm is typical of high myopia.
- Pathological myopia refers to the occurrence of pathological changes in a high myope, the most typical being a posterior staphyloma.
- Other signs of myopia include disc changes such as a large, pale disc, high CDR, temporal crescent, disc pit, disc tilt, disc coloboma and macular changes such as MH, foveoschisis, subretinal hemorrhage, lacquer cracks, foster Fuchs spots, CNVM, focal atrophy; peripheral changes, such as retinal degeneration, lattice, paving stone, atrophic retinal holes, WWOP, HSTs, tessellated or tigroid fundus, and diffuse chorioretinal atrophy. None of these, however, is specific for myopia.

Q.16. What are the systemic conditions associated with RRD?

Ans. *See* Table 2.

Q.17. Why is the configuration of SRF important?

Ans. Because SRF spreads in a gravitational fashion and its shape is governed by anatomic limits (ora and optic nerve), it can be used to locate the primary break. Knowledge of Lincoff rules is imminent as these rules indicate the location of the retinal break.

Q.18. What are the factors promoting SRF into the break?

Ans.
- Ocular movements
- Gravity
- Vitreous traction, at the edge of the break
- PVD

Q.19. What is Lincoff rules?

Ans. SRF usually spreads in a gravitational fashion and its shape is governed by

anatomical limits and the location of the primary retinal break. If the primary break is located superiorly, SRF first spreads inferiorly on the same side of the break and then spreads superiorly on the opposite side of the fundus.
- A shallow inferior RD in which SRF is slightly higher on the temporal side points to a primary break on that side.
- A primary break at 6 o'clock will cause inferior RD with equal fluid levels.
- In a bullous inferior RD, the primary break usually lies above the horizontal meridian.
- If a primary break is in the upper nasal quadrant, the SRF will revolve around the optic disc and then rise on the temporal side until it is level with the primary break.
- A subtotal RD with a superior wedge of attached retina points to a 1° break located in the periphery nearest its highest borders.
- When the SRF crosses the vertical midline above the primary break near 12 o'clock the lower edge of the RD corresponds to the side of the break.

Q.20. What is vitreoretinal traction?
Ans. It is the force exerted on the retina by structures originating in the vitreous.
Types:
- *Dynamic:* It is induced by rapid eye movement, where there is a centripetal force toward the vitreous cavity. Responsible for retinal tears and RRD.
- *Static:* Independent of ocular movements and plays an important role in the pathogenesis of tractional RD and proliferative vitreoretinopathy.
  It may be:
  - *Tangential:* Epiretinal fibrovascular membranes
  - *Anteroposterior traction:* Contraction of fibrovascular membranes
  - *Bridging (trampoline) traction:* Contraction of fibrovascular membranes, which stretch from one part of the posterior retina to another or between vascular arcades, which tends to pull the 2 involved points together.

Q.21. How do you differentiate between the three types of RD?
Ans. *See* **Table 1**.

Q.22. Differentiate clinically between CD and RD
Ans.
- RD is gray, and CD is brown.
- RD has undulating motions, while CD may have "jiggly" movements.
- USG shows the typical double peaked sign of a membrane arising from the equator till ora.

Q.23. What are the factors governing visual function following surgical reattachment?
Ans.
- *Macular involvement:* If the macula has been involved the prognosis is poorer.
- *Duration:* Typically, a macular detachment <7 days is believed to have good visual prognoses. The patient may achieve the pre-RD visual acuity. Detachment beyond 10 days usually had poor outcomes.
- Height of macular detachment.
- Age >60 years negatively affect visual restoration.

Q.24. What are the indications for segmental circumferential buckling?
Ans.
- Multiple breaks located in 1 or 2 quadrants and varying distance
- From ora serrata
- Anterior breaks
- Wide breaks, dialysis, and giant tears.

Q.25. What are the indications for encircling buckle (360°)?
Ans.
- Break involving 3 or more quadrants
- Extensive RD without detectable breaks particularly in eyes with hazy media
- Lattice degeneration, snail track degeneration involving 3 or more quadrants
- Along with vitrectomy
- Multiple breaks
- Pseudophakia and aphakia

Q.26. What are the steps in scleral buckling surgery?
Ans.
- Preliminary examination
- 360° peritomy

- Traction (bridle) sutures around the recti
- Inspection of sclera
- Localization and marking of the break
- Cryotherapy
- Scleral buckling
- Drainage of SRF
- Intravitreal air or BSS injection followed by reinspection
- Closure of the peritomy

Q.27. What are the indications for subretinal fluid (SRF) drainage?

Ans.
- Difficulty in localization of retinal breaks in bullous detachments
- Long-standing RD as SRF is viscous
- Bullous RD
- As part of DACE procedure
- Glaucomatous cyclitis
- Resurgeries

Q.28. What are the methods of SRF drainage?

Ans. *Prang:* Here digital pressure is applied till the central retinal artery is occluded and the choroidal vasculature is blanched. Then full thickness perforation is made with a 27-G hypodermic needle to drain SRF. Air is injected to form the globe.

Cut down: Radial sclerotomy is made beneath the area of the deepest SRF. Mattress suture may be placed across the lips of the sclerotomy. The prolapsed choroidal knuckle is examined with a +20D lens for large choroidal vessels. After ruling this out, light cautery is applied to the knuckle to avoid bleeding, and the knuckle is perforated with a 25-gauge hypodermic needle.

Q.29. What are the advantages of SRF drainage?

Ans. It provides immediate contact between the sensory retina and RPE with the flattening of the fovea. If this contact is delayed, the stickiness of RPE wears off and adequate adhesion may not occur, resulting in nonattachment of the retina.

Q.30. What are the precautions taken before drainage of SRF?

Ans.
- Examine the fundus to make sure, SRF has not shifted
- Avoid vortex vein
- IOP should not be elevated (it may cause retinal incarceration).

Q.31. How to choose a site for drainage?

Ans. The most dependent retinal area is, the horizontal median as it is generally devoid of vortex vessels, just behind muscle insertions, preferably nasal site to avoid macular complications. Superior sites should be avoided for the risk of macular bleeds. Cryotherapy sites and break sites are to be avoided; draining under the planned buckle area is suitable.

Q.32. How do you know that SRF drainage is completed?

Ans. By the presence of pigments.

Q.33. What are the complications of SRF drainage?

Ans.
- Choroidal hemorrhage
- Ocular hypotony
- Iatrogenic break
- Retinal incarceration
- Vitreous prolapse
- Damage to long posterior ciliary arteries and nerves
- Endophthalmitis
- Subretinal bleed. Just after drainage, IO must be done to rule this out. If present, immediate building of IOP with head tilt must be done. If the still bleed reaches beneath the macula, gas injection with positioning or immediate vitrectomy should be considered.

Q.34. What are the indications for internal tamponade in scleral buckling?

Ans.
- Superior break
- Hypotony
- Retinal folds
- Fish mouthing
- Posterior breaks
- Subretinal bleed
- DACE procedure.

Q.35. Who are the best candidates for pneumatic retinopexy?

Ans.
- A detachment caused by a single break, in superior 8 clock hours
- The break should not be >1 clock hour
- Multiple breaks but within 1–2 clock hours of each other

Table 3: Commonly used vitreous substitute.

Gas	Expansion	Nonexpansible concentration	Average duration	Volume used for PR
SF6	2x	20%	10–14 days	0.5 mL
C3F8	4x	12%	30–45 days	0.35 mL
Air	Nonexpansible	–	5–7 days	0.8 mL

- Free of systemic disease (rheumatoid arthritis) (who can maintain position)
- Phakic patients
- Total PVD.

Q.36. What are the principles of pneumoretinopexy?
Ans. Intraocular gases keep the retinal break closed by the following properties:
- Mechanical closure and thus RPE pump removes excessive SRF
- Surface tension
- Buoyancy.

Q.37. What are the substances used as vitreous substitutes in RD surgery?
Ans.
- *Intraocular gases:*
  - *Nonexpansile:* Air, SF6: Air mixture, C3F8: Air mixture
  - *Expansile:* SF6, C3F8 **(Table 3)**
- Silicone oil
- Perfluorocarbon liquids (PFCL)

Q.38. What are different surgical options for RRD and compare them?
Ans. *See* **Table 1**.

Q.39. What is the difference between fresh and old RD?
Ans. *See* **Table 4**.

Q.40. What is the pathogenesis of traumatic RD?
Ans. *See* the chapter on traumatic RD.

Q.41. How to draw an RD chart?
Ans. *See* **Figure 1**.

Q.42. What are the disadvantages of silicone oil?
Ans. The major disadvantage is the need for a second surgery for removal. Complications include emulsification of oil causing media opacification, glaucoma, corneal edema, BSK, and cataract amongst others. It has been noted that aphakic patients do not do well with long-term silicone oil. The silicone oil study suggested the use of oil in children and other patients noncompliant with positioning and in eyes with large breaks and hypotony. Otherwise, results with C3F8 were comparable.

Table 4: Features of fresh and old RD.

Fresh RD	Old RD
• Loss of choroidal pattern • *Retina:* Convex configuration, corrugations • Fluid extending up to ora serrata • Slightly opaque with dark blood vessels • Moves freely with eye movements	• Demarcation lines • Immobile retina • Very thin atrophic retina • Secondary intra-retinal cysts • Tobacco dust • Advanced PVR

(PVR: proliferative vitreoretinopathy; RD: retinal detachment)

Q.43. What is PVR?
Ans. *Proliferative vitreoretinopathy:* This is dedifferentiation followed by proliferation, migration, and then fibrotic metaplasia of progenitor cells, such as RPE cells, glial cells, and Müller cells. The most common theory states that RPE cells exposed to vitreous as in an open break are responsible for the same. They migrate to form epiretinal membranes and subretinal bands. RD is not a prerequisite of PVR, and it may form in attached retinas as well.

Q.44. What are classification systems for PVR?
Ans. Three important classification systems include retina society classification,

silicone oil study classification, and then the updated retina society classification system. *See* **Tables 5 to 8**.

Q.45. How can PVR be managed?
Ans. Medical management for prevention includes the use of steroids, antineoplastic drugs, such as daunorubicin, use of heparin, and other drugs like tetracyclines. These have not proven to be beneficial.

Surgical management peeling of mature membranes, removal of subretinal membranes, using PFCLs, and performing relaxing procedures, such as retinotomies and retinectomies.

Q.46. Discuss prophylactic management of RD.
Ans. Normally, HSTs should always be treated. As per theory holes and other lattice degenerations need to be treated only if there is symptomatic PVD or it is a fellow eye of a patient. Patients with a family history, high myopia, undergoing cataract surgery, or any other predilection need to be informed regarding the same, before opting for treatment. Methods of prophylaxis may be laser delimitation or cryotherapy.

Q.47. What is subclinical RD?
Ans. It is a break surrounded by minimal SRF. Different definitions may be found. One definition says SRF <1 DD around a break no part of which is posterior to the equator. Another definition says SRF <2 DD, no part of which is >1 DD posterior to the equator. Such patients can be managed by walling off the RD till ora or by laser delimitation around the SRF. Cryotherapy may be done in selected cases.

Table 5: Retinal Society proliferative vitreoretinopathy classification.

Grade (stage)	Characteristics
A	Vitreous haze, vitreous pigment clumps
B	Wrinkling of the inner retinal surface rolled edge of a retinal break, retinal stiffness, vessel tortuosity
C	Full-thickness retinal folds in
C-1	One quadrant
C-2	Two quadrants
C-3	Three quadrants
D	Fixed retinal folds in four quadrants
D-1	Wide funnel shape
D-2	Narrow funnel shape (anterior end of funnel visible by indirect ophthalmoscopy)
D-3	Closed funnel (optic nerve not visible)

Table 6: Silicone study classification system for proliferative vitreoretinopathy.

Grade	Features
A	Vitreous haze, vitreous pigment clumps
B	Inner retinal wrinkling, rolled edge of retinal breaks
CP	
P1: 1 quadrant (1–3 clock hours)	Starfolds and/or diffuse contraction in posterior retinal and/or subretinal membrane in posterior retina
P2: 2 quadrants (4–6 clock hours)	
P3: 3 quadrants (7–9 clock hours)	
P4: 4 quadrants (10–12 clock hours)	
CA	Circumferential and/or perpendicular and/or anterior traction in anterior retina
A1: 1 quadrant (1–3 clock hours)	
A2: 2 quadrants (4–6 clock hours)	
A3: 3 quadrants (7–9 clock hours)	
A4: 4 quadrants (10–12 clock hours	

Table 7: Updated proliferative vitreoretinopathy grade classification by Machemer.

Grade	Features
A	Vitreous haze, vitreous pigment clumps, pigment clusters on the inferior retina
B	Wrinkling of the inner retinal surface, retinal stiffness, vessel tortuosity, rolled and the irregular edge of a retinal break, decreased mobility
CP 1–12	Posterior to the equator, focal, diffuse, or circumferential full-thickness folds, subretinal strands
CA 1–12	Anterior to the equator, focal, diffuse, or circumferential full-thickness folds, subretinal strands, anterior displacement

Table 8: Silicone study classification of contraction type in proliferative vitreoretinopathy.

Type number	Contraction type	Location of PVR	Summary of clinical signs
1	Focal	Posterior	Star fold
2	Diffuse	Posterior	Confluent irregular retinal folds in the posterior retina; the remainder of retina drawn posterior; optic disc may not be visible
3	Subretinal	Posterior	"Napkin ring" around the disc, or "Clothesline" elevation of the retina
4	Circumferential	Anterior	Irregular retinal folds in the anterior retina; series of radial folds more posteriorly; peripheral retina within vitreous base stretched inward
5	Perpendicular	Anterior	The smooth circumferential fold of the retina at the insertion of the posterior hyaloid
6	Anterior	Anterior	The circumferential fold of the retina at the insertion of the posterior hyaloid pulled forward; through the peripheral retina anteriorly; ciliary processes stretched with possible hypotony; the iris retracted

Q.48. What are the basic principles of vitrectomy for RD?

Ans. These include performing a central vitrectomy, inducing PVD, and complete peripheral vitreous dissection followed by SRF drainage. This is followed by retinopexy around all retinal breaks and finally, a vitreous substitute is inserted. All membrane removal is done before fluid air exchange and SRF drainage.

Q49. What are the causes of pediatric RD?

Ans. The causes are trauma, ROP, FEVR, hereditary syndromes, high myopia, coloboma, coat disease, IOFB, previous surgery, etc.

Q50. What are the causes of failed surgery?

Ans. Major causes include missed/new retinal breaks and PVR. Additionally, in buckling, optimum break buckle relationship, and in vitrectomy optimum tamponade and positioningares are required. Poor drainage and poor retinopexy are other causes of failure or relapses.

BIBLIOGRAPHY

1. Azad R, Azad SV, Takkar B. Basics of Vitrectomy. New Delhi: Thieme Medical and Scientific Publishers Pvt. Ltd; 2016.
2. Kanski JJ, Bowling B. Clinical Ophthalmology: a Systematic Approach: Expert Consult, 7th edition. Philadelphia: W B Saunders Co Ltd; 2011.
3. Ryan SJ. Retina: Expert Consult Premium, 5th edition. United States: Elsevier Health Sciences; 2012.

AGE-RELATED MACULAR DEGENERATION

Ritu Nagpal, Shipra Singhi, Raghav Ravani

■ INTRODUCTION

Age-related macular degeneration (ARMD or AMD), is a degenerative disease of persons above the age of 50 years that is characterized by the following abnormalities in the macula:[1]
- Presence of at least intermediate-size drusen (63 µm or larger in diameter)
- Retinal pigment epithelium (RPE) abnormalities such as hypopigmentation or hyperpigmentation
- Reticular pseudodrusen
- *Presence of any of the following features*: Geographic atrophy of the RPE, choroidal neovascularization (exudative, wet), polypoidal choroidal vasculopathy, or retinal angiomatous proliferation.

Visual acuity is not a factor in the disease definition or classification scheme. In the postgraduate examination, it can be given as a long case.

■ HISTORY

Chief Complaints

ARMD can present with:
- Gradual painless loss of vision in the eye (dry ARMD)
- Sudden loss of vision (wet ARMD)
- Shadows, distorted vision, difficulty in discerning colors, decreased contrast, slow recovery of visual function after exposure to bright light, and slow reading may accompany the loss of vision.
- Central scotomas—shadows or missing areas of vision may be present (positive scotoma).

History of Present Illness

Those with nonexudative macular degeneration may be asymptomatic or notice a gradual loss of central vision, whereas those with exudative macular degeneration often notice a rapid onset of vision loss.

History of Past Illness

History of previous anti-VEGF injections, laser, PDT, and low vision aid may be there. AMD is multifactorial in etiology and is thought to involve a complex interaction between polygenic, lifestyle, and environmental factors. The various risk factors should be identified on history and include the following:
- Age is the major risk factor.
- *Race:* Late AMD is more common in white individuals than those of other races.
- *Heredity:* Family history is important; the risk of AMD is up to three times as high if a first-degree relative has the disease.
- Variants in many genes have been implicated in AMD risk and protection such as the complement factor H gene *CFH*, which helps to protect cells from complement-mediated damage, and the *ARMS2* gene on chromosome 10. Genes related to lipid metabolism are also thought to be important.
- Smoking roughly doubles the risk of AMD.
- Hypertension and other cardiovascular risk factors.
- *Dietary factors:* High fat intake and obesity may be promoted.
- Aspirin may increase the risk of neovascular AMD. Though the evidence is limited, if an individual at high risk requires an antiplatelet agent it may be sensible to consider an alternative to aspirin.
- *Other factors:* Such as cataract surgery, blue iris color, high sunlight exposure, and female gender are suspected, but their influence remains less certain.

Family History

Family history may be there.

Past Surgical History

Rule out any past intravitreal surgery.

EXAMINATION

General examination/specific systemic examination should be carried out to rule out any systemic risk factors as described above.

Ocular Examination

- *Eyebrow:* Brow-ptosis may occur due to aging.
- *Eyeball:* Generally normal.
- *Lid:* Senile ptosis, dermatochalasis may be present (due to aging).
- *Conjunctiva:* Generally normal.
- *Cornea:* Arcus senilis may be present (due to aging).
- *Sclera:* Usually normal.
- *Anterior chamber:* Usually normal.
- *Iris:* Increased risk of AMD in people with blue or light iris color compared with those with darker iris pigmentation.
- *Pupil:* Usually normal.
- *IOP:* Usually normal.
- *Gonioscopy:* Usually normal.
- *Lens:* Senile cataract, another comorbidity is found due to aging factors.
- *Anterior vitreous:* Liquefied vitreous, mostly age-related and may be present.
- *Fundus:* Stereoscopic fundus examination is the best method for examining a patient with suspected choroidal neovascularization (CNV). A fundus contact or noncontact lens in conjunction with slit lamp biomicroscopy should be utilized for the examination. For those less comfortable with the noncontact fundus macular lenses, a fundus contact lens is the easiest to use. The following findings should be looked for.
- *Dry ARMD:*
  - *Drusen:* Age-related drusen are rare before the age of 40 but are common by the sixth decade. Numerous intermediate—large soft drusen; may become confluent. Drusen is positively associated with the size of lesions and the presence or absence of associated pigmentary abnormalities. The distribution is highly variable, and they may be confined to the fovea, encircle it, or form a band around the macular periphery (**Fig. 1**). They may also be seen in the peripheral and midperipheral fundus.
  - *Pigment epithelial abnormalities:* Focal hyper- and/or hypopigmentation of the RPE is associated with a significantly higher likelihood of progression to late AMD with visual loss.
  - Sharply circumscribed areas of *RPE atrophy* associated with variable loss of the retina and choriocapillaris atrophy.
  - *Geographic atrophy*, enlargement of atrophic areas, within which larger choroidal vessels may become visible and pre-existing drusen disappear (**Figs. 2 and 3**). Visual acuity may be severely impaired if the fovea is involved. Rarely, CNV may develop in an area of GA.
  - *Dystrophic calcification* may develop in all types of drusen.
  - *Drusenoid RPE detachment* may occur. Drusenoid PED develops from confluent large soft drusen and is often bilateral. Shallow elevated pale areas with irregular scalloped edges.

High-risk characteristics of drusen for the development of CNV include Soft type, large size, greater than five in number, confluent, and presence of RPE stippling, and family history of wet AMD or other eye wet AMD. These risk factors have been used by the AREDS to formulate a 5-year risk of developing wet AMD.

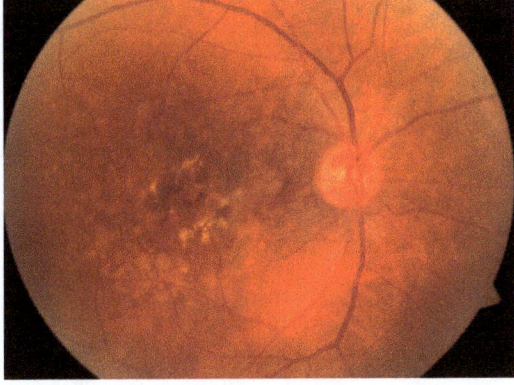

Fig. 1: Clinical photograph of dry AMD. Both soft and hard drusens are present.

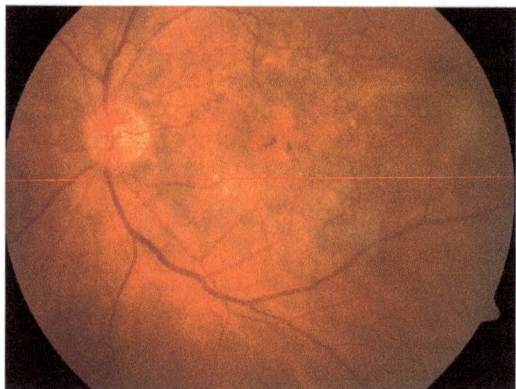

Fig. 2: Clinical photograph of geographic atrophy.

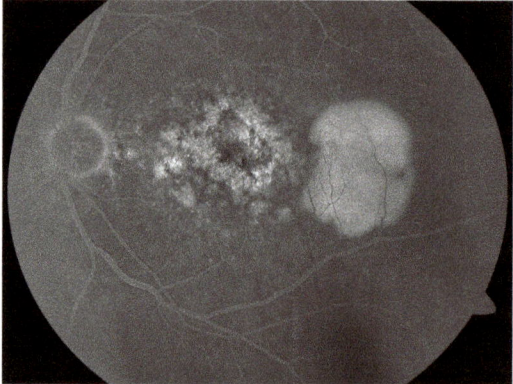

Fig. 3: FFA of geographic atrophy with large temporal PED. (FFA: fundus fluorescein angiography; PED: pigment epithelial detachment)

Wet ARMD Neovascular

- *CNV:* It can be occult or classic CNV **(Table 1)**.
  - It appears as a gray–green or pinkish-yellow lesion. Associated medium–large drusen are a typical finding in the same or fellow eye.
  - Signs of CNV include subretinal fluid, hard exudates, subretinal hemorrhage or intraretinal hemorrhage, pigmented subretinal lesions, and sub-RPE fluid.
  - Localized subretinal fluid, sometimes with cystoid macular edema may be present.
  - Intra- and subretinal lipid deposition, sometimes extensive.
  - Hemorrhage is common, e.g., subretinal, preretinal/retrohyaloid, or vitreous (breakthrough bleed can occur in to vitreous).
  - Serous and/or hemorrhagic detachment of the sensory retina or RPE may occur.
  - *Serous PED:* An orange dome-shaped elevation with sharply delineated edges, often with a paler margin of subretinal fluid. Multiple lesions may occur. An associated pigment band may indicate chronicity. Associated blood, lipid exudation, chorioretinal folds, or irregular subretinal fluid may indicate underlying CNV.
  - *Fibrovascular PED* is much more irregular in outline and elevation than serous PED. This is regarded as a form of wet AMD

Table 1: FFA and ICG findings in ARMD.

Clinical condition	FFA	ICG
Classic CNV	Well-demarcated boundaries, discerned during transit, late leakage often obscuring boundaries	Similar to FFA but less well delineated. ICGA demonstrates CNV as a focal hyperfluorescent "hot spot" or "plaque"
Occult CNV: Fibrovascular PED (FVPED)	*Stippled hyperfluorescence:* Irregular elevation of RPE, boundaries may or may not be well-demarcated, persistent staining or leakage of fluorescein at 10 minutes	*Stippled hyperfluorescence*
Serous PED	A well-demarcated oval area of hyperfluorescent pooling that increases in intensity but not in area with time; an indentation (notch) may signify CNV	An oval hypofluorescent area with a surrounding hyperfluorescent ring

Contd...

Contd...

Clinical condition	FFA	ICG
Drusenoid PED	Early diffuse hypofluorescence with patchy relatively faint early hyperfluorescence, progressing to moderate irregular late staining	Hypofluorescence predominates
Hemorrhagic PED	Dense masking of background fluorescence, but overlying vessels are visible	Similar to ICG
Basal laminar drusen	Hyperfluorescence early and gives an appearance of a "starry night"	
Hard exudates	Window defects with early hyperfluorescence and fading of fluorescence in late frames	
Soft exudates	Early hypofluorescence or hyperfluorescence with no late leakage	
RPE tear/rip	The fluorescein angiogram shows blocked fluorescence in the area of scrolled RPE and hyperfluorescence in the area without RPE	
Idiopathic polypoidal choroidopathy (IPC)	Hyperfluorescent dilated complexes of choroidal vessels (branching vascular networks) that leak in the later phases of the angiograms. These dilated complexes look like polyps or grapes	Hyperfluorescent nodules and a network of large choroidal vessels with surrounding hypofluorescence appear in the early phase. The polyp-like swellings rapidly begin to leak. The previously darker surrounding region becomes hyperfluorescent by the late phase
Geographical atrophy	Autofluorescent hyperfluorescent on angiography due to transmission defect and staining	
RAP	FFA is usually similar to occult or minimally classic CNV but may show focal intraretinal hyperfluorescence	ICGA is diagnostic in most cases, showing a hot spot in mid and/or late frames, and frequently a perfusing retinal arteriole and draining venule ('hairpin loop' when linked)

(ARMD: age-related macular degeneration; CNV: choroidal neovascularization; FFA: fundus fluorescein angiograms; ICG: indocyanine green; IGGA: indocyanine green angiography; PED: pigment epithelial detachment)

and should not be confused with serous/drusenoid PEDs.
- *Hemorrhagic PED:* Sub-RPE or subretinal blood is found **(Fig. 4)**.
- Fibrovascular disciform scar
- *Retinal pigment epithelial tear/rip:* An RPE tear may occur at the junction of attached and detached RPE. Tears may occur spontaneously, following laser (including PDT), or after intravitreal injection. Older patients and large irregular PEDs associated with CNV are at higher risk. A crescent-shaped pale area of RPE dehiscence is seen, next to a darker area corresponding to the retracted and folded flap. An RPE tear is readily identifiable as a sharply demarcated area of bare choroid with a straight, linear edge. This straight, linear edge corresponds to the location of the associated retracted, scrolled RPE.

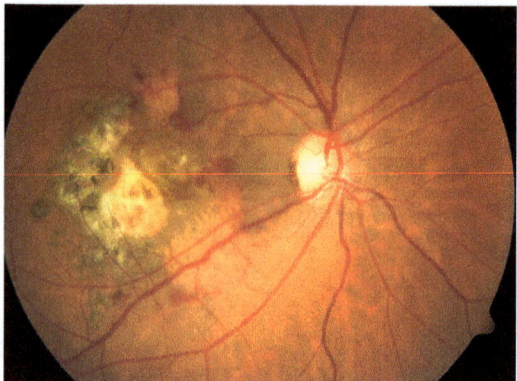

Fig. 4: Clinical photograph of wet AMD showing disciform scar with subretinal bleed.

- *Retinal angiomatous proliferation (RAP):* It is an atypical form of neovascular AMD. The presence of small central macular hemorrhages, sometimes punctiform, associated with edema in an eye with soft drusen, is highly suggestive of RAP in its initial stages. The following lesions suggest RAP in AMD:
    - Small multiple hemorrhages, pre, intra, or subretinal, normally not observed in macular neurosensory detachments with choroidal neovascularization.
    - Tortuous, dilated retinal vessels, sometimes showing retino-retinal anastomoses.
    - Telangiectasias
    - Microaneurysms
    - Sudden disappearance of a retinal vessel that appears to have moved deeper.

Hard exudates around the retinal lesion. Earlier CNV was classified into type 1—sub-RPE and type 2—subretinal with sub-RPE. RAP now has been labeled as type 3 CNV.

Idiopathic polypoidal choroidopathy (IPC): This is another atypical form of neovascular AMD in which highly exudative lesions with steep-walled hemorrhagic pigment epithelial detachments are seen most typically adjacent to the optic disc, but can occur anywhere within the macula and even outside the macula.

■ DIFFERENTIAL DIAGNOSIS

- *Nonexudative macular lesions mimicking AMD:* Several conditions feature lesions similar to age-related drusen
    - *Doyne honeycomb retinal dystrophy* (malattia leventinese and autosomal dominant radial drusen) is an uncommon condition in which fairly characteristic drusen appear during the second or third decades.
    - *Pattern dystrophy (PD):* It affects the macula and can be mistaken for nonexudative AMD. The most common types of PD seen are adult vitelliform macular dystrophy (AVMD) and less commonly butterfly-shaped pattern dystrophy. Differentiating AVMD from AMD can be difficult. Fundus autofluorescence imaging especially when combined with OCT is helpful in distinguishing PD from AMD. Fluorescein angiography can show a typical *"corona sign"* in AVMD, and the branching lines seen in butterfly-shaped PD are associated with a hyperfluorescence distributed in the area of the deposits, which does not show leakage throughout the phases of the angiogram.
    - *Cuticular drusen,* also known as grouped early adult-onset or basal laminar drusen tend to be seen in relatively young adults. The lesions consist of small (25–75 µm) yellowish nodules that tend to cluster and increase in number with time and can progress to serous PED. FA characteristically gives a *'stars in the sky'* appearance. The condition has been linked to a variant of the *CFH* gene.
    - *Type 2 membranoproliferative glomerulonephritis* is a chronic renal disease that occurs in older children and adults. A minority of patients develop bilateral diffuse drusen-like lesions. The *CFH* gene has again been implicated.
- *Exudative macular lesions mimicking AMD*
    - Diabetic maculopathy
    - High myopia
    - Inflammatory CNV
    - Angioid streaks and chorioretinal inflammatory conditions such as presumed ocular histoplasmosis.

INVESTIGATIONS

- *Ultrasonography:* USG is useful in cases of media haze for fundus evaluation.
- *Fluorescein angiography (FA):* This is central to diagnosis and management. **Table 1** has for various findings for it. FA is used to diagnose CNV (**Figs. 5 and 6**) and to plan and monitor the response to laser photocoagulation or PDT. Current indications include:
  - Diagnosis of CNV before committing to anti-VEGF treatment; FA should usually be performed urgently on the basis of clinical suspicion. To detect the presence of and determine the extent, type, size, and location of CNV. If verteporfin PDT or laser photocoagulation surgery is being considered, the angiogram is also used as a guide to direct treatment.
  - To detect persistent or recurrent CNV following treatment.
  - To assist in determining the cause of visual loss that is not explained by the clinical examination.
  - As an adjunct to diagnosis of an alternative form of neovascular AMD such as PCV and RAP.
  - Localization for extrafoveal photocoagulation, or guidance for PDT.
  - Monitoring response to therapy.

CNVs can be detected and categorized either as classic or occult or a combination of the two, depending on the leakage patterns they present at various time points on the angiogram. This differentiation was imperative for laser treatments where well-defined margins for treatment decisions were necessary.

Classic CNVM—present as discrete, early hyperfluorescence with late leakage of dye into the overlying neurosensory RD. A lacy pattern within the CNVM is most often not observed in exudative AMD. Only 12% of newly diagnosed patients with exudative AMD present with classic CNV.

Occult CNVM—are categorized into two basic forms, late leakage of undetermined source and fibrovascular PEDs.

Late leakage of an undetermined source (LLUS) manifests as regions of stippled or ill-defined leakage into an overlying neurosensory RD without a distinct source focus that can be identified on the early frames of the angiogram.

Fibrovascular PEDs present as irregular elevation of RPE, which is associated with stippled leakage into an overlying neurosensory RD in the early and late frames of the angiograms. Fibrovascular PEDs can be differentiated from serous PEDs, which show more rapid homogeneous filling of the lesion in the early frames without leakage in the late frames of the angiogram. Serous PEDs typically show smooth and sharp hyperfluorescent contours.

Stereoscopic fluorescein angiography is indicated to determine the extent, type, size, and location of CNV. ICG is useful when assessing patients with macular hemorrhage or suspected of having retinal angiomatous proliferative

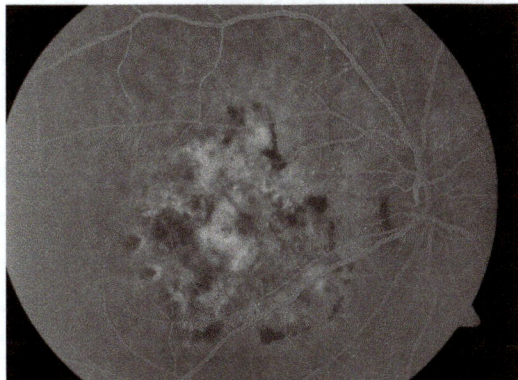

Fig. 5: FFA of wet AMD with disciform scar with subretinal bleed.

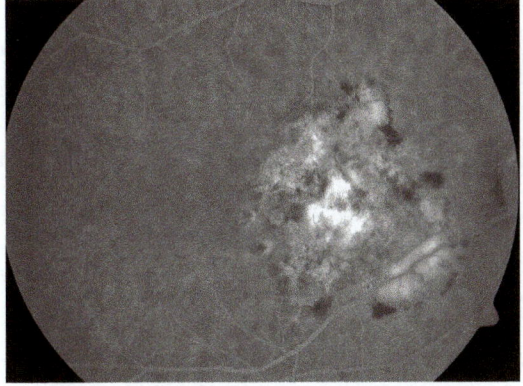

Fig. 6: Late phase FFA of wet AMD of Figure 5, confirms the presence of leakage.

lesions, idiopathic polypoidal choroidopathy, or nonvascularized versus vascularized PEDs.

- *OCT:* High-resolution OCT, such as spectral domain OCT, is mandatory for diagnosis and monitoring response to therapy **(Fig. 7)**. With enhanced depth imaging OCT (EDI OCT) and swept-source OCT choroidal evaluation have opened up new windows as has OCT angiography. The CNVM can be charted out and the response to therapy measured. On OCTA, various types of CNVMS have been seen Sea fan-like, spider-like, medusa head pattern, poorly defined, etc. For different findings see **Table 2 and Figures 8 and 9**.

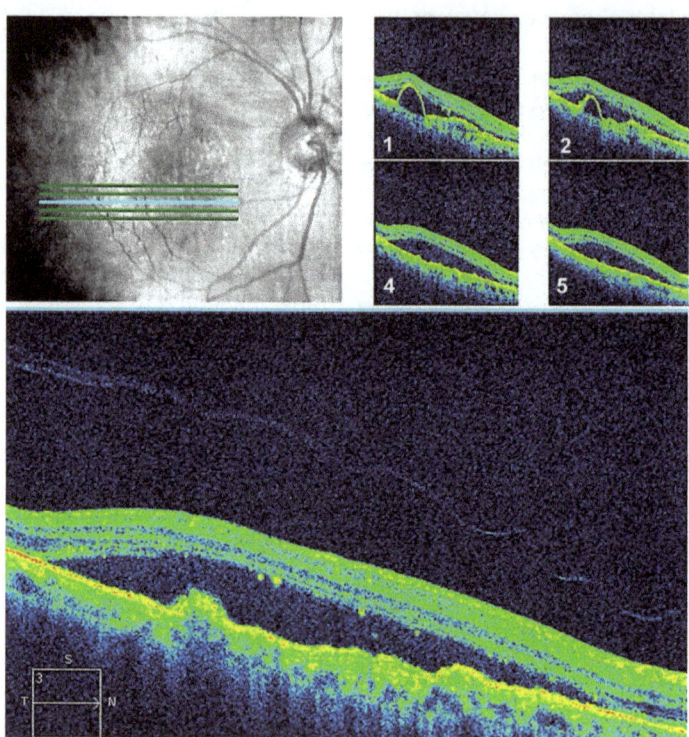

Fig. 7: OCT collage of a patient with PED, CNVM complex, and subretinal fluid. (CNVM: choroidal neovascularization membrane; OCT: optical coherence tomography; PED: pigment epithelial detachment)

Table 2: OCT in ARMD.

Clinical condition	OCT findings
Classic CNV	Classic CNV presents on OCT as a fusiform thickening and disruption of the RPE-BM-CC complex. Some CNV is anterior to it but in contact with it
Occult CNV	Occult is characterized by a focal, irregular poorly defined enhanced reflectivity anterior to choroid. Hyperreflectivity extends from above to below the RPE with no separation line
CME	On OCT images is seen as hyporeflective, dark spaces within retinal tissue
RPE detachments	Highly reflective tissue beneath the dome of the RPE detachment (OCT shows the separation of the RPE from the Bruch membrane by an optically empty area. CNV may be indicated by a notch between the main elevation and a second small mound)

Contd...

Contd...

Clinical condition	OCT findings
Double RPE detachments	Separated by notch rest similar to RPE detachments
Fibrovascular PED	Less uniform than a serous PED; both fluid and fibrous proliferation are shown, the latter as irregular scattered reflections
Drusenoid PED	OCT shows homogeneous hyper-reflectivity within the PED, in contrast to optically empty serous PED. There is commonly no subretinal fluid
RPE tears	Loss of the normal dome shape of the RPE layer in the PED, with hyper-reflectivity of the folded RPE
PCV	Cup-shaped RPE elevations and choroidal angiomatous lesions. Hemorrhagic and serous detachments of the retina and the RPE also can be seen
RAP	Initial signs that correspond to stage 1 (intraretinal vascularization) consist of a focal area, usually extrafoveal, with increased retinal reflectivity that is not associated with epiretinal, intraretinal, or subretinal changes or changes in the retinal thickness. When RAP reaches the subretinal space and merges with the RPE, a serous detachment of the RPE usually develops (stage 2 or CNV). In well-developed cases, there may be retinal choroidal anastomoses (stage 3 or CNV)
Drusen	• RPE excrescences overlying reflective material consistent with drusen • Saw-toothed configuration or bunching of the RPE • Discrete nodular drusen which actually disrupts as opposed to distorting the RPE
Outer retinal tubulations	Roundish hyporeflective spaces, often around the margin of GA
Outer retinal corrugations	Basal laminar deposit Basal linear deposit

(ARMD: age-related macular degeneration; CME: cystoid macular edema; CNV: choroidal neovascularization; OCT: optical coherence tomography; PED: pigment epithelial detachment; RPE: retinal pigment epithelium)

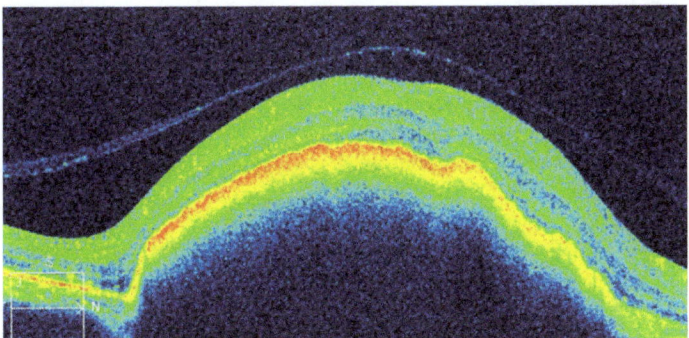

Fig. 8: OCT of a large PED. Note the notches in the PED. (OCT: optical coherence tomography; PED: pigment epithelial detachment)

- *Amsler grid:* The Amsler grid is a useful test for detecting the early visual symptoms of exudative AMD in patients with high-risk AMD. Each box on the grid represents 1° of the visual field. Thus, the *Amsler grid tests the central 10°* of the visual field beyond fixation. The patient is asked to fixate on the central black dot and to note whether surrounding lines are wavy, missing, or obscured by scotomas (dark areas). If these findings are present, the patient should

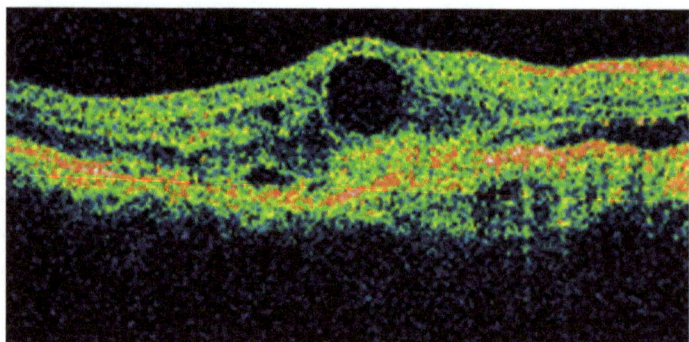

Fig. 9: A time domain OCT of a patient with disciform scar and cystoid retinal spaces.

be instructed to seek attention urgently with his or her ophthalmologist as it is likely that the cause is neovascular AMD. There are limits to Amsler grid testing which includes the cortical completion phenomenon, crowding phenomenon, and lack of forced fixation.

- *Preferential hyperacuity perimeter (PHP):* A newly developed computer-automated, three-dimensional, threshold, Amsler grid visual field test has been shown to be useful in the earlier detection of AMD. The central 14° is tested in about 5 minutes.
- *SLO microperimetry:* SLO microperimetry has found impaired rod photoreceptor function and photopic sensitivity respectively in areas of increased FAF in the junction zone, which underscores abnormalities associated with increased fundus autofluorescence.
- *Fundus autofluorescence (FAF):* FAF imaging in patients with GA is characterized by a decreased signal with sharp borders corresponding to the area of atrophy on conventional retinography.

■ CLASSIFICATION

See **Tables 3 to 5**.

Classification of CNVM

Angiographic

The terminology used to describe CNV on FA is derived from the Macular Photocoagulation Study (MPS):

- *Classic CNV* (20%) fills with dye in a well-defined "lacy" pattern during early transit subsequently leaking into the subretinal space

Table 3: Clinical classification of age-related macular degeneration (AMD).

Category	Definition, based on the presence of lesions within two-disc diameters of the fovea in either eye
No apparent aging changes	• No drusen • No AMD pigmentary abnormalities
Normal aging changes	• Only drupelets • No AMD pigmentary abnormalities
Early AMD	• Medium drusen (>63 μm but <125 μm) • No AMD pigmentary abnormalities
Intermediate AMD	• Large drusen (>125 μm) • Any AMD pigmentary abnormalities
Late AMD	Neovascular AMD and/or any geographic atrophy

Table 4: Classification of age-related macular degeneration.

Non-neovascular (DRY)	Neovascular (WET)
• Drusen • Focal hyperpigmentation • Nongeographic atrophy • Geographic atrophy	• Choroidal neovascularization • Disciform scarring

Table 5: AREDS classification.

Class	AREDS category	Features
No AMD	1	No or few small drusen (<63 μm in diameter). Represented the control group of (AREDS)
Early AMD	2	Combination of multiple small drusen, few intermediate drusen (63–124 μm in diameter), or mild RPE abnormalities
Intermediate AMD	3	Any of the following features: • Numerous intermediate drusen • At least one large druse (≥125 μm in diameter) • Geographic atrophy not involving the center of the fovea

Advanced AMD	4	One or more of the following (in the absence of other causes) in one eye:
		• Geographic atrophy of the RPE involving the foveal center.
		• Neovascular maculopathy that includes the following:
		  – CNV
		  – Serous and/or hemorrhagic detachment of the neurosensory retina or RPE
		  – Retinal hard exudates (a secondary phenomenon resulting from chronic intravascular leakage)
		  – Subretinal and sub-RPE fibrovascular proliferation
		  – Disciform scar (subretinal fibrosis)

(AREDS: age-related eye disease study; CNV: choroidal neovascularization; RPE: retinal pigment epithelium)

over 1–2 minutes, with late staining of fibrous tissue. Most CNV is subfoveal, extrafoveal being defined as ≥200 μm from the center of the FAZ on FA.
- *Occult CNV* (80%) is used to describe CNV when its limits cannot be fully defined on FA. Variants are fibrovascular PED and "late leakage of an undetermined source" (LLUS).
- *Predominantly or minimally classic* CNV is present when the classic element is greater or <50% of the total lesion respectively.

Topographic

The location of well-demarcated CNVs was broken into three categories:
1. *Extrafoveal:* CNV is 200 microns or more from the foveal center.
2. *Juxtafoveal:* CNV is between 1 micron and 199 microns from the foveal center.
3. *Subfoveal:* CNV is under the foveal center.

■ MANAGEMENT

The management guidelines have been described in **Table 6**.

Management of Dry AMD

Most vases need observation only. Prophylaxis for the prevention of complications includes the following:
- *Antioxidant supplementation:* Age-related eye disease study (AREDS), now known as AREDS1 and AREDS2 has proven the efficacy of such therapy.

Indications:
– *Extensive intermediate:* (≥63–125 μm) drusen
– At least one large (≥125 μm) drusen
– GA in one or both eyes
– Late AMD in one eye (greatest benefit in AREDS1)

AREDS1 formulation included antioxidant vitamins—500 mg of vitamin C; 400 IU of vitamin E; 15 mg of β-carotene; 80 mg of zinc oxide and 2 mg of cupric oxide. This formulation has been shown to reduce the risk of developing advanced AMD and the associated visual loss by as much as 25%, over 5 years, in individuals with moderate to high risk of ARMD (AREDS categories 3 and 4). These findings were accompanied by a 19% reduction

Table 6: Management of ARMD.[1]

Major category	Recommended treatment	Diagnoses eligible for treatment
Non-neovascular AMD	Observation	• Early AMD (AREDS category 2) • Advanced AMD with bilateral subfoveal geographic atrophy or disciform scars
	Antioxidant supplements as recommended in AREDS2 reports	• Intermediate AMD (AREDS category 3) • Advanced AMD in one eye (AREDS category 4)
Neovascular AMD	Aflibercept intravitreal injection 2.0 mg	Macular CNV
	Bevacizumab intravitreal injection 1.25 mg	Macular CNV
	Ranibizumab intravitreal injection 0.5 mg	Macular CNV
• Less commonly • Used treatments for neovascular AMD	PDT with verteporfin as recommended in the TAP and VIP reports	• Macular CNV, new or recurrent, where the classic component is >50% of the lesion and the entire lesion is ≤5,400 μm in greatest linear diameter • Occult CNV may be considered for PDT with vision <20/50 or if the CNV is <4 MPS disc areas in size when the vision is >20/50 • Juxtafoveal CNV in select cases
	Laser photocoagulation as recommended in the MPS reports	• May be considered for extrafoveal classic CNV, new or recurrent • May be considered for juxtapapillary CNV

(AMD: age-related macular degeneration; AREDS: age-relate eye disease study; CNV: choroidal neovascularization; MPS: macular photocoagulation study; PDT: photodynamic therapy; TAP: treatment of age-related macular degeneration with photodynamic therapy; VIP: verteporfin in photodynamic therapy)

in the risk of moderate vision loss (loss of three or more lines on the visual acuity chart), at 5 years.

However, high zinc doses are potentially associated with genitourinary tract problems; β-carotene can increase the incidence of lung cancer in current and former smokers. AREDS2 looked at adjusting the β-carotene and zinc components, and also whether additional or alternative supplements could enhance outcomes.[2]

Recommended daily supplementation based on AREDS2 includes:
- Vitamin E (400 IU)
- Vitamin C (500 mg)
- Lutein (10 mg)
- Zeaxanthin (2 mg)
- Zinc (25–80 mg; the lower dose may be equally effective)
- Copper (2 mg; this may not be required with the lower zinc dose).

Risk factors modification should be addressed, e.g., smoking, ocular sun protection, cardiovascular, and dietary.

An Amsler grid should be provided for home use, with advice to self-test on a regular basis, perhaps weekly, and to seek professional advice urgently in the event of any change, when imaging (e.g., OCT and FA) should be performed to rule out progression to neovascular AMD. This might be of increased importance following cataract surgery.

Provision of low vision aids for patients with significant visual loss and certification as visually impaired if available as this may facilitate access to social and financial support.

Management of Wet Age-related Macular Degeneration

Antivascular Endothelial Growth Factor

Indications of anti-VEGF include the following:
- All CNV subtypes respond to anti-VEGF therapy, but the benefit is only likely in the presence of active disease.
- Active disease includes fluid or hemorrhage, leakage on FA, an enlarging CNV membrane, or deteriorating vision judged likely to be due to CNV activity.
- An eye with almost any level of vision may benefit, although better VA at presentation is associated with a better visual outcome.

Anti-VEGF agents: See **Table 1** in the chapter on proliferative diabetic retinopathy (PDR).

Aflibercept (Eylea) is a recombinant fusion protein that binds to VEGF-A, VEGF-B, and placental growth factor (PlGF). The advantage is the maintenance regimen consists of one injection every 2 months in contrast to the monthly injections recommended with ranibizumab and bevacizumab. In addition, it is more efficacious than Lucentis due to its increased affinity to bind the receptors. The standard dose is 2 mg in 0.05 mL; an induction course of three injections is given at monthly intervals.

Ranibizumab (Lucentis): Ranibizumab is a humanized monoclonal antibody fragment developed specifically for use in the eye, though is derived from the same parent mouse antibody as bevacizumab (see next). It nonselectively binds and inhibits all isoforms of VEGF-A. The usual dose is 0.5 mg in 0.05 mL.

Bevacizumab (Avastin): In contrast to ranibizumab, bevacizumab is a complete antibody originally developed to target blood vessel growth in metastatic cancer deposits. Its use for AMD and other indications is "off label"; it is very much cheaper than ranibizumab and aflibercept. Clinical trials suggest comparable results to ranibizumab in efficacy and safety. The dose of bevacizumab is usually 1.25 mg/0.05 mL.

Pegaptanib (Macugen): Pegaptanib sodium was the first anti-VEGF agent approved by regulatory authorities for ocular treatment; the results are similar to outcomes with PDT, and its use is now extremely limited.

Photodynamic Therapy

Photodynamic therapy (PDT) is useful for eyes with subfoveal CNV **(Table 6)**. Verteporfin is a light-activated compound preferentially taken up by dividing cells including neovascular tissue. It binds to LDL receptors and upon reaction to light produces singlet oxygen residues. It is infused intravenously followed by the delivery of laser light of a wavelength of 689 nm to the CNV lesion as a single spot with a diameter 1,000 μm larger than the greatest linear diameter of the lesion. When activated by a diode laser it causes thrombosis.

Laser

Thermal argon or diode laser ablation of CNV is now rarely used, though may still be suitable for the treatment of small classic extrafoveal membranes well away from the macular center, and possibly some cases of PCV and RAP.[1]

Other Therapies

Various treatment modalities have been tried with variable success. These are transpupillary thermotherapy (TTT), teletherapy (EBRT), brachytherapy (Plaque Radiotherapy), anecortave acetate (an angiostatic steroid), small interfering RNA (siRNA), vatalanib (inhibitor of all known VEGF receptor tyrosine kinases), squalamine lactate (an antiangiogenic amino sterol derived from cartilage of the dogfish shark, action includes blockade of cell membrane ion transporters that regulate cell function by controlling pH and metabolism. Sphingomab (monoclonal antibody targeted against sphingosine-1-phosphate, which has been implicated in angiogenesis, scar formation, and inflammation), volociximab (a chimeric monoclonal antibody that inhibits the functional activity of α5ß1 integrin, a protein found on activated endothelial cells, and prevent angiogenesis), designed ankyrin repeat proteins (DARPins) (genetically engineered antibody mimetic proteins that are a potent VEGF inhibitor), sirolimus (rapamycin), infliximab (a monoclonal antibody that binds and neutralizes tumor necrosis factor-alpha), eculizumab (complement inhibitors), Pigment epithelial-derived growth factor (PEDF), brimonidine, antioxidant eye drops, alprostadil (choroidal blood perfusion enhancers), maculoplasty (overall tissue engineering attempt to reestablish the normal subretinal anatomy), Macular translocation (moving the neurosensory retina of the fovea in one eye with recent-onset subfoveal CNV to a new location before the occurrence of permanent retinal damage, may allow it to recover or to maintain its visual function over a healthier bed of RPE-Bruch's membrane-choriocapillaris complex), gene therapy, stem cells.

Management of Poor Vision

Low vision aid refers to an optical device that improves or enhances residual vision by magnifying the image of the object at the retinal level. Nonoptical aids also work as LVAs as they may help in enhancing visual performance.[3]

VIVA QUESTIONS

Q.1. What is the rate of progression of CNV?
Ans.
- Progress rapidly irrespective of its initial location and extent at a mean rate of 18 μm/day.
- Disciform scars with fibrous tissue or geographic atrophy represent the end stages of both types of CNV.

Q.2. What is drusen?
Ans. *Drusen* (singular: druse) are extracellular deposits located at the interface between the RPE and Bruch membrane. The material of which they are composed has a broad range of constituents and is thought to be derived from immune-mediated and metabolic processes in the RPE. Their precise role in the pathogenesis of AMD is unclear but is positively associated with size. The earliest pathological changes are the appearance of basal laminar deposits (BlamD) and basal linear deposits (BlinD). BlamD consists of membrano-granular material and foci of wide-spaced collagen between the plasma membrane and basal lamina of the RPE. BlinD consists of vesicular material located in the inner collagenous zone of Bruch's membrane.

Q.3. Discuss the high-risk characteristics of drusen for development of CNV.
Ans. High-risk characteristics of drusen for the development of CNV include: soft type, large size, greater than five in number, confluent, and presence of RPE stippling.

Q.4. Discuss the high-risk characteristics for development of CNV.
Ans. Systemic risk factors associated with CNV include increased age, Caucasian race, and smoking. Ocular risk factors associated with increased risk of CNV include large drusen, confluent drusen, hyperpigmentation, and hypertension.

Q.5. What is the median rate of enlargement of GA?
Ans. GA continues to enlarge over time with a median rate of enlargement over 2 years of 1.8 MPS disc areas. The prevalence of GA increases with age, being half as common as CNV at age 75, and more common than CNV in older age groups. GA is bilateral in more than half of the people with this condition.

Q.6. What is bionic eye/Argus II?
Ans. Designed for patients who are blind due to diseases, such as retinitis pigmentosa and AMD. Relies on the patient having a healthy optic nerve and a developed visual cortex. The prosthesis consists of—a digital camera built into a pair of glasses—a video processing microchip built into a handheld unit—a radio transmitter on the glasses—a receiver implanted above the ear—a retinal implant with electrodes on a chip behind the retina. The camera captures an image Send the image to a microchip converts the image to electrical impulses of light and dark pixels—Send the image to a radiotansmitter—it transmits pulses wirelessly to the receiver and sends impulses to the retinal implant by a hair-thin implanted wire—The stimulated electrodes generate electrical signals that travel to the visual cortex.[1]

Q.7. What is an implantable miniature telescope?
Ans. An implantable miniature telescope is implanted into one eye only (typically the nondominant or poorer-seeing eye).

It generates a 20–24° field of vision. The FDA approved the implantable miniature telescope (IMT) in 2010 for patients 75 years and older with stable severe-to-profound vision impairment (20/160 to 20/800) caused by bilateral end-stage AMD.

Q.8. Name some low vision aids.

Ans. *Optical devices:* Hand-held telescopes, mounted telescopes, intraocular LVA (IO-LVA) NEAR, spectacles—prismatic ½ eyes—bifocals, magnifiers.
Absorptive lenses: Tinted lenses, photochromatic lenses, polarization glasses, filters—corning CPF, younger PLS—visual field enhancement devices, Fresnel Prisms, Gottlieb field expanders, reverse telescopes, hemianopic mirrors.
Nonoptical: Lighting, contrast enhancement, increasing size of object, auditory aids.
Electronic magnifiers: CCTV, large print computers.
Orientation and mobility LVA: Canes, guide dogs, electronic orientation devices, GPS
Newer technology LVA: E-readers, smartphones, tablets.

■ REFERENCES

1. American Academy of Ophthalmology. Preferred Practice Pattern® Guidelines. [online] Available from https://www.aao.org/education/about-preferred-practice-patterns [Last accessed February, 2024].
2. Age-Related Eye Disease Study Research Group. A randomized, placebo-controlled, clinical trial of high-dose supplementation with vitamins C and E, beta carotene, and zinc for age-related macular degeneration and vision loss: AREDS report No. 8. Arch Ophthalmol. 2001;119(10):1417-36.
3. Maniglia M, Cottereau BR, Soler V, Trotter Y. Rehabilitation Approaches in Macular Degeneration Patients. Front Syst Neurosci. 2016;10:107.

INTERMEDIATE UVEITIS

Raghav Ravani, Karthikeya R, Harathy Selvan, Atul Kumar

■ INTRODUCTION

As per its anatomical definition, intermediate uveitis (IU) is defined as an inflammation involving the anterior vitreous (hyalitis), ciliary body (posterior part of ciliary body), and peripheral retina.[1]

■ NOMENCLATURE

Various names were used to describe the condition including chronic cyclitis, vitritis, cyclochorioretinitis, pars planitis, intermediate uveitis, peripheral uveoretinitis, etc.[1] Recently, as per the SUN (Standardization of Uveitis Nomenclature, IUSG*) working group's guidelines,[2] IU refers to the subset of uveitis wherein the major site of inflammation is vitreous and there is an associated infection or systemic disease. The term pars planitis refers to the "idiopathic" subset of intermediate uveitis occurring in the absence of any associated infection or systemic disease.

Pars planitis forms the majority subset of intermediate uveitis, as high as 70–80%.

Also, note that the involvement of vessels in the form of peripheral vascular sheathing and cystoid macular edema (CME) does not change the nomenclature or classification.

Intermediate uveitis is usually given as a long case or a short case in the exams.

■ HISTORY

Chief Complaints

The condition may have minimal symptoms. Unlike anterior uveitis, the symptoms are bilateral more than unilateral, and often asymmetrical. Also, the disease may present with its complications, such as CME, vitreous membranes, glaucoma, and cataract. The usual presenting complaints are:
- *Floaters:* The most common (due to snowballs, membranes, vitreous opacification)
- Blurring of vision (chronic, painless—due to CME, cataract)

*International Uveitis Study Group
- Loss of vision (sudden, painless due to glaucoma, spillover uveitis, secondary RRD)—rarely
- Noted during routine fundus evaluation.

History of Present Illness

- Intermediate uveitis tends to affect young individuals with a bimodal distribution, i.e., affecting two age groups, 5-15 years and 20-40 years, equally affecting males and females. Some reports from India put it as the most common subtype of uveitis in children, whereas others report it as the least common.
- Unlike anterior uveitis, it has an insidious onset.
- The most common presenting symptoms are floaters.
- Associated pain, redness, and watering are usually absent or may be present in children with associated anterior uveitis. These are usually minimal when present and often seen as spillover anterior uveitis.
- The patient may have a history of similar episodes in the past with remissions or may have a chronic history without remissions.
- Patients may complain of chronic worsening of vision or a sudden worsening of vision in a background of long-standing history.

History of Past Illness

Past medical and surgical history must include careful history to rule out the systemic associations or etiological causes of intermediate uveitis. There may be a past history of associations of intermediate uveitis as well (i.e., sarcoidosis, TB, multiple sclerosis, etc.) Even in the absence of symptoms, leading questions must be asked for commonly associated disorders as IU may be the primary presentation **(Flowchart 1)**.

Family History

Intermediate uveitis though not hereditary has been seen reported in families. It is associated with HLA DR-15 and HLA DR-51 alleles. IU is seen in families with common HLA haplotypes. Also, note that HLA DR-15 is associated with multiple sclerosis and thus may suggest a predisposition of it in patients with IU with HLA DR-15 positivity.

■ EXAMINATION

General Examination

Detailed systemic examination is warranted to know any associated conditions like sarcoidosis, TB, multiple sclerosis, signs of tick bite, or Lyme disease. The following conditions are associated with IU **(Flowchart 1)**.

Ocular Examination

Visual acuity: The visual acuity is usually normal in early cases. The patient may have vision acuity of 6/6 with floaters being the only complaint. The main cause of decreased visual acuity in IU is the development of cystoid macular edema (CME). Other causes of dimness of vision include the development of cataract, dense vitreous membranes/opacities, epiretinal membrane (ERM), VH from neovascularization, and tractional or RRD.

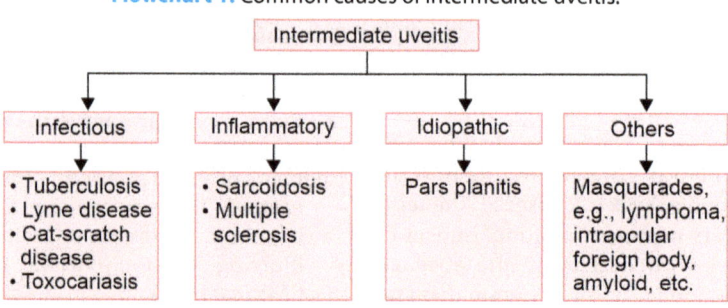

Flowchart 1: Common causes of intermediate uveitis.

Table 1: Grading of anterior chamber cells as per standardization of uveitis nomenclature (SUN) workshop (2004) consensus.	
The cells are counted in a dark background of an undilated pupil in a slit of 1 mm × 1 mm	
Grade	Number of cells/field
0	<1 cells
0.5+	1–5 cells
1+	6–15
2+	16–25
3+	26–50
4+	>50

Table 2: National Eye Institute grading of vitreous haze as adapted by the standardization of uveitis nomenclature (SUN) working group.	
Grade	Description
4+	The optic nerve head is not visualized
3+	Optic nerve head hazily visualized
2+	Retinal vessels are visualized better. Optic nerve head hazy
1+	Vitreous cells and haze are present but the optic nerve head and retinal vessels clearly visualized
0.5+	Some media haze is present, and nerve fiber layer striations are not able to be visualized. But disc and retinal vessels are seen distinctly
0	No inflammation, normal fundus view

Eyeball: Squint may be present but is a consequence of complications of disease due to loss of fusion.

Lid/conjunctiva/cornea/sclera are usually within normal limits (WNL). There may be aponeurotic ptosis or in rare cases enophthalmos as a side effect of previous treatment in the form of periocular steroid injections. Scleritis may be present; the disease is then called sclerouveitis. Keratic precipitates (KPs) may be present; in fact, IU is characterized by KPs that may be central rather than the typically inferior Arlt's triangle KPs of anterior uveitis.

Anterior chamber: It may show a variable number of spill-over anterior chamber cells/flair. These should be carefully documented as per SUN classification **(Table 1)**.

Pupil: Pupil is circular as there is no or minimal anterior chamber reaction, and usually no synechiae. Pupillary reflexes are usually within normal limits unless complicated by retinal detachment, which is rare.

IOP: A rise in IOP may occur, especially as a complication in IU due to steroid use or secondary glaucoma. A rise in IOP in uveitis is also associated with increasing age, duration since diagnosis, and active inflammation. IOP may be low in case of severe reaction and formation of cyclitic membrane.

Lens: Cataract may occur in 50–60% of cases and is one of the causes of decreased vision in IU. A posterior subcapsular cataract is the most common cataract associated, however, even anterior subcapsular cataract may be found. Cataract in IU may be due to chronic inflammation or long-term steroid treatment or glaucoma medications (especially cholinergic agents) used in the treatment of uveitis and uveitic glaucoma. Retrolental space should be carefully examined for cells, which is pathognomic for present/past anterior vitreous inflammation. However, the presence of these cells does not indicate active disease. Vitreous haze should be noted and graded **(Table 2)**. Increasing vitreous haze is a sign of activity and decreasing vitreous haze is a sign of response.

Vitreous: Vitreous is the major site of inflammation in intermediate uveitis. Thus inflammatory cells mainly accumulate in the vitreous cavity in the form of retrolental cells, and vitreous membranes, which may condense as "snow-balls" or may settle down inferiorly over the retina or pars plana as "snow-banking" leading to variable degrees of vitreous haze. 'Snowballs' appear as yellow-white condensations in midvitreous, especially inferiorly.

"Snow-banking" depicts more severe inflammation. "Snow-banking" appears like exudates over the pars plana, especially inferiorly, but may be seen all around. Scleral indentation or use of a Goldmann three-mirror contact lens may be required to view the peripheral retina and pars plana. Sometimes vitreous haze may be severe enough to obscure the view of the fundus preventing further examination. Early PVD may be seen.

Fundus: If media clarity permits, examination of the retina must be done carefully in all cases of intermediate uveitis. The fundus findings include:
- Tortuosity of vessels
- Involvement of peripheral retinal vasculature in the form of sheathing (e.g., periphlebitis)
- Neovascularization, which is usually peripheral near the area of snow-banking
- Peripheral vitreous traction and hole formation due to contraction of inflammatory membranes may be seen
- Retinal detachment has also been reported as a complication of intermediate uveitis
- Peripheral choroiditis may also be seen, though severe choroidal involvement indicates a review of clinical diagnosis.

DIFFERENTIAL DIAGNOSIS

- Vitreous membranes
- Vitreous degeneration
- Leukemia
- Lymphoma
- Endophthalmitis
- Panuveitis
- Amyloidosis
- Old VH

INVESTIGATION

Systemic Evaluation

As previously mentioned, many infections and systemic conditions are associated with intermediate uveitis (IU). A careful history, ocular examination, and ancillary/laboratory tests should be carried out to search for the etiology or associated condition. The test may include:
- Complete blood count with differential count and ESR
- Purified protein derivative skin test (PPD) (Mantoux test)
- Chest X-ray (to look for evidence of pulmonary TB or sarcoidosis)
- Serum angiotensin-converting enzyme levels
- Gallium scan
- MRI brain
- Lyme titers and western blot—if high suspicion and in endemic areas.

The list is very large and should be based on a tailored work-up **(Flowchart 1)**. In the Indian subcontinent, TB should be ruled out in all cases. Masquerades should be considered whenever applicable.

Ocular Investigation

- *Ultrasonography (USG) B-scan:* To be done to rule out complications like retinal detachment in cases where intense inflammation leads to severe media haze preventing fundus evaluation. It may also help to rule out conditions masquerading as intermediate uveitis like intraocular tumors.
- *Ultrasound biomicroscopy (UBM):* To demonstrate pars plana exudates when clinical examination is difficult in the presence of media opacities.
- *OCT:* To document the presence of cystoid macular edema, especially in patients with complaints of the dimness of central vision **(Fig. 1)**. It can be used as a guide to therapy.

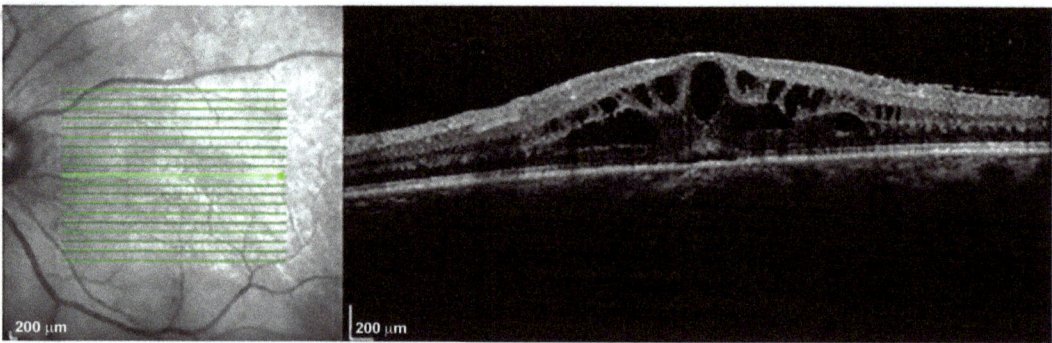

Fig. 1: OCT image depicting cystoids macular edema.

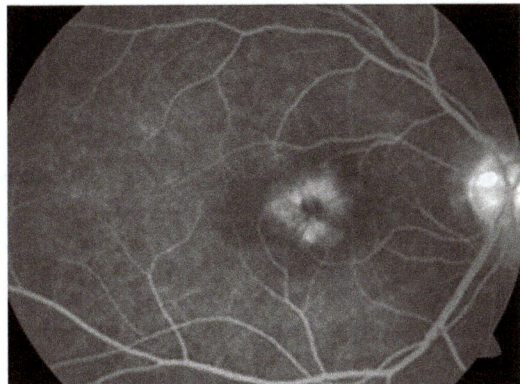

Fig. 2: FA image showing macular leakage of dye in CME.
Note: The petaloid configuration.

Choroidal thickness should also be monitored once treating concomitant choroiditis. Later on, epiretinal membranes (ERMs) and tractional changes can also be seen in studying the virtual reality (VR) interface.
- *Fluorescein angiogram* shows the presence of peripheral capillary nonperfusion, peripheral neovascularization, presence of retinal vasculitis and petaloid **(Fig. 2)** and honeycomb leakage suggestive of cystoid macular edema (CME). Fluorescein angiography may also be helpful for follow-up after cryotherapy or laser photocoagulation treatment.
- *Ultrawide imaging* helps in documenting peripheral changes. Ultrawide-field fluorescein angiography may also help in documenting peripheral CNP areas and the presence of peripheral neovascularization.

■ COMPLICATIONS

- Cataract
- Glaucoma
- Cystoid macular edema
- Epiretinal membrane
- VH
- Retinal detachment
- Rarely, optic disc edema

■ MANAGEMENT

If an etiology has been identified on investigation, treatment depends on the cause. In cases where no specific etiology has been identified, the following are the management options. Mild cases without CME may be managed conservatively by observation. A four-step approach for the treatment of intermediate uveitis was proposed by Kaplan.[3] It should be remembered that every case may not need treatment. In the absence of media haze (<grade 1), in cases with only a few inferior snowballs and the presence of complications like CME, just meticulous frequent observations may suffice.

The following are the management options:
- *Step 1:* Infections should always be ruled out if planning for steroids. Periocular steroids may be considered as an initial treatment modality, especially in uniocular conditions. Subtenon injection is the most common route for depot corticosteroids. Another route for local therapy includes intravitreal corticosteroid injection. In case of failure of depot steroids and bilateral cases, systemic corticosteroids could be considered. In cases with CME, periocular steroids help by maintaining a constant influx of steroids. The presence of CME should indicate an alerting sign warranting aggressive therapy as it may lead to permanent visual loss. Throughout therapy, patients should be monitored for ocular and systemic side effects of steroids, which can be debilitating at times. Dietary supplementation for calcium should also be considered.

  A more recent advancement is the use of sustained-release steroid implants, such as Ozurdex and Retisert. These have now been approved for ocular use in noninfectious uveitis. They work well in isolated ocular disease, but complications should be monitored. The recently conducted multicenter uveitis steroid treatment (MUST) study has shown good results with fluocinolone implants when compared to systemic therapy.
- *Step 2:* Peripheral retinal ablation over a snow bank near the pars plana region may be considered in case of nonresponse to peribulbar steroids. This may be done either using cryopexy (double-freeze thaw technique) or peripheral scatter photocoagulation, especially in cases with peripheral neovascularization. This may help

decrease the risk of bleeding and regression of neovascularization. Recent studies indicate the primary role of cryotherapy as a first measure also. However, this treatment may lead to a temporary worsening of the disease as well.
- *Step 3:* Pars plana vitrectomy with induction of PVD and peripheral laser is helpful in cases resistant to previous modalities and in whom immunosuppressive therapy may be contraindicated. This is particularly helpful in cases with decreased vision due to severe media haze with vitreous membrane, in cases with VH, in cases with nonresponding CME, or in cases complicated with retinal detachment/ERMs.
- *Step 4:* Systemic immunomodulatory therapy is of special benefit in bilateral disease. Chronic or frequently relapsing cases may benefit due to lesser steroid dependence. Further, voclosporin [Lux Uveitis Multicenter Investigation of a New Approach to Treatment (LUMINATE study)] is showing promise as a steroid-sparing agent.

Note: The treatment plan may not necessarily follow the step-wise approach and a combination of one or more modalities may be considered as per individual cases to achieve early remission or decrease the duration of corticosteroids.

VIVA QUESTIONS

Q.1. What is the most common presenting symptom in the case of intermediate uveitis?
Ans. The patients most commonly present with symptoms of floaters in the case of intermediate uveitis.

Q.2. What are the causes of vision loss in the case of intermediate uveitis?
Ans. Cystoid macular edema (CME) is the most common cause of dimness of vision. Other causes include:
- *Cataract:* Especially posterior subcapsular cataract
- *Epiretinal membrane:* This may lead to distortion of vision and if severe, dimness of vision.
- Media haze due to intense vitritis leading to vitreous veils/membranes.
- *VH:* Secondary to peripheral neovascularization.
- *Retinal detachment:* Tractional or RRD.

Q.3. What are the other causes of ocular inflammation with "white" eye?
Ans. Apart from intermediate uveitis, other causes include:
- Fuchs heterochromic iridocyclitis
- Juvenile rheumatoid arthritis
- Posner–Schlossman syndrome
- Kawasaki disease

Q.4. What are the causes of intermediate uveitis?
Ans.
- *Infectious conditions:*
    - TB (*Mycobacterium tuberculosis*) (especially in endemic countries like India)
    - Syphilis (*Treponema pallidum*)
    - Toxoplasmosis (*Toxoplasma gondii*)
    - Toxocariasis (*Toxocara canis*)
    - Lyme's disease (*Borrelia burgdorferi*) (in endemic areas)
    - Cat-scratch diseases (*Bartonella henselae* and *Bartonella quintana*)
    - Human T-lymphotropic virus type 1 (HTLV-1)
- *Noninfectious conditions:*
    - Sarcoidosis
    - Multiple sclerosis
    - Intraocular lymphoma
- Idiopathic/pars planitis

Q.5. Describe Kaplan's four step management for intermediate uveitis.
Ans. It is as described above in the text.

Q.6. Discuss the differential diagnoses of IU.
Ans. *Causes of media haze:* Old vitreous haze (VH), ocular lymphoma, amyloidosis, endophthalmitis, *Candida* infections, *Propionibacterium acnes* endophthalmitis, leukemia, acute retinal necrosis (ARN), and intense vitritis due to other causes such as toxoplasmosis.

Q.7. Discuss steroid implants.
Ans. *See* the above and a chapter on DME.

Q.8. What are the side effects of steroids?

Ans. *Ocular side effects:* Cataract, glaucoma, activation of viral keratitis (topical), fungal corneal ulcer, central serous chorioretinopathy.

Systemic side effects: Cushingoid state, diabetes, hypertension, osteoporosis, peptic ulcer disease, sodium, and water retention, worsening of psychosis, menstrual irregularities, weight gain, thromboembolism, muscle weakness, aseptic necrosis of femoral head, pancreatitis, easy bruisability, convulsions, etc.

REFERENCES

1. Vitale AT, Zierhut M, Foster CS. Intermediate uveitis. In: Foster CS, Vitale AT (Eds). Diagnosis and treatment of uveitis. Philadelphia: WB Saunders and Company; 2002. pp. 844-57.
2. Jabs DA, Nusenblatt RB, Rosenbaum JT; Standardization of Uveitis Nomenclature (SUN) Working Group. Standardization of uveitis nomenclature for reporting clinical data. Results of the First International Workshop. Am J Ophthalmol. 2005;140(3):509-16.
3. Kaplan HJ. Intermediate uveitis (pars planitis, chronic cyclitis): a four-step approach to treatment. In: Saari KM (Ed). Uveitis Update. Amsterdam: Experta Medica; 1984. pp. 169-72.

CHOROIDAL MELANOMA

Karthikeya R, Raghav Ravani, Prateek Kakkar, Atul Kumar

INTRODUCTION

Uveal melanoma is a rare form of melanoma accounting for <3% of the primary malignant melanomas in the body. This includes anterior uveal melanoma (which includes iris melanoma) and posterior uveal melanomas (which include ciliary body melanoma and choroidal melanoma). In this chapter, we will focus only on choroidal melanoma. Choroidal melanoma is the most common uveal melanoma (90%) and also the most common primary intraocular tumor in an adult. It has an incidence of about 5 cases per million population per year in the West. Like other melanomas, it is much less commonly seen in India as compared to the West. In the West, it is seen 150 times more frequently in Caucasians as compared to the blacks.

HISTORY

The presenting clinical features of a case of choroidal melanoma are highly variable.[1,2]

Chief Complaints

Patients with choroidal melanoma are usually picked up incidentally. Symptoms are often absent, with the tumor detected by chance on routine fundus examination. When symptoms do occur, they can be variable depending on the tumor characteristics such as location, size, proximity to the macula, proximity to the optic nerve, and presence or absence of overlying retinal changes. Anteriorly located masses present later and are usually larger in size and more advanced at the time of diagnosis while posteriorly located tumors present early due to visual symptoms. Gradual painless diminution of vision is the most common presentation and is usually due to the presence of an exudative retinal detachment or a cystoid macular edema. An intelligent patient can also report a scotoma or a field loss. Subfoveal growth can cause a central scotoma or can cause a refractive error. Very rarely, patients may present with severe eye pain due to involvement of the posterior ciliary nerves or sudden onset of loss of vision due to VH subsequent to the tumor involving a large retinal or choroidal vessel. Photopsias can occur due to the subretinal location of the tumor. Presentation with loss of weight and appetite, bony pain, and headache may suggest an advanced disease with metastasis.

History of Present Illness

Choroidal melanoma usually presents in patients over 60 years of age in the West. However, in the Asian population, it is noted to occur early at around 45 years. Males are affected slightly more frequently than females. Note the duration and progression of symptoms. Rapidly changing symptoms in a patient with exudative RD may be a uveitic entity. Eliciting a history of pain, redness, and photophobia is also important for the same reason. Symptoms in the contralateral eye are also less likely to occur—choroidal melanoma is only rarely multicentric and extremely rarely bilateral.

History of Past Illness

History of previous medical and surgical illnesses is important to document and rule out other differentials of a choroidal mass or exudative RD such as tuberculoma, hypertension, metastases, Vogt–Koyanagi and Harada's disease, and other posterior uveitic entities. History of mass lesion anywhere else in the body should be specifically sought for to rule out a metastases to the eye of a primary elsewhere or a metastases of the choroidal melanoma. Choroidal melanoma is rarely inherited or familial—it is a sporadic malignancy. Relevant systemic history should be elicited when deciding on other differential diagnoses **(Table 1)**.

■ EXAMINATION

General Examination

Should include an examination of the general condition of the patient—to look for pallor, icterus, lymphadenopathy, cachexia, other palpable masses in the neck or abdomen, pathological fractures, etc. which may indicate distant metastases. In the skin examination, look for nevi, atypical nevi, cutaneous melanocytosis, and freckles—all of which are risk factors for the development of uveal melanoma.

Ocular Examination

- *Visual acuity:* As discussed above, visual acuity may be decreased in certain presentations of melanoma.
- *Eyeball and lids:* Look for proptosis, chemosis, and restriction of movements—all of which suggest an extraocular extension of the melanoma.
- *Conjunctiva:* A sentinel vessel might be observed in cases of ciliary body melanoma or an anteriorly located choroidal melanoma. It is a dilated tortuous anterior ciliary artery in the quadrant of the tumor which supplies the tumor of its blood supply.
- *Cornea:* Corneal edema may be present if there is a co-existing glaucoma.
- *Sclera:* Nevus of Ota (oculocutaneous melanocytosis) is a risk factor for choroidal melanoma. It presents as unilateral slate-gray pigmentation of the sclera, uvea, orbit, periocular skin, meninges, etc. Also, look for any scleral thinning/uveal show which may indicate a scleral extension of the tumor.
- *Iris/Pupil:* Iris nevus is a risk factor for uveal melanoma (Iris melanoma > choroidal melanoma). Choroidal melanoma with extension into the ciliary body or primary ciliary body melanoma causes a variety of abnormalities in the angle and anterior chamber—irregular anterior chamber depth, localized peripheral anterior synechiae, etc. Rarely choroidal melanoma with extensive exudative RD can cause NVG. Also, note iris color—light iris is a risk factor for choroidal melanoma.
- *IOP:* Choroidal melanoma can cause NVG. Ciliary body extension can cause glaucoma by destruction/infiltration of the trabecular meshwork.
- *Lens:* Localized cataract can occur in anteriorly placed tumors which impinge upon the lens or tumors with ciliary body extension.
- *Vitreous:* Look for cellular infiltration of the anterior vitreous—if present indicate an inflammatory pathology.
- *Fundus:* A distant direct ophthalmoscopy examination may reveal a dark shadow in the area of the mass, a ciliary body mass on the other hand may obliterate the red reflex together. Choroidal melanomas are usually seen as dome-shaped masses smoothly arising from the underlying choroid varying in size from <3 mm to large tumors over 15 mm in base diameter. The height of the tumor is more important as a differentiating feature from benign nevus **(Tables 2 and 3)**. When they break through the Bruch's membrane they take the classically described collar-stud appearance or mushroom appearance. They can arise anywhere in the fundus either de-novo or from a pre-existing choroidal

Table 1: Differentiating choroidal melanoma from other mass-like choroidal pathologies.

Character-istic	Choroidal melanoma	Choroidal nevus	Choroidal metastasis	Circumscribed choroidal hemangioma	Choroidal osteoma	Congenital hypertrophy of RPE	Optic disc melanocytoma	Posterior scleritis
Age/Sex	5th decade and above	Adolescence	Elderly	30–50 years	10–30 years, 90% female	Congenital	30–40 years	30–50 years, female
Laterality	Unilateral	Unilateral	20% bilateral	Unilateral	20% bilateral	Mostly unilateral	Unilateral	Unilateral
Location	Posterior pole or periphery	Posterior to equator	Posterior pole	Within 2DD from ONH	Juxtapapillary/circumpapillary	Peripheral	ONH	Peripheral/posterior pole
Symptoms	Occasional visual loss	Asymptomatic	Occasional visual loss	Occasional visual loss	Occasional visual loss	Asymptomatic	Enlarged blind spot	Pain
Clinical appearance	• Amelanotic or darkly pigmented • Dome/mushroom-shaped • Shifting SRF + • Overlying orange pigment	• Amelanotic to darkly pigmented, flat, <5 DD, • Overlying drusen (50–80%), • Rare: Orange pigment/SRF/CNV	• Amelanotic or pale • Broad-based with variable thickness • Overlying RPE changes • Often extensive SRF	Orange-red, <5 DD, RPE changes, and SRF +	Yellow-white to orange, well-demarcated, pseudopod margins, RPE changes, vascular spider, occasional CNV	Jet black, rarely amelanotic, well-defined, flat to ovoid, overlying amelanotic lacunae	Jet black to brown, fibrillated margin, choroidal nevus can be associated	Yellowish or the same color as adjacent RPE, concentric choroidal folds

Contd...

Contd...

Character-istic	Choroidal melanoma	Choroidal nevus	Choroidal metastasis	Circumscribed choroidal hemangioma	Choroidal osteoma	Congenital hypertrophy of RPE	Optic disc melanocytoma	Posterior scleritis
Fluorescein Angiography	Early hyperfluorescence with late leakage and stippling	Hypofluorescence unless drusen/RPE changes	Diffuse late leak	Early prearterial hyperfluorescence of large choroidal vessels, late staining/leakage	Irregular fluorescence with late staining	Hypofluorescence with hyperfluorescence of lacunae	Hypofluorescence, late ON hyperfluorescence is possible	Hyperfluorescent mottling with multiple pinpoint areas of leakage
Ultrasonography	• Low-medium reflectivity, Kappa sign • Regular internal structure • Choroidal excavation, "hollowing", subjacent shadowing	<2 mm thick variable reflectivity	• Flat/multinodular • High irregular internal reflectivity	Homogenous medium-high internal reflectivity	• High initial spike (low gain) • Acoustic shadowing	Flat	Slight elevation, irregular height reflectivity	High internal reflectivity, thickened sclera, and choroid, fluid in subtenon space (T-sign)

Table 2: Differentiating a choroidal melanoma from a choroidal nevus.

Characteristic	Choroidal nevus	Choroidal melanoma
Age	Any age, discovered on screening	Sixth or seventh decade
Symptom	More likely to be asymptomatic. But can cause vision loss due to SRF, CME, or CNVM	More likely to be symptomatic. Symptoms described above
Margins	Well defined	Poorly defined or abruptly elevated edges
Elevation	Tends to be flat (<2 mm)	>2 mm
Drusen	More likely	Less likely
Depigmented halo	Characteristic	Absent
Orange pigment	Less likely	More likely
Subretinal fluid	Less likely	More likely
Overlying RPE changes	Likely	Likely
Growth	Very slow (0.5 mm in a decade)	Rapid (Over 1–2 years)

Table 3: Showing the definitions used in COMS.

COMS	Apical height	Largest basal diameter
Small tumor	1.5–2.4 mm	5–16 mm
Medium-sized tumor	2.5–10 mm	≤16 mm
Large sized tumor	>10 mm	>16 mm
(COMS: collaborative ocular melanoma study)		

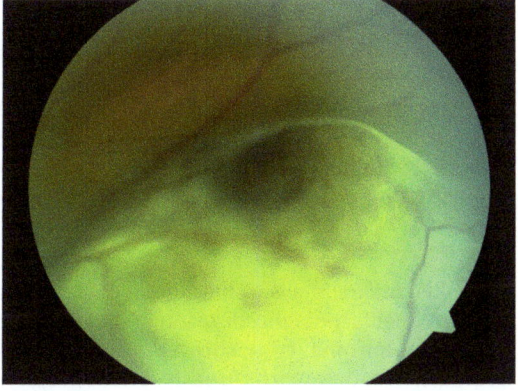

Fig. 1: A pigmented choroidal melanoma with surrounding subretinal fluid and orange pigmentation over it.

nevus. They are usually pigmented in most of the cases (about 85% of the cases) but about 15% are amelanotic—which means they do not show any melanin clinically. The color per se could vary from dark brown to tan **(Fig. 1)**. About 5% of the tumors are diffusely infiltrative without any nodular mass. About 60% of the tumors are located within 3 mm of the optic disc or fovea. They could be bilobular or multilobular and could even be multicentric.

The retinal pigment epithelium (RPE) overlying the tumor often shows stress changes such as drusen, mottling, areas of atrophy, pigment epithelial detachment, etc. owing to the deprivation of normal choroidal circulation to the RPE due to the presence of the tumor. Orange pigment on the melanoma is an important sign to differentiate it from the benign choroidal nevus and represents the accumulated melanin and lipofuscin in the RPE cells after phagocytosis of the cellular debris of the melanocytes. The overlying neurosensory retina may also show chronic degenerative changes such as cystoid spaces, schitic cavities, and CME.

Exudative RD is commonly associated with choroidal melanoma and is again an important differentiating feature from choroidal nevus **(Table 2)**. The exudative RD may be so bullous it can sometimes hide the tumor under it and appear like an RRD. Typically, the subretinal fluid is seen surrounding the mass and largely spread fluid indicates a possibility of choroidal metastasis. Associated intra and subretinal hemorrhage is

B-mode ultrasonography can help detect tumors and detail the internal characteristics in cases of exudative detachment and hazy media. It can help in measuring the size, extent, and spread and in ruling out differentials. The characteristic findings are: (1) homogenous internal structure with low to medium reflectivity; (2) choroidal excavation; (3) shadowing of the subjacent choroidal structures; (4) an acoustically empty zone at the base (acoustic hollowing). A "collar stud" appearance is highly suggestive of choroidal melanoma. It will also define the area of RD.

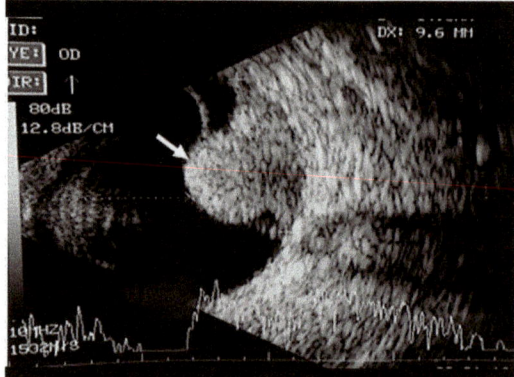

Fig. 2: Combined ultrasonography A- and B-scan showing a mushroom-shaped mass arising from the choroid with surrounding subretinal fluid and homogenous internal reflectivity. A-scan shows moderate spikes. There is acoustic hollowing toward the base of the tumor.

generally a sign of the development of CVNM in a long-standing dormant melanoma. Vitreous hemorrhage and massive subretinal hemorrhage can occur in melanoma owing to erosion of a large retinal/choroidal vessel by the tumor or due to necrosis of a part of the tumor.

■ INVESTIGATION

Choroidal melanoma is a clinical diagnosis that is aided by ancillary diagnostic testing. Collaborative ocular melanoma trial showed that clinical evaluation along with fundus photography, ultrasonography, and fluorescein angiography is 99% accurate in diagnosing choroidal melanoma.

Ultrasonography

Ultrasonography **(Fig. 2)** is the most useful investigative modality in the diagnosis of choroidal melanoma.[3] A standardized ultrasonography has a diagnostic accuracy of >95%. On A scan, Ossoinig described four cardinal acoustic hallmarks of malignant melanoma: (1) A regular internal structure with similar height of the inner tumor spikes or regular decrease in height (positive angle kappa sign); (2) low to medium reflectivity; (3) solid consistency; and (4) echographic sign of vascularization with a fast, spontaneous, continuous, flickering vertical motion of single tumor spikes.

Fluorescein Angiography

Fluorescein angiography (FA) is not diagnostic and adds limited information to the diagnosis. It helps in ruling out hemorrhagic lesions such as a ruptured retinal arterial macroaneurysm or peripheral choroidal neovascularization, which generally blocks fluorescence. Choroidal melanomas on fluorescein angiography show their intrinsic vasculature different from the overlying retinal vasculature and this is called "dual circulation". There may be early stippling and late leakage and staining. There are no pathognomic signs on angiography for choroidal melanoma.

Indocyanine Green Angiography

Indocyanine green angiography (ICG) angiography better delineates the extent of mass since the infrared red waves are used to penetrate the RPE well. They can also pick up choroidal neovascularization. It helps in differentiating a melanoma from a choroidal hemangioma, the latter shows a washout of dye.

Fundus Autofluorescence

Intense diffuse or confluent hyperautofluorescence is seen in melanoma.

Optical Coherence Tomography

The OCT (EDI) may be useful in detecting tumors <3 mm in size which are difficult to pick up on clinical examination and ultrasonography. It is also helpful in confirming the presence of subretinal fluid in small doubtful lesions. The presence of subretinal fluid shifts the diagnosis more toward melanoma than toward choroidal nevus.

Secondary retinal changes like CME, and atrophic changes are often evident overlying the lesion. Recently, due to the enhanced choroidal imaging, OCT characteristics of melanoma and other choroidal tumors have been defined, the focus being on the shape and edge of the tumor and the internal vascularity. Still like FA, these features are not conclusive of a differential diagnosis.

CT Scan

Melanomas appear hyperdense on CT scanning with moderate contrast enhancement. It is useful for the evaluation of metastasis.

Magnetic Resonance Imaging

For ocular diagnoses, an MRI is more useful than a CT scan. On MRI, melanomas (like retinoblastoma) are hyperintense to vitreous on T1 and hypointense to vitreous on T2. It is also useful in assessing extraocular spread and in ruling out some of the differentials.

Tissue Diagnosis

When clinical methods and noninvasive investigative modalities fail to conclusively prove or rule out the diagnosis of a melanoma, tissue diagnosis by a fine needle aspiration a transscleral biopsy or a bimanual biopsy with chandelier assisted 25-G vitrectomy system may be useful. One should be careful of port/aspiration site spread, and cryotherapy should be considered at the entry sites. Also, if the diagnoses are proven to be melanoma, the earliest possible further management (like enucleation should) be done to avoid tumor spread. A lymph node biopsy or that of another site of spread may also be done if appropriate.

Systemic Investigations

It is directed principally toward detecting metastatic spread. Hepatic transaminases and alkaline phosphatase are the basic screening tests since the liver is the most common site of metastasis. If these enzymes are elevated CT scan of the abdomen or ultrasonography can be considered. PET-CT scan should be considered if available as metastasis was believed to be the rule (Zimmerman's hypothesis), even after successful excision of the tumor. Other sites of systemic spread include bone marrow, skin, brain, and lungs.

■ DIFFERENTIAL DIAGNOSIS

Since the clinical manifestation and appearance of the tumor are highly variable, numerous differentials need to be considered in the case of choroidal mass. **Table 1** summarizes the differentials in a tabular form.

■ MANAGEMENT

Treatment in the case of choroidal melanoma depends on the size and extension of the tumor, the life expectancy of the patient, and the visual potential of the eye. Treatment is tailor-made for each patient.

Observation

Increasingly the trend in ocular oncology is to treat smaller melanomas to reduce the risk of metastasis. But observation still has a role, especially in tumors <2.5 or 3 mm in height and <10 mm in diameter which are very slow growing, or in tumors in whom an unequivocal diagnosis of choroidal melanoma could not be reached. Also, in patients with limited life expectancy or untreatable conditions, observation might be a prudent choice.

Enucleation

Enucleation is the classic treatment modality for large melanomas or melanomas with poor visual potential or extensive spread within and outside the globe. The COMS also suggested enucleation for "large" tumors (see below). Additional precautions must be taken in the form of performing an indirect ophthalmoscopy after draping the parts to confirm the correct eye is enucleated. In large tumors, preenucleation radiotherapy may not provide additional mortality benefits. If there is extrascleral extension, the entire tumor should be removed en bloc to reduce the risk of residual disease. All treatment modalities developed subsequently to preserve the globe and salvage some useful visions are compared against enucleation in terms of mortality and metastasis.

Episcleral Plaque Brachytherapy

Brachytherapy is done by suturing an Iodine-125 or Ruthenium-106 plaque to the sclera over the area of the tumor. This may be used for medium-sized tumors with some potential for salvaging vision and <15 mm in basal diameter and up to 10 mm in height. Survival is similar to that following enucleation. Complications include cataracts, papillopathy (with or without NVD), and radiation retinopathy. About 25% of the patients develop iris neovascularization.

External Beam Radiotherapy

Melanomas are radioresistant. To radiate them using conventional external-beam radiotherapy techniques would require a high radiation dose and this subsequently leads to severe complications. Modern techniques of delivering precise high-dose radiation like proton beam irradiation and stereotactic radiotherapy can be used for tumors that are unsuitable for brachytherapy due to their large size or posterior location. These techniques cause minimal damage to the adjacent tissues. Their efficacy is similar to brachytherapy.

Transpupillary Thermotherapy and Photodynamic Therapy

These modalities can be used to treat smaller lesions. In some reports, double fluence (100 J/cm^2) and double duration (166s) of PDT have been used. While TTT is more useful in pigmented tumors, PDT is useful in amelanotic tumors.

Surgical Management

Melanomas can be removed through the scleral approach or through pars plana vitrectomy. In the scleral approach, the tumor is removed en-bloc with the surrounding choroid and overlying sclera if involved. In the pars-plana approach, the tumor is removed in piecemeal through a vitreous cutter (endoresection). These procedures are technically difficult and are indicated in carefully selected tumors that are too thick for radiotherapy but less than about 16 mm in diameter. The results are difficult to compare as long-term follow-up is needed to disprove systemic spread. Orbital exenteration is rarely done for melanoma with orbital extension because the disease has generally reached an advanced stage with extensive metastasis by this time. A nonconventional approach should be considered where visual/eyeball salvation is possible.

Systemic Chemotherapy

Systemic chemotherapy is used only in cases with metastatic disease.

VIVA QUESTIONS

Q.1. What are the risk factors for choroidal melanoma?

Ans. Risk factors include fair skin, lighter iris color, blonde hair, chronic sunlight exposure, choroidal or iris nevus, nevus of Ota, atypical nevus syndrome, multiple nevi, exposure to arc welding, uveal melanocytoma and BRCA-1 associated protein 1 (BAP1) mutation. The exposure to sunlight although hypothesized and believed widely, has not been proven by epidemiological studies.

Q.2. What is the diagnostic accuracy of ultrasonography in diagnosing choroidal melanoma?

Ans. Combined A- and B-scans have a diagnostic accuracy of over 95% in diagnosing choroidal melanoma. (COMS showed that clinical diagnosis which included clinical examination, fundus photography, and ultrasonography was 99% accurate in diagnosing choroidal melanoma).

Q.3. What are the histopathological features of choroidal melanoma?

Ans. Calender in 1931 developed a histopathological classification system for uveal melanomas depending on the most prominent cell type in a tumor. This included tumor is classified as:
- Spindle cell subtype A
- Spindle cell subtype B
- Epithelioid type
- Fascicular type and
- Mixed type.

There were inherent limitations in this system and therefore this classification was

revised in 1983 by McLean who classified uveal melanomas as follows:
- Spindle cell melanoma (composed of spindle B cells)
- Epithelioid cell melanoma and
- Mixed types of melanoma.

McLean did not classify Spindle A cells as malignant. They are fusiform cohesive cells that form choroidal nevus. Spindle B cells are also fusiform but are plumper and have poorly defined margins. Epithelioid cells are round or pleomorphic, noncohesive cells with large nuclei, prominent mitotic figures, and defined borders. There are also intermediate cells—intermediate between spindle and epithelioid. These cell types and other histopathological features can only be detected on enucleation or block resection specimens. Needle biopsy and tumor removal in piecemeal are difficult to type.

Choroidal melanomas arise de novo from the melanocytes in the uveal tissue. They can also arise from a choroidal nevus (in which case histopathology may show spindle A cells) or a melanocytoma. Immunohistochemical markers of melanoma are S-100 and HMB-45.

Q.4. What are the prognostic factors of choroidal melanoma?

Ans. Tumor size is the most important prognostic factor.[4,5] Several studies have shown that large tumors have the highest 5-year mortality rate—53%, while small and medium-sized tumors have a mortality rate of 16 and 32% respectively. Tumor histology is another important prognostic factor. Epithelioid tumors had a 10-year mortality of 72–100% while spindle A tumors had a 10-year mortality of 11–19%. Modern histopathological prognostic markers are indices such as the number of epithelioid cells per HPF and inverse standard deviation of nucleolar area. Extrascleral extension is another important prognostic marker—5-year survival is poor if there is extrascleral extension. Anteriorly located tumors present much later and therefore have a poorer prognosis. Among medium-sized tumors, posteriorly located tumors have a poorer prognosis since it is difficult to provide brachytherapy to more posterior sites. Ciliary body invasion of choroidal tumors indicates a poor prognosis. Tumors recurrent after brachytherapy or external radiotherapy also behave poorly. Tumor genetic characteristics such as somatic mutations in the *BAP1* gene are also linked to a greater chance of metastasis.

The liver, bone, and lung are the common sites of metastasis. At presentation, only about 1–2% of patients have detectable metastases, but mortality is up to 50% at 10 years.

Q.5. What is a diffuse infiltrating choroidal melanoma?

Ans. It is a variant of choroidal melanoma which does not present as a tumorous mass but shows lateral growth in the choroid and presents with exudative RD. It has been defined as a tumor <5 mm in height and occupying >25% of the uveal tract. It accounts for about 5% of all the choroidal melanomas. It is difficult to diagnose because of the absence of the tumor and the presence of an exudative RD. It generally has a poor prognosis.

Q.6. What is a collaborative ocular melanoma study?

Ans. Collaborative ocular melanoma study (COMS) is a National Eye Institute sponsored multicentric three-armed study started in 1985. The first arm studied the natural history of small choroidal melanoma. The other two arms were randomized control trials evaluating treatment options for medium and large-sized tumors. Iodine-125 brachytherapy was compared against enucleation for medium-sized tumors and enucleation alone was compared to enucleation preceded by external beam radiotherapy in large tumors. The definitions of small, medium, and large tumors are summarized in **Table 3**.

The natural history arm recruited 204 patients. Six deaths occurred due to metastatic melanoma. The 5-year tumor-specific mortality rate was 1%. The medium-sized tumor trial showed that there was no statistically significant difference in the mortality rates of patients treated with enucleation and iodine-125 brachytherapy. The risk of treatment failure in the case of brachytherapy was 10% and was increased in patients with thicker tumors and patients with posterior tumors. In the large-sized tumor trial, pre-enucleation brachytherapy was not found to significantly affect survival.

Q.7. What is Zimmerman's hypothesis?
Ans. Zimmerman, McLean, and Foster in 1978 hypothesized in their paper that enucleation may accelerate metastases. This was based on their observation of a peak in the mortality rates 2 years postenucleation which after 6 years stabilized to the preenucleation rates. They hypothesized that tumor manipulation during surgery caused dissemination of the tumor causing a spike in metastasis and mortality. Based on this they also suggested high vigilance during enucleation for uveal melanoma and preenucleation radiotherapy.[6]

Subsequent epidemiological studies have also shown a post-therapeutic spike (spike after any form of treatment to the melanoma—enucleation, brachytherapy, or proton beam radiotherapy) in the mortality rates in accordance with the observation made by Zimmerman et al. The current understanding of this phenomenon is that it involves host-tumor interaction and host-immune mechanisms. Also, there could be a role played by antiangiogenic mediators such as angiostatin produced by the primary melanoma which may have growth inhibitory effects on the micrometastases. Removal/treatment of the primary tumor alters the host immune response and the antiangiogenic signals from the primary tumor and causes micrometastases to progressively grow and cause mortality. Therefore, surgery *per se* is not the cause of the increased postenucleation mortality but the treatment of the tumor is.

Q.8. What are the pros and cons of endoresection of tumors, and what are the results?
Ans. Endovitreal resection of medium to large-sized choroidal melanomas (limited to the globe) has been reported by multiple authors. The advantages of this procedure are globe preservation, preservation of some visual function, removal of the tumor in its entirety, abundant sample for histopathology and genetic studies, avoiding radiation complications, and photocoagulation of microscopic elements under direct observation. The disadvantages of this procedure are the theoretical risk of tumor seeding and metastasis (although the MIVS systems with the trocar and cannula entry have been shown to be safe), the need for hypotensive anesthesia, the demand more skill, need for multiple surgeries. The reported results are good, comparable to other globe salvaging procedures in terms of metastasis. Survival data is as yet limited.[7]

▮ REFERENCES

1. Ryan SJ, Schachat AP, Wilkinson CP, Hinton DR, Sadda SR, Wiedemann P. Ryan's Retina, 7th edition. Amsterdam: Elsevier Health Sciences; 2012.
2. Savar A, Esmaeli B. Management of primary eyelid cancers. In: Esmaeli B (Ed). Ophthalmic Oncology. New York: Springer; 2011. pp. 113-4.
3. Ossoinig KC. Standardized echography: basic principles, clinical applications, and results. Int Ophthalmol Clin. 1979;19(4):127-210.
4. Kaliki S, Shields CL. Uveal melanoma: relatively rare but deadly cancer. Eye (Lond). 2016;31(2):241-57.
5. Margo CE. The Collaborative Ocular Melanoma Study: An Overview. Cancer Control. 2004;11(5):304-9.
6. Singh AD, Rennie IG, Kivela T, Seregard S, Grossniklaus H. The Zimmerman-McLean-Foster hypothesis: 25 years later. Br J Ophthalmol. 2004;88(7):962-7.
7. Venkatesh P, Gogia V, Gupta S, Shah BM. 25 Gauge Endoresection for Moderate to Large Choroidal Melanoma. Indian J Surg Oncol. 2015;7(3):365-7.

SHORT CASES

CHERRY-RED SPOT

Rajesh Pattebahadur, Brijesh Takkar

■ INTRODUCTION

Cherry-red spot (CRS) is an important finding suggestive of a large group of diseases. Among these diseases, diagnosis of metabolic disorders helps in prognosticating the condition, while early diagnosis of conditions such as central retinal artery occlusion (CRAO) helps in early management and salvaging the permanent loss of vision.[1]

■ HISTORY

Chief Complaints

As stated earlier CRS is not a disease, a patient with history of metabolic disorder may show CRS on fundus examination. Also, a case of sudden diminution of vision (CRAO) or ocular contusion will have CRS on fundus examination.

History on Present Illness

The patient's age of presentation will have different sets of complaints and different sets of diagnosis. In pediatric age group, patient may show hepatosplenomegaly, bone changes, neurological changes, ascites, myoclonic jerk, and mental retardation. Whereas in adults, history of trauma to eye can be present or sudden diminution of vision (CRAO) may be there.

Medical History

Past medical history of hypertension, dysostosis multiplex (DM), hypercoagulable states, sickle cell, atherosclerosis, cardiac valvular disease, sepsis, and intravenous drug abuse may be there.

Family History

Family history is important in cases with metabolic disorders associated with the CRS.

■ EXAMINATION

Systemic Examination

Detailed examination may reveal systemic findings of the underlying cause, in a case of CRS.
- *Cardiovascular system:* Patient may be having hypertension along with valvular heart disease.
- *Abdominal system:* Hepatosplenomegaly is important finding suggestive of severe metabolic abnormalities. Along with this ascites can also be seen.
- *Neurological system:* Delayed response, mental retardation, myoclonic jerks, and hypotonia are important findings.
- *Respiratory system:* Interstitial pneumonia can be present.
- Along with these other features include coarse facies, bone changes.

Ophthalmic Examination

Following points must be recorded:
- Uncorrected and best corrected visual acuity
- Globes are generally aligned.
- Eyelids are generally within normal limit.
- Conjunctiva does not show any specific finding but in cases of ocular trauma may show bleeding or tear in conjunctiva.
- Corneal clouding can be seen, typical of underlying systemic diseases.
- Anterior chamber is usually within normal limit. Angle recession can be seen in cases of severe ocular trauma. Iridodialysis, lens subluxation, post-traumatic cataract are a few findings which suggest the ocular trauma as a cause for the CRS.
- Distant direct ophthalmoscopy may not reveal any specific finding unless there is cataract.

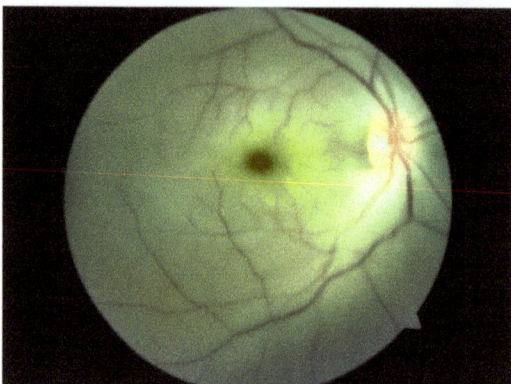

Fig. 1: Fundus photograph of cherry-red spot in a case of central retinal artery occlusion (CRAO).

Indirect Ophthalmoscopy

- Detailed examination should include cup disc ratio, neuroretinal rim, arteriovenous ratio, and foveal reflex.
- The CRS is visualized as a bright to dull red spot at the center of macula, surrounded and bordered by a grayish white or yellowish halo (**Fig. 1**).

DIFFERENTIAL DIAGNOSIS

As said earlier the underlying cause has to be identified. The common causes are:
- *Bilateral CRS:* Metabolic disorders, drug toxicity (quinine, dapsone, methanol, and carbon monoxide) and Leber's congenital amaurosis.
- *Unilateral CRS:* CRAO, orbital contusions, macular hole with retinal detachment, lamellar macular hole, and macular hemorrhage.

The CRS is more commonly associated with CRAO in adults. The age, health of patient, history of trauma or vascular disease and unilaterality of lesion may help to distinguish it from the metabolic disorders. In such instances providing emergency management and treating the underlying disorders or risk factors constitute vital therapeutic interventions.[1,2]

In children with CRAO hemoglobinopathies such as sickle cell disease, hypercoagulable states such as antiphospholipid antibodies and vasculitis due to systemic lupus erythematosus are more common causes, whereas in adults two-thirds of all patients with CRAO have associated hypertension, one-fourth have carotid occlusive disease, diabetes or cardiac valvular disease or a combination. Bilateral involvement is rare and suggestive of arteritic disease.[1,2]

MANAGEMENT

Treatment involves treating the underlying cause. CRAO, an ophthalmic emergency, should be treated within 24 hours. Ocular massage can be tried to dislodge the obstructing emboli using. Other options include medical and surgical lowering of intraocular pressure, carbon dioxide rebreathing, steroids (in vasculitis), vasodilator drugs, hyperbaric oxygen, antifibrinolytic drugs, barbiturate coma, free radical scavengers and antioxidants have been tried with variable results. The CRS resolves in due course with resolution of edema, however, optic atrophy ensues.[1,2]

VIVA QUESTIONS

Q.1. What is cherry-red spot (CRS)?
Ans. It is a clinical sign seen in the context of thickening and loss of transparency of posterior pole of the retina. The CRS is visualized as a bright to dull red spot at the center of macula, surrounded and accentuated by a grayish white or yellowish halo. Its color is due to the pigment epithelium and choroid, and therefore may demonstrate color variability according to the race.[1]

Q.2. What is differential diagnosis for CRS?
Ans. *See* **Box 1**.

Q.3. What are the causes of CRS-like lesions and pseudo-CRS?
Ans. Certain illnesses are associated with macular lesions resembling a CRS. These include:
- Adult Niemann–Pick disease (ring of perifoveal crystalloid deposits)
- Gaucher's disease (atypical macular CRS)
- Lactosyl ceramidosis (increasing redness of macula)
- Sea blue histiocyte syndrome (perifoveal yellowish white scintillating granules in doughnut-shaped pattern)

Box 1: Differential diagnosis of cherry-red spot.
- Central retinal artery occlusion (CRAO)
- Orbital contusion
- Orbital ischemia
- Tay–Sachs disease
- Sandhoff's disease
- Sialidosis
- Infantile Niemann–Pick disease type IA
- GM1 gangliosidosis
- Metachromatic leukodystrophy
- Goldberg's disease
- Gaucher's disease (infantile form), Hurler's syndrome
- Mucopolysaccharidosis VII
- Hallervorden–Spatz syndrome
- Batten–Mayou; Vogt–Spielmeyer syndrome
- Spranger's disease
- Cryoglobulinemia
- Leber's congenital amaurosis
- Drugs—quinine, carbon monoxide, methanol and dapsone toxicity

Conditions such as macular hemorrhage or macular hole with retinal detachment could be considered as pseudo-CRS, because the abnormality is in the foveola rather than parafoveal area.

Q.4. What is the pathophysiology of CRS?

Ans.
- The retina has around 1 million ganglion cells.
- However, macular region (foveola, in particular) is almost devoid of these cells.
- Diseases associated with accumulation of storage material (such as glycolipids or sphingolipids) in the retinal cellular layers result in swelling and loss of transparency of the multilayered ganglion cells giving it a "white" appearance.
- The foveola, the thinnest part of the retina being devoid of ganglion cells, retains its relative transparency allowing the normal choroidal vasculature to be seen through it.
- These histological features result in the appearance of the central red area (normal foveola) that is surrounded by dull halo resulting from attenuation of transparency of the surrounding area.
- Later in the course of the disease, ganglion cell death makes the spot less prominent. Atrophy of retinal nerve fiber layer and optic atrophy may also follow.
- In *CRAO* the fundoscopy reveals a diffuse retinal arteriole constriction often with visible emboli or blood flow segmentation. The fovea retains its blood supply via the choroidal circulation while the surrounding retina appears milky white due to infarction, intracellular edema, cellular necrosis, and cellular debris accumulation.
- The CRS seen in *methanol poisoning* is due to macular cystoid edema and in *quinine poisoning* due to retinal edema.
- In *macular hemorrhage*, blood which is darker red than the retina contributes to the CRS appearance.

Q.5. Which are predisposing conditions for the CRAO?

Ans. Conditions that predispose to CRAO include retinal emboli due to endogenous or exogenous source; hypertension, diabetes mellitus, carotid occlusive disease, cardiac valvular disease, atheromatous vascular disease, arteriosclerotic vascular disease, vasculitic syndromes (temporal arteritis, SLE, etc.), blood dyscrasias (e.g., sickle hemoglobinopathy), hypercoagulable states (e.g., antiphospholipid antibodies), sepsis and DIC, vasospasm, vascular compression, cervical trauma with carotid artery dissection, intravenous drug use and migraine.

Q.6. How to diagnose and manage the CRS?

Ans. *In pediatric age group:* Metabolic diseases constitute the most common cause for CRS. The exact metabolic or storage disease can be diagnosed on the basis of age of onset, associated manifestations, inheritance pattern.

In newborns:
- Hepatosplenomegaly with vacuolated lymphocytes would suggest GM1 gangliosidosis, Niemann–Pick disease type IA or early infantile galactosialidosis.

- An additional finding of coarse facies, bone changes, edema with ascites would favor GM1 gangliosidosis or early infantile galactosialidosis; interstitial pneumonia and neurologic deterioration would suggest Niemann-Pick disease type IA disease.

In infancy:
- Exaggerated neuronal response, hepatosplenomegaly, myoclonic jerks, hypotonia, and neuroregression would suggest a diagnosis of GM2 gangliosidosis type 1 (Tay-Sachs disease) or type 2 (Sandhoff's disease).
- Whereas hepatosplenomegaly with bone changes would favor a diagnosis of late infantile galactosialidosis.
- In late childhood, blindness and progressive myoclonic jerks suggest sialidosis (CRS myoclonus syndrome) whereas bone changes, dysmorphism, angiokeratoma, corneal opacities and psychomotor retardation would suggest juvenile galactosialidosis.

Several inherited metabolic diseases have no definitive treatment. However, early diagnosis allows for appropriate counseling and prenatal diagnosis (for example, determination of levels of hexosaminidase A and B levels in Sandhoff's disease).

REFERENCES

1. Suvarna JC, Hajela SA. Cherry-red spot. J Postgrad Med. 2008;54:54-7.
2. Chen H, Chan AY, Stone DU, Mandal NA. Beyond the cherry-red spot: Ocular manifestations of sphingolipid-mediated neurodegenerative and inflammatory disorders. Surv Ophthalmol. 2014;59(1):64-76.

CENTRAL SEROUS CHORIORETINOPATHY

Vaishali Ghanshyam Rai, Ashish Markan, Raghav Ravani

INTRODUCTION

Central serous chorioretinopathy (CSCR) is a maculopathy characterized by idiopathic circumscribed serous retinal detachment, usually confined to the central macula. It is a favorite short case for PG examinations.

HISTORY

Demography

Central serous chorioretinopathy typically affects middle-aged individuals in the 30-50 years age range.[1,2] Males are much more commonly affected than females, accounting for 72-87.5% of CSCR patients. The incidence in men was approximately six times higher than in women. Younger patients usually have unilateral involvement, while older patients are more likely to have bilateral involvement in CSCR. CSCR is more prevalent in Asians as compared to Caucasians and Africo-Americans.

Chief Complaints

The patient can present with following:
- Recent unilateral painless diminution of vision is the most common symptom. Often the patient's complaint is one of transiently seeing a dark spot in the center of the visual field in one eye, with or without metamorphopsia.
- Unilateral metamorphopsia is the classic symptom.
- Patients may also present with unilateral blurred vision, micropsia, impaired dark adaptation, color desaturation, reduced contrast sensitivity, and a relative scotoma.

Past History

Following points must be noted:
- History of any emotional stress.
- History of *smoking*
- History of *type A personality* is important
- History *long-term steroid* use in any form, e.g., oral, inhaler or topical
- History of pregnancy in female patients

- History of any organ transplant in the past should be taken.
- History of similar complaints in past is important to rule out recurrent CSCR.

■ EXAMINATION

General Examination

Look for the presence of any disease requiring chronic steroid intake. Also, look for signs of steroid toxicity.

Ocular Examination

Visual Acuity

- Visual acuity ranges from 20/15 (6/5) to 20/200 (6/60) but averages 20/30 (6/9).
- The visual acuity may *improve with hyperopic correction*.

Anterior Segment

It is usually normal.

Posterior Segment

- *Acute form of CSCR:*
  - Oval yellow-gray elevations at parafoveal or macular area may be seen **(Fig. 1)**. These are generally less than one-fourth of a disc diameter in size and are surrounded by a faint grayish halo.
  - Absence of the normal foveal light reflex.
  - The subretinal fluid is usually clear, but granular or fibrinous deposits may be present in the subretinal space. The accumulation of granular/fibrinous material between the RPE and the neurosensory retina increases with the duration of symptoms. Subretinal fluid usually resolves within 3 months.
  - Abnormalities of the RPE present as one or more yellow spots or a small pigment epithelial detachment (PED).
  - The fellow eye may show evidence of either concurrent or previously resolved CSCR, manifested as focal areas of retinal pigment epithelium rarefaction or small asymptomatic retinal pigment epithelium detachments. Bilateral involvement occurs in approximately 20% of patients.
  - Recurrence of CSCR can be seen in 40–50% of patients in long course. A patient can have recurrent focal leaks or progress inexorably to the more visually threatening chronic CSCR.
- *Chronic CSCR*
  - It is characterized by persistence of subretinal fluid for >3 months and associated with presence of diffuse or multifocal, irregular retinal pigment epitheliopathy. It is also known as diffuse retinal pigment epitheliopathy (DRPE). Clinical examination can reveal the presence of gravitational tracts in the retina. Recently, multifocal posterior pigment epitheliopathy (MPPE) has also been described with multiple leaks with large amounts of SRF. Subretinal fibrosis and choroidal neovascular membranes (CNVMs) may ensue as complications.
  - The retinal detachments tend to be shallow and more diffuse than in the classic form and with amorphous subretinal deposits. Subretinal lipid that typically appears as discrete, hard-edged, subretinal accumulations at the borders of a neurosensory detachment can be seen.
  - More often bilateral and may occasionally present with gravitational tracts a term used for oblong, vertical patches of RPE hypopigmentation that extend inferiorly. These tracts are produced by subretinal fluid of high specific gravity sinking toward

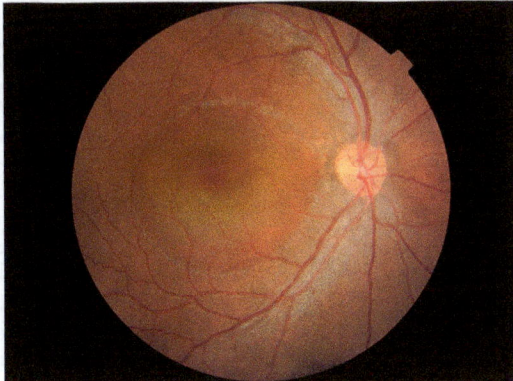

Fig. 1: Fundus photograph of a case of CSR.

the inferior fundus and dissecting its way through the subretinal space.
- *Recurrent CSCR:* It is defined as a new episode of acute CSCR within 12 months of resolution of previous episode. Reported recurrence rate is 19–51%.
- Rare forms
  Bullous form of CSCR:
  - Rarely CSCR can present as a bullous, inferior nonrhegmatogenous peripheral retinal detachment. Atrophic tracts of the RPE extending inferiorly to the serous retinal detachment can be seen in such cases.
  - It is often associated with subretinal fibrinous exudates and shows the phenomenon of subretinal fluid shifting position with changes in posture.
  - More common in Japan, and patients with history of organ transplant
  Neovascular CSCR: Rarely as a complication of chronic CSCR.

■ DIFFERENTIAL DIAGNOSIS

Central serous chorioretinopathy must be differentiated from a neural retinal detachment secondary to:
- *Subretinal choroidal neovascularization (CNV):* CNV presents with thickening at the level of the RPE, notched PEDs and subretinal or subpigment epithelial blood that are absent in CSCR. In addition, there will be coexistent ocular findings related to the generation of new blood vessel growth in eyes with CNV. Indocyanine green angiography of subretinal choroidal neovascularization usually reveals only one area of hyperfluorescence that progressively enlarges during the later frames of the study.
- *Tumors and infiltrative conditions* (leukemia, amelanotic melanoma, or metastatic disease) these lesions generally have a different color than the surrounding normal choroid; USG would show thickening of the choroid serous PEDs are absent.
- *Inflammatory (posterior scleritis or Harada's disease):* There will be signs of intraocular inflammation such as iritis or vitritis, and other signs such as patches of yellowish discoloration in the posterior pole, papillitis, thickening of the choroid on USG. These should always be considered for chronic and multifocal cases.
- *Polypoidal choroidal vasculopathy:* Indocyanine green angiography of polypoidal choroidal vasculopathy demonstrates small-caliber, polypoidal choroidal vascular lesions and no areas of choroidal hyperpermeability.
- *Optic disc pit:* The optic nerve pathology is visible on ophthalmoscopy. There are no leaks on fluorescein angiography. OCT can show the tract connecting to optic nerve head along with splitting of retinal layers, at times with an impending macular hole.

■ INVESTIGATION

Fundus Fluorescein Angiography

- Fundus fluorescein angiography is not required routinely but is a good practice for documenting the baseline disease, in chronic forms and when suspecting other disorders.
- Fundus fluorescein angiography classically shows dye from the choroid leaks through a focal RPE defect and pools in the subretinal space **(Figs. 2 and 3)**. In >75% of patients, this pooling occurs within 1 disc diameter of the fovea, very common in the superior nasal area.
- Fundus fluorescein angiography findings can be described as *"smokestack leak"* or the more common *"inkblot leak"* patterns. Multiple leaks may be seen in multifocal disease.

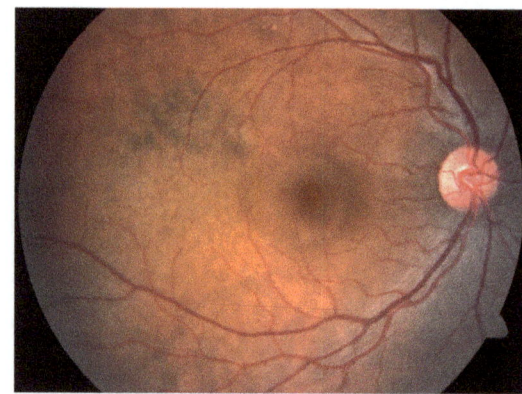

Fig. 2: Fundus photograph of a patient of CSR. Note the fluid accumulation beneath the fovea and the superior-temporal pigment mottling.

Indocyanine Green Angiography

- Earlier considered gold standard, choroidal ischemia and dilatation of larger choroidal vessels and hot spots corresponding to leaking areas can be seen.
- Staining appears in the midphase of the indocyanine green angiography (ICGA) and fades in the late phase.
- Features of venous obstructive choroidopathy, increased choroidal hyperpermeability, asymmetry of choroidal outflow, and morphological alterations at vortex vein ampullae have been reported on ultrawide field ICG angiography in recent studies.
- Pick-up CNVMs when doubtful.

Optical Coherence Tomography

- Demonstrate the presence of subretinal fluid and pachyvessels in the choroid (**Fig. 4**).
- Helps to quantify and follow the amount and extent of subretinal fluid and to demonstrate thickening of the neurosensory retina.
- Dark spot sign in cases of acute fibrinous CSCR.
- Helps in diagnosis of doubtful cases.
- Choroidal OCT imaging can reveal pachychoroid epitheliopathy in both eyes, now considered a precursor of CSR.
- Posteriorly loculated fluid in choroid can also be seen on choroidal imaging.

Optical Coherence Tomography Angiography

- OCTA in CSCR has shown altered superficial and deeper choroidal vasculature in acute and chronic eyes.
- Detection of CNVMs in chronic cases of CSCR.

■ TREATMENT

Observation

Majority of cases of central serous chorioretinopathy (CSC) resolve spontaneously over a period of 3–4 months. Most often, as per conventional teaching, the initial treatment of choice is observation. If the patient is using corticosteroids, these should be discontinued if medically possible. The patient must be advised

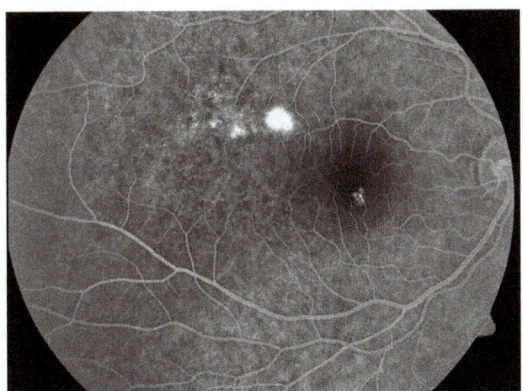

Fig. 3: Fluorescein angiography (FA) picture of the patient in Figure 1. Large ink blot leak can be seen. Staining is also visible in the area of pigment mottling.

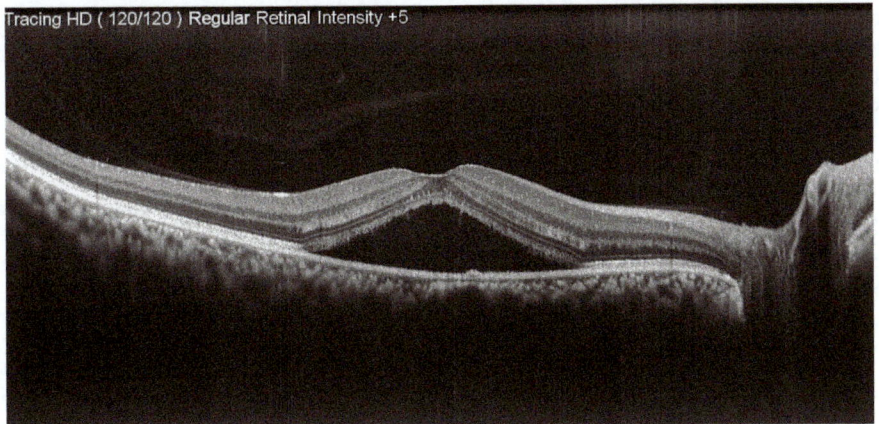

Fig. 4: OCT image showing subretinal fluid.

to avoid tobacco and smoking. Patients with type A personality should be addressed by lifestyle modification and stress management.

Acetazolamide

Systemic acetazolamide treatment promotes the resorption of subretinal fluid and case reports suggest that it may reduce subretinal fluid in CSCR. However, there is no evidence that treatment promotes healing of the retinal pigment epithelium (RPE) lesion, long-term preservation of visual function, or a reduced rate of recurrence.

■ ANTICORTICOSTEROID THERAPY

Mineralocorticoid receptors have been implicated in pathogenesis of CSCR. As a result, mineralocorticoid antagonist such as eplerenone has been tried in several studies with variable results. A recent RCT (VICI trial) has shown no role of eplerenone in management of CSCR.

Laser Photocoagulation

- Indications:
    - Extrafoveal leaks which fail to improve after 4-6 months.
    - Demonstrate permanent changes from CSCR in the other eye.
    - Demonstrate multiple recurrences.
    - *Occupational:* Require improved vision for work.
- Laser photocoagulation is applied to the site of fluorescein leakage. The technique of laser photocoagulation involves using a green-wavelength laser to produce a light scar over the focal RPE leak.
- Typically, 6-12 laser burns of 50-200 μm spot size at 0.1-second duration, and 75-200 mW are used. Permanent RPE change is induced at the site of the laser scar.
- Treatment should be avoided if the leak occurs within 300 μm of the center of the foveal avascular zone.

Photodynamic Therapy

- Photodynamic therapy has been used to treat chronic CSC (defined as >6 months' duration of disease) with diffuse compensation of the RPE and lacking focal FA leak. However, recent evidence from East Asia supports its role in acute uncomplicated CSR as well, especially when done at low fluence.
- Photodynamic therapy is a treatment that is more effective with a lower complication rate for patients with subfoveal or juxtafoveal leaks.

Transpupillary Thermotherapy

Few studies suggest that this treatment may accelerate the resolution of CSC, but long-term safety and efficacy are not known.

Others: Several other modalities have been described.[3]

- The beta-adrenergic receptor blocker propranolol and the mixed alpha and beta-adrenergic receptor blocker labetalol.
- Mifepristone as an antagonist of progesterone and glucocorticoid receptors.
- Ketoconazole is an adrenocorticoid antagonist that has been shown to lower endogenous cortisol.
- Intravitreal bevacizumab has been investigated for treatment of CSR; theoretically, the antipermeability characteristics of this antibody to vascular endothelial growth factor (VEGF) may allow for reduced leakage, favoring resorption of the exudative retinal detachment in CSR.
- *Aspirin:* Plasminogen activator inhibitor-1 (PAI-1) is increased in CSCR, and aspirin is effective in lowering PAI-1 levels and platelet aggregation.
- Rifampicin is another drug that has been tried for CSR, though the evidence level is low.

VIVA QUESTIONS

Q.1. What are the risk factors associated with CSCR?

Ans. *See* **Table 1**.

Q.2. What is the clinical course and outcome of CSCR?

Ans. The visual prognosis is good in the majority of cases of CSCR. The majority of patients suffer no significant permanent visual loss. Although visual acuity usually

Table 1: Risk factors and associations with central serous chorioretinopathy.	
Systemic conditions	*Type A personality, emotional stress:* • Pregnancy • Organ transplantation • Systemic lupus erythematosus • Tobacco and alcohol use • Membranoproliferative glomerulonephritis type II • *Helicobacter pylori* infection • Gastroesophageal reflux disease • Systemic hypertension
Medications	*Corticosteroids:* • Antihistamines • Sildenafil citrate • Psychopharmacologic medications • Amphetamine • Antacids and antireflux medications • Sympathomimetics • Antibiotics

improves, patients may continue to have persistent metamorphopsia probably due to a photoreceptor misalignment causing a *Stiles–Crawford effect*.

Q.3. Mechanism of action of acetazolamide in CSCR.

Ans. It helps in absorption of the subretinal fluid by inhibiting carbonic anhydrase pump located in the RPE and creating a localized acidic milieu.

Q.4. Hypothesis for pathogenesis of CSCR.

Ans. Choroidal circulation anomaly of the middle choroidal layers leading on to focal choroidal ischemia, choroidal edema which sets up a vicious cycle. This leads to accumulation of fluid in the choroid, formation of PEDs which eventually give way to cause leakage and manifest as SRF. Choroidal imaging confirms this by demonstrating pachychoroid epitheliopathy, localized choroidal fluid, and increased compensatory vascularity. Recent studies have evaluated the role of venous obstructive choroidopathy in pathogenesis of CSCR.

Q.5. Histopathological classification.

Ans. *Type 1:* Only neurosensory detachment
Type 2: Neurosensory with pigment epithelium detachment.

Q.6. What are the indications for treatment of CSR?

Ans. *See* chapter for answer.

■ REFERENCES

1. Liew G, Quin G, Gillies M, Fraser-Bell S. Central serous chorioretinopathy: a review of epidemiology and pathophysiology. Clin Exp Ophthalmol. 2013;41(2):201-14.
2. Ross A, Ross AH, Mohamed Q. Review and update of central serous chorioretinopathy. Curr Opin Ophthalmol. 2011;22(3):166-73.
3. Iacono P, Battaglia Parodi M, Falcomatà B, Bandello F. Central serous chorioretinopathy treatments: a mini review. Ophthalmic Res. 2016;55:76-83.

DIABETIC MACULAR EDEMA

Brijesh Takkar, Dhaval Patel, Ashish Markan

■ INTRODUCTION

Macular edema is an important cause of decrease in vision in cases with diabetes mellitus (DM). Determination of diabetic macular edema (DME) is important for ophthalmologists for the early treatment and visual rehabilitation. DME is very frequently kept as short case or a spotter.

■ HISTORY

Chief Complaints

A known case of DM will give a history of diminution of vision and other macular symptoms such as scotoma or distorted vision. The patient may also give a history of inadequate control of the blood sugar levels, or recent fluctuation in blood sugar levels or even recent change in diabetic medication. Sometimes, DME may be picked up on routine diabetic screening without symptoms, especially when noncenter involving. Also, such patients often present after referral by an endocrinologist with minimal visual symptoms.

Past History

In this condition, there should always be a parallel focus on the systemic features apart from a meticulous ocular workup. Past history of DM, hypertension, coronary artery disease, asthma, diabetic nephropathy should be recorded. Conditions such as pregnancy and dyslipidemia are other risk factors and should always be carefully recorded. History of use of insulin and the type of antidiabetic drugs should be recorded as they influence macular findings and treatment outcomes.

Importantly, the record of past fundus examinations with grade of diabetic retinopathy recorded in last visits is essential.[1-3] If any treatment, e.g., laser or intravitreal injections was given in past, then detailed record, including the number of setting of PRP, time since last panretinal laser photocoagulation (PRP), and number of intravitreal injections given, should be noted.

Family History

The family history of DM should be recorded. It is essential to ask for family history because DM has familial inheritance. Each relative having DM should undergo the fundus examination according to the type and duration since diagnosis.

■ EXAMINATION

Systemic Examination

Since DM is a disease affecting various systems of the body, detailed examination of cardiovascular, central nervous system, respiratory system, renal system, should be done to rule out any comorbidity associated with diabetic retinopathy DR.

Ophthalmic Examination

Uncorrected visual acuity and best corrected visual acuity should be noted.

Eyeball may not show any specific finding. But it is not uncommon for a patient of DM to have cranial mononeuropathy. If such mononeuropathy is present, the patient will have corresponding squint.

Eyelids—blepharitis can be seen in patients of DM; lid edema may indicate nephropathy.

Conjunctiva does not show any specific finding, signs of dryness may be seen as a complication of neuropathy and chronic conjunctivitis may be present.

Cornea—diabetic neuropathy can lead to neurotrophic keratopathy. So, assessment of corneal sensation is important. Dryness and epitheliopathy may be noticed on slit-lamp examination.

Anterior chamber and angle—neovascularization of iris (NVI) must always be ruled out.

Lens—status should be noted, since macular edema can be precipitated or aggravated by cataract surgery and may cause decrease in visual acuity. Snowflake cataract is typically seen in uncontrolled young diabetics.

Vitreous body should be examined for any hemorrhage or pigments. Asteroid hyalosis is a known association of DM and can preclude fundus examination.

IOP measurement is important to rule out glaucoma, open-angle glaucoma (OAG) is a known association.

Fundus Examination

Documentation of details of disc finding should be done, including the cup disc ratio, neuroretinal rim, arteriovenous ratio, foveal reflex along with evidence of vitreomacular adhesion (VMA), retinal thickening, hard exudates, microaneurysms, and soft exudates. One should perform a careful peripheral retinal examination for features of proliferative diabetic retinopathy (PDR) and slit-lamp biomicroscopy examination is a must for classifying the macular edema **(Fig. 1)**.

■ DIFFERENTIAL DIAGNOSIS

- Retina vein occlusion
- Ruptured macroaneurysm
- Irvine–Gass syndrome

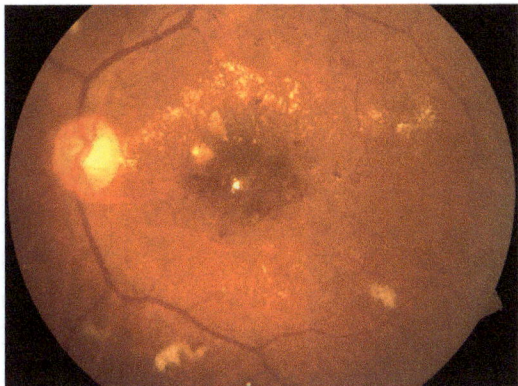

Fig. 1: Fundus photograph depicting diabetic macular edema (DME). Hard exudates can be seen along with retinal thickening within the central area. Other signs of nonproliferative diabetic retinopathy (NPDR) can also be seen.

- Radiation retinopathy
- Hypertensive retinopathy
- Subfoveal choroidal neovascularization.

CLASSIFICATION

- The diabetic retinopathy study (DRS) first gave the term DME. Later, the early treatment diabetic retinopathy study (ETDRS) defined clinically significant macular edema as presence of:
  - Retinal edema is located at or within 500 μm of the center of the macula.
  - Hard exudates at or within 500 μm of the center if associated with thickening of adjacent retina.
  - A zone of thickening larger than 1 disc area if located within 1 disc diameter of the center of the macula.
  To characterize the severity of macular edema and for treatment guidelines, the term clinically significant macular edema (CSME) is used.
- The international classification system classifies DME as mild, moderate, or severe, depending on proximity of retinal thickening to the foveal center.
- Based on fundus fluorescein angiography (FFA), DME may be classified as focal, diffuse, or ischemic.
- Recently, Diabetic Retinopathy Clinical Research (DRCR) network has classified it as a center involving DME (CI-DME) and non-CI-DME. C1-DME is defined as retinal thickening in the macula that involves the central subfield zone (1 mm in diameter), whereas NCI-DME is defined as retinal thickening in the macula that does not involve the central subfield zone (1 mm in diameter).

INVESTIGATIONS

Fluorescein Angiogram

The fluorescein angiogram (FA) is used to identify areas of increased vascular permeability, for example, leaking microaneurysms or capillary beds, and to evaluate retinal ischemia. Leakage on the angiogram does not necessarily indicate retinal edema since extracellular edema requires that the rate of fluid ingress into the retina (i.e., as indicated by leakage on the FA) exceeds the rate of fluid clearance from the retina (e.g., via the RPE pump).

Clinically significant macular edema (CSME) is further classified into *focal* or *diffuse*, depending on the leakage pattern seen on the fluorescein angiogram (FA). In *focal CSME*, scattered points of retinal hyperfluorescence are present on the FA due to focal leakage. The source of this focal leakage is microaneurysms. It is hypothesized that leaking microaneurysms are the cause of retinal thickening. Commonly, these leaking microaneurysms are surrounded by circinate rings of hard exudates. The exudates are lipoprotein deposits in the outer retinal layers.

In *diffuse DME*, areas of diffuse leakage are noted on the FA due to intraretinal leakage from a dilated retinal capillary bed and/or intraretinal microvascular abnormalities (IRMA), and/or (in severe cases) from arterioles and venules without discrete foci of leaking microaneurysms (**Fig. 2**). There may be associated cystoid macular edema. Cystoid macular edema results due to fluid accumulation, primarily in the outer plexiform layer.

Ischemic maculopathy (**Fig. 3**) in presence of large capillary nonperfusion (CNP) areas, macular collaterals, and foveal avascular zone (FAZ) changes such as irregular shape, increased size with pruned arterioles.

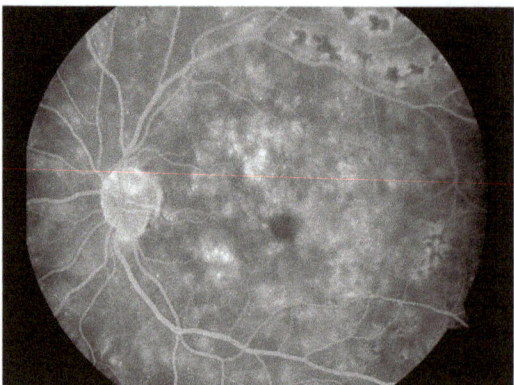
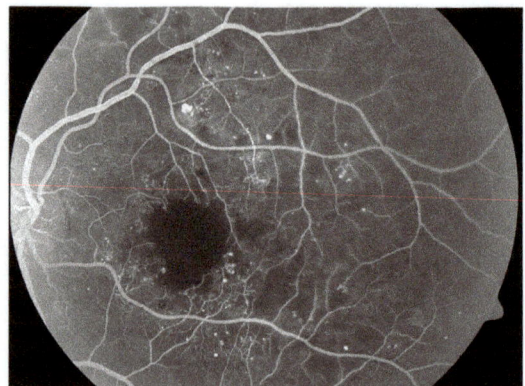

Fig. 2: Fluorescein angiography (FA) picture of diffuse diabetic macular edema (DME). Diffuse leaks with few scattered microaneurysms can be seen. Peripheral laser marks are also visible.

Fig. 3: Fluorescein angiography (FA) picture of macular ischemia. Distortion of FAZ with increased size is seen, irregular borders are accompanied by pruned vasculature.

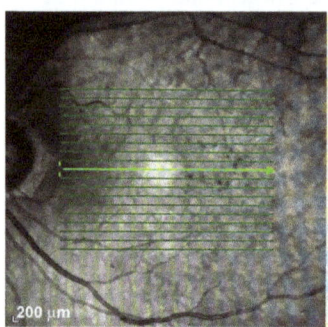
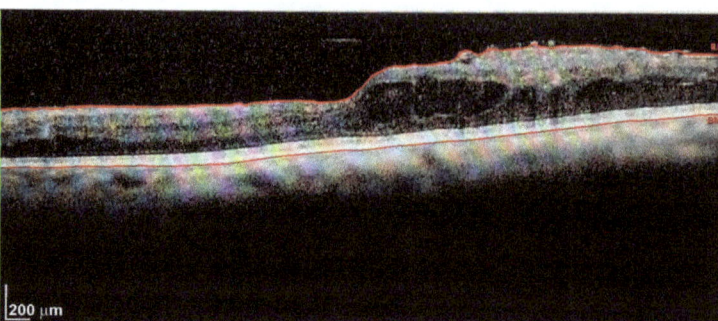

Fig. 4: Optical coherence tomography (OCT) picture of hemifield DME. Large cystoids spaces are visible in middle retinal layers.

Optical Coherence Tomography

The optical coherence tomography (OCT) has been used for high-resolution imaging of the retina and detection of increased retinal thickness (**Fig. 4**). There are several studies done for the use of OCT in case the of CSME. OCT can be used for measuring macular volume, determining central retinal thickness, and determining the type of edema. Recently, distortion of inner retinal layers has been described for ischemic DME.

Hyperreflective foci are also seen in DME. Choroidal thickness is under evaluation for DME with special focus on treatment-induced changes.

Patterns of OCT findings associated with CSME:
- Spongiform
- Cystoid
- Sensory detachment
- VMT
- TRD and mixed

Macular thickness map is a specific protocol used for analysis of macular thickness on OCT that measures in nine thickness sectors centered on fovea in three rings of diameter of 1, 3, and 6 mm.

Compared to clinical examination, OCT is a more sensitive and specific method for macular evaluation. It is an excellent tool for follow-up and deciding treatment endpoints, prognosis, and measuring response to therapy.

OCT biomarkers for poor prognosis in a case of DME:
- Disorganization of the retinal inner layers (DRIL)

- External limiting membrane (ELM) and ellipsoid zone (EZ) disruption
- Hyperreflective foci in retina and choroid
- Bridging retinal processes
- Associated vitreomacular traction

OCT has several advantages as a retinal imaging technique:
- It is noninvasive (no injection of dye involved) and well tolerated.
- It is highly sensitive and specific for retinal thickness measurement.
- It clearly reveals the presence and extent of vitreomacular traction.
- Other investigations such as OCTA are useful for visualizing FAZ, microaneurysms, capillary density, and choroidal changes.

Ultrawide imaging and VR interface enhancement with OCT is under investigation for use in DME. These are currently under investigation but are expected to play important roles in deciding treatment protocols soon.

Multifocal electroretinography (MFERG) and microperimetry: These are more research tools.

■ MANAGEMENT

Medical Therapy

This includes:
- Strict control of diabetes, hypertension, and hypercholesterolemia
- Diet modification
- Weight loss
- Exercise.

Controlling systemic parameters are extremely important. High-grade evidence in support has been given by DCCT, UKPDS, ACCORD, and FIELD trials. The standard of treatment for CSME has been focal laser photocoagulation in the days of ETDRS with 50% prevention of moderate visual loss at the end of 2 years **(Table 1)**. Conventionally, in "focal" CSME, a focal laser pattern is used to treat leaking microaneurysms identified on the FA that contribute to the retinal edema. In "diffuse" CSME, intraretinal leakage is noted on the FA from dilated retinal capillary beds or intraretinal microvascular abnormalities (IRMA) without isolated, discrete foci of leakage. Modified ETDRS macular grid laser was advocated for managing DDME (*See* **Table 1** for details).

Table 1: Different laser procedures for diabetic macular edema.

Parameters	Focal laser	Classic grid laser	Modified grid laser
Wavelength	Argon green, double frequency Nd:YAG		
Duration	100 ms		
Spot size	50 µm	50 µm	
Power	80 mW (titrated according to requirement)	50 mW (titrated according to requirement)	
Interburn distance	–	2 burns	
Intensity of burn	Grade 2–3 (dirty white)/ blanching or darkening of microaneurysms	Grade 1–2 (Faint white)	
Area of laser	Based on FA findings and location of microaneurysms. Central ring is spared	Laser burns are given at 500 µm from the center of macula to all microaneurysm within 3,000 µm	Laser burns are given at 500 µm from the center of macula in a C-pattern sparing papillomacular bundle. Can be done up to 2 DD from the center of macula
Follow-up	1 week, 1 month, 4-month (FFA)	1 week, 1 month, 4-month (FFA)	1 week, 1 month, 4-month (FFA)

Pharmacotherapy

Up till anti-VEGF intravitreal treatment came to the fore, laser was standard of care for managing CSME. While this still holds true for non-center involving DME, current evidence states that intravitreal anti-VEGF provides more effective treatment for CSME than monotherapy with laser or steroid in center involving edema. This conclusion has been drawn from long-term results of a study from diabetic retinopathy clinical research (DRCR) network, which found monthly loading therapy with ranibizumab followed by as needed (also called *pro re nata or* PRN schedule) maintenance to have best results in center involving DME vis-a-vis early laser, only laser and steroid injection. 5-year data has confirmed these results. Though repeated intravitreal injections have the financial constraints and obviously can lead to untoward ocular complications, the final visual acuity and macular anatomy is better than managing with laser monotherapy. As discussed above for ETDRS, laser chiefly halted moderate visual loss, but did not improve acuity. Triamcinolone injections have poorer results as well as more complications than anti-VEGF.

Other notable studies on anti-VEGF are READ, RISE, RIDE, BOLT, RESTORE, and RESOLVE studies. Further, DRCR has analyzed aflibercept for DME and found it to be useful in patients with worse initial visual acuity; da Vinci study is another notable study. A newer analyzed drug is steroid implant-dexamethasone (BEVORDEX study) and fluocinolone (FAME study). Basic advantage of implants is frequency of injections with noninferior results. Typically, they are useful in the presence of hard exudates and may be for macular ischemia.

Combined Therapy

These therapies may be combined, the most fruitful example is combination of ranibizumab with deferred laser.

Surgical Management

Pars plana vitrectomy (PPV) for removal of VMT may be considered. The posterior hyaloid is removed along with any posterior cortical vitreous strands to the foveal edge and any visually significant epiretinal membrane. 50% of eyes will have a reduction in central subfield thickness to <250 μm. As per the DRCR net study, only 28–49% of such eyes will have improvement of visual acuity, and between 13 and 31% may have worsening of visual acuity. The effectiveness of PPV for DME in the absence of VMT is unclear. ILM peeling has been evaluated as a treatment for chronic DME as well as primary treatment with differing outcomes.

Treating Refractory DME

Though no fixed definition is quotable, commonly used dictum is failure of response to therapy with multiple anti-VEGF and, at least, one sitting of laser. The available options for management include checking diagnoses, checking systemic control, and ruling out anatomical causes. Steroids, higher frequency, or dosing of anti-VEGF, change in anti-VEGF drug peripheral laser, surgery, and newer molecules such as tyrosine kinase-based therapies (TIME study), angiopoietin and AGE inhibitors may be tried.

Managing Macular Ischemia

Outcomes remain bad. Often these patients have poor systemic control. Lasers and anti-VEGF are relative contraindications in presence of ischemia. These patients may benefit from peripheral laser and steroids/implants.

Pseudophakic ME and DME

Differentiation may be difficult, presence of microaneurysms typically indicate DME while late disc stippling indicates Irvine–Gass syndrome.

In patients with DME, simultaneous treatment with intravitreal injections is indicated for prevention of exacerbation following cataract surgery.

VIVA QUESTIONS

Q.1. What is the basic pathogenesis of DME?
Ans. Breakdown of inner and outer blood retinal barrier, anatomical disturbance of the VR interface, blood flow changes such as hyperviscosity and other changes such as retinal neuropathy.

Table 2: Comparison of dexamethasone implant and fluocinolone acetonide.

Parameters	Dexamethasone implant (Ozurdex)	Fluocinolone acetonide (Iluvien)
Formulation	Biodegradable implant	Nonbiodegradable implant
Dose	0.7 mg	0.19 mg
Duration of action (months)	≤6	24–36
Efficacy (15-ETDRS-letter BCVA gain at 3 years)	18.4–22.2 (% patients)	28.7–27.8% (% patients)
IOP rise	34–36%	37–45%
Cataract	64–67%	81–88%
Incisional glaucoma surgery	0.3–0.6%	4.8–8.1%

Note: The values are from two studies FAME (fluocinolone acetonide for macular edema) and MEAD (dexamethasone intravitreal implant in patients with diabetic macular edema). Lower complications (in the range given in table) were associated with lower dose [i.e., dexamethasone intravitreal implant 0.35 mg vs. 0.7 mg; fluocinolone acetonide low-dose intravitreal implant (0.2 μg/day vs. 0.5 μg/day)].[4]

Q.2. Differentiate between different anti-VEGF agents.

Ans. *See* table of chapter on proliferative diabetic retinopathy (PDR).

Q.3. What are steroid implants used for DME management?

Ans. *See* **Table 2**.

Q.4. What was the conclusion of ETDRS regarding DME?

Ans. ETDRS had defined CSME. It also defined moderate visual loss as loss of 15 letters or more, or doubling of visual angle, over two visits spread 4 months apart. ETDRS concluded that lasering CSME prevented moderate visual loss in 50% of patients till 2 years of follow-up. Visual gain was however seen in roughly around 15% of the patients.

REFERENCES

1. American Academy of Ophthalmology Retina/Vitreous Panel. (2016). Preferred Practice Pattern® Guidelines. Diabetic Retinopathy. [online] Available from: www.aao.org/ppp [Last accessed February, 2024].
2. Nentwich MM, Ulbig MW. Diabetic retinopathy—ocular complications of diabetes mellitus. World J Diabetes. 2015;6(3):489-99.
3. Heng LZ, Comyn O, Peto T, Tadros C, Ng E, Sivaprasad S, et al. Diabetic retinopathy: pathogenesis, clinical grading, management and future developments. Diabet Med. 2013;30(6):640-50.
4. Dugel PU, Bandello F, Loewenstein A. Dexamethasone intravitreal implant in the treatment of diabetic macular edema. Clin Ophthalmol. 2015;9:1321-35.

EPIRETINAL MEMBRANE

Dhaval Patel, Brijesh Takkar

INTRODUCTION

An epiretinal membrane (ERM) is a sheet-like fibrocellular structure that develops on or above the surface of the retina. Epiretinal membrane (ERM) can be given as a short case or spot case for ophthalmoscopy examination.

HISTORY

Chief Complaints

- *Loss of vision:* Ranges from no symptoms at all to severe visual dysfunction, usually progressive and painless.

- Metamorphopsia is common, due to distortion of the sensory retina.
- Early stages hamper monocular function, while late stages cause binocular disturbance also.
- Patients with idiopathic ERM may also give history suggestive of acute posterior vitreous detachment (PVD) in recent past preceding the ERM-related symptoms.

Past History

A careful past history can often point toward the probable underlying cause. Following things must be recorded carefully:
- Trauma
- Previous retinal tears
- Retinal detachment
- Retinal vascular occlusive diseases
- Ocular inflammatory diseases
- Vitreous hemorrhage
- Diabetic retinopathy

Past Surgical History

- Previous history of intraocular surgery may or may not be present.
- Photocoagulation or cryotherapy can also be the cause of ERM.

■ EXAMINATION

Ocular Examination

- Uncorrected and best corrected visual acuity (UCVA and BCVA) should be recorded, Amsler grid or M charts may be used to document metamorphopsia.
- Anterior segment examination can often be normal. Signs of previous intraocular surgery or trauma or inflammation must be examined carefully.
- *Vitreous:*
  - Posterior vitreous detachment (PVD) is present in the most eyes (75–90%) with idiopathic ERMs, although it is not a prerequisite.
  - Signs of degenerative vitreous may be seen.
- *Fundus:*
  - An irregular or glistening light reflex from the retinal surface may be the only sign in asymptomatic patients, similar to cellophane maculopathy **(Fig. 1)**.
  - In more advanced cases, in symptomatic patients with actual contraction or shrinkage of the membrane, distinct retinal findings can be appreciated, such as retinal striae radiating from the center of the ERM, retinal vessels straightened toward the membrane center, or tortuosity of retinal vessels and dilated retinal veins **(Fig. 2)**. Wrinkling of the retina may be noted.
  - Pigmentary changes indicate chronicity of the disease with poorer prognoses.

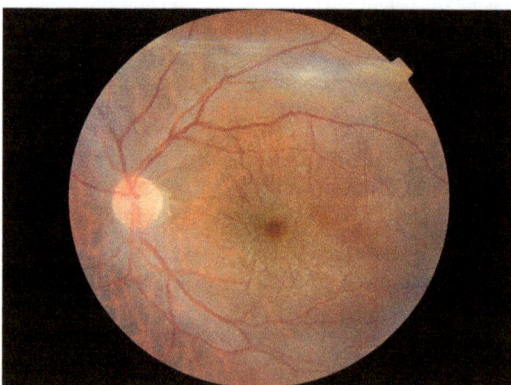

Fig. 1: Fundus photograph of early stage ERM with minimal distortion of retinal vessels. Absence of signs of chronicity and retinal distortion indicates good prognoses.

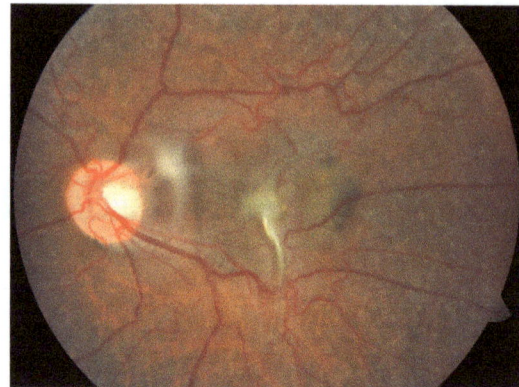

Fig. 2: Thick mature epiretinal membrane (ERM). Gross distortion of retina and pigmentary changes are visible. Such membranes ensue poor prognosis.

- A pseudohole can also be there.
- Peripheral examination should always be done for retinal breaks.
- Gass Grading System is useful in describing the clinical findings.
    - *Grade 0:* Cellophane maculopathy—an irregular translucent sheen is present in early ERM, best detected using green (red-free) light.
    - *Grade 1:* Crinkled cellophane maculopathy—membrane thickens and contracts, becomes more obvious and causes mild distortion of blood vessels.
    - *Grade 2:* Macular pucker—distortion of blood vessels, marked retinal wrinkling, and striae and obscuration of underlying structures.

■ DIFFERENTIAL DIAGNOSIS

- *Vitreomacular traction (VMT):* OCT and careful 90D examination can rule out VMT, though both may be present simultaneously.
- *Epiretinal proliferation (ERP):* It is a fibrocellular tissue found on the inner surface of the retina and is usually associated with lamellar macular holes (LMH), full-thickness macular holes (FTMH), and ERM **(Table 1)**.

Table 1: Differences between ERM and ERP.

	ERP	ERM
1.	An isoreflective space-filling material over the retinal surface, often delimited by a thin highly reflective line	Hyperreflective layer often irregularly over the inner surface of the retina
2.	It drapes over the epiretinal surface, tightly following the underlying retinal contour	There is space between it and the underlying RNFL, in some cases
3.	EPR does not have strong contractile properties	ERM has contractile properties causing striae of the inner retinal surface as well as vascular tortuosity

- *Cystoid macular edema (CME):* Presence of cystic spaces and absence of characteristic distortion of blood vessels helps in differentiating this entity.
- *Macular hole or pseudohole:* Watzke-Allen test and red beam test and in doubtful cases OCT can differentiate this entity.

■ INVESTIGATION

Following investigative modalities are useful in ERM:

Ocular Coherence Tomography

- By far, the modality of choice.
- Ocular coherence tomography (OCT) provides good visualization of the vitreoretinal juncture and shows the membrane on the retinal surface as a hyper-reflective structure **(Fig. 3)**.
- Ocular coherence tomography (OCT) also may play a role in preoperative and postoperative evaluation of surgery for ERMs by indicating prognostic markers.
- It also helps in differentiating detaching vitreous cortex from ERM, differentiating pseudoholes, and true lamellar holes.
- Disruption of the outer most hyper-reflective bands, previously termed IS-OS junction, may be associated with a worse visual outcome following surgery. However, recent focus for prognostication is now shifting toward the inner retinal layers.
- Enhancement of the VR interface by vitreous windowing helps in studying it on detail using OCT.

Fluorescein Angiography

- Not required routinely.
- Anatomic features of retinal distortion may be better seen on FA, such as straightened retinal vessels, retinal vascular tortuosity, foveal ectopia, and macular dragging.
- Fluorescein leakage and macular edema secondary to ERM traction-induced vascular leakage also may be assessed.
- One of the important roles of FA is to detect the presence of other retinal pathology, such as a choroidal neovascular membrane (CNVM).

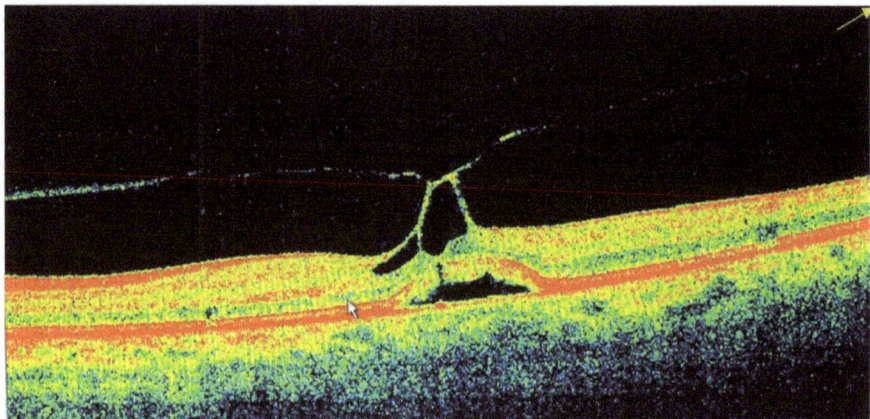

Fig. 3: Ocular coherence tomography (OCT) picture of vitreomacular traction (VMT) with fine epiretinal membranes (ERM). An impending full thickness macular hole is visible.

■ CLASSIFICATION

The different classification systems used for ERM are as follows:

Standard Classification

- *Idiopathic:*
  - Age-related/PVD related
  - Up to 20% are bilateral
- *Secondary associations:*
  - Vascular disease (diabetic retinopathy, CRVO)
  - Inflammatory disease (posterior uveitis)
  - Trauma
  - Retinal surgery (RD surgery, laser photocoagulation, cryotherapy)
- *Iatrogenic*
  - *Postoperative:* Cataract/retinal detachment/silicone oil/retinopexy/laser or cryotherapy.

Gass clinical grading system: It has been described in the examination section.

Foos Classification

- *Simple ERM:* Incidental without contraction features or associated ocular disease.
- *Intermediate ERM:* Thicker than simple ERMs and contain contraction features and pigment.
- *Complex ERM:* Present after retinal detachment surgery or after trauma and may be secondary to other ocular conditions.

Traction retinal detachments may develop as a result of contraction of such membranes.

International vitreomacular traction study (IVTS) group optical coherence tomography (OCT)-based anatomic classification system for diseases of the vitreomacular interface (VMI) has been described in **Table 2** of chapter on macular hole.

Other classification systems based on OCT and confocal scanning loser ophthalmoscopy (CSLO) are also notable, but not in common clinical use.

■ MANAGEMENT

The management options for ERM have been described below:

Observation: It is always advisable to have a short period of observation before embarking upon surgery. In early stages with good visual acuity (e.g., better than 6/12), absence of visually disturbing symptoms and if membrane is nonprogressive observation is the rule. Spontaneous resolution of symptoms can occur due to separation of the ERM from the retina as a previously incomplete PVD completes and also sometimes in secondary cases.

Medical management with enzymatic vitreolysis: Use of ocriplasmin (microplasmin) has been described by MIVI-TRUST trials. In this trial 27% vitreomacular adhesion (VMA) resolved as compared to 10% in placebo. But given the expenses and nonavailability is currently not preferred.

Surgical intervention with pars plana vitrectomy and epiretinal membrane peeling: Indications for surgery:
- High visual requirements (occupation, young age)
- VA <20/60
- Associated CME or tractional detachment.
Whether internal limiting membrane (ILM) peeling should be combined with ERM removal or not is controversial, one of the schools of thought indicates lesser recurrences while the other is based on neuronal damage caused by the ILM peel itself. Intraoperative OCT is now commercially available and may be seen to have a greater role in future (PIONEER study). Long-term results, up to 5 years, have revealed low recurrence rates with ILM peeling but with associated progressive thinning of regional macular thickness. See the chapter on macular hole for discussion on surgical technique and vital dyes.

VIVA QUESTIONS

Q.1. How do epiretinal membranes (ERM) develop?

Ans. A dehiscence of the internal limiting membrane allows retinal glial cells [predominant cellular constituent, probably derived from the indigenous posterior hyaloid membrane (PHM) cell population (laminocytes), myofibroblasts and fibroblasts] to proliferate along the retinal surface. Contraction of these membranes causes cellophane maculopathy or macular pucker. Detachment of the posterior vitreous is present in almost all eyes. PVD may be responsible for inducing microretinal breaks.

Q.2. What is the chance of recurrence after surgery?

Ans. Recurrence of the membrane after PPV is uncommon. Reported recurrence rates are low, with visually significant recurrences up to 5%.

Q.3. What is VMA?

Ans. As per definition, it refers to largely attached cortical vitreous with some areas of detachment not causing retinal structural changes. In contrast, VMT causes tractional disturbance in the retinal architecture and in the presence of symptoms it termed VMT syndrome. VMA is more likely to have a smooth contour rather than ERM. The terminology and classification system for different diseases of the vitreomacular interface (VMI) has been described in **Table 2** of chapter on macular hole.

■ BIBLIOGRAPHY

1. Albert DM, Miller JW, Azar DT. Albert and Jakobiec's Principles and Practice of Ophthalmology; 2008.
2. Bowling B. Kanski's Clinical Ophthalmology: A Systematic Approach, 8th edition. Edinburgh: Elsevier; 2015.
3. Ryan SJ, Schachat AP, Wilkinson CP, Hinton DR, Sadda SR, Wiedemann P. Retina; 5th edition. Elsevier Health Sciences, 2012.

FUNDAL COLOBOMA

D Satyasudha, Ruchir Tewari, Atul Kumar

■ INTRODUCTION

Coloboma (plural—colobomata) is derived from Greek word "koloboma" meaning mutilated or curtailed. Walther introduced the term "coloboma." Coloboma of the fundus is a congenital ocular malformation, which generally results from failure of the fetal or choroidal fissure to close during 5-7th week of fetal life, at 7-14 mm stage. This is the period between the invagination of the optic vesicle and the closure of fetal fissure. Closure starts at the equator of eye/ciliary body region and continues anteriorly and posteriorly. A coloboma may extend from the iris margin to the optic disc and involve one or more defects along line of fusion. Any ocular structure can be involved including cornea, iris, ciliary body, zonules, choroid, retina and optic disc or optic nerve.[1-3]

Coloboma can be unilateral or bilateral, the latter being seen in 60–70% of cases. Bilateral colobomas are usually inherited in an autosomal dominant fashion with variable penetrance. Recessive inheritance has also been reported. If fetal fissure fails to close posteriorly, then a coloboma affecting the retinal pigment epithelium, neurosensory retina or choroid may occur. Typical coloboma occurs in the inferonasal quadrant. There can be associated with apparent lens coloboma due to persistence of mesodermal vascular remnants that prevent development of zonules in that area leading to flattening of the lens edge. Mutation in *PAX6* gene has been reported in association with syndromic forms of colobomata.

■ HISTORY

Chief Complaints

Usual history is of a child or young adult presenting with diminution of vision for distance. In some cases, parents may present complaining about small size or different shape of eye. Sometimes presence may be noted only at time of complications such as cataract or retinal detachment (RD).

Presenting Complaints

The visual loss is typically painless detected on routine examination in a child or suddenly due to its complications. This would vary from case to case. In severe cases, the child may present with nystagmus, microphthalmos or even inability to follow objects. With concomitant iris defects, the presentation may be for cosmetic reasons. In peripheral colobomas, the visual acuity is spared but other complications may be the cause of presentation.

Past History

This is rather necessary as syndromic association is well-defined and actually may even be the reason for presentation. Typical syndromes have been discussed later.

Family History

Analysis of pedigree charts is mandatory to identify inheritance patterns. Genetics has been discussed later in the chapter.

■ EXAMINATION

Visual Acuity

It varies depending on the type and laterality of coloboma. Peripheral colobomas sparing macula usually have better visual acuity than those involving macula. Similarly, unilateral colobomas may have accompanying refractive error that may lead to anisometropic amblyopia with consequent poor visual acuity, even when macula is spared.

Motility and Eyeball

Usually, not associated with ocular motility defects. Unilateral cases may have a history of long-standing squint. Nystagmus/nystagmoid movements may be noted. Microphthalmos may also be seen.

Lids and Conjunctiva

Usually, unaffected unless in syndromic association.

Cornea

Usually, pear shaped in cases with iris involvement.

Iris and Pupils

"Keyhole" pupil due to associated iris coloboma **(Fig. 1)**. Iris coloboma may be typical/atypical, complete/incomplete/partial/total.

Lens

There can be nuclear sclerosis of varying degrees with associated cortical component, with associated zonular coloboma inferiorly **(Fig. 2)**. True lens colobomas are rare, albeit to surface ectoderm origin of the lens vis-a-vis the coloboma.

Intraocular Pressures

Usually normal, can be low in cases of RD or thigh in those associated with glaucoma.

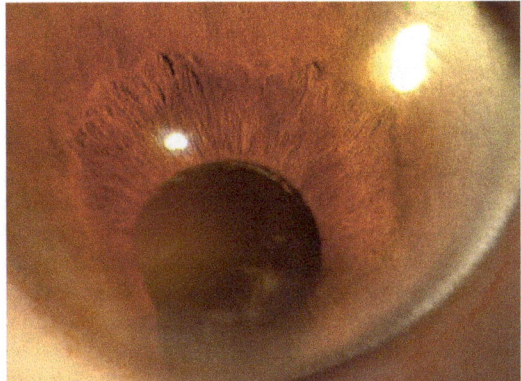

Fig. 1: "Keyhole" pupil due to associated iris coloboma.

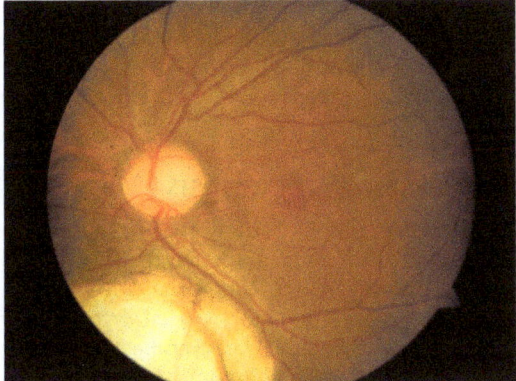

Fig. 3: Fundal coloboma with sparing of disc and macula (type 3 coloboma).

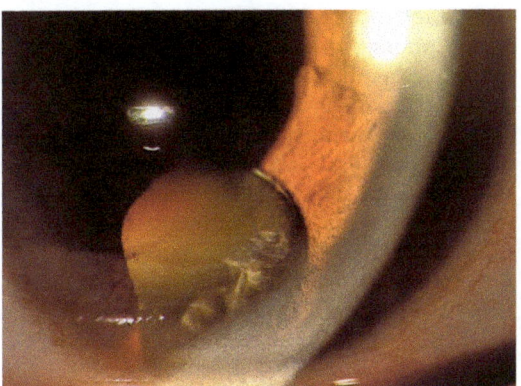

Fig. 2: Nuclear sclerosis with associated zonular coloboma inferiorly.

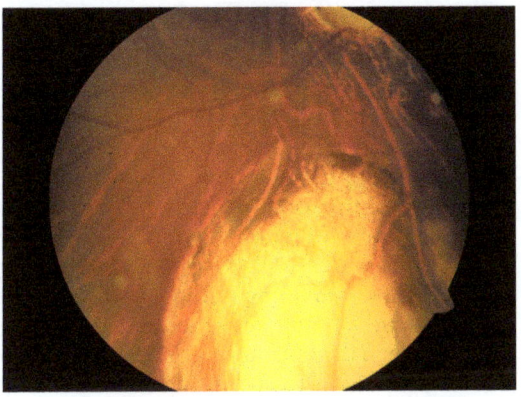

Fig. 4: Choroidal excavation in the area of the coloboma with overlying retinal vessels.

Fundus Examination[4-6]

Following findings must be noted:
- On ophthalmoscopic examination, the white background of the sclera usually showing a glistening white sheen replaces normal color of the fundus **(Fig. 3)**.
- Typically, coloboma is oval.
- Usual location is downward and inward.
- Posterior end frequently stops short of the disc (see classification later).
- Anterior end sometimes reaches forward beyond the limits of ophthalmic examination, due to involvement of the ciliary body region as well.
- Sometimes the defect can be relatively small, round, or transversely oval, or several isolated defects can be scattered along the line of fissure.
- Edges are usually cleanly cut and frequently pigmented.
- Floor of the coloboma is usually depressed below the level of the rest of the fundus.
- Two types of vessels can be seen, retinal vessels that dip down into the coloboma as they pass from the normal fundus and choroidal vessels, more tortuous and broader lying at a deeper level **(Fig. 4)**.

Macular colobomas are atypical coloboma; with causation different form that of the choroidal coloboma. Peripheral examination must be conducted for presence of peripheral retinal breaks and retinal degenerations. Scleral depression may be necessary for areas not visible to the eye as such. One must look for retinal breaks at the edge of the coloboma also. While total RD may be seen, sometimes it is present only in the colobomatous area.

■ DIFFERENTIAL DIAGNOSIS

Choroidal colobomas may be confused with infective conditions such as toxoplasmosis in macular cases and Zika virus infections in predisposed patients. Pathological myopia may also have staphylomas with scleral ectasia giving false appearance of a coloboma. Causes of large chorioretinal atrophy areas should also be kept in mind (also see viva questions).

■ INVESTIGATIONS

Systemic investigations should be done for syndromes as applicable. Genetic tests may also be needed. In hazy media, ultrasonography (USG) is necessary for charting the coloboma and identifying RD. Although not compulsory, OCT, with its enhanced penetration, is a handy adjunctive investigation, which is currently more of a research tool. It helps in identifying retinal breaks, examining changes at the edge of coloboma, though still not advocated for routine clinical use. VER may have a prognostic value and be useful in surgical decision making in long standing cases of RD.

■ MANAGEMENT

Amblyopia

Uniocular coloboma not involving the macula can be associated with refractive errors that need prompt correction to avoid development of amblyopia. In cases with bilateral coloboma, severe refractive errors may lead to ametropic amblyopia. Such cases, again, are good candidates for correction of refractive errors.

Family and Genetic Screening

Some cases of coloboma may be associated with genetic variations. Family history, including close relatives, may be helpful in identifying such cases. Genetic screening and genetic counseling in such cases may help. Other associated anomalies arising due to the defective genes may be picked up in unsuspecting family members that may be amenable to treatment.

Retinal Detachment

Retinal detachment is a known and frequent complication of choroidal colobomas. Colobomas may present with different forms of retinal detachments (see viva questions). Prophylactic role of laser photocoagulation to coloboma edges is proven effective in decreasing chances of retinal detachment. Laser photocoagulation may be performed at the earliest possible time. Surgery for retinal detachment usually involves pars plana vitrectomy, endolaser photocoagulation and silicone oil tamponade. Most of the cases have a retinal break in and around the edge of the coloboma. Use of an encircling element is controversial, though, may be advocated in cases with significant proliferative vitreoretinopathy. These cases usually have poor surgical outcomes after silicone oil removal with high re-detachment rates that may necessitate long-term oil tamponade and oil exchanges instead of removal to maintain retinal attachment. Buckling surgery has poor outcome in cases where the primary break is in the colobomatous region. It may be used in cases where a peripheral primary break is causative.

Cataract

Earlier onset of cataract is a known finding in colobomas. Most common type of cataract detected is nuclear sclerosis, being seen in almost half of cases. A distinct type of linear cataract may also be seen in the area of coloboma. As these eyes may be associated with microphthalmos and microcornea, different surgical techniques such as scleral tunnel phacoemulsification have been advocated in such cases. Use of capsular tension rings to stabilize the area of coloboma has also been described. Implantation of intraocular lens in cases with apparent small eye is aided with ultrasound biomicroscopy to measure the sulcus size.

Choroidal Neovascularization

Though rare, development of choroidal neovascularization developing at the edge of the coloboma has been described in literature. Use of both photodynamic therapy and anti-VEGF agents have been described in such cases.

VIVA QUESTIONS

Q.1. What is the embryological defect in a case of coloboma?

Ans. Following points must be remembered:
- Cranial end of differentiating CNS forms neural folds
- Optic pits appear at 21 days of life, on each side of neural grove
- Optic grooves (recognizable by 4 weeks) in neural folds
- Neural ectoderm evaginates from each groove toward surface (recognized by 25th day) as optic vesicles.
- Optic vesicle is connected to forebrain by optic stalk.
- Surface ectoderm overlying optic vesicle thickens forming lens placode—lens pit—lens vesicle.
- Optic vesicle invaginates forming double layered optic cup; lens vesicle gets pinched off by 4th week, lies in the optic cup.
- Margins of the optic cup do not grow over inferior part of the lens, showing a deficiency in this part known as choroidal/fetal fissure (usually closes by 6th week, failure to close by 6–7th week results in typical coloboma).
- Outer layer of the optic cup forms retinal pigment epithelium, inner layer forms neurosensory retina.

Q.2. What are the various types of coloboma?

Ans. The different types are as follows:

Iris coloboma
- Typical/atypical iris coloboma
  - *Typical coloboma* is in the inferonasal quadrant as this is the site of closure of embryonic fissure
  - *Atypical coloboma:* Located anywhere other than inferonasal quadrant
- Complete/incomplete iris coloboma
  - *Complete coloboma:* Full thickness defect involving both pigment epithelium and iris stroma.
  - *Total:* Extending to iris root (keyhole pupil)
  - *Partial:* Involving pupillary margin (oval pupil)
- *Incomplete coloboma:* Partial thickness defect involving either pigment epithelium or iris stroma.
  - Wedge shaped
  - Demonstrated by transillumination
- Lens coloboma—misnomer as it is actually zonular coloboma that manifests as flat lens surface visible through pupillary defect.
- Posterior segment coloboma—retinochoroidal coloboma
- Optic nerve coloboma

Lid colobomas have been discussed in relevant chapter. They should not be confused with ocular coloboma as involved embryonic layers are different.

Q.3. What is the pathophysiology of choroidal coloboma?

Ans.
- In eyes with defective closure of fetal fissure, inner layer destined to form neurosensory retina grows faster than outer layer destined to form retinal pigment epithelium, leads to eversion.
- Gradual displacement of retinal pigment epithelium, leading to development of double layer of photoreceptors facing each other.
- Absence of retinal pigment epithelium.
- Since choroid development is influenced by retinal pigment epithelium, choroid is absent in areas of coloboma.

Q.4. What is the histopathology of coloboma and colobomatous border?

Ans. *Histopathology of coloboma:*
- Sclera is thinned by loss of its inner layers, ability for ectasia increases.
- Absence of choroid and choriocapillaris *Hermann Schubert, described the histopathology of the colobomatous border.*

- Retina splits into two layers near the margin of the coloboma. The split in the layers of the retina has been identified at the level of inner nuclear or outer plexiform layer or both.
- The inner layer continues as the *intercalary membrane* onto the coloboma, while the outer layers turn back, become disorganized, and fuse with the retinal pigment epithelium.
- The choroid is terminated as a distinct pigmented layer peripheral to the point of reversal. The junction where this reversal occurs has been termed "*locus minoris resistentiae.*"
- The intercalary membrane progressively becomes thinner as it is traced centrally.

Q.5. What are the various systemic associations with coloboma?

Ans. There are many syndromes, decreasing the specificity of coloboma as an association. For example,
- *CHARGE syndrome:* Colobomatous microphthalmos, heart defects, atresia (choanal), retarded growth, genital anomalies, and ear anomalies.
- *AICARDI syndrome:* Retinal cystic dysplasia, occipital encephalocele, polydactyly, pulmonary hypoplasia.
- *WARBURG syndrome:* Hydrocephalus, agyria, retinal dysplasia.
- Goltz syndrome
- Basal cell nevus syndrome
- Meckel–Gruber syndrome
- Trisomy 13 (Patau), 18 (Edward)
- 13 q deletion syndrome
- Cat eye syndrome, Rubinstein–Taybi syndrome
- Posterior fossa malformations hemangiomas-arterial anomalies-cardiac defects-eye (PHACE) syndrome.

Q.6. Differential diagnosis of various colobomata.

Ans. *Iris coloboma:*
- Iatrogenic—postsurgery
- Traumatic—open globe injury
- Congenital—sporadic, familial, syndromic.

Choroidal coloboma:
- *Retinal scars:* Toxoplasma, toxocara
- *Congenital anomalies:* Torpedo maculopathy, staphyloma

Disc coloboma:
- *Excavated disc anomalies:* Coloboma, morning glory syndrome, peripapillary staphyloma, optic disc pit.

Q.7. What are the various classifications of fundal coloboma?

Ans. *See* **Tables 1 and 2**.

Q.8. What is the incidence of retinal detachment in patients with coloboma?

Ans. Incidence of rhegmatogenous retinal detachment in patients with retino-choroidal coloboma is 23–40%.

Q.9. What are the various locations of retinal breaks in coloboma?

Ans. Breaks can occur at two locations:[7]
- At the locus minoris resistentiae
- In the intercalary membrane:
  - 63.8% of breaks are located within 2-disc diameter (DD) of the margin of coloboma and rest in the central portion of the coloboma.
  - 54.1%—breaks at margin
  - 24.7%—within coloboma
  - 8.2%—macula

Various clinical situations depending on the combination of the breaks:
- Break at the locus minoris resistentiae only—cannot lead to retinal detachment.

Table 1: Ida Mann classification.	
I	Above the disc
II	Superior border of the disc
III	Below the disc (separated from the optic disc by normal narrow area of retina)
IV	Isolated disc coloboma (inferior crescent below the disc)
V	Peripheral with normal retina above and below (isolated gap in the line of fissure)
VI	Pigmentary disturbance
VII	Extreme peripheral coloboma

Table 2: Lingam Gopal classification (1996); types of optic disc involvement in fundus coloboma.

I	Disc outside the fundus coloboma and totally normal (27.8%)
II	Disc outside the fundus coloboma and abnormal (10.4%)
III	Disc outside the fundus coloboma and independently colobomatous (8.9%)
IV	Disc within the fundus coloboma and normal (5%)
V	Disc within the fundus coloboma and colobomatous (44.3%)
VI	Disc shape not identified; blood vessels emanating from superior aspect of the large fundus coloboma

Note: High myopia is more common in types I–III with better visual acuity. Microphthalmos is more common in types IV–VI.

- Break in the intercalary membrane only—detachment of intercalary membrane only.
- Break in both intercalary membrane and the locus minoris resistentiae—leads to clinical retinal detachments.
- Breaks in the normal peripheral retina alone—the retinal detachment will be seen to stop short of the colobomatous border.
- Breaks in the peripheral retina and the locus minoris resistentiae but no break in the intercalary membrane—the retinal detachment will be seen to extend into the colobomatous area.
- Breaks in peripheral retina, locus minoris resistentiae, intercalary membrane-total retinal detachments.

Q.10. Why is it difficult to localize breaks in colobomatous area?

Ans. It is difficult to localize breaks in colobomatous area because of:
- Little contrast in colobomatous area due to absence of choroid and RPE
- Thinned out retina
- Nystagmus
- Ectatic sclera

Q.11. What is the pattern of retinal breaks and detachments in coloboma?

Ans.
- *Type I:* Retinal detachment does not extend into coloboma.
- *Type II:* Retinal detachment extends into coloboma to a variable extent with or without retinal detachment outside coloboma.
  - *IIA: Subclinical*—restricted to coloboma
  - *IIB:* Visible break within coloboma
  - *IIC:* Visible break both within and outside coloboma
  - *IID:* Break only in peripheral retina
  - *IIE:* Break not visible

Q.12. What are the causes of low vision in coloboma?

Ans. Following can be the causes:
- Refractive error
- Subluxated lens
- Optic disc anomalies
- Macular involvement
- Retinal detachment
- Cataract
- Choroidal neovascular membrane

Q.13. What are the various complications associated with retinochoroidal coloboma?

Ans. *Complications*:[8]
- Retinal detachment
- Cataract/lens subluxation
- Amblyopia
- Anisometropia
- Sensory strabismus
- Subretinal neovascularization
- Secondary glaucoma

Q.14. What is the management of retinal detachments in retinochoroidal coloboma?

Ans. *It includes following:*
- Prophylactic laser photocoagulation posteriorly along the edge of the coloboma for prevention of detachment.
- Proper localization of breaks—if breaks are outside the coloboma with an RD not extending into coloboma then buckling surgery may be indicated.

- Vitrectomy—for all retinal detachments where breaks are at the margin or inside colobomatous region.

Q.15. Role of prophylactic laser photocoagulation in fundal coloboma.

Ans. It reduces the incidence of rhegmatogenous retinal detachment. A recent study[8] highlighted the importance of prophylactic laser in coloboma for prevention of retinal detachment. They reported prevalence of retinal detachment to be 2.9% in laser treated eyes compared with 24.1% in untreated eyes with a total prevalence of 17.9%.

Q.16. Which laser is preferred?

Ans. Diode laser is preferred over argon because of less damage to retinal nerve fiber layer owing to deeper penetration. Currently frequency doubled Nd:YAG (532 nm) green laser is laser of choice for all retinal photocoagulations.

Q.17. How are various types of coloboma lasered?

Ans.
- *Type 1 (Ida Mann):* Laser spots are applied initially along the superior margin of the coloboma and then continued along the whole nasal margin. Temporal margin is lasered inferior to the presumed inferotemporal vascular arcade and superiorly up to the superotemporal arcade sparing the macula.
- *Type 2 (Ida Mann):* Laser spots are applied starting from nasal to the optic disc. The nasal margin is lasered. Temporally, laser is performed inferior to the presumed inferotemporal vascular arcade.
- *Type 3 (Ida Mann):* Margins of the coloboma are lasered sparing the area within the temporal vascular arcade and nasally up to 0.5 mm from the disc.
- *Type 5 (Ida Mann):* Coloboma is surrounded by three rows of laser.

Q.18. Why is buckling difficult in retinochoroidal coloboma?

Ans. External buckling is difficult in retinochoroidal coloboma because of:
- Difficulty in identifying breaks in intercalary membrane.
- Impossibility of creating adhesion around breaks due to absence of choroid and retinal pigment epithelium.
- Posterior location of breaks.

Q.19. Why is PPV preferred?

Ans. Pars plana vitrectomy is preferred because of:
- Ease of identifying breaks in the intercalary membrane with more certainty.
- Removal of traction
- Closure of breaks or sealing off colobomatous regions with laser retinopexy.

REFERENCES

1. Duke-Elder S (Ed). System of ophthalmology. St. Louis: CV Mosby. 1963;3:465-9.
2. Duke-Elder S (Ed). System of ophthalmology. St. Louis: CV Mosby. 1963;3:472-81.
3. Onwochei BC, Simon JW, Bateman JB, Couture KC, Mir E. Ocular colobomata. Surv Ophthalmol. 2000;45(3):175-94.
4. Gopal L, Badrinath SS, Kumar KS, Doshi G, Biswas N. Optic disc in fundus colobama. Ophthalmology. 1996;103(12):2120-6; discussion 2126-7.
5. Gopal L, Badrinath SS, Sharma T, Parikh SN, Shanmugam MS, Bhende PS, et al. Surgical management of retinal detachments related to coloboma of the choroid. Ophthalmology. 1998;105(5):804-9.
6. Lingam G. Pattern of blood vessels in eyes with coloboma. Indian J Ophthalmol. 2013;61(12):743-8.
7. Gopal L, Badrinath SS, Sharma T, Parikh SN, Biswas J. Pattern of retinal breaks and retinal detachments in eyes with choroidal coloboma. Ophthalmology. 1995;102(8):1212-7.
8. Uhumwangho OM, Jalali S. Chorioretinal coloboma in a paediatric population. Eye. 2014;28:728-33.

GIANT RETINAL TEAR

Ashish Markan, Brijesh Takkar

■ INTRODUCTION

A giant retinal tear (GRT) is a full-thickness neurosensory retinal break that extends circumferentially around the retina for three or more clock hours. It accounts for around 1.5% of rhegmatogenous retinal detachments (RRD). Most GRTs are idiopathic (55–66%). The most common predisposing factors for the development of a GRT are trauma (4–31%), hereditary vitreoretinopathies (14.5%), and high myopia (9.7%).[1] It can be given as a short case in postgraduate examinations.

■ HISTORY

Epidemiology/Demography

Giant retinal tears have a significant male preponderance, between 65 and 91%. The mean age of patients ranges from 30 to 53 years of age. Right eyes appeared to be more frequently affected, with most studies reporting a right eye incidence of 48 to 67%. GRTs have been estimated to be the cause of the RD in 0.5–8.3% of cases in adults. In contrast, in the pediatric population (16 years or younger), the prevalence is higher and is between 18 and 31.7%.[1]

Chief Complaints

The patient usually presents with sudden loss of vision in eye, flashes, floaters, and photopsia. It may be associated with dull ocular pain due to inflammation.

History of Present Illness

The sudden loss of vision in eye is commonly associated with floaters; presentation can be unilateral or bilateral. It may be rapidly progressive. History of associated trauma or use of high power glasses must be recorded in such cases.

History of Past Illness

Past history of trauma, cryo may be there. There may be history of recent ocular surgery such as scleral fixated intraocular lens (SFIOL) or phakic intraocular lens (IOL) in an already predisposed patient.

Family History

Family history may be there (Marfan, Stickler, Ehlers–Danlos syndrome).

Past Surgical History

Past history of intraocular surgery may be there. Conventionally, GRTs would be found at the edge of heavy cryo burns.

■ EXAMINATION

Systemic Examination

Giant retinal tear (GRT) may be associated with Wagner, Stickler, and Marfan syndrome.

Ocular Examination

Visual acuity: Visually, acuity is commonly very low with inaccurate PR in large GRTs due to massive receptor dysfunction, especially in displaced flaps.

Eyeball: Eyeball may appear large in high myopic patient.

Lid: Lids are generally normal except signs of previous trauma such as scar.

Conjunctiva: Conjunctiva is generally normal.

Cornea: It may be large and corneal thinning may be there (Myopia).

Sclera: Scleral thinning may be there (blue sclera in collagen vascular disease). Globe tenderness can be elicited in presence of inflammation.

Anterior chamber (AC): AC may be deep in high myopic eyes. AC inflammation is frequent in cases of GRT.

Iris: Iridodialysis or atrophy may be there in cases of previous trauma.

Pupil: An eccentric pupil may be there in Marfan's syndrome.

Intraocular pressure (IOP): There is usually hypotony in cases of GRT. This is a characteristic feature of GRTs and is observed due to rapid egress of fluid via the exposed choroidal circulation.

Gonioscopy: Angle recession or cyclodialysis may be there in case of trauma.

Lens: Lens may be subluxated or dislocated. Zonular dialysis may be there. Phacodonesis may be present there in cases of Marfan's syndrome or Ehlers–Danlos syndrome or trauma. When the tear involves retina with patent vasculature, vitreous hemorrhage may develop.

Anterior vitreous: There may be presence of vitreous pigments (Shaffer's sign) or hemorrhage. Shaffer's sign/tobacco dusting is seen in virtually all patients with GRT.

Fundus: To examine retina in cases of displaced flaps **(Fig. 1)**, patient positioning may be adjusted accordingly (*Note:* In virtually all patients with a GRT, the tear is either partially or completely inverted. The posterior flap of the tear may invert over the optic disc or even the whole macula, making it difficult to assess the full extent of the associated RD. For inverted and mobile GRT, positioning of the patient appropriately may unfold the tear, facilitating a more accurate examination). Choroidal detachment and multiple tears are very common. Following points must be noted:
- Vitreous syneresis/liquefaction, posterior vitreous detachment (PVD)
- Extent of tear (in degrees or clock hours), location of tear (postoral, equatorial, or posterior)
- Lattice or other degenerations

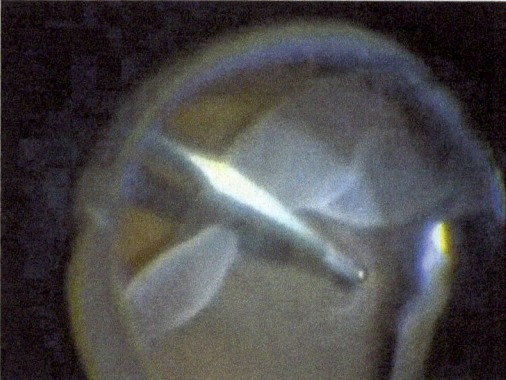

Fig. 1: Intraoperative photograph of a GRT stabilized partially with PFCL. Note the large flap of the retinal tear that has fallen over the retina. Underlying bare choroid is also visible.

- Proliferative vitreoretinopathy (PVR)/macular pucker (*Note:* PVR is a well-recognized feature of GRTs. The large surface area of exposed RPE increases the propensity for the liberation of RPE cells and subsequent PVR).
- Retinal detachment; extent of retinal detachment (total or subtotal), retinal tear flap if displaced or mobile.

Fellow eye must be examined carefully to look for myopic changes, lattice, vitreous condensation, white without pressure (WWOP) changes, retinal breaks, giant retinal tear, and retinal detachment. Up to 50% of fellow eyes may be predisposed to RD.

Classification of Giant Retinal Tear (Tables 1 and 2)

Schepens Classification (Based on Etiology)
- Idiopathic
- Traumatic
- Lattice related
- Iatrogenic

■ DIFFERENTIAL DIAGNOSIS

Giant retinal dialysis: A retinal dialysis is a circumferential retinal disinsertion at the ora serrata, frequently secondary to blunt trauma. The differentiating points are discussed in **Table 3**.

■ INVESTIGATIONS

Ultrasonography (USG) is useful in the presence of media haze precluding fundus evaluation.

Table 1: Scott classification (based on location of GRT).

1.	Equatorial	Most common
2.	Equatorial with posterior extension	
3.	Oral	Least common

Table 2: Based on configuration.

1.	GRT without retinal detachment
2.	GRT with retinal detachment with posterior flap (unrolled, rolled or inverted)
3.	GRT with retinal detachment with associated radial rips at or within the tear margin

Table 3: Differences between GRT and GRD.

Giant retinal tear	Giant retinal dialysis
Break may extend beyond the posterior limit of the vitreous base insertion	The break is located anterior to the posterior limit of the vitreous base insertion
Vitreous attached to anterior flap	Vitreous attached to posterior flap hence the tear is prevented from rolling over or inverting
PVD is usually present	PVD is usually absent
Massive preretinal vitro proliferation and macular pucker is present	PVR not massive, macular pucker is rare
Radial posterior tear extensions can be there	Absence of the radial posterior tear extensions
Vitreoretinal surgery is needed	Rarely needed; RD surgery is generally successful

(PVD: posterior vitreous detachment; PVR: proliferative vitreoretinopathy)

Ultrawide image documentation may be considered. Systemic diseases should be screened in cases of GRT.

■ MANAGEMENT

It should be aggressive. One may consider preoperative local steroids if delay is expected. Traditionally, primary scleral buckling and buckle pneumatics have been considered for early GRT. Vitrectomy is now generally preferred. In the preperfluorocarbon liquids (PFCL) era, prone position fluid-air exchange and retinal tacks have been used. PFCLs have over all revolutionized typically a GRT-RD surgery by acting as the "Third hand." Management of GRT depends on the extent and associated PVR changes.[2]

Conventional Protocol

- *GRT without displacement:* Treatment is by either cryopexy or laser (contiguous and at edge of tear reaching up to or at edge
- *GRT with displacement, mobile postflap:*
  - Extent <180°—scleral buckling (DACE)
  - Extent ≥180°—vitreoretinal (VR) surgery

- *GRT with everted/rolled up posterior retinal flap with or without star folds/macular pucker:* Treatment—vitreoretinal surgery.

Other Indications of Vitreoretinal Surgery

- Opaque media (lenticular opacity, vitreous hemorrhage)
- Retained intraocular foreign body (RIOFB)
- Retinal and vitreous incarceration (trauma)

It should however be remembered that in today's era, vitrectomy is generally preferred for GRT-related RD.

Role of silicone oil: Generally, preferred except in early stages. Silicon oil restores and holds flap in position until the time retinopexy occurs. It also counters the occurrence of postoperative PVR.

Role of perfluorocarbon liquids: PFCL is a great help by helping in undisplacing the retinal flap and keeping it in position until retinopexy is done. It acts as the third surgical hand. In highly complicated cases, surgeons have left PFCL *in situ* to attain attachment, and performed silicone oil exchange as a secondary procedure. There after 3–5 rows of endolaser are placed to hold the flap in position. For SRF drainage, PFCL silicone oil exchange, or PFCL-air, followed by Air-PFCL exchange is done. Particularly, the edge of the GRT has to be kept dried during this maneuver.

Role of lensectomy: Lensectomy has to be done in following cases—
- Increased risk of development of cataract within 2 years
- Subluxation of lens
- Presence of PVR especially in anterior PVR to get access to vitreous base region.

Surgical Objectives

- Vitrectomy, PVD, and restoration of folded flap to original position
- Remove PVR, may remove the anterior retinal flap, and manage edge of GRT
- Retinopexy under PFCL
- To drain all SRF
- To hold flap in position until retinopexy adhesion occur

Management of Fellow Eyes

Cryotherapy: It is indicated in all retinal holes, small dialysis and small retinal tears located anterior to equator.

Photocoagulation: All retinal holes, and small retinal tears located posterior to equator should be photocoagulated.

Scleral buckling: Large retinal tears, multiple retinal tears, and tears associated with vitreous hemorrhage.

Prophylactic Scleral Buckle in High-risk Eye

The following characteristic puts the patient at high-risk of having GRT:
- High myopia >10 diopters
- Increasing white without pressure (WWOP)
- Increasing vitreous base condensation

Role of Pneumatic Retinopexy

Expansible gases with increased longevity are indicated in cases of small GRT and cooperative patient with good compliance. Its advantages are—it avoids complication of VR surgery, and the procedure is relatively simple and easy. However, the chances of failure are high and chances of slippage of flap are higher than silicon oil.

Role of Vitrectomy with Scleral Buckle

This is a highly debated topic. Scleral buckle would help by supporting vitreous base and decreasing tractional forces. On the other hand, it may result in flap slipping and fish mouthing.

Complications of surgery: Complications of GRT surgery are summarized in **Table 4**.

Prognosis: Primary and final anatomical success is from 70% to over 90%, but <50% of patients will achieve 20/40 or better acuity. Poor visual prognosis factors[3] are macular detachment, hypotony, pseudophakia/aphakia, high grade PVR, GRT >180°, poor visual acuity at presentation, and persistent retinal detachment.[1]

VIVA QUESTIONS

Q.1. GRT definition.
Ans. A giant retinal tear (GRT) is a full-thickness neurosensory retinal break that extends circumferentially around the retina for three or more clock hours in the presence of a posteriorly detached vitreous.

Q.2. Differences between GRT and GRD.
Ans. *See* **Table 3**.

Q.3. What is the risk of developing RD in fellow eye?
Ans. The incidence of bilateral nontraumatic GRT at presentation ranges between 0 and 21%. The fellow eye is also at risk of developing an RD unrelated to a GRT. The rate of fellow eye RD ranges from 6 to 42%.[1]

Q.4. Classification of GRT.
Ans. *See* **Tables 5 and 6**.

Q.5. Syndromes associated with GRT.
Ans. *See* **Table 7**.

Q.6. Most common complications.
Ans. *See* **Table 4**.

Q.7. Role of PFCL.
Ans. *See* text.

Q.8. Indications of lensectomy in GRT.
Ans. *See* text.

Table 4: Complications of GRT surgery.

Intraoperative	- Slippage (around 3–15%) - Vitreous hemorrhage - Retinal folds - Rolled edge
Postoperative	- Recurrent retinal detachment (40–50%) - Cataract (40–50%) - Macular pucker - Hypotony (IOP ≤ 5 mm) - Corneal decompensation - Vitreous hemorrhage - Hyphema - Phthisis bulbi

(GRT: giant retinal tear)

Table 5: GRT classification (based on extent).

GRT I	<180°
GRT II	180–270°
GRT III	>270–<360°
GRT IV	360°

(GRT: giant retinal tear)

Table 6: GRT classification (based on PVR severity).

GRT I	Without displacement
GRT II	With displaced; mobile posterior retinal flap
GRT III	With everted or rolled up posterior retinal flap
GRT IV	With everted or rolled up posterior retinal flap and star fold/macular pucker

(GRT: giant retinal tear)

Table 7: Etiology of GRT.

Ocular	Systemic
Idiopathic (75–80%)	Stickler's syndrome
Traumatic (10–20%)	Marfan's syndrome
Myopia	Ehlers–Danlos syndrome
Lattice degeneration	
Previous retinal	
Cryotherapy	
Intravitreal surgery	

(GRT: giant retinal tear)

Q.9. Pathogenesis of idiopathic GRT.

Ans. Central vitreous liquefaction followed by vitreous condensation and formation of equatorial membranes, transequatorial forces lead to formation of large break at posterior edge of vitreous base, as if a zipper has opened.

Q.10. Most common associations of GRT.

Ans. The most common predisposing factors for the development of a GRT are—trauma (4–31%), hereditary vitreoretinopathies (14.5%), and high myopia (9.7%).[1-3]

■ REFERENCES

1. Shunmugam M, Ang GS, Lois N. Giant retinal tears. Survey Ophthalmol. 2014;59(2):192-216.
2. Ambresin A, Wolfensberger TJ, Bovey EH. Management of giant retinal tears with vitrectomy, internal tamponade, and peripheral 360 degrees retinal photocoagulation. Retina. 2003;23:622-8.
3. Al-Khairi AM, Al-Kahtani E, Kangave D, Abu El-Asrar AM. Prognostic factors associated with outcomes after giant retinal tear management using perfluorocarbon liquids. Eur J Ophthalmol. 2008;18:270-7.

POSTERIOR SEGMENT CYSTICERCOSIS

Harika Regani, Karthikeya R, Yamini Attiku, Atul Kumar

■ INTRODUCTION

Ocular cysticercosis is most commonly caused by *Cysticercus cellulosae*, the larval form of the *Taenia solium* (pork tapeworm), though other species may also be involved. It is endemic in tropical areas such as Sub-Saharan Africa, India, Latin America, and East Asia. The posterior segment is involved in approximately 68% cases.[1] In the posterior segment, vitreous cavity is the most commonly involved site followed by subretinal space.[2]

Posterior segment cysticercus is discussed here, which can be a short case/spotter in the examination with specific questions.

■ HISTORY

Chief Complaints

The patient is typically a young male and presents with diminution of vision. An aware patient can also complain of scotoma due to the presence of a cyst, retinal detachment, or scarring. Pain during ocular movements can occur if optic nerve is involved or there is concomitant extraocular infection.

History of Present Illness

Onset may be sudden or insidious depending on the presentation. It could be painful and associated with redness (particularly dying cyst causes severe inflammation and vitritis) or painless (in case of retinal detachment or submacular scarring). The presentation is usually unilateral but can be bilateral in cases of disseminated cysticercosis. Most commonly affected are patients from lower socioeconomic strata due to poor hygienic practices and food habits (contaminated fruits and vegetables with tapeworm ova). Patient may be vegetarian by diet.[2]

History of seizures, headache, vomiting, subcutaneous nodules need to be elicited in patients suspected of cysticercosis. The central nervous system (CNS) and skin involvement are more common than ocular involvement. It is rather very common to have CNS involvement in cases of ocular cysts, while solitary ocular cysts per se are less common. Overall, CNS manifestations are most frequent, up to 90% in some descriptions.[1]

Past and family history are usually not significant in such cases.

■ EXAMINATION

Systemic Examination

In general, any organ system may be affected.
- Thorough work-up of the CNS (motor, sensory, and all cranial nerves) for any signs of focal neurological deficit.
- *Musculoskeletal system:* Palpate major muscle masses (forearm, arm, thighs, and legs) for evidence of cysts in the muscle belly.
- Skin examination for subcutaneous nodules.

Ocular Examination

Adnexal and orbital examination and its findings are covered elsewhere in the book: Particularly subconjunctival cysts should be looked for, even in absence of findings such as proptosis and ocular movement disorders.

Vision: Best-corrected visual acuity with projection of rays is recorded in both the eyes. Vision can be very poor in cases with severe vitritis or retinal detachment but can also be surprisingly well maintained in a few cases.

IOP: It can be normal or decreased (uveitis) or increased (neovascular glaucoma).

Anterior segment: It can show evidence of active inflammation (AC cells, flare, keratic precipitates) or past inflammation [old keratic precipitates (KPS), flare, pigments on endothelium, frank endotheliitis]. Occasionally, a cysticercus can migrate into the anterior chamber from the posterior chamber through zonules.

Posterior segment: The cyst can be found subretinally (80% of the time being at the posterior pole, or anywhere in the fundus), in the vitreous and rarely on the optic disc. Sometimes multiple or dumbbell shaped cysts (half in vitreous and half subretinal) may also be encountered.

Gross examination of the cyst: Globular, elongated or oval, milky white transilluminant cyst with translucent wall and a white, opaque, dot-like area at one end, which indicates the position of the scolex **(Fig. 1)**. This is typical for a live cyst. On illumination of the cyst with a bright light, such as that of the indirect ophthalmoscope, the cyst shows undulating movements of the cyst wall, which is movement of the cyst wall due to a mobile scolex. The size of the cyst may vary from 0.5 to 3 cm in diameter.

Posterior segment findings:
- *Subretinal cysts:* May vary in size from 3 to 6 DD
- *RPE disturbances:* Because of presence or migration of the cyst through the subretinal space, which causes mild inflammation and subsequent RPE changes. Sometimes they may represent the site of access to subretinal space from the choroid.
- Intraretinal hemorrhage.
- *Vascular sheathing:* Thought to be immune mediated reaction to the antigens of the cysticercus.
- Retinal detachment.
  - Rhegmatogenous (Rhema being the site of exit of the cysticercus from the subretinal space)

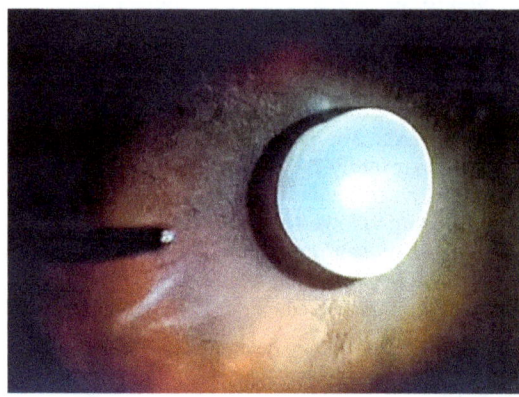

Fig. 1: Intraoperative photo of an intravitreal cyst along with its scolex. Presence of scolex is diagnostic for the parasite.

- *Tractional:* Due to proliferation of the cells over the retina caused due to inflammation.
- Submacular/subretinal scarring.
- *Severe vitritis and a picture like endogenous endophthalmitis:* Due to a dying cyst which leaks contents into the surrounding vitreous which are strongly antigenic.
- *Calcified cyst/granuloma:* A dead cyst can get calcified and may lead to a granuloma formation.

DIFFERENTIAL DIAGNOSES

In presence of mobile cysts with scolex, the diagnosis is rather straightforward. Dead cysts may cause difficulty. Else other diagnoses of retinal cysts-old RD, hamartomas, retinal mass versus calcified cyst, dropped lens as a USG finding in hazy media, ciliary body cyst, etc.

INVESTIGATIONS

Head imaging should always be done, regardless of symptoms (see above). Following investigations are carried out:
- *Complete blood count:* To look for eosinophilia.
- *Stool examination:* To find the eggs or proglottids of the worm.
- *Ultrasonography:* Cyst can be seen as a sonolucent area with well-defined anterior and posterior margins. An echo dense, curvilinear, highly reflective structure is present within the cyst corresponding to the scolex. USG is better than CT for the detection of the scolex. High amplitude spikes correspond to the cyst wall and the scolex. The scolex shows a high amplitude spike due to presence of calcareous corpuscles. Presence of high reflective scolex within a clear cyst is diagnostic of cysticercus.
- *CT scan:* Nonenhanced circular area of low attenuation with tiny areas of increased attenuation within the lesion. This confirms the diagnosis and helps to rule out neurocysticercosis.
- *MRI brain:* If neurocysticercosis is suspected.
- *ELISA:* Rarely helpful. Positive for anticysticercal antibodies (cystic lesions without a scolex with positive ELISA for anticysticercal antibodies is diagnostic).

MANAGEMENT

In cases of neurocysticercosis, ophthalmic examination should be first done to rule out cysticercosis before starting the patient on cysticidal drugs. Starting cysticidal drugs in the presence of an intraocular live cysticercus can lead to disastrous consequences by leading to severe intense inflammation and eventual loss of eye. Therefore, in cases with neurocysticercosis and intraocular cysticercosis, ocular management should precede neurological management, albeit without delay.

Intraocular cysts are best managed by surgical removal.[2,3] They are the treatment of choice in the modern era. Historically, the cysts used to be removed in-toto using large sclerotomies, but the current best practice is to rapidly lyse the cyst *in vivo* and aspirate the cyst contents with the vitrector using high suction and high cut rate. In toto removal has the advantage of allowing a histopathological documentation.

Dead cyst or dying cyst with severe inflammation is best managed by steroids. Anterior segment cysts may be managed by using viscoexpression.

VIVA QUESTIONS

Q.1. What is the life cycle of cysticercosis?
Ans. In the life cycle of *Taenia solium*, man is the definitive host where sexual reproduction occurs, and the eggs are produced. Man acquires *Taenia* infection by eating raw or undercooked pork infested with the cysticerci. These cysticerci exvaginate in the stomach, attach to the intestinal wall through scolex and develop into the adult worms. Adult tapeworms develop, (up to 2 to 7 m in length and produce <1,000 proglottids, each with approximately 50,000 eggs) and reside in the small intestine for years.

The eggs/proglottids excreted in the excreta are ingested by the intermediate hosts, pigs, in whom the eggs hatch in the stomach, pierce the stomach, reach skeletal muscle through blood and lead to cysticercus formation. The life cycle is complete when human consumes raw or undercooked pork. This cycle usually does not lead on to ocular involvement unless autoinfection occurs with the human ingesting eggs or retrograde peristalsis.

Typically, cysticercosis of humans occurs when man acts as an accidental intermediate host and consumes vegetables (salad) contaminated with eggs of the *Taenia solium*.[4]

Q.2. How do the cysticerci reach the posterior segment?

Ans. Cysticercosis is caused by the ingestion of the eggs of *Taenia solium* or by reflux of gravid proglottids in a patient with taeniasis from lower intestines into stomach and their subsequent excystment. The embryos hatched out of the eggs penetrate the walls of the stomach, reach bloodstream, and lodge at sites with high blood circulation such as the eye, skeletal muscle, skin, heart, and brain. It reaches the orbit through the ophthalmic artery and the posterior segment through the posterior ciliary arteries. It penetrates the choriocapillaris and reaches the subretinal space. Macula has been noted to be the preferred site for the lodgment of the cysticercus possibly due to the rich blood supply. From the macular subretinal space, it can enter the vitreous cavity through a break in the overlying neurosensory retina. When this migration occurs, the defect in the retina, thus, formed can give rise to rhegmatogenous retinal detachment or more commonly, this site heals with a scar due to the inflammation associated with the cysticercus migration and leads to an area of scarring in the retina. An alternate route of entry for cysticercus into the vitreous cavity has been hypothesized to be directly from the retinal blood vessel or the ciliary body.[2]

Q.3. When does cysticercus lead to inflammation?

Ans. A live cysticercus has mechanisms to evade the host immune system and only causes mild inflammation. A dying cyst, however, has faltered immune evading mechanisms, develops micro leaks in the cyst wall and leads to severe inflammation. This is the reason why a patient with live intraocular cysticercosis requires treatment for removal of cyst even if he is 6/6 at the time of presentation, and not cysticidal therapy. A dead cyst does not incite significant inflammation and may not be removed.

Q.4. What is the prognosis of a case of intraocular cysticercosis?

Ans. Prognosis depends on the presentation of the condition. An uncomplicated intravitreal live cysticercosis can be managed with pars plana vitrectomy with cyst lysis and aspiration with good outcomes (if no preexisting macular scar). In cases with retinal detachment, prognosis is guarded. In cases with subretinal cysticercosis, macular scarring, tractional retinal detachment prognosis is guarded.[3]

■ REFERENCES

1. Duke-Elder S (Ed). Cysticercosis. System of ophthalmology. St. Louis: CV Mosby; 1978. p. 40.
2. Sharma T, Sinha S, Shah N, Gopal L, Shanmugam MP, Bhende P, et al. Intraocular cysticercosis: clinical characteristics and visual outcome after vitreoretinal surgery. Ophthalmology. 2003;110(5):996-1004.
3. Azad S, Takkar B, Roy S, Gangwe AB, Kumar M, Kumar A. Pars plana vitrectomy with in vivo cyst lysis for intraocular cysticercosis. Ophthalmic Surg Lasers Imaging Retina. 2016;47(7):665-9.
4. Junior L, Perera CA. Ocular cysticercosis. Am J Ophthalmol. 1949;32(4):523-48.

CATARACT IN SILICONE OIL-FILLED EYES

Sagnik Sen, Esha Agarwal, Raghav Ravani, Atul Kumar

■ INTRODUCTION

Silicone oil with its biomechanical properties of buoyancy, surface tension, and viscosity is a very good agent for endotamponade and has been used along with pars plana vitrectomy especially in complicated rhegmatogenous retinal detachments, old detachments with proliferative vitreoretinopathy changes, giant retinal tears, endophthalmitis, etc. But, at the same time silicone oil implantation has been associated with its own set of changes in the eye when kept for a long time, namely, oil in the anterior chamber, emulsification, cataract in phakic eyes, glaucoma, and keratopathy. Management of cataract in silicone oil-filled eyes is different from senile cataract not only due to difficulty in getting the true biometry in these patients but also due to the anatomical challenges.

■ HISTORY

Chief Complaints

Usually, recurrent loss of vision following vitrectomy or in some cases no gain in vision following vitrectomy.

History of Presenting Illness

The history is generally straightforward; there is usually the history of gain in vision following vitreoretinal surgery followed by gradual diminution of vision. In most of the cases cataract develops within a year of vitrectomy, before or following its extraction. However, some patients can present within days or weeks with total cataract—in such cases iatrogenic damage to the lens capsule should be suspected. It is important to take a detailed history of the nature of the vitreoretinal pathology and the extent of previous surgery as they have a direct bearing on the success or complexity of the phacoemulsification procedure and its overall visual benefit to the patient.

Past History

History of trauma, detailed history of the vitreoretinal procedure, and pathology for determining the visual prognosis.

Family History

This is usually not significant to workup.

■ EXAMINATION

Eyeball, lids and adnexa should be examined as in any other case.

Cornea: One should look for band-shaped keratopathy (BSK), corneal pigments and corneal opacity, which may have been incurred during the vitrectomy.

Scleral and episcleral scarring should be noted and recorded.

Anterior chamber: Oil bubbles inside the anterior chamber (hyperoleon sign; **Fig. 1**) and signs of emulsification are common.

Pupil: Pupil dilation, regularity, and neovascularization of the iris (NVI) should be noted. Direct light reflex in the index eye or consensual reflex of the other eye may be used as good prognostic indicators.

Lens: Presence of iridophacodonesis indicating compromised zonules, lens subluxation, anterior

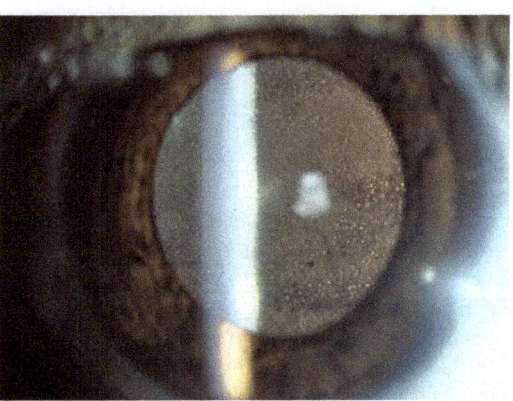

Fig. 1: Oil bubbles stuck behind the lens.

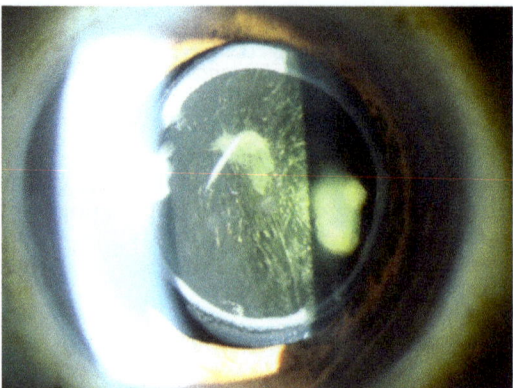

Fig. 2: Slit-lamp photograph depicting posterior capsule plaque behind the IOL after phacoemulsification. Such plaques may be later tackled with laser capsulotomy.

capsular plaque, posterior capsular plaque/defect (**Fig. 2**). Cataract should be graded as in any other case. Sometimes emulsified oil bubbles may be found stuck to the anterior or posterior capsule.

Fundus should be carefully examined especially to know the optic nerve status and the integrity of macula. One should refer to preoperative retinal findings and intraoperative findings for determining prognosis if retina cannot be examined due to media haze.

■ DIFFERENTIAL DIAGNOSIS

It includes other causes of vision loss following vitreoretinal surgery: Secondary glaucoma, band-shaped keratopathy, refractive error, retinal complication such as RD, epiretinal membrane, cystoid macular edema, retinal toxicity, optic neuropathy.

■ INVESTIGATIONS

B-scan Ultrasonography

One should remember that due to the differing sound speed in oil, the eyeball appears to be large and enhanced depth mode should be utilized. In eyes with advanced cataract, fundus evaluation with an indirect ophthalmoscopy may not be feasible and an assessment using a B-scan should be made. Here the imaging is best carried out in sitting position to determine inferior RDs as well. In addition to that, careful evaluation of the posterior capsule by ultrasound B-scan can be done if direct visualization is not possible. If the ultrasound shows an abnormally large lens thickness or an out-pouching of the posterior lens surface, a defect in the posterior lens capsule should be suspected.

Biometry

Biometry should be performed for IOL power calculation. However, axial length measurement in an oil filled eye is a big challenge. In ultrasonography, due to change of velocity of sound in different viscosity, axial length measurements also vary as compared to normal vitreous in silicone oil-filled eyes. Velocity of sound in physiological vitreous filled phakic eye is 1,532 m/s. Velocity of sound in oil is slower, being 987 m/s in oil of viscosity 1,000 cSt, causing measured axial length to be longer in oil-filled eyes.

Determining the length of the anterior chamber, lens, and vitreous cavity separately and adding these values together can calculate the true AL.

AL = ACD + LT + VCD (AL = axial length; ACD = anterior chamber depth; LT = lens thickness; VCD = vitreous cavity depth).

Theoretically, the velocity of sound in silicone oil of viscosity 1,000 centistokes compared with the velocity of sound in vitreous humor decreases by a factor of 0.64 (987 m/s ÷ 1532 m/s). It is, therefore, possible to calculate the true depth of the vitreous cavity (VCDoil × 0.64) and hence the true AL.

The conversion factor of 0.71 multiplied by the measured axial length has been reported by Murray[1] to correct for the apparent increase in axial length induced by silicone oil of viscosity 1,300 cSt.

Other alternative methods include partial coherence interferometry (IOL Master, Zeiss), which is preferred over ultrasonography to calculate the axial length of the silicone oil filled eye. It should be remembered that light speed is not affected to a level significant enough to cause falsifications in AL calculation as in USG. Axial length of the fellow eye can be used in certain cases in which axial length measurement of the oil filled eye is not possible. Previous records if available can also be used especially if scleral explants have not been used. Intraoperative retinoscopy has also been used for IOL power calculation.

Specular Microscopy

In the postvitrectomized eyes, the corneal endothelium is often compromised especially in those cases where silicone oil is present in the anterior chamber, so it is important to perform specular microscopy in these patients.

Anterior segment OCT (ASOCT) may also be used to analyze PC when appropriate to document integrity of the PC.

■ TREATMENT

Cataract surgery, typically using phacoemulsification and intraocular lens implantation, is recommended for individuals with visually significant lens opacities. Phacoemulsification with IOL implantation can be performed safely in post-vitrectomized eyes.[2] Patients who need both cataract surgery and silicone oil removal can undergo either a combined or two-step surgical approach. Most of the studies show similar visual outcome and complication rates with both the approaches; however, combined surgery offers the advantages of a single surgical event and a faster visual rehabilitation.[3] Silicone IOLs should be avoided. In presence of PC defect oil bubbles are suddenly seen in AC. Frequent AC wash may be needed during surgery for removing the emulsified oil, and AC tends to collapse often, as oil tends to rise in supine position. Capsulorhexis may be difficult to plaques and retroillumination-assisted maneuvers are typically difficult due to poor glow. The capsular opening tends to run out. Use of viscocohesive should always be considered.

VIVA QUESTIONS

Q.1. What is the incidence of cataract following vitreoretinal surgery with silicone oil injection in phakic patients?

Ans. All eyes with silicone oil injection inadvertently undergo cataract formation in almost 100% cases. The incidence of development of visually significant cataract ranges from 8 to 80% for nuclear sclerotic cataract and 4–34% for posterior subcapsular cataract (PSC) in various studies.[4,5] Although, early removal of oil has been associated with a decreased risk of cataract formation, however, cataracts have been reported even months after oil removal.

Q.2. What are the common morphologies of cataract seen in oil-filled eyes?

Ans.
- Posterior subcapsular feathery opacity, seen in early postoperative periods.
- Development of posterior fibrous pseudometaplasia and finally posterior subcapsular cataract and posterior capsular plaque.
- Formation of lens vacuoles in posterior part of lens.
- Early lens opacities leading to nuclear sclerosis, with or without brunescence.
- Rapid progression of nuclear sclerosis to white cataract with hypermaturity, often leading to leaking of proteins and uveitic changes.

Q.3. Which is the most common type of cataract seen in oil-filled eyes?

Ans. Progressive nuclear sclerosis is the most common type followed by posterior subcapsular cataract in the young patients.

Q.4. What are the various risk factors for development of cataract in post-vitrectomized eyes?

Ans.
- Older age.
- Degree of preoperative nuclear sclerosis
- Intraoperative lens touch
- Diabetic retinopathy
- Silicone oil injection.

Q.5. What is the pathomechanism of cataract formation in oil-filled vitrectomized eyes?

Ans. However, the exact cause of cataract formation in oil filled eye is not known entirely. However, it has been postulated that altered metabolism at the lens-oil interface and direct oil induced toxicity may be responsible, both leading to oxygen stress to the lens proteins leading to their oxidation. Also, increased oxygen exposure to the lens following vitrectomy, lens toxicity from intraocular irrigating solution, intraoperative lens touch by surgical instruments, use of intravitreal steroids during vitrectomy, removal of barrier function provided by the vitreous, permeability changes in lens capsule, uveitis were the various other reported causes of cataract formation following vitrectomy.[6,7]

Q.6. What are the various refractive changes seen in aphakic and phakic patients following silicone oil injection?

Ans. Refractive state in silicone oil-filled eyes depends on the extent of oil fill inside the vitreous cavity and the shape of the anterior oil surface. In aphakics, the anterior surface is convex; hence acting similar to the crystalline lens and due to the induced myopia may bring these eyes toward emmetropia. However, in phakic eyes, this anterior surface being concave and refractive index of oil being higher than that of the crystalline lens, the oil acts as a minus lens rendering the eye hypermetropic. These myopic and hypermetropic shifts have been on an average close to 6D. Further changes may occur depending on whether or not an encirclage was used during vitreoretinal surgery.

Q.7. What are the fallacies in measuring axial length using A-scan ultrasound and other methods to measure axial length in silicone oil-filled eyes?

Ans. Refer to the chapter above.

Q.8. Which type of IOL should be preferred in silicone oil filled eye?

Ans. As silicone oil can interact with various intraocular lens biomaterials with a potential of reducing the optical quality of the lens, the type of IOL used becomes an issue. It has been postulated that it is the hydrophobia of silicone oil, which influences its interaction with intraocular lenses. The more hydrophobic a lens biomaterial is the more the adherence of silicone oil; the more hydrophilic, the less the adherence. Interaction of silicone oil was seen maximal with silicone lenses, so they should be best avoided. Acrylic lenses or polymethyl methacrylate (PMMA) lenses can be successfully used. As convex-plano lens with the plane surface facing posteriorly induces minimal refractive change, they are preferred in silicone oil-filled eyes.

Q.9. How to choose an appropriate IOL power in silicone oil-filled eyes?

Ans. Silicone oil due to its higher index of refraction (1.40) as compared to vitreous behaves like an intraocular minus lens in pseudophakia. Therefore, without appropriate power adjustment, significant hyperopic overcorrection would be expected. The more curvature or power incorporated in the posterior surface of the lens, the greater is the postoperative error. The convex-plano lens with the plane surface facing posteriorly induces minimal refractive change.

The following formulas have been suggested by Patel (1995) and Meldrum[8] to find the additional IOL power to be added to the calculated IOL power to arrive at the power of IOL to be implanted in a silicone oil-filled eye:

Additional IOL power = $\{(Ns-Nv)/(AL-ACD)\} \times 1,000$

Ns: Refractive index of silicone oil (1.4034)
Nv: Refractive index of vitreous (1.336)
AL: Axial length in millimeters
ACD: Anterior chamber depth in millimeters.

Table 1: Surgical difficulties and intraoperative complications.

Cornea	Peripheral corneal injury-stripped Descemet's membrane
Anterior chamber	• Fluctuations in AC depth • Infusion deviation syndrome
Iris	Prolapse miotic pupil
Lens	• Tears in rhexis margin • Marked zonular laxity/dehiscence • Posterior capsular plaque • Unplanned posterior capsulorhexis • Posterior capsule rupture • Unplanned AC intraocular lens (IOL)
Posterior segment	• Nuclear drop/dropped lens fragment • Suprachoroidal hemorrhage
Others	Conversion from topical to intracameral anesthesia

Table 2: Early and late postoperative complications.	
Cornea	• Moderate-to-severe corneal edema • Pseudophakic bullous keratopathy
Anterior chamber	• IOP spike • Wound leak
Iris	• Chronic postoperative iritis • Irregular pupil • Rubeosis iridis
Lens	• Incorrect intraocular lens power • Intraocular lens decentration or dislocation • Capsulorhexis contraction • Posterior capsular opacification
Posterior segment	• New or persistent macular edema • Retinal detachment

Q.10. What are the various surgical difficulties and intraoperative and postoperative complications in silicone oil-filled eyes?

Ans. Surgical difficulties and intraoperative complications are summarized in **Table 1**.[2] Early and late postoperative complications are summarized in **Table 2**.[2]

REFERENCES

1. Murray DC, Durrani OM, Good P, Benson MT, Kirkby GR. Biometry of the silicone oil-filled eye: II. Eye. 2002;16:727-30.
2. Grusha YO, Masket S, Miller KM. Phacoemulsification and lens implantation after pars plana vitrectomy. Ophthalmology. 1998;105(2):287-94.
3. Krepler K, Mozaffarieh M, Biowski R, Nepp J, Wedrich A. Cataract surgery and silicone oil removal: visual outcome and complications in a combined vs. two step surgical approach. Retina. 2003;23(5):647-53.
4. Melberg NS, Thomas MA. Nuclear sclerotic cataract after vitrectomy in patients less than 50 years of age. Ophthalmology. 1995;102:1466-71.
5. Novak MA, Rice TA, Michels RG, Auer C. The crystalline lens after vitrectomy for diabetic retinopathy. Ophthalmology. 1984;91:1480-4.
6. Holekamp NM, Shui YB, Beebe DC. Vitrectomy surgery increases oxygen exposure to the lens: a possible mechanism for nuclear cataract formation. Am J Ophthalmol. 2005;139:302-10.
7. Petermeier K, Szurman P, Bartz-Schmidt UK, Gekele F. Pathophysiology of cataract formation after vitrectomy. Klin Monbl Augenheilkd. 2010;227:175-80.
8. Shamnas HJ. IOL lens power calculation: Ultrasound measurement of the challenging eye. Slack Incorporated. New Jersey: Thorofare; 2004. pp. 113-23.

SILICONE OIL-INDUCED SECONDARY GLAUCOMA

Ashish Markan, Esha Agarwal, Raghav Ravani, Atul Kumar

INTRODUCTION

Silicone oil (polydimethylsiloxane) is a linear synthetic polymer made of repetitive Si-O units and is used as an internal tamponade agent in vitreoretinal surgeries. First introduced by Paul Cibis in 1960s, it has become an important adjunct in vitreoretinal surgery. Secondary glaucoma can occur at any time in the postoperative period and may range from mild and transient to severe and sustained resulting in vision loss.

HISTORY

Chief Complaints

Patients are generally asymptomatic. However, few cases may present with acute pain, redness, blurred vision, and colored halos following vitrectomy.

History of Presenting Illness

As most of these patients are asymptomatic, most of the cases will be detected with glaucoma/high intraocular pressure (IOP) on follow-up.

Some patients may develop very high IOPs in immediate/late postoperative period and may present with complaint of nausea, vomiting, pain, redness, and blurred vision. The patient can present with these symptoms within hours or years after surgery. Some cases present with history of gradual painless loss of vision following vitreoretinal surgery.

Past History

Detailed history of vitreoretinal pathology for which surgery was done, history of preexisting glaucoma, trauma, any history of steroid intake in past or present and its mode and duration should be taken. Other eye history should also be recorded, as that of other risk factors of glaucoma. OT notes may be reviewed for amount of oil fill if available.

Family History

Family history of glaucoma is important, as patients with positive family history can be steroid responders.

■ EXAMINATION

Eyeball, lids and adnexa should be examined as in any other case.

Cornea: Corneal edema and bullous keratopathy are suggestive of raised IOP. Any band-shaped keratopathy, corneal pigments and corneal opacity should be documented.

Scleral and episcleral scarring with special concern to its site and extent should be noted, it is especially important if one is planning trabeculectomy.

Anterior chamber: AC depth should be carefully examined as patients with pupillary block glaucoma or malignant glaucoma will present with shallow AC. Presence of any AC cells, flare, hyphema, emulsified oil **(Fig. 1)** or oil globules in anterior chamber should be noted as it helps in knowing the etiology.

Angle: Gonioscopy should be performed to look for emulsified oil in angle (superior angle), NVI, PAS, increase pigmentation, and angle recession. These patients are prone to surgical failure.

Intraocular pressure measurement: IOP should be measured using Goldmann applanation tonometer.

Iris: Pupillary ruff atrophy, sphincter tear, NVI, and any iridotomy and its patency if present should be noted.

Pupil: Direct and consensual light reflex should be checked as it gives the gross idea of optic nerve status.

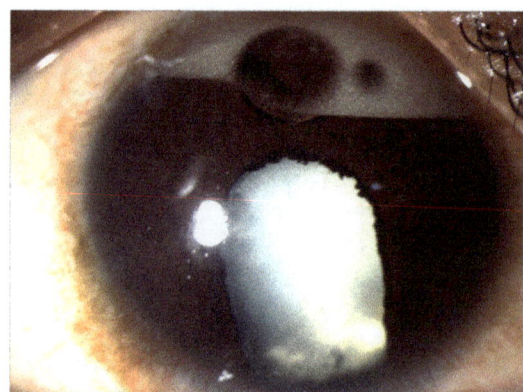

Fig. 1: Hyperoleon—along with bubbles of silicone oil. These bubbles induce fibroses in the angle leading onto glaucoma.

Lens: Aphakic, phakic, or pseudophakic status as well as presence of any subluxation should be documented.

Fundus should be carefully examined especially to know the optic nerve status (vertical cup disc ratio, neuroretinal rim, bayonetting, baring of circumlinear vessels, pallor) and the integrity of macula. A retinal examination should be performed keeping in mind the original indication of surgery and OT notes, and findings carefully documented.

■ INVESTIGATIONS

Pachymetry

As variation of central corneal thickness (CCT) in normal corneas can lead to falsely higher-pressure readings with thicker corneas and falsely lower with thinner corneas, it is important to measure CCT to know the corrected IOP.

Visual Fields

Static perimetry (HVF/Octopus) should be performed wherever possible as it helps in diagnosing as well as in detecting progression of glaucoma. If HVF/Octopus is not possible due to poor vision, Goldmann visual field should be performed.

B-scan Ultrasonography

It should be performed if media is hazy and fundus evaluation is not possible by indirect ophthalmoscopy. It can also be used to detect glaucomatous cupping of 0.7 or greater in eyes in which optic nerve cannot be examined due to media haze.

RNFL-OCT may be done, scanning laser based or otherwise. Comparisons with unaffected fellow eye are helpful to loss of NRR.

■ MANAGEMENT

Treatment is directed toward treating the etiology (see viva questions). If planning for surgery, oil removal should be considered in cases with emulsification.

Medical Therapy

- Corticosteroids and cycloplegics are indicated to reduce the inflammation. Aqueous suppressants are generally preferred to reduce the IOP. Hyperosmotic agents can be used for short-term control of IOP.
- Success rate of medical therapy in controlling high IOP in silicone oil-filled eyes varies from 30 to 78% in various studies.[1,2]

Prophylactic Peripheral Iridectomy

Inferior peripheral iridectomy (PI) described by Ando[3] helps to prevent pupillary block glaucoma in aphakic. As silicone oil floats superiorly (specific gravity 0.97), an iridectomy (ideal size 150–200 μm) done at 6 o'clock position prevents pupillary block by allowing aqueous passage from the posterior to the anterior chamber. Superior PI is done in cases where heavy silicone oil is used.

However, postoperative closure of the PI has been reported in about one-third of eyes undergoing silicone oil surgery. If the PI is not patent, treatment involves reopening the peripheral iridectomy, either with a YAG laser or surgically. If the cause is a blockage by fibrin or clot, injection of tissue plasminogen activator (tPA) into anterior chamber has been reported with success.

Selective Laser Trabeculoplasty

Selective laser trabeculoplasty (SLT) may be considered as a treatment option for the patients with open-angle glaucoma (OAG) secondary to emulsified SO which are not at high risk for progressive glaucomatous damage to save time before more invasive surgical interventions are performed.[4] It acts by activating the macrophages loaded with SO and remodeling the extracellular matrix in the trabecular meshwork by releasing cytokines, hence increasing trabecular outflow. Typically, recurrences are seen needing alternative therapy in due course.

Silicone Oil Removal

The benefit of early SO removal before the emulsification was demonstrated to be effective for IOP regulation in higher proportion of the eyes. However, the late removal of emulsified SO does not necessarily prevent the development of glaucoma as prolonged contact of emulsified silicone oil with trabecular meshwork causes organic changes in the endothelium and collagen component of trabecular meshwork leading to its collapse and sclerosis. Furthermore, SO removal itself can cause IOP elevation by several mechanisms; Firstly, due to edema of the trabecular meshwork because of postoperative inflammation. Secondly, the mechanical impact of balanced salt solution during silicone oil removal may split the silicone oil droplets into much smaller drops, which are more likely to obstruct the trabecular meshwork.[5] Therefore, whether oil removal helps or not is still a matter of debate.

Filtration Surgery

Conventional filtration surgery has a limited role and success rate in the management of glaucoma after pars plana vitrectomy and silicone oil injection.[6] Trabeculectomy in these eyes is also technically difficult because of conjunctival scarring from previous retinal surgeries. Increased postoperative inflammation and emulsified silicone oil may lead to blockage of internal ostium and trabeculectomy failure. Inferior trabeculectomy is not advisable as it carries high risk of endophthalmitis.

Glaucoma Drainage Device

Glaucoma drainage implants offer a good surgical option and have better surgical outcomes as compared to trabeculectomy in oil-filled eyes.

However, oil migration can occur through the tube into subconjunctival space inciting an inflammatory reaction and its failure.

Cyclodestructive Procedures

Transscleral photocoagulation can be used to control IOP in oil-filled eyes, but as it carries a risk of visual loss, it is generally reserved for cases with poor visual outcome.

VIVA QUESTIONS

Q.1. What is the incidence of secondary glaucoma following vitreoretinal surgery with silicone oil injection?

Ans. The true incidence of glaucoma after silicone oil injection is difficult to ascertain from the literature. First reported by Cibis, the incidence of high IOP intraocular pressure ranges from 2.2 to 56% in various studies,[7,8] depending on the definition of elevated IOP and the time considered.

In the silicone study, 8% of the cases that underwent SO tamponade experienced glaucoma at 36-month follow-up.

Q.2. What are the various risk factors for development of glaucoma in post-vitrectomized eyes?

Ans. Following are the risk factors for developing silicone oil-induced glaucoma:
- Preexisting glaucoma
- Diabetes
- Trauma
- Aphakia
- Oil in the anterior chamber
- Emulsification of the oil
- Use of low viscosity silicone oils as compared to high viscosity oils
- Heavy silicone oils
- Duration of oil tamponade.

Q.3. What is the pathomechanism of glaucoma in oil-filled vitrectomized eyes?

Ans. Several mechanisms have been proposed for secondary glaucoma following the use of silicone oil in vitreoretinal surgeries:

Early postoperative rise in IOP
- Pupillary block
- Migration of silicone oil into the anterior chamber with consequent mechanical impediment to filtration
- Inflammation
- Overfill
  - Absolute
  - Relative—due to increase choroidal thickness
- Preexisting glaucoma.

Late postoperative rise in IOP
- Infiltration of the trabecular meshwork by silicone bubbles
- Chronic inflammation
- Synechial angle closure
- Rubeosis iridis
- Migration of emulsified and non-emulsified silicone oil into the anterior chamber
- Idiopathic open-angle glaucoma.

Q.4. What is the ideal site of peripheral iridectomy in silicone oil-filled eyes?

Ans. It should be inferior at 6 o'clock, peripheral and not >2 mm because larger more centrally located inferior iridectomy may allow silicone oil to enter the anterior chamber, creating a form of reverse pupillary block with a deep anterior chamber.

Q.5. State whether silicone oil removal helps in controlling IOP in oil-filled eyes.

Ans. *See* discussion in chapter above.

Q.6. What are the causes of failure of trabeculectomy in silicone oil-filled eyes and ways to prevent it?

Ans. Scleral and episcleral scarring from previous surgery and increased postoperative inflammation are the main causes of trabeculectomy failure in oil-filled eyes. Emulsified oil droplets may block the ostium/bleb. Use of antimetabolites (MMC or 5-FU) during trabeculectomy, making large ostium, performing cyclodialysis combined with trabeculectomy may decrease the chance of failure.

Q.7. What are the other causes of glaucoma after VR surgery?

Ans. Tight explants, steroid induced, gas overfill, improper concentration of gas, NVG, malignant glaucoma, lens intumescence, inflammatory, choroidal hemorrhage, etc.

Q.8. How can one prevent migration of silicon oil into anterior chamber in patients with aphakia and aniridia?

Ans. This can be done by placing retention sutures (grid-like suture) in place of an iris-lens-diaphragm, using a non-absorbable 10-0 polypropylene "Prolene" monofilament suture with a long 16-mm needle.

■ REFERENCES

1. Honavar SG, Goyal M, Majji AB, Sen PK, Naduvilath T, Dandona L. Glaucoma after pars plana vitrectomy and silicone oil injection for complicated retinal detachments. Ophthalmology. 1999;106:169-76.
2. Al-Jazzaf AM, Netland PA, Charles S. Incidence and management of elevated intraocular pressure after silicone oil injection. J Glaucoma. 2005;14(1):40-6.
3. Ando F. Intraocular hypertension resulting from pupillary block by silicone oil. Am J Ophthalmol. 1985;99(1):87-8.
4. Alkin Z, Satana B, Ozkaya A, Basarir B, Altan C, Yazici AT, et al. Selective laser trabeculoplasty for glaucoma secondary to emulsified silicone oil after pars plana vitrectomy: a pilot study. Biomed Res Int. 2014;13:469163.
5. Pastor S. Cyclophotocoagulation: A report by the American Academy of Ophthalmology. Ophthalmology. 2001;108(11):2130-8.
6. Nguyen QH, Llyod MA, Huer DK, Baerveldt G, Minckler DS, Lean JS, et al. Incidence and management of glaucoma after intravitreal silicone oil injection for complicated retinal detachments. Ophthalmology. 1992;99:1520-6.
7. Unosson K, Stenkula S, Törnqvist P, Weijdegård L. Liquid silicone in the treatment of retinal detachment. Acta Ophthalmol (Copenh). 1985;63(6):656-60.
8. de Corral LR, Cohen SB, Peyman GA. Effect of intravitreal silicone oil on intraocular pressure. Ophthalmic Surg. 1987;18:446-9.

POSTERIOR DISLOCATED LENS

Shipra Singhi, Brijesh Takkar

■ INTRODUCTION

Posterior dislocation of lens is one of the worst complications of cataract surgery. Rarely cases of spontaneously dislocated lens can also be seen in clinical practice. Such cases are commonly given as short cases. These may include lens drop/IOL drop/lenticular fragment drop/subluxation of lens/decentered intraocular lens (IOLs).

■ HISTORY

Chief Complaints

The usual presenting symptoms are loss of vision, floaters, pain, and redness of the affected eye.

History of Present Illness

The patient may present with sudden loss of vision in eye after trauma or no visual gain after intraocular surgery or gradual visual loss in disorders associated with slow zonular dehiscence. There may be complaints related to recent inflammation. In the cases where subluxation preceded dislocation, there may be history of diplopia/edge effect related astigmatism.

History of Past Illness

History of trauma, intraocular surgery, coloboma, pseudoexfoliation syndrome, or systemic diseases associated with ectopia lentis must be ruled out.

Family History

Family history may be there in cases of ectopia lentis (Marfan, homocystinuria, sulfite oxidase deficiency syndrome, hyperlysinemia, and focal dermal hypoplasia) and coloboma.

Past Surgical History

Recent history of cataract surgery may be there in case of IOL dislocation or lenticular fragment dislocation.

EXAMINATION

General Examination/Specific Systemic Examination

A thorough systemic examination is carried out when ectopia lentis is supposed to be the underlying cause.

Ocular Examination

Visual acuity: Uncorrected visual acuity (UCVA), best corrected visual acuity (BCVA) both undilated and dilated (especially in cases of decentered IOLs/partially subluxated lens) should be checked as final management depends on the same.

Eyeball: Large eyeball is seen in high myopic patient while small eyeball may be seen in cases of coloboma. Nystagmus or squint may be present in cases of coloboma.

Lid: Lid findings are usually normal.

Conjunctiva: Scar may be present in case of previous surgery. Ciliary as well as diffuse conjunctival congestion can be there due to associated inflammation.

Cornea: Cornea may be pear shaped in coloboma. Krukenberg spindle may be present in pseudoexfoliation. Corneal edema or Descemet folds may be present in cases with history of recent complicated cataract surgery. This finding is extremely important in deciding the timing of surgery. In cases of lens drop during phacoemulsification, the wound might have been extended in an attempt to deliver the nucleus, in such cases careful examination (with fluorescein staining) has to be done to ensure proper wound closure. In addition, any vitreous twig extending to corneal wounds must be ruled out.

Sclera: Scleral thinning may be there in cases of connective tissue disorders (e.g., blue sclera in collagen diseases) and pathological myopia. In cases of nucleus drop following small incision cataract surgery (SICS) careful examination of the wound integrity must be done.

Anterior chamber (AC): AC may be deep in high myopic eyes or shallow in pseudoexfoliation. Anterior chamber cell and flare may be present (more in case of dislocated crystalline lens). ACD should be checked as an ACIOL may be implanted during rehabilitation. Presence of vitreous in AC must be ruled out by careful slit-lamp examination. If vitreous is touching corneal, endothelium there is a chance of corneal decompensation, in such cases the decision to go ahead with surgery has to be expedited.

Iris: Iridodialysis (in trauma) or atrophy may be there. Transillumination test is positive in pseudoexfoliation syndrome. Iridodonesis is common in such cases.

Pupil: Pupillary abnormalities that can be seen in such cases include eccentric pupil in Marfan's syndrome, and a poorly dilating pupil in pseudoexfoliation syndrome. Size of the pupil must be evaluated, vis-a-vis. secondary IOL implantation.

Intraocular pressure (IOP): IOP may be raised in case of inflammation or pseudoexfoliation.

Gonioscopy: Angle recession or cyclodialysis may be there in case of trauma. Dense pigmentation of the angles is seen in pseudoexfoliation.

Lens: IOL may or may not be present, depending on initial management by the phaco surgeon. It is necessary to look for presence and status of the capsular rim, as the best option is a sulcus IOL implant for rehabilitation. One should carefully look for presence of the anterior vitreous in pupil plane/AC or otherwise.

Fellow eye: Lens may be subluxated or dislocated in bilateral diseases. Broken zonules or zonular dialysis may be there. Pseudoexfoliation material may be present over anterior lens capsule. A posterior polar cataract may be present, partially explaining the complicated surgery in the other eye. Traumatic cases would generally have a normal fellow eye. In cases of pseudophakia in the other eye, look for evidence of posterior capsular rent (PCR) in the other eye; that may suggest a posterior polar cataract as the predisposing factor for lens drop.[1,2]

Anterior vitreous: Presence of vitreous pigments also known as tobacco dusting or Shaffer's sign may be there (*Note*: Shaffer's sign is one of the characteristic signs of rhegmatogenous retinal detachment, however, both trauma and surgery can produce this sign).

Distant direct examination: On distant direct examination in fellow eye may reveal subluxation or dislocation. There will be a poor glow in the aphakic eyes and characteristic crescent reflex is seen in cases of subluxation in the other eye.

Fundus: Indirect ophthalmoscopy is the most important examination. Dislocated lens **(Fig. 1)** or IOL **(Fig. 2)** may be entangled into vitreous/vitreous base or may be situated inferiorly. The location depends on the status of vitreous degeneration. One should look for vitreous hemorrhage, status of PVD, retinal tear, its extent (in degrees or clock hours), location of tear, retinal detachment, extent of retinal detachment (total or subtotal), macular edema. In myopia or Marfan's disease, there may be accompanying signs of vitreoretinal degeneration.

In case of lens drop, size of fragment must be noted as up to 20% sized fragments may be traditionally left alone. Only cortical drop can be managed easily with steroid therapy and inflammation control. Grade of nuclear sclerosis must be noted, harder lens would need fragmentation while softer lens is amenable to cutter dissection. In cases of IOL drop, it should be noted if the IOL is rigid or foldable, broken, or intact. If IOL power is suitable, the IOL may even be repositioned in the sulcus.

Fellow eye: One should look for posteriorly dislocated lens, myopic changes, lattice, retinal tear, and retinal detachment in the fellow eye.

■ DIFFERENTIAL DIAGNOSIS

Usually, the cases are straightforward. In patients with media haze, however, ultrasonography (USG) finding can have differentials such as endophthalmitis, cysticercosis, IOFB, etc.

■ INVESTIGATIONS

Axial length and keratometry or optical biometry (if possible) is done, if secondary IOL implantation is planned.

Ultrasonography

Ultrasonography is done in presence of media haze.
- *Ultrasonography appearance of dropped nucleus:* Seen as a biconvex body, which may be mobile or fixed. Lens fragment usually produces vitritis that can be seen as multiple mild-moderate amplitude spikes.
- *USG appearance of dropped IOL:* Appears similar to a foreign body showing high reflectivity and shadowing effect behind it.

■ UBM

UBM is useful in cases of angle recession, and for sulcus assessment.

Specular Count

It is done for evaluation of corneal endothelium, and it is necessary for complicated surgeries.

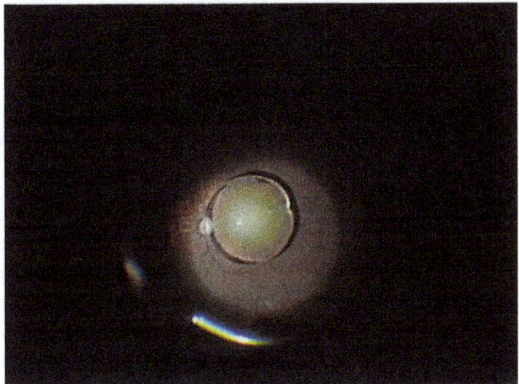

Fig. 1: Intraoperative photograph depicting dropped sclerotic lens over the posterior pole. Note nuclear sclerosis.

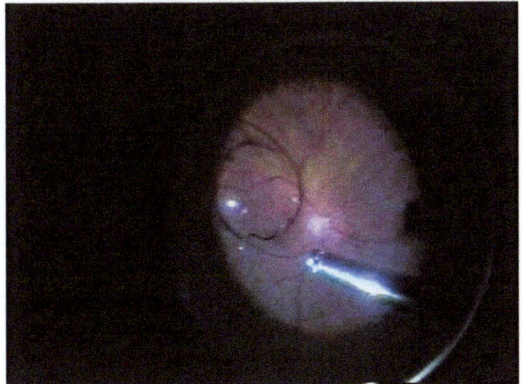

Fig. 2: Intraoperative photograph of dropped rigid IOL. The haptics are being freed of vitreous.

Optical Coherence Tomography

Optical coherence tomography (OCT) is done to rule out CME, only if suspected.

■ MANAGEMENT

The management of dropped nucleus begins at the time of first surgery itself.

Recommendations for Anterior Segment Surgeon

- Attempt lens fragment removal if only accessible.
- Perform anterior vitrectomy to avoid vitreous prolapse in limbal wound.
- Insert PCIOL or ACIOL whenever possible (unless fragment is very hard and later limbal extraction is planned).
- Close wound in standard fashion and ensure watertight closure.
- All vitreous and viscoelastic must be removed completely.
- Postoperative medication must include intensive steroid for inflammation control (both systemic and topical), cycloplegics and antiglaucoma medication. Include topical hypertonic saline drops if corneal edema is present.
- Refer to posterior segment surgeon as soon as possible.

Conservative Therapy

For smaller nuclear fragments and cortical drop, conservative management may be planned. Though in the era of safe vitrectomy, usually surgery is recommended. Until the time surgery is awaited, delayed, or planned, careful control of IOP, inflammation and corneal edema should be planned, along with regular posterior examinations.

Lens Removal (Phacofragmentation)

Surgical removal is preferred within 2 weeks after original cataract surgery.

Indications of surgery includes following:
- Nuclear size >2 mm or >25%
- Inflammation not responding to treatment by 1–2 weeks despite optimum therapy. Nucleus is full of antigens that can incite inflammation.
- Persistently raised IOP despite medical therapy.
- Retinal detachment, retinal tear, endophthalmitis, and other complications.

Factors affecting the technique of removal of lens includes:
- Size of lens
- Matter-nuclear or cortical
- Time since surgery
- Presence of inflammation

Surgery

Two routes can be used-either limbal or pars plana. The various techniques that can be used include vitrectomy cutter (for cortical matter); Ultrasonic fragmentation (for grade 2/3 hardness of nucleus); mechanical crushing between two instruments; limbal extraction of hard nuclear fragment (advanced grades/brunescent cataract). However, with modern day vitrectomy machines, vitrectomy with fragmentation is the preferred technique.

Role of Perfluorocarbon Liquid (PFCL)

It floats nucleus anteriorly and decreases complication. Chattering in the vitreous cavity is rather frequent. Perfluorocarbon liquid (PFCL) helps in management of such small pieces as well, while preventing macular damage. Additionally, PFCL also prevents ultrasonic energy-induced damage to the retinal cells.

Prognosis

Careful case selection and timing of surgery along with postoperative care results in better prognosis. Around 60–80% patients achieve a visual acuity of >20/40 with proper care.[3]

Other types of posterior surgeries: Torsional fragmentation, four-port vitrectomy with chandelier, limbal vitrectomy with electrical cutter, PFCL levitation and removal through limbus for hard cataracts, using micro vitreoretinal knife (MVR) for lens elevation.

■ INTRAOCULAR LENS DISLOCATION

Inadequate posterior capsular support from capsular/zonular rupture due to trauma is usually the basis of intraocular lens (IOL) dislocation. It can be early or late.

Early Dislocation

Completely dislocated PCIOL usually occurs in first week. Placing the IOL on anterior hyaloid through posterior capsule rupture or spontaneous IOL haptic rotation can cause early dislocation.

Late Dislocation

Late dislocation is less common. Trauma or spontaneous loss of zonular support as in pseudoexfoliation syndrome or laser capsulotomy (after YAG capsulotomy dislocation of IOL, characteristically foldable IOL dislocate due to release tension from fibrosis) can cause late dislocation.

Intraocular Lens Removal

Three different approaches are followed IOL removal, IOL removal with IOL exchange or IOL removal with IOL repositioning. For IOL repositioning capsular rim should be at least, six clock hours/180° in which three clock hours should be intact inferiorly. Best way to judge is retroillumination.

Indications for Removal

Mobile IOLs with attached vitreous cortex can typically cause complications and should be removed. In addition, IOLs stuck over the posterior poles causing visual dysfunction need removal. Conventionally immobile IOLs away from posterior pole with detached cortical vitreous have been left *in situ*. However, again, in today's era of safer vitrectomy, most IOLs are removed.

Other Indications

Substantial intraocular inflammation, CME, retinal detachment, vitreous in wound/attached to iris.

Surgery involves vitrectomy, PVD induction, PFCL injection, freeing the IOL from all vitreous tags, grasping the IOL at optic-haptic junction, careful removal through the limbus while maintaining IOP and protecting endothelium. Secondary IOL may be placed, wound closed and vitrectomy completed with PFCL removal. Complications are similar to lens drop.

VIVA QUESTIONS

Q.1. What are predispositions to complicated cataract surgery, and what are the signs for posterior polar cataract?
Ans. *See* chapter on posterior polar cataract.

Q.2. Management of PCR during phacoemulsification with prevention of nucleus drop.
Ans. It is important to recognize risk factors for complicated surgery before beginning the cataract surgery. See risk factors above.

Next the surgeon should recognize the presence of PCR early (see chapter on polar cataract). Further management should depend on the size of PCR, size of lenticular fragments pending for emulsification, and surgeon's ability. If drop is imminent, it would be wiser to enlarge the wound using appropriate viscoelastics and deliver out the lenticular fragments manually.

See recommendations for anterior segment above in chapter.

Q.3. What are the causes of ectopia lentis?
Ans. *See* the chapter on ectopia lentis.

Q.4. Discuss management of dropped lens.
Ans. This has been discussed above.

Q.5. What is optimum timing for management of dropped lens during phacoemulsification?
Ans. There are two opinions on this. Immediate surgery at the time of the drop has the advantage of a single surgery with less patient anxiety and quicker rehabilitation. Later surgery after corneal edema and inflammation control has the advantage of better and easier surgery planned IOL rehabilitation and already loosened vitreoretinal attachments. However, most surgeons believe if cornea is clear enough to allow for surgery and vitreoretinal expert is available, it is better to go for immediate surgery.

Q.6. How to rehabilitate an aphakic patient?
Ans. Spectacle, contact lens, and secondary IOLs (SFIOL/ACIOL/sulcus IOL/iris-fixated IOLs) are the options. Surgery

may be deferred if poor visual function is anticipated. See relevant chapters for discussion.

■ REFERENCES
1. Aasuri MK, Kompella VB, Majji AB. Risk factors for and management of dropped nucleus during phacoemulsification. J Cataract Refract Surg. 2001;27(9):1428-32.
2. Khokhar S, Soni A, Pangtey MS. Risk factors for and management of dropped nucleus after phacoemulsification. J Cataract Refract Surg. 2002;28(8):1310.
3. Ryan SJ, Schachat AP, Wilkinson CP, Hinton DR, Sadda SR, Wiedemann P. Retina. 5th edition. Elsevier Health Sciences, 2012.

STARGARDT DISEASE

Aswini Kumar Behera, Ruchir Tewari

■ INTRODUCTION

Stargardt disease, or fundus flavimaculatus (fundus flavimaculatus is the term designated for the phenotypic presentation of Stargardt disease in which "flecks" are distributed throughout the fundus) is an inherited form of juvenile macular degeneration.[1] It causes progressive vision loss usually to the point of legal blindness. It is the most common childhood-inherited macular dystrophy. It is commonly kept as a short case in postgraduate examination.

■ HISTORY

Symptoms

The disease is bilateral and symmetric, though asymmetric presentations may be seen. Main symptom is loss of visual acuity. Complaints of diminution of vision may first be recognized as early as 5 years but may even be seen as late as 50 years or more. Very early onset patients usually have a fairly severe *ABCA4* genotype and more sensitive foveal cones.

History of Presenting Illness

Apart from painless, gradual in onset vision loss, other symptoms include:
- Wavy vision/metamorphopsia
- Central scotoma
- Blurring
- Impaired color vision
- Difficulty in adapting to dim lighting
- Photophobia
- Slow dark adaptation

Vision is most noticeably impaired when the macula (center of retina and focus of vision) is damaged, leaving peripheral vision more intact. Peripheral visual fields also tend to stay stable.

Family History

This is extremely important. Typically, autosomal recessive pattern may be traced on pedigree analysis.

Genetics

Stgd (Stargardt disease) 1: Most common form of mutation in Stargardt disease. It is the recessive form caused by mutations in the *ABCA4* gene.

Stgd 3: Seen in dominant form of Stargardt disease caused by mutations in the *ELOVL4* gene.

Stgd 4: Autosomal dominant transmission. *PROM1* gene-heterozygous mutation.

Disease spectrum is determined largely by the total amount of residual *ABCA4* function.[2]

■ EXAMINATION

Systemic Examination

Systemic examination may not reveal findings in isolated ocular disease and are typically absent.

Ocular Examination

Visual acuity: Best corrected visual acuity should be recorded. Refractive errors may be seen. Loss of visual acuity can be as mild as 20/30 or as severe as 20/200.

Examination of anterior segment, eyeball, lid adnexa, and orbit usually does not show any findings.

Posterior segment: While 90 D examination is a must for macular examination, peripheral examination with 20 D/28 D lens should also be done. Peripheral lesions such as retinal degenerations and pigmentary changes may be associated with macular dystrophy. Typical findings include:
- Abnormal fundus appearance that is incidentally discovered.
- Light-colored flecks at the level of the retinal pigment epithelium—*more elongated than round.*
- *Pisciform (fish-tail):* Two adjacent flecks form an obtuse angle.
- Many different fleck configurations.
- *Fairly reliable diagnostic sign:* Relative sparing of the peripapillary retinal pigment epithelium (RPE).
- Uniform vermillion or light-brown color to the fundus with complete obscuration of the underlying choroidal details.
- Frank RPE atrophy is commonly seen in the center of the macula and the bases of these atrophic lesions have a metallic sheen **(Fig. 1)**.
- "Beaten-bronze" appearance.
- Choroidal neovascular membranes (CNVMs) and subretinal bleeding may be seen as complications.

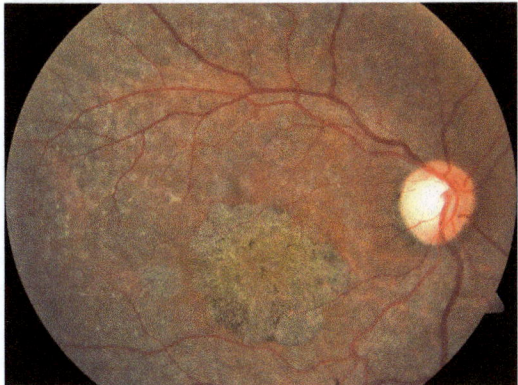

Fig. 1: Macular atrophy and flecks in a case of macular dystrophy. Note the pigment mottling and temporal disc pallor.

There is interplay of three factors:
1. Severity of *ABCA4* genotype (determines rate at which toxic bisretinoids are formed in the photoreceptors).
2. Relative sensitivity of the foveal cones to the genotype.
3. Relative sensitivity of the retinal pigment epithelium to the genotype.

■ DIFFERENTIAL DIAGNOSIS

Differentials of Bull's eye maculopathy:
- Stargardt diseases
- Cone and cone-rod dystrophy
- Chloroquine retinal toxicity
- Age-related macular degeneration (ARMD)
- Chronic macular hole
- Central areolar choroidal dystrophy
- Olivopontocerebellar atrophy
- Ceroid lipofuscinosis

Other macular dystrophies should be kept as differential diagnosis.

■ INVESTIGATIONS

Autofluorescence

Due to lipofuscin deposits, hyper-autofluorescence may be elicited. However, diagnostic reliability is low as some patients can have hypo-autofluorescence also. Amount/density of autofluorescence may be utilized in follow-up also.[3]

Fundus Fluorescein Angiography Finding

- Complete masking of the choroidal circulation.
- With angiography, the dye-filled retinal vessels lie upon a completely hypofluorescent background that results in a finding variously known as a dark, silent, or masked choroid.[4]

Optical Coherence Tomography

Optical coherence tomography (OCT) can reveal the extent of outer retinal loss and RPE atrophy and it can also distinguish the anatomic level of flecks with accuracy. Choroidal layer changes have also been studied, though concrete evidence is lacking. Choriocapillaris may be lost. Late stages reveal thinned out macula and may catch CNVMs or SRF.

Electrophysiology

As full-field ERG represents a mass response of all photoreceptors, it is typically normal in patients with Stargardt disease. Cone and rod functions may be affected in severe *ABCA4* genotypes.[5] Multifocal electroretinogram (mfERG) is a sensitive tool in detecting very early involvement in even clinically normal cases. A significant decrease in ERG wave form amplitudes is noted in all rings, even the most peripheral eccentricity group 10–31°, although the change from normal goes on decreasing as we move from central to peripheral eccentricity rings.

Visual Field Testing

Visual field testing in Stargardt patients is often normal in early disease stages.

Over time, relative central scotomas develop which progress to absolute central scotomas. Color vision and contrast sensitivity may be done for progressions or as ancillary tests, but do not add to diagnosis.

■ MANAGEMENT

There is currently no proven treatment for this disease. Since a primary defect in *ABCA4*-associated retinal disease is an accumulation of toxic bisretinoids in the RPE and photoreceptors, drugs that modulate the visual cycle (e.g., Isotretinoin and fenretinide), have been investigated for their potential to slow the formation of these toxic products.

Gene therapy and cell replacement may be upcoming treatment modality.

Visual Rehabilitation

Low vision aids (LVA)—such as magnifying glasses may be helpful in cases with macular atrophy.

Patient Counseling

- Stargardt patients should be encouraged to maintain good sun protection, as exposure to bright light can lead to the formation of all-transretinal in photoreceptors and contribute to lipofuscin accumulation.
- Avoidance of cigarette smoking or avoidance of high-dose vitamin A supplements, including AREDS vitamins, because of their potential to increase the formation of bisretinoids in the retina.
- Sibling screening and genetic counseling is important.
- These patients should be kept on follow-up for documenting progression and treating complications.

VIVA QUESTIONS

Q.1. Name few macular dystrophies.
Ans. *See* Table 1.

Q.2. What are differential diagnoses of Bull's eye maculopathy?
Ans. *See* the section on differential diagnosis.

Q.3. What is Stargardt-like dominant macular dystrophy (SLDMD)?
Ans. *Stargardt-like dominant macular dystrophy (SLDMD).*
- Autosomal dominant
- Chromosome 6

Table 1: Common examples of macular dystrophy.

Macular dystrophy	Gene	Chromosome	Pattern
Best macular dystrophy	BEST1	11	AD/AR
Stargardt disease	ABCA4	1	AR
Stargardt-like dominant macular dystrophy	ELOVL4	6	AD
Pattern dystrophy	PRPH2	6	AD
Sorsby fundus dystrophy	TIMP3	22	AD
Autosomal dominant radial drusen	EFEMP1	2	AD

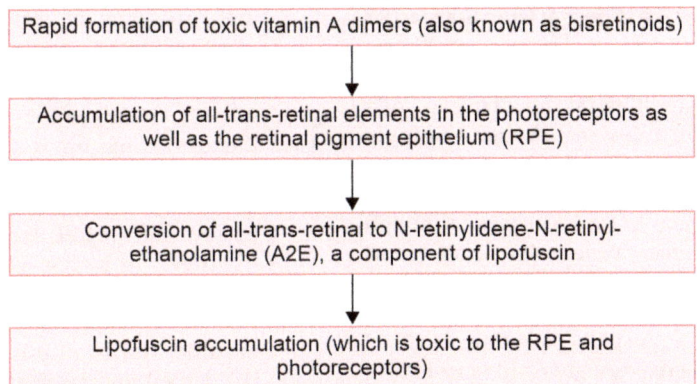

Flowchart 1: Pathophysiology of Stargardt disease.

- *Elovl4 gene:* Elongation of very long chain fatty acids-4
- Most characteristic features of this disease are circular zone of RPE atrophy, a pigmented spot beneath the fovea, and a ring of flecks just beyond the margin of the atrophy
- ERG is usually normal.

Q.4. What are the fundus findings in Stargardt disease?

Ans. *See* above.

Q.5. What is the pathophysiology of Stargardt disease?

Ans. *See* **Flowchart 1**.

Q.6. What is Fishman classification of Stargardt disease?

Ans. *See* **Table 2**.

Q.7. What is fundus flavimaculatus?

Ans. Fundus flavimaculatus and Stargardt disease are varied clinical presentation of the same disease process and belong at both ends of the clinical spectrum. Pure Stargardt disease presents with macular involvement and pure fundus flavimaculatus presents with multiple mid peripheral "fleck" lesions with preservation of macular region. In most cases, a mixed presentation is usually seen. In general, patients with extensive extramacular flecks have poorer long-term visual prognosis than patients with only macular involvement.

Table 2: Fishman classification of Stargardt disease.

Stage 1	• *Fundus:* Pigmentary change in macula, "beaten-bronze" appearance • *ERG:* Normal
Stage 2	• *Fundus:* Flecks beyond 1 DD from margin of fovea, extending beyond arcade • *ERG:* Normal. • Prolonged period of dark adaptation
Stage 3	• *Fundus:* Diffuse flecks and choriocapillary atrophy at macula • *ERG:* Subnormal cone and rod amplitude • Central field defect as well as peripheral/midperipheral field impairment
Stage 4	• *Fundus:* Diffuse flecks and extensive RPE atrophy throughout the fundus • *ERG:* Reduced cone and rod amplitude Peripheral field—moderate-to-extensive restriction

Q.8. What are fleck lesions?

Ans. These are accumulations of lipofuscin seen at the RPE level. They are usually more elongated than drusens and may connect with each other forming a net-like branching pattern. Different shapes, size, color, and location can be seen. They may remain stable in number and location with preservation of visual acuity or may grow in size leading to widespread atrophy and decline in vision.

Q.9. What is best dystrophy? What are it stages? How is it different from Stargardt?

Ans. Best disease is a juvenile onset vitelliform macular dystrophy that is characterized by classic single bilateral macular egg yolk-like vitelliform lesions, though, multiple lesions involving the posterior pole may be seen. It has an autosomal dominant mode of inheritance in typical cases, although autosomal recessive inheritance as well as adult onset has been described. The classic lesions typically appear in early childhood, though are not usually picked up as visual acuity remains very good till very late in the disease process. Different stages for the lesions are described but the disease may not follow specific staging pattern.

Stages:
- Previtelliform
- Vitelliform
- Pseudohypopyon
- Vitelliruptive
- Atrophic

On SD-OCT, the vitelliform lesions represent accumulation of hyper-reflective material in the subretinal space. Full field ERG is typically normal. EOG is a specific investigation for Best disease. An Arden ratio of <1.5 is said to be characteristic of Best disease.

Cases with Best disease differ from Stargardt disease in many ways:
- Presence of a well-defined yellow lesion at the macula
- Maintained visual acuity till late stages
- Absence of flecks
- Electrooculogram (EOG) <1.5 with normal ERG
- Characteristic SD-OCT with presence of subretinal hyper-reflective material.

It may become difficult to clinically distinguish the two in cases with atrophic Best disease as only well-defined central atrophy might be present in such cases. EOG may be diagnostic in such cases. Also, autosomal dominant inheritance with presence of lesions in otherwise asymptomatic relatives may help in diagnosis.

Q.10. What is Arden's ratio?

Ans. Electrooculogram is a measure of the difference in standing potential of the eye between the cornea that is electrically positive and the RPE that is electronegative. As there is much variation in EOG amplitudes, a ratio known as the Arden ratio, which represents ratio between the maximal height of potential in the light (light rise) and minimal potential in the dark (dark trough) is used to quantify the EOG values. Most of the responses are manifested due to photoreceptor activity and RPE. Electrooculogram is a specific investigation for Best disease. A highly abnormal EOG with normal ERG is diagnostic of Best disease.

REFERENCES

1. Hadden OB, Gass JD. Fundus flavimaculatus and Stargardt's disease. Am J Ophthalmol. 1976;82:527-39.
2. Cremers FP, van de Pol DJ, van Driel M, den Hollander AI, van Haren FJ, Knoers NV, et al. Autosomal recessive retinitis pigmentosa and cone-rod dystrophy caused by splice site mutations in the Stargardt's disease gene ABCR. Hum Mol Genet. 1998;7:355-62.
3. Lois N, Halfyard AS, Bird AC, Holder GE, Fitzke FW. Fundus autofluorescence in Stargardt macular dystrophy-fundus flavimaculatus. Am J Ophthalmol. 2004;138:55-63.
4. Jayasundera T, Rhoades W, Branham K, Niziol LM, Musch DC, Heckenlively JR. Peripapillary dark choroid ring as a helpful diagnostic sign in advanced Stargardt disease. Am J Ophthalmol. 2010;149:656-60.e2.
5. Schindler EI, Nylen EL, Ko AC, Affatigato LM, Heggen AC, Wang K, et al. Deducing the pathogenic contribution of recessive ABCA4 alleles in an outbred population. Hum Mol Genet. 2010;19:3693-701.

TRAUMATIC RETINAL DETACHMENT

Priyanka Ramesh, Shreyas Temkar, Dheepak Sundar, Atul Kumar

■ INTRODUCTION

Traumatic retinal detachment accounts for 12% of all rhegmatogenous retinal detachment (RD) and is the most common cause of rhegmatogenous RD (RRD) in children. RD can occur both following open globe and closed globe injury. In closed globe injury, the detachment is following a retinal tear or dialysis, whereas in an open globe injury, the retinal detachment is due to vitreous traction following vitreous prolapse or direct injury-related break.[1]

■ HISTORY

Sometimes it is easy to link trauma to RD, whereas sometimes the patient may try to hide the history or may even have forgotten it. The onus is on the ophthalmologist to identify the precipitating event in the latter case.

Chief Complaints

The patient can present in following ways:
- Sudden onset of field loss and diminution of vision.
- Incidental RD may also be detected while managing for other manifestations of trauma.

It is usually seen in young male patients with definitive history of trauma either blunt or penetrating. Patients can present either immediately following trauma or can present until usually about 2 years following trauma.

History of Presenting Illness

Detailed history about when the trauma occurred, the mode of injury has to be taken. In addition, following points must be enquired:
- History of any surgical intervention such as corneal/scleral perforation repair has to be noted.
- If a patient is presenting late after trauma, then the previous ocular findings, visual acuity has to be reviewed. This may help in case wise prognostication. Children typically present late after trauma. All these points become very crucial in a medicolegal case.
- History of trauma should always be ruled out on leading questions in unexplained ophthalmic cases.

Past History

History of any surgical procedures done before the trauma or for its management has to be taken. History of recurrent trauma may indicate patient abuse or even self-mutilation (mentally challenged) or poor functional status of vision.

Family History

In doubtful cases, family history of retinal disorders must be inquired for.

■ EXAMINATION

Systemic Examination

History of loss of consciousness, ENT bleeds, and seizures have to be evaluated in case of multiple injuries. In cases of polytrauma, other system involvement has to be assessed. These patients would require multidiscipline management.

Ocular Examination

Visual acuity: Best-corrected visual acuity of both eyes with projection of rays has to be checked.

While pure retinal detachment may cause inaccurate PR rarely, it can be present in post-traumatic cases, which suggest concomitant optic nerve damage and hence poor visual prognosis.

Eyeball: Presence of squint, ocular movement restrictions, enophthalmos, discontinuity in the orbital rim has to be checked to rule out any orbital trauma. It is not uncommon to see signs of blow out fractures.

Lids, conjunctiva: May show signs of trauma. There may be lid laceration or subconjunctival hemorrhage. Complex lacerations may need a plastic surgical review.

Sclera: In fresh cases, one should always look at the integrity of the globe and rule out the presence of any scleral rupture. In doubtful delayed cases, a thorough examination should be done as posterior as possible for signs of old repaired scleral wounds.

Cornea: In fresh cases, there may be a corneal laceration and in old cases, there might be scars of previously operated corneal laceration or of a self-sealed corneal wound. Limbal scars are common in blunt trauma-related open globe injury.

Anterior chamber: In acute injury there might be hyphema in the anterior chamber. Detailed examination must be done to check for any signs of inflammation-like cells and flare.

Iris: There might be associated iridodialysis, which appears as a D-shaped pupil and best confirmed on a distant direct examination. The iris may also show presence of sphincter tears and traumatic mydriasis, which causes anisocoria. Sphincter tears may also be seen.

Gonioscopy: It is necessary to do gonioscopy in all patients with trauma to rule out angle recession. Findings must always be compared with the other eye. There will be increased width of the ciliary body band and increased pigmentation. Cyclodialysis can also be picked up on gonioscopy.

Lens: It can be cataractous ranging from total cataract to posterior subcapsular variety, typically the rosette cataract. There can also be associated subluxation/dislocation of the lens. These patients will have phacodonesis and iridodonesis. One should keenly examine for presence of the Vossius ring.

Pupillary reactions: Direct and consensual reflexes must be checked in both eyes and swinging torch light test must be done for relative afferent pupillary defect (RAPD). In case the affected eye has traumatic mydriasis or there is obscuration of the pupil due to hyphema then the consensual in the other eye becomes a very important predictor of an intact optic nerve.

Intraocular pressure (IOP): In the presence of retinal detachment, the IOP is usually low, but in the presence of angle recession or increased inflammation, there might be raised IOP.

Posterior segment: The idea is two pronged—identify signs of trauma and work-up for RD. The vitreous cavity may show the presence of vitreous hemorrhage in acute cases. If the posterior segment details are obscured due to vitreous hemorrhage, an ultrasonography (USG) of the posterior segment is required to rule out retinal detachment.

If the fundus is visible, then the fundus has to be examined thoroughly to look for:
- All retinal breaks have to be localized.
- Indentation indirect ophthalmoscopy has to be done to check for dialysis and vitreous base avulsion.
- Retinal dialysis is typical for blunt trauma; SN is pathognomonic while IT is most common.[2,3]
- Other indicative breaks include giant retinal tear (GRT), ragged margin multiple tears, etc. As such, any kind of break may be seen. Work-up should be done for retinal detachment. Young patients with delayed presentation will have chronic RD often with signs of proliferative vitreoretinopathy (PVR) (**Fig. 1**).
- Other signs of trauma such as commotio retinae, subretinal bleed, choroidal rupture, macular hole should be looked for.[4]
- Optic disc must be evaluated for presence of traumatic optic neuropathy or for glaucomatous changes.
- Other eye examination is necessary for satisfying Cox's postulates in doubtful cases.

See **Table 1** for posterior segment signs of trauma.

DIFFERENTIAL DIAGNOSIS

See chapter on RD. Specifically in a patient with GRT differentials such as myopia, iatrogenic and

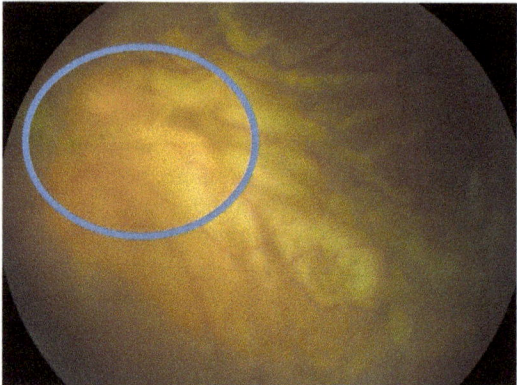

Fig. 1: PVR in a case of traumatic RD. Note the encircled peripheral retinal fold.

Retina

Table 1: Posterior segment signs of trauma.

Closed globe injury	Open globe injury
• Vitreous base avulsion • Retinal tears (dialysis, horseshoe tears, operculated holes, and tears with ragged margins) • Retinal detachment • Commotio retinae • Macular hole • Choroidal rupture • Subretinal bleed and submacular hemorrhage • Vitreous hemorrhage • Choroidal hemorrhage • Posteriorly dislocated lens/IOL • Retinitis sclopetaria • Traumatic optic neuropathy • Optic nerve head avulsion	• Scleral rupture/penetration • Retinal tears • Retinal detachment • Proliferative vitreoretinopathy • Retained intraocular foreign body • Endophthalmitis

idiopathic, and in patients with retinal dialysis, inferior temporal retinal dialysis of young should be kept in mind (see discussion). Ragged margin breaks may also be due to viral retinitis-related necrosis.

■ INVESTIGATIONS

USG B scan: It can be used to rule out RD in patients where the visualization of the retina is hampered. It can show vitreous incarceration in few cases. USG is also useful to rule out presence of retained intraocular foreign body.

X-ray orbit: Used to rule out orbital fractures or any retained intraocular foreign body.

Optical coherence tomography: It may be done for concomitant macular changes due to trauma.

Visual evoked response (VER): It is useful in cases of old RD and those in which traumatic neuropathy is suspected.

■ MANAGEMENT

Medicolegal cases need proper documentation while a multidepartment approach may be needed. Other concomitant manifestations of trauma may need management. See chapter of RD for detailed management and figures. In patients with blunt trauma, it is necessary to rule out retinal dialysis. PVD is typically absent in these patients. Prognostication is of the essence as these patients typically need recurrent surgeries and have poor outcomes. Complications such as postoperative glaucoma and cataract are frequent.

In patients with open globe injury, it is necessary to secure the wound in the coats.

VIVA QUESTIONS

Q.1. What are the mechanical changes in the globe following blunt trauma?

Ans. *Changes occur in four phases:*
1. Compression
2. Decompression
3. Overshooting
4.. Oscillations

Blunt trauma typically causes anteroposterior compression with equatorial expansion of the globe.

Q.2. What are the types of retinal breaks seen following blunt trauma and what is the mechanism of breaks?

Ans. Blunt trauma (ocular contusion) results in numerous types of breaks such as retinal dialysis, horseshoe tears, giant retinal tears (GRT), operculated holes, and macular hole. These breaks can be due to coup injury causing breaks at the site of trauma or counter coup, opposite the site of trauma and are usually located predominantly in the vitreous base region. Breaks caused by retinal necrosis occur slowly and show ragged, uneven edges.

Q.3. What is the definition of retinal dialysis and what is the most common location of dialysis following trauma?

Ans. Retinal dialysis is defined as disinsertion of the retina from the nonpigmented epithelium of the ciliary body at the ora serrata. It accounts for 8–14% of the retinal detachments. GRT and dialysis account for 69% of all traumatic detachments.

Most common location is inferotemporal accounting for 66% of cases. This is because the inferotemporal quadrant is least protected based on orbital anatomy. Superonasal location is the most pathognomonic of trauma. Weidenthal and Schepens reported that nasal retina has greater susceptibility to traumatic retinal dialysis secondary to its narrow vitreous base. The mean size of post-traumatic dialysis is around 2.4 clock hours.

Q.4. When does retinal detachment occur following trauma?

Ans. Retinal detachment immediately following trauma is rare and in general the detachment progresses slowly occurring weeks to months following trauma. This is because of the presence of formed vitreous in young patients. Following points must be remembered:
- 12% detachments are identified immediately.
- 30% detachments are identified within 1 month.
- 50% detachments are identified within 8 months.
- 80% detachments are identified by 24 months.

GRT following trauma usually shows a rapid progression.

Q.5. What is the mechanism of retinal detachment following open globe injury?

Ans. In the presence of open globe injury, the vitreous is incarcerated in the wound and there is fibrous ingrowth along the vitreous scaffold. There is also breakdown of blood retinal barrier, which initiates an inflammatory response causing proliferation of pigment epithelial cells, fibroblasts, and glial cells. These produce collagenous extracellular matrix, which causes contraction. This causes traction on the peripheral retina, rolling forward at the vitreous base and junction of the ora. Over weeks, the proliferation progresses and causes cyclitic membrane, epiretinal membrane, and retro retinal membrane. There can also be abrupt PVD causing retinal breaks.

Q.6. What are the seven rings of trauma?

Ans. Blunt trauma can result in injury to various tissues of the eye. Seven rings of tissues affected by blunt trauma to the eye are:
- Tears in Sphincter pupillae—seen as disruption of pupillary margin on slit lamp.
- Iridodialysis—seen as dehiscence of iris from the sclera with a D-shaped pupil.
- Angle recession—characterized by separation of circular muscle fibers from longitudinal fibers of ciliary body. There is posterior displacement of the iris and widening of ciliary body band on gonioscopy. It is always important to confirm this finding by comparing with the fellow eye.
- *Cyclodialysis:* Separation of ciliary body attachment from scleral spur. This can result in hypotony.
- Trabecular meshwork tears.
- Zonular dialysis resulting in subluxation of the crystalline lens.
- Retinal dialysis—disinsertion of the retina from nonpigmented epithelium of ciliary body at the ora serrata.

Inferotemporal quadrant is most commonly involved but superonasal dialysis is pathognomonic of trauma.

Q.7. What are the posterior segment signs of trauma?

Ans. *See* **Table 1**.

Q.8. What are the Cox's postulates for traumatic retinal detachment?

Ans. In some cases it is difficult to differentiate between spontaneous retinal detachments from those occurring due to trauma. Cox, Schepens, and Freeman gave certain postulates, which could point toward occurrence of retinal detachment from trauma. They include:
- Unilateral retinal detachment preceded by ocular contusion.
- Objective signs of contusion in the affected eye.

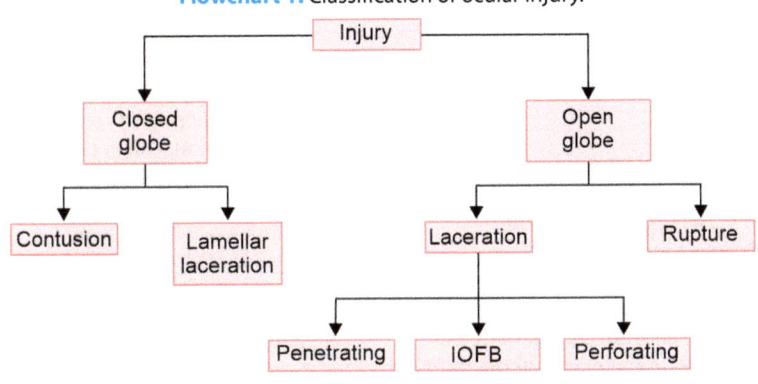

Flowchart 1: Classification of ocular injury.

(IOFB: intraocular foreign body)

- Absence of visible vitreoretinal degeneration of the types known to cause retinal breaks in both the affected and fellow eyes.

Q.9. What is inferior temporal dialysis of young?

Ans. The patient is typically young male and has unilateral or bilateral retinal dialysis in the inferior temporal area. Sometimes other changes such as WWOP, retinal cystic degeneration, and pigmentation/holes may be there. The causation is related to abnormal development of the inferior temporal pars plana, which normally develops the last. This is an important differential of a case of traumatic RD with retinal dialysis.

Q.10. Tell in brief about BETT classification.

Ans. This system utilizes definitions that refer to the entire globe, not to a specific tissue. This solves the problem of using confusing terms with respect to individual tissues.

Flowchart 1 showing clinical classification of injuries based on BETT system.

BETT system also defines these injuries as follows:
- *Eye wall:* Sclera and cornea
- *Closed globe injury:* No full-thickness wound of eye wall
- *Open globe injury:* Full-thickness wound of the eye wall
- Contusion no wound of the eye wall. The damage may be due to direct shock wave by the object (e.g., choroidal rupture), or to changes in the shape of the globe (e.g., angle recession)
- *Lamellar laceration:* Partial-thickness wound of the eye wall
- *Rupture:* Full-thickness wound of the eye wall, caused by a large blunt object
- *Laceration:* Full-thickness wound of the eye wall, caused by a sharp object
- *Penetrating injury:* An entrance wound is present.
- *IOFB:* One or more foreign objects are present.
- *Perforating injury:* Both an entrance and an exit wound are present.

Based on the Birmingham Eye Trauma Terminology, injured eyes are categorized by four parameters:
- *Type* (based on the mechanism of trauma):
  Closed globe injury
  – Concussion
  – Lamellar laceration
  – Superficial foreign body
  – Mixed
- *Open globe injury*
  – Rupture
  – Penetration

- Perforation
- Retained intraocular foreign body
- Mixed
- *Grade* (based on visual acuity at presentation):
  - VA >20/40
  - VA 20/50–20/100
  - VA 19/100–5/200
  - VA 4/200–light perception
  - No light perception
- *Pupil:*
  - Positive afferent pupillary defect
  - Negative afferent pupillary defect
- *Zone* (based on the extent of the injury):
  - Cornea and limbus
  - Up to 5 mm from limbus
  - >5 mm from limbus

REFERENCES

1. Campbell DG. Traumatic glaucoma. In: Shingleton BJ, Hersh OS, Kenyon KR (Eds). Eye Trauma. St Louis: Mosby. 1991.
2. Zion VM, Burton TC. Retinal dialysis. Arch Ophthalmol. 1980;98:1971-4.
3. Cox MS, Schepens CL, Freeman HM. Retinal detachment due to ocular contusion. Arch Ophthalmol. 1966;76:678-85.
4. Regillo CD. Basic and Clinical Science Course, Section 12: Retina and Vitreous. American Academy of Ophthalmology; 2012.

CHAPTER 5

Neuro-ophthalmology and Strabismus

LONG CASES

THIRD CRANIAL NERVE PALSY

Adarsh Shashni, Shipra Singhi

■ INTRODUCTION

Cranial nerve (CN) palsies can be given as long case in examination. The third CN supplies majority of extraocular muscles (MR, SR, IR, IO), levator palpebrae superioris (LPS), and contains pupillomotor fibers. Lesion involving the superior and inferior branches of oculomotor nerve results in a down and out eyeball position with limitation of elevation, adduction, and depression in abduction. Most of the cases are acquired. Following discussion is primarily on acquired palsy.

■ HISTORY

Chief Complaint

A case of third nerve palsy may present with following:
- Diplopia
- Deviation of eyes
- Limitation of movements
- Drooping of eyelid
- Diminution of vision for near, head posture, face turn, facial asymmetry, protrusion of eye, chemosis

History of Present Illness

Age at Onset

It is important to note the age of onset to differentiate between congenital and acquired form. At times a close observation of old photographs may be helpful. Age <50 years warrants urgent imaging to rule out ICSOL.

Mode of Onset

Acute onset of diplopia or deviation warrants immediate neuroimaging to rule out life-threatening conditions, hence, the type of onset is extremely important to note.

Diplopia

It is the presenting symptom in majority of cases. Primarily seen as horizontal and vertical binocular diplopia. It must be remembered that patients due to ptosis may not volunteer diplopia. It may also be absent in patients with long-standing disease with early age of onset resulting in suppression.

Pain

Headache, localized pain in the orbit, and periorbital region can be there suggestive of orbital inflammatory disease like Tolosa–Hunt syndrome. Aneurysm of posterior communicating artery can be associated with severe pain or headache. Ischemic mononeuropathy [e.g., diabetes mellitus (DM)] can be associated with variable degree of pain.

Poor Visual Acuity, Abnormal Head Posture, and Facial Asymmetry

Presence of these suggests congenital nature of the disease.

Glare

Rarely a dilated pupil (due to involvement of pupillomotor fibers).

Associated Symptoms

Although rare, patient may complain of difficulty in reading, protrusion of eye, chemosis, headache, pain, vomiting. Patient may present with other neurological symptoms like contralateral hemiparesis in Weber's syndrome, contralateral tremors in Benedict syndrome, and ipsilateral ataxia in Nothnagel syndrome.

History of Past Illness

A careful past history is helpful in identifying the probable cause of third nerve palsy. Important causes include etiologies for oculomotor palsy: vasculopathic process [diabetes, hypertension, CAD (coronary artery disease)], trauma, compression (e.g., aneurysm, ICSOL) and/or infiltrative (e.g., leukemia), inflammatory, infection, demyelinating disease, toxic (e.g., chemotherapy).

Similar episodes in past must be enquired. Recurrent third nerve palsy can occur in DM, aneurysm, and ophthalmoplegic migraine.

Past Surgical History

History of any previous neurosurgical procedure must be recorded.

Family History and Birth History

In cases of congenital third nerve palsy, both of these histories are important.

■ EXAMINATION

General Examination/Specific Systemic Examination

A complete evaluation should be performed to rule out any associated neurological symptoms, headache, jaw claudication (giant cell arteritis), and symptoms of ear disease, such as reduced hearing and persistent ear discharge. Any other signs of trauma should be examined. Neurological examination must include other CNs and the peripheral nervous system. In a child, an otorhinolaryngological review may be sought.

Ocular Examination

Visual Acuity

Distance and near visual acuity (VA) should be recorded after lifting the ptotic eyelid. Near VA can be particularly reduced due to mydriasis and loss of accommodation. It may be reduced due to amblyopia in congenital or early-age onset third CN palsy. VA must be checked with and without glasses.

Face

Head posture: Head posture is taken to position the eye away from direction of action of paralytic muscles so as to minimize the deviation which can be fused to avoid diplopia. So, for left third CN palsy—face turn to right with head tilt to left with chin elevation.

Facial asymmetry should be noted in congenital cases. This can be assessed by measuring the lateral canthus to angle of mouth distance and comparing with that of other side.

Palpebral fissure asymmetry—measurement of palpebral fissure should be done using transparent ruler in primary gaze, in adduction and abduction and depression to rule out aberrant regeneration.

Eyeball

- Palsy of medial rectus (MR), superior rectus (SR), inferior oblique, and inferior rectus results in the unopposed action of their antagonist extraocular muscles, lateral rectus (LR) and superior oblique (SO). Thus, resulting

in the characteristic down (due to SO) and out (due to LR) position of the eyeball **(Fig. 1)**.
- There can be complete or partial absence of the extraocular movements depending on the extent of involvement (paresis/palsy). There is limitation of elevation (SR and IO), depression (IR) and adduction (MR) **(Fig. 2)**.
- Intorsion results from an intact SO, which increases on attempted downgaze.
- To check the trochlear nerve function, patient is requested to attempt to look down and outward. The examiner then observes the presence of incyclotorsion during this movement. The movements of the nasal limbal vessels should also be observed for the torsional movements.
- In case of partial third CN, palsy the deficit of adduction, supraduction, and infraduction should be apparent even if partially paralyzed. One can also check for saccades which will be floating in direction of action of paretic muscles.
- In very mild cases, latent deviation or phoria can be elicited by Maddox rod or alternate

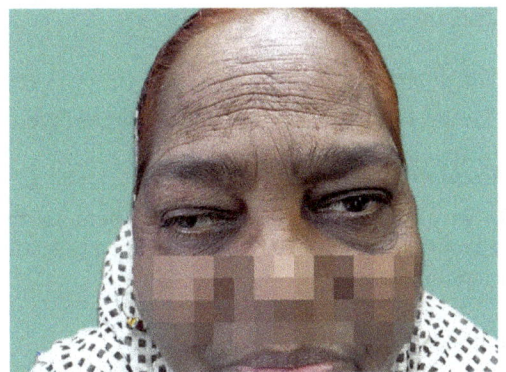

Fig. 1: Characteristic "down and out" position of the eyeball in third nerve palsy.

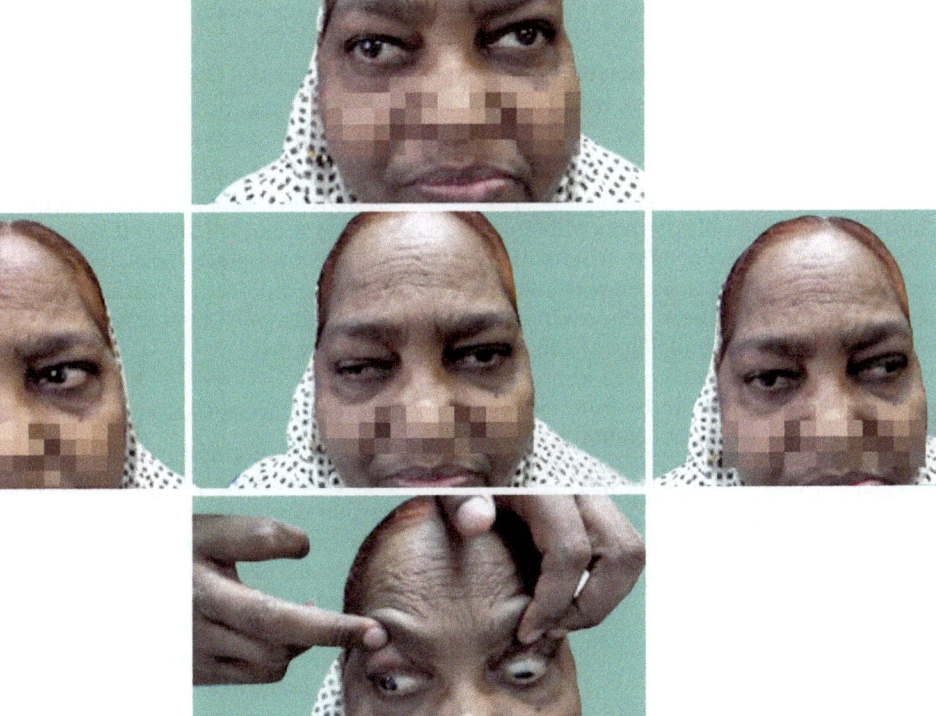

Fig. 2: Limited elevation (SR), depression (IR), and adduction (MR) in third nerve palsy.

cover testing (exo- and hypodeviation) to dissociate the two eyes and interrupt fusion).

Lid

Ptosis is usually severe and to evaluate the ocular motility, upper lid will have to be raised by the examiner (or an assistant). If there is ptosis, one must look for lid fatigue or lid twitch (kindly see myasthenia short case) because these might indicate myasthenia gravis. Lagophthalmos should be checked in all such cases. Aberrant regeneration to LPS from extraocular motor nerve fibers should be checked which might improve ptosis on attempted duction movements of the respected involved recti muscles (e.g., pseudo von Graefe sign—lid retraction seen on attempted downgaze). Aberrant regeneration is important to document as it helps in guiding the surgical management.

Conjunctiva

Conjunctival injection or chemosis can be present in cases of lymphoma and thyroid dysfunction.

Cornea/Sclera/Iris

Usually normal, corneal sensation should be checked in all cases of CN palsy, which may be lost in orbital inflammatory disease.

Pupil

Third CN palsy generally presents with anisocoria more prominent in daylight. This sluggish or absent reaction to light is there due to involvement of parasympathetic fibers that originate in the Edinger–Westphal subnucleus of the third CN complex. Aberrant regeneration to pupil should also be checked. This can be from ciliary body resulting in light near dissociation (tonic pupil) or from extraocular motor nerve fibers which can be assessed by checking pupillary constriction on attempted duction (e.g., if from MR than on attempted adduction).

IOP/Lens/Vitreous

This is usually normal.

Fundus

Usually normal; however always rule out papilledema [raised intracranial tension (ICT)], any vasculitis, vascular disease, and choroidal fold (orbital mass lesions).

Special Tests for Squint/Third Nerve Palsy

Measurement of deviation (kindly *see* the chapter of 6th nerve palsy and esotropia).

Convergence

This will be absent if the MR muscle is paralyzed.

Accommodation

In pupil involving lesions, the fibers to the ciliary body are also involved causing a defective accommodation.

Binocular Function

Binocular function should be assessed after neutralization of deviation. This is usually absent especially in congenital and early-age onset third CN palsy with large angle of deviation. Those with late onset and in partial third CN palsy binocular function are usually intact.

Worth Four-dot Test

The test uses red and green glasses for dissociation and can be used for both distance and near. The test can differentiate between binocular single vision (BSV), suppression, and anomalous retinal correspondence (ARC). If the patient sees two red and three green lights, it suggests presence of diplopia, and if the patient sees either red or green color lights only, then it suggests suppression of the either eye.

Bagolini Striated Glasses

The Bagolini glasses consist of fine striations that converts the point source of light into line perpendicular to striations. The test is used to differentiate between BSV, suppression, and ARC.
- *Double Maddox rod test*
- Red and green Maddox rods, with the cylinders vertical, are placed one in front of either eye.
- Each eye will therefore perceive a more or less horizontal line of light.
- In the presence of cyclodeviation, the line perceived by the paretic eye will be tilted and therefore distinct from that of the other eye.

- One Maddox rod is then rotated until fusion (superimposition) of the lines is achieved.
- The amount of rotation can be measured in degrees and indicates the extent of cyclodeviation.

Diplopia Charting

- *Diplopia charting using red-green glasses:* It is done by using red-green glasses and projecting a streak of light on a screen testing the patient at 1 m (see 6th nerve palsy)
- *Synoptophore:* The synoptophore simultaneously presents the stimuli to both the eyes by compensating for the angle of squint.

Applications:
- Detects suppression, ARC, and binocular function in cases of manifest squint
- Measures horizontal, vertical, and torsional deviations in the cardinal positions of gaze, thus aiding in surgical planning
- *Hess chart:* The findings of Hess chart vary in different stages of paralytic squint. The paralytic eye shows a constricted field whereas the contralateral eye shows overaction and a larger field.

For example, in a patient of left third nerve palsy—the area enclosed on the left chart is much smaller than that on the right.
- Left exotropia—note that the fixation spots in the inner charts of both eyes are deviated laterally. The deviation is greater on the right chart (when the left eye is fixating), indicating that secondary deviation exceeds the primary, typical of a paretic squint.
- Left chart shows underaction of all muscles except the LR.
- Right chart shows overaction of all muscles except the MR and inferior rectus, the "yokes" of the spared muscles.
- In inferior rectus palsy, observing intorsion on attempted depression can only assess the function of the SO muscle. Observing a conjunctival landmark using the slit lamp best performs this. Hess charting in case of left third nerve palsy

Forced Duction Test

The forced duction test (FDT) is an attempt by the examiner to move a patient's eye farther in a given direction than the patient can move it. Topical anesthetic is placed on the appropriate limbal location (generally 180° away from the duction limitation) with a small cotton swab and the limbal conjunctiva is grasped firmly with a toothed forceps. The patient is asked to rotate the eye fully in the direction of the limited duction. An attempt is then made by the examiner to rotate the eye beyond the position attained by the patient while avoiding globe retraction. Care must be taken not to abrade the cornea. Patients who have pure nerve palsy exhibit no restriction to full movement by the examiner; patients who have pure restriction (dysthyroid orbitopathy, entrapment of ocular contents after blowout fracture) exhibit restricted movements (sometimes termed a positive FDT). Some patients initially have pure nerve palsy, but contracture of the antagonist muscle results in secondary mechanical restriction of movement. Suction cup devices have been developed for examiners who are wary of using toothed instruments at the limbus; a cotton swab may be a sufficient tool in some patients.

Active Force Generation Test

Active force generation test (AFGT) may be used to evaluate the ability of a muscle to move the eye against a resisting force. The forceps is placed at the limbus of the anesthetized (topical) globe in the meridian of the muscle whose duction is limited and the patient requested to rotate the eye in the direction of the limited duction. The examiner judges through the forceps the relative amount of force generated. Strain gauges have been devised that enable quantitation of this force. In case of positive AFGT, strengthening surgical procedures can be done on involved paretic muscle (e.g., resection or plication). If negative the involved muscle should be left untouched.

Aberrant Regeneration (Oculomotor Synkinesis)

Regrowth of damaged nerve fibers following complete or severe third nerve palsy results in change in the action of muscles supplied by the third nerve. Aberrant regeneration usually occurs after trauma, tumor, or an aneurysm that has resulted in the breach of endoneural sheath. It may occur from weeks to months after the onset of the third nerve paresis. Aberrant regeneration is known to involve pupil, LPS, and to other extraocular muscles.

■ INVESTIGATION

- Acute onset paralytic squint always warrants an immediate neuroimaging unless the physician is certain about the diagnosis.
- Neuroimaging is indicated in following cases of acquired third CN palsy—all cases with age <50 years; age >50 years, if patient has headache, nausea, vomiting, other neurological signs and symptoms, involvement of pupil, ocular pain, proptosis, papilledema, loss of corneal sensation, history of trauma, nonresolving or worsening cases and lastly a willing patient.
- Remember, majority (around 60%) of cases are idiopathic and of presumed microvascular lesions in older patients. However, a wide range of life-threatening causes (e.g., aneurysm) can be there hence a low threshold should be adopted for neuroimaging.
- CT angiography is usually the preferred modality by most physicians. Newer modalities such as magnetic resonance imaging (MRI) brain and orbits with venography can provide additional information.
- Vascular risk factor assessment [erythrocyte sedimentation rate (ESR), C-reactive protein (CRP), complete blood count (CBC), blood sugar, lipid profile, blood pressure, homocysteine levels, etc.] similar to that for retinal arterial disease should be done to rule out microvascular causes.
- Other investigations like lumbar puncture and vasculitis profile consisting of c-ANCA, p-ANCA, anti-ds-DNA antibodies may be required in patients with suspected rare etiologies like syphilis, Lyme disease or giant cell arteritis, and vasculitis related third nerve palsy.

■ MANAGEMENT

Observation

- Appropriate in presumed microvascular cases; majority of case shows signs of recovery at 2 weeks and recover by 3-6 months.
- In patients with partial or recovering ptosis uniocular occlusion helps to avoid diplopia.

- Temporary prisms may be useful for smaller deviations.
- Young children should be treated with alternate patching to prevent amblyopia.

Surgical Treatment

- Surgical management should be planned after stabilization of the paralysis. One should wait for at least 6-12 months before planning the surgical management.
- The aim is to provide binocular fusion in at least primary position and if possible in downgaze and to correct vision limiting or cosmetically annoying upper lid ptosis.
- For surgical purpose, it can be divided into three groups:
  1. Complete third CN palsy—supramaximal LR recession, periosteal fixation of LR, transposition of LR to MR, Scott procedure, Peter's procedure (SO to MR)
  2. Partial third CN palsy—MR resection and LR recession (adjustable procedure for cooperative patient), vertical transposition of SR and IR to MR, surgeries on SR and IR for correction of vertical deviation.
  3. Aberrant regeneration to LPS—to do surgery on the normal eye which takes the advantage of fixation duress for correction of ptosis, and same side surgery may worsen the same
- *Scott procedure:* Transposition of the insertion of the SO tendon to a point anterior and medial to the insertion of the SR muscle without trochleotomy combined with large recessions of the LR muscle and, occasionally, recession-resection procedures of horizontal rectus muscles of noninvolved eyes can result in a satisfactory cosmetic outcome and alignment in primary position in some cases.

Botulinum Toxin

Its role in the management of acute or chronic third nerve paresis has not been adequately investigated. In patients with prolonged recovery time botulinum toxin injection in the uninvolved LR muscle prevents the muscle contracture.

Permanent Prism

It is used, as an alternative to surgery, to get rid of troublesome but mild residual deviation.

VIVA QUESTIONS

Q.1. What are the causes of isolated third nerve palsy?

Ans. *Microvascular disease (ischemic mononeuropathy):* Diabetes and hypertension are the most common etiologies of third nerve palsy

Aneurysm of the posterior communicating artery at its junction with the internal carotid [remember ischemic mononeuropathy is usually associated with pain in the periorbital region, and pupil is often spared (75% of cases) in spite of significant restriction of motility. In contrast, pain is variably present in aneurysm and pupillary involvement is almost always present in spite of less severe restriction of motility].

- *Trauma,* both direct and secondary to subdural hematoma with uncal herniation, can produce isolated third nerve palsy.
- *Miscellaneous* uncommon causes include tumor, infections like Lyme disease and syphilis, and vasculitis associated with sarcoidosis, collagen vascular disorders, and giant cell arteritis.

Q.2. What are the causes of recurrent isolated third nerve palsy?

Ans. Episodes of third nerve dysfunction with spontaneous recovery over 3–6 months can occur in:
- Ophthalmoplegic migraine
- DM
- Aneurysm
- Raised ICT

Q.3. What are the causes and localization of third CN palsy?

Ans. This is summarized in **Table 1**

Q.4. What is the importance of pupil sparing nerve palsy?

Ans. Pupillary involving third nerve palsy is usually associated with *"surgical" lesions* like aneurysms, uncal herniation, and space-occupying lesions. Pupil is characteristically involved due to compression of the pial

Table 1: Causes and localization of third cranial nerve palsy.

Level of lesion	Etiology	Manifestations
Nuclear portion	Infarction hemorrhage neoplasm abscess	• Paralysis of the contralateral SR • Bilateral ptosis • Ipsilateral IR, MR, IO palsy • Patients with damage to the oculomotor nuclear complex need not have ipsilateral pupillary dilation, but when involved, it indicates dorsal rostral damage
Fascicular midbrain portion	Infarction hemorrhage neoplasm abscess	• Lesions at this level can produce complete or incomplete palsies • Lesion at the superior cerebellar peduncle (Nothnagel's syndrome) presents ipsilateral third nerve palsy and cerebellar ataxia. • Lesions at the red nucleus (Benedikt's syndrome) are characterized by ipsilateral third nerve palsy and contralateral involuntary movement • Lesion at the cerebral peduncle (Weber's syndrome) produces ipsilateral third nerve palsy and contralateral hemiplegia • Isolated dysfunction of either the superior and inferior division

Contd...

Contd...

Level of lesion	Etiology	Manifestations
Fascicular subarachnoid portion	• Aneurysm • Infectious meningitis—bacterial, fungal/parasitic, viral • Meningeal infiltrative • Carcinomatous/lymphomatous/leukemic infiltration, granulomatous inflammation (sarcoidosis, lymphomatoid granulomatosis, Wegener granulomatosis) • Ophthalmoplegic migraine	• CN III palsy with fixed dilated pupil in case of surgical lesion • CN III palsy without pupil involvement in case of medical disease
Fascicular cavernous sinus portion	• Tumor—Pituitary adenoma, meningioma, craniopharyngioma, metastatic carcinoma Pituitary apoplexy (infarction within existing pituitary adenoma) • Vascular • Giant intracavernous aneurysm carotid artery—cavernous sinus fistula • Carotid dural branch—cavernous sinus fistula cavernous sinus thrombosis • Ischemia from microvascular disease in vasa nervosa • Inflammatory—Tolosa–Hunt syndrome (idiopathic or granulomatous inflammation)	• Most commonly associated with other cranial nerves dysfunctions • It presents as paresis of oculomotor, trochlear, and abducens nerves with associated maxillary division of trigeminal nerve, producing pain
Fascicular orbital portion	• Inflammatory—orbital inflammatory pseudotumor, orbital myositis endocrine (thyroid orbitopathy) • Tumor (e.g., hemangioma, lymphangioma, meningioma)	• Lesions within the orbit are associated with visual loss, ophthalmoplegia and proptosis • Third nerve ophthalmoplegia can be associated with trochlear and abducens nerves palsies • It is important to remember that at the orbit the oculomotor nerve divides into superior (SR, LPS) and inferior division (IR, MR, pupillomotor fiber). This can cause partial oculomotor nerve palsies

blood vessels supplying the superficially located pupillary fibers (parasympathetic fibers).
- Pupillary sparing usually suggests an underlying "medical" lesion such as hypertension and diabetes. The microangiopathy involves the vasa nervorum, resulting in ischemia of the main trunk of the nerve.
- However, it must be remembered exceptions can be there. Pupillary involvement may develop a few days after the onset of diplopia in case of aneurysm as it gradually expands. In few cases such as basal meningitis and uncal herniation pupillary involvement may be the only sign of third nerve palsy, so mild pupillary signs may be clinically significant in such cases. Pupil involvement may not be helpful in children to differentiate the underlying causes of third nerve palsy.

Q.5. What is the course of third CN?
Ans. Nucleus at the level of the superior colliculi ventral to the Sylvian aqueduct
↓
Fasciculus (efferent fibers) passes from the third nerve nucleus through the red nucleus and the medial part of cerebral peduncle
↓
Basilar part starts as a series of "rootlets" that leave the midbrain on the medial aspect of the cerebral peduncle, before coalescing to form the main trunk
↓
Pierces the dura lateral to posterior clinoid process to enter the cavernous sinus
↓
Superior orbital fissure, in the annulus of Zinn
↓
Divides in two divisions, superior and inferior

Superior division of third nerve supplies the LPS and SR muscles, whereas *inferior division* of third nerve supplies the MR, the inferior rectus, and the inferior oblique

The branch supplying the inferior oblique also carries with it the preganglionic parasympathetic fibers from the Edinger–Westphal subnucleus, and innervates the ciliary muscle and the sphincter pupillae.

Q.6. Enumerate the subnuclei of third nerve nucleus complex.
Ans.
- *Levator subnucleus is unpaired* and supplies *both levator muscles.* Lesions limited to levator subnuclei, hence results in bilateral ptosis.
- SR *subnuclei are paired.* Each of the subnuclei supplies the *contralateral SR.* Nuclear third nerve palsy thus affects the contralateral SR.
- *The subnuclei of MR, inferior rectus, and inferior oblique are paired* and innervate the respective *ipsilateral muscles.*

Q.7. What are the childhood causes of third nerve (oculomotor) palsy?
Ans. Trauma; subdural hematoma
- Neoplasm
- Ophthalmoplegic migraine
- Postoperative cause
- Meningitis/encephalitis/viral or post-upper respiratory tract infection/varicella-zoster virus
- Aneurysm
- Orbital cellulitis
- Sinus disease
- Mesencephalic cyst
- Poison

SIXTH CRANIAL NERVE PALSY

Shipra Singhi, Swati Phuljhale

■ INTRODUCTION

The sixth nerve nucleus is located in the pons. The sixth nerve contains only somatic efferent fibers. Runs a long course from the brainstem to the LR muscle, through the superior orbital fissure and into the orbit through the middle part of superior orbital fissure and then to LR. The VI CN supplies the LR muscle only. A lesion affecting the nerve will result in defective abduction of the eye. Sixth nerve has the longest subarachnoid course of all the CN, which makes it vulnerable to injury at many levels. Due to close association between sixth nerve and seventh nerve (facial) in the brainstem, there may be involvement of seventh nerve also in some cases.[1,2]

■ HISTORY

Chief Complaint
A case of sixth nerve palsy can present in following ways:
- Inward deviation of eyes
- Diplopia in acquired cases
- Face turn on the same side amblyopia may be present in congenital cases
- Patient may complain of headache and hearing problem, depending on the location of involvement of sixth nerve.

History of Present Illness

Points that must be noted in history are described in the following text.

Age at Onset

Patient has history of deviation of eye inward and limitation of movement toward outward. The congenital sixth nerve palsy is present since birth. In acquired type, the onset can be at any age, depending upon the underlying cause. Previous photographs help in the documentation of strabismus. Deviation may be large or small.

Mode of Onset

Acute onset of diplopia or deviation warrants immediate neuroimaging to rule out life-threatening conditions, hence, the type of onset is extremely important to note.

Diplopia

Patient usually complains of horizontal diplopia, which characteristically worsens in the lateral gaze and distance fixation (direction of the action of paralyzed muscle).

Head Posture

Face turn on the ipsilateral side is present. Face turn is seen in acquired cases. Face turn in congenital cases may prevent amblyopia and maintain BSV.

Past History

Any history of febrile disease such as viral or bacterial, DM, raised ICT, trauma or cerebral palsy must be asked for. Adult—History of DM, hypertension, thyroid disease, other diseases (duration, treatment), trauma, and medication taken must be enquired for.

Past Surgical History

History of any previous neurosurgical procedure must be recorded as it gives a clue about diagnosis.

■ EXAMINATION

Systemic Examination

Examination of CNs and the peripheral nervous system should be performed by the appropriate specialist if essential. It is important to examine specifically for V, VII, and VIII nerve to locate the site of lesion, particularly, at the level of cerebellopontine angle. Moreover, the fasciculus of VII nerve forms a bend around the VI nerve nucleus before emerging from the pons, and thus in a case of nuclear VI nerve palsy the VII nerve involvement is frequently seen.

Ocular Examination

Visual Acuity

Affected eye fails to fixate properly due to the presence of a marked esodeviation. Long-standing convergent squint particularly in congenital cases results in amblyopia causing and a reduced VA.

Abnormal Head Posture

Patient acquires a head posture toward the affected side to minimize diplopia.

Ocular Motility

- The unopposed action of MR results in esotropia in the primary position (as shown in **Figure 1**, right eye sixth nerve party with right esotropia in primary gaze). The esodeviation (and symptomatic description) characteristically worsens for distance than near fixation.
- Limitation of abduction is characteristically on the side of the lesion (**Figure 2** shows limitation of adduction in right eye in right sixth nerve palsy).
- Normal adduction of the affected eye is seen (as shown in **Figure 3** in case of right sixth nerve palsy).

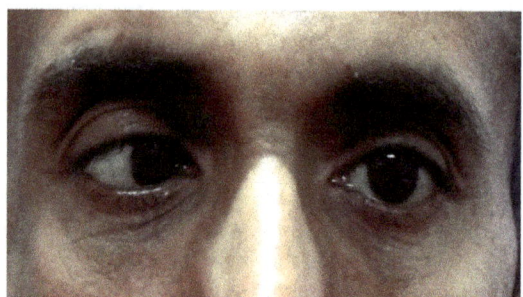

Fig. 1: Esotropia of right eye in primary position in a case of right sixth nerve palsy.

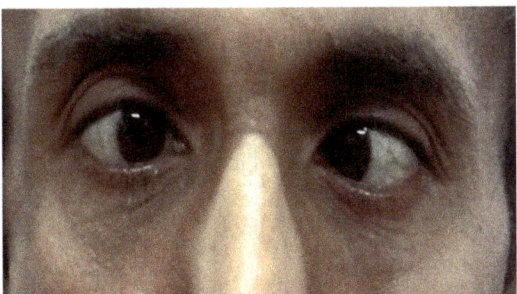

Fig. 2: Limitation of adduction in right eye in right sixth nerve palsy.

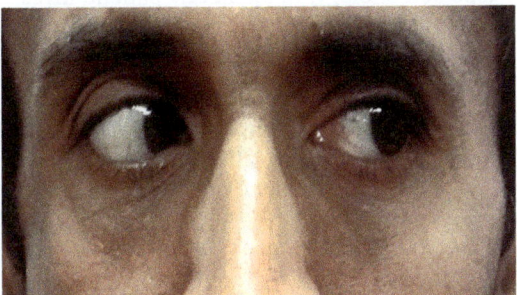

Fig. 3: Normal adduction of the right eye in a case of right sixth nerve palsy.

Lid: It is usually normal.

Conjunctiva: Conjunctival injection or chemosis can be present in cases of lymphoma and thyroid dysfunction.

Cornea/sclera/iris: Usually normal; corneal sensation may be reduced in acoustic neuroma. It is first sign in acoustic neuroma while first symptom is hearing loss.

Pupil: It is usually normal.

IOP/lens/vitreous: Usually normal

Fundus: Papilledema may be present due to raised ICT.

Special Tests

Cover test: Cover test reveals esodeviation that is greater for distance. The cover test should be done both with and without a head posture. It should be done in all nine gazes, at least in dextroversion and levoversion to look presence of incomitance.

The amount of deviation will always be more in the direction of the involved muscle. Similarly, the cover test should be done with either eye fixing to differentiate the primary (fixing with the normal eye) and secondary deviation (fixing with affected eye). In all paralytic strabismus, the secondary deviation is always more than the primary deviation.

Past pointing: Presence of past pointing indicates recent onset. It can be tested by asking the patient to point with his finger the object viewed by the paretic eye (hand–eye coordination) with a septum not allowing him to have a visual feedback to correct the coordination due to paresis. In the presence of paresis extrainnervation is required for a movement in the direction of field of action of the paretic muscle which is perceived by the brain as if the object is located farther than it is, giving extrainnervation to the hand for pointing. This causes past pointing. For example, paretic right LR palsy requires more innervation to fixate an object in dextroversion causing past pointing.

Diplopia charting: The subjective deviation is recorded by asking the subject to quantify the separation between the double images, which are dissociated by red–green glasses. This is repeated in all the nine diagnostic positions. In paralytic strabismus, the separation is maximal in the field of action of the paretic muscle. Using a slit, horizontal for vertical strabismus, and vertical for horizontal strabismus, one can also know the subjective cyclotropia. Three points to be remembered are:
1. Maximum separation is in the direction in which the muscle acts most (field of action).
2. The image that appears farthest belongs to the deviating eye.
3. The image is displaced in the direction of action of the paralyzed muscle.
   In case of LR, palsy image shifts outward.

Binocular function: In the presence of a head posture, binocular function is usually normal for near fixation. Fusion may have been lost in patients with extensive head trauma. Binocular function can be assessed with any of the following tests; Worth four-dot test, Bagolini striated glasses, Maddox rod, and synoptophore.

Hess charting: On Hess charting the eye with paralysis demonstrates a smaller constricted

field; the contralateral eye shows overaction of its muscles. Following points must be remembered while interpreting:
- Affected eye has a smaller chart with maximum restriction in the direction of action of paretic muscle
- Overacting yoke muscle of the contralateral eye shows larger chart, with maximum expansion in the direction of action of the yoke muscle.
- Each square in the chart is of 5°. Hence, an approximate estimate of angle of deviation can be made by measuring the degree of disparity between template and plotted point in any position of gaze.

Force duction test (FDT): The FDT is done to look in mechanical restriction due to MR. Under the topical anesthesia, the examiner passively moves the patient's eye in the direction opposite to that in which mechanical restriction is suspected. For example, in a case of right LR limitation, there may be contracture of right medical rectus. After the topical anesthesia, the medial limbal conjunctiva is grasped firmly with a toothed forceps and the globe is lifted up from the orbit. The patient is asked to look in abduction so that the MR is relaxed. The examiner then tries to passively move the eye in abduction. Care must be taken not to abrade the cornea. If examiner can successfully manage to move the eye until the lateral limbus touches the lateral canthus that means that there is no mechanical restriction and the motility defect is clearly caused by paralysis of the LR muscle. And if resistance is encountered, it means that the FDT is positive, mechanical restrictions do exist medially which may be due to contracture of the MR muscle, conjunctiva, or Tenon's capsule. Important causes for MR contracture include thyroid eye disease, entrapment of medial contents after fracture, myositis, and cysticercosis. Some patients initially have pure nerve palsy, but contracture of the antagonist muscle results in secondary mechanical restriction of movement. FDT can be falsely negative if the globe is not lifted out of the orbit while performing the test for recti muscle and if not depressed inside the orbit while performing the test for oblique muscles.

Active force generation test: AFGT may be used to evaluate the ability of a muscle to move the eye against a resisting force. After topical anesthesia, the paralytic muscle is held with the fixation forceps and the patient is asked to look in the direction of the limited duction; the amount of force generated by the muscle is felt as a tug by the examiner. The test should be repeated in the other eye for the comparison of the forces.

■ DIFFERENTIAL DIAGNOSIS

Refer to **Table 1**.

■ MANAGEMENT

Investigations are tailored depending on the suspected etiology. In an elderly patient, investigations to rule out diabetes, hypertension, dyslipidemia, and CAD should be done.

The indications for neuroimaging are:
- VI nerve palsy along with involvement of other CNs, such as V, VII, and VIII, is suggestive of lesion at brainstem and cerebellopontine angle
- VI nerve and presence of disc edema (pseudolocalizing sign)

Table 1: Differential diagnosis of sixth nerve palsy.

Diseases	Features
Duane's retraction syndrome	Difficulty on abduction and adduction with eyelid retraction
Graves' orbitopathy (TED)	Proptosis + decreased ability of eye movement + diplopia
Orbital trauma	Orbital fracture + muscle swelling + eye restriction + diplopia
Infantile esotropia	Esotropia + limit in abduction (improve after doll's head maneuver) + IO overaction + nystagmus + vertical deviation
Spasm of the near reflex	Triad of intermittent: esotropia + accommodative spasm + miosis
Myasthenia gravis	Muscle restriction, diplopia, and ptosis
High myopia	Can lead to progressive loss of abduction

- Isolated VI nerves palsy in patient with <60 years of age
- No improvement or if worsening seen within 6 weeks of onset in cases of ischemic nerve palsy
- Development of other neurological signs in patients with systemic risk factors

Observation

Since most of the idiopathic and microvascular lesions recover on their own it is advisable not to jump to surgery immediately. In meantime the aim is to avoid diplopia.

Occlusion: Use of frosted gasses in spectacles, occluder patches for spectacles, pirate patches, occluder contact lenses, etc. are the various methods employed for patching depending upon the patient's demands and comfort.

Prismatic (e.g., temporary Fresnel stick-on) for correction of diplopia can be done if deviation is of small angle. Alternate patching should be advised to prevent amblyopia especially in young children.[1,2]

Botulinum toxin injection: To prevent contracture of the antagonist muscle, botulinum toxin can be injected as a temporary measure. It also helps to assess residual function of the paralytic muscle and facilitates prismatic correction in patients with large deviation.

Surgery should be considered at least after 6–12 months from onset.[1,2] The aim of the surgery is to correct diplopia and head posture.

Partial palsy (paresis), adjustable MR recession, and LR resection in the affected eye can be performed in patients with residual LR function and positive AFGT.

Complete palsy: Complete palsy of LR is managed by transposition of the superior and inferior recti to positions above and below the affected LR muscle. This may or may not be coupled with weakening of the ipsilateral MR depending on FDT. If FDT is positive then one should recess the MR to release the globe. In such cases where MR recession is required, a partial tendon transposition is done instead of full tendon. Disinsertion of three recti muscles in the same sitting increases the risk of anterior segment ischemia. Various types of transposition surgeries are described

Table 2: Investigations in sixth nerve palsy.

Forced duction test (FDT)	For diagnosing the presence of mechanical restriction of ocular motility
Force generation test (FGT)	• To assess muscle strength of an extraocular muscle • To differentiate paretic from restrictive strabismus
Magnetic resonance imaging (MRI)	Provides greater resolution of the orbits, cavernous sinus, posterior fossa, and cranial nerves
Cerebrospinal fluid (CSF)	Helps diagnose disease affecting the brain and spinal cord if vasculitis is suspected clinically
Erythrocyte sedimentation rate and/or C-reactive protein	Helps detect inflammation associated with conditions such as infections, cancers, and autoimmune diseases

for the sixth nerve palsy; Hummelsheim (full tendon transposition of superior and inferior recti to LR), Jensen (tying of the inferior half the LR belly with the temporal half of the inferior rectus belly and tying of the superior half of the LR to the temporal half of SR.

■ INVESTIGATION

Refer to **Table 2** for investigations.

VIVA QUESTIONS

Q.1. What is the course of sixth nerve?

Ans. Sixth nerve nucleus lies in pons at the floor of the fourth ventricle

↓

Fasciculus of sixth nerve leaves the brainstem ventrally at the pontomedullary junction.

↓

Basilar part of the nerve then enters prepontine basilar cistern, and traverses up close skull base. Anterior inferior cerebellar artery crosses the nerve here

↓

Dorello canal (underneath the petroclinoid ligament)
↓
Intracavernous part intercavernous sinus
↓
Superior orbital fissure
↓
Intraorbital part enters orbit
↓
LR muscle

Q.2. What are the causes of sixth nerve palsy?

Ans. Causes of sixth nerve palsy are summarized in **Table 3**. The four most common causes were idiopathic (26%), hypertension alone (19%), coexistent diabetes and hypertension (12%), and trauma (12%).

Table 3: Causes of sixth nerve palsy.

Causes	Examples	
Congenital		• Birth trauma • Infection (maternal) • Hereditary causes • Anomalies of lateral rectus development • Moebius syndrome
Acquired	Children	• Space-occupying lesions • Infections, bacterial or viral • Trauma • Raised intracranial pressure • Decompensated esophoria • Infantile esotropia with cross fixation • Duane's retraction syndrome
	Young adults	• Trauma • Space-occupying lesions • Postviral inflammation • Multiple sclerosis • Diabetes • High myopia • Ophthalmoplegic migraine
	Older adults	• Vascular • Hypertension • Diabetes • Space-occupying lesions • Senile lateral rectus weakness

Q.3. What is false localizing sign?

Ans. Raised intracranial pressure may cause stretching one or both sixth nerves due to their long intracranial course or the compression against the petrous tip, in this situation sixth nerve palsy that may be bilateral, is a false localizing sign.

Q.4. What is management of diplopia?

Ans. Diplopia can be managed by advising monocular occlusion, fogging of glasses, prismatic (e.g., temporary Fresnel stick-on) and opaque contact lenses especially in patients with microangiopathic and idiopathic causes. Most of the patients (up to 90%) recover spontaneously, over weeks to several months. Alternate patching should be advised to young children to prevent amblyopia.

Q.5. How will you do diplopia charting?

Ans. Refer to third nerve palsy.

Q.6. How will you do Hess/Lees charting?

Ans. Refer to third nerve palsy.

Q.7. What is relationship of sixth nerve with other structures in cavernous sinus?

Ans. Third, fourth, and the first division of the fifth CN pass through the lateral wall of cavernous sinus. The sixth nerve is the most medially situated and runs through the substance of the sinus in close relation to the internal carotid artery. Occasionally, intracavernous sixth nerve palsy is accompanied by a postganglionic Horner syndrome (Parkinson syndrome) due to damage to the paracarotid sympathetic plexus.

Q.8. Can a patient present with isolated nuclear sixth nerve palsy?

Ans. Nuclear sixth nerve presents as horizontal gaze palsy, where there is limitation of abduction due sixth nerve nucleus involvement as well as adduction limitation on contralateral side due to lack of impulse to contralateral MLF. Convergence may be preserved in such cases, e.g., facial (seventh) nerve fibers wrap around the sixth nerve nucleus, so ipsilateral lower motor neuron (LMN) facial nerve palsy is also common. Isolated sixth nerve palsy is never nuclear in origin.

Q.9. What is Foville syndrome?
Ans. *Etiology:* Foville syndrome (inferior medial pontine/dorsal pontine syndrome) is most commonly associated with vascular microangiopathic causes and space-occupying lesions.
Clinical features: Sixth nerve paresis, ipsilateral V, VII, VIII CN palsy, ipsilateral Horner's syndrome, and horizontal conjugate gaze palsy

Q.10. What is Millard–Gubler (ventral pontine) syndrome?
Ans. Millard–Gubler, also known as ventral pontine syndrome, is most commonly associated with vascular diseases, demyelinating, and space-occupying lesions.
Clinical features: These are ipsilateral sixth nerve palsy, contralateral hemiplegia, and ipsilateral LMN facial nerve palsy.

Q.11. What is the muscle function test/how to differentiate total or partial sixth nerve palsy?
Ans. Refer to **Table 4**.

Table 4: Total versus partial sixth nerve palsy.

Tests	Finding
Forced generation test	Residual lateral rectus function—feel a tug on forceps
Botulinum toxin injection into a contracted medial rectus	If abduction past midline—partial LR palsy
Saccadic velocity analysis	• Mild paresis—varies from 40°/s • Complete paralysis—slow lateral saccades (160°/s)
Electromyography	• Record action potential in LR muscle • Increased signal in attempt to abduction → residual LR function

■ REFERENCES

1. Walsh and Hoyt's Clinical Neuro-ophthalmology. Philadelphia: Lippincott Williams & Wilkins; 2005.
2. Azarmina M, Azarmina H. The six syndromes of the sixth cranial nerve. J Ophthalmic Vis Res. 2013;8(2):160-71.

FOURTH CRANIAL NERVE PALSY

Gunjan Saluja, Shipra Singhi, Patil Mukesh Prakash

■ INTRODUCTION

Fourth CN is the thinnest and longest CN (75 mm) and the only CN that comes out from the dorsal aspect of the brainstem. It is the only CN, which crosses completely to the opposite side. This originates from the contralateral nucleus. The IV CN supplies the contralateral SO muscle. Its nucleus lies at the level of the inferior colliculus. Any lesion affecting the nerve may result in difficulties of depression in adduction, incyclotorsion and abduction of the eye. Acute-onset vertical diplopia, along with characteristic contralateral head tilt, usually indicates fourth nerve palsy. Peripheral lesions cause ipsilateral and nuclear lesions contralateral SO weakness. In postgraduate examinations, it may come as a long case.

■ HISTORY

Chief Complaint

A case of fourth nerve palsy may present with following:
- Sudden hypertropia
- Diplopia
- Head posture
- Although amblyopia may be associated in congenital cases, it is rarely seen in presence of a head posture.

History of Present Illness

Following points must be recorded:

Age at Onset

It is important to note the age of onset (to differentiate between congenital and acquired form).

Inspection of previous photographs may be useful for the documentation of head posture.

Diplopia

Vertical diplopia which is worse in downgaze is a characteristic symptom in acquired cases. Since diplopia is worse in downgaze, it usually associated with difficulty in climbing stairs or reading.

Post-traumatic SO palsy often bilateral and these patients may complain of torsional diplopia in downgaze.

Past History

Past history should include following:
- Any history of febrile disease (viral or bacterial), DM, space-occupying lesions
- Since trauma is the most important cause of fourth nerve palsy, it should always be ruled out, particularly blow to the dorsal aspect of midbrain.
- In adults, history of DM, hypertension, thyroid disease, and myasthenia gravis, other diseases (duration, treatment), trauma, and medication should be taken.

Past Surgical History

History of any previous neurosurgical procedure must be recorded.

Birth History

A complete birth history beginning from gestational history, birth trauma, type of delivery, forceps or vacuum-assisted birth, and birth weight should be elucidated. History of trauma, fall, and central nervous system (CNS) infections during neonatal period should also be taken.

Family History

History of strabismus in the parents or siblings may be positive. It shows autosomal dominant inheritance.

■ EXAMINATION

General Examination/ Specific Systemic Examination

A thorough review of systems should be conducted, including enquiry about trauma, diabetes, hypertension, etc. and symptoms of viral illness. Neurological examination must include other CNs and the peripheral nervous system.

Ocular Examination

Visual Acuity

Vision may be reduced in congenital cases due to amblyopia. VA must be checked with and without glasses.

Facial Asymmetry and Abnormal Head Posture

- A compensatory head posture avoids diplopia. The functions of SO muscle include intorsion, depression, and abduction. To compensate for each of these, there is a characteristic head posture. For example, in a case of right SOP the held tilt would be toward left shoulder to compensate for intorsion, chin depression is present to compensate for depression action and there will be face turn to same side to compensate for abduction. In bilateral cases since intorsion and abduction of both the eyes is affected there's no head tilt or face turn, unless the involvement is asymmetrical. Facial asymmetry in form of (plagiocephaly) causes congenital weakening of SO muscle. The premature fusion of coronal axis on one side causes posterior placement of trochlea, thus making SO muscle more parallel to the coronal than the sagittal axis (de-sagittalization). The posterior placement of trochlea causes laxity of the SO tendon thus reducing all of its action.
- Bilateral cases have chin depression. Usually there is no head tilt or turn except in asymmetric involvement.
- Congenital torticollis (tight sternocleidomastoid) should be excluded in patients with persistent abnormal head posture even after surgery for trochlear nerve palsy.

Lid

If there is ptosis, one must look for third nerve involvement.

Conjunctiva

Conjunctival injection or chemosis can be present in cases of lymphoma and thyroid dysfunction.

Cornea/Sclera/Iris

Usually normal, corneal sensation should be checked in all cases of CN palsy.

Pupil

It is usually normal. It may be mydriatic in third nerve palsy.

IOP/Lens/Vitreous

Usually normal.

Special Examination of Squint

Cover Test

All the strabismus examination should be performed after correcting the compensatory head posture. A latent deviation exists if a compensatory abnormal head posture is adopted. When the test is repeated with the head straight, the deviation will increase and may become manifest. The affected eye shows a hyperdeviation and an associated esodeviation.

There will be hypertropia of the affected eye which increases on opposite gaze and same side head tilt, also known as Park's three step test.

Park's Three-step Test

The test is illustrated with the example of left superior oblique paresis (SOP). It should be noted that the test is only for identifying the paralyzed cyclovertical muscle.

Step 1: To assess which eye is hypertropic in the primary gaze **(Fig. 1A)**.

In case of left hypertropia, the following muscles could be involved:
- Depressors of the left eye, i.e., SO and inferior rectus causing hypertropia of left eye
- Elevators of the right eye, i.e., the SR or inferior oblique causing hypotropia of right eye

Step 2: To assess which lateral direction has worse hypertropia **(Fig. 1B)**.

If the left hypertropia increases on right gaze, it implicates a left SO or right superior rectus (RSR) involvement.

Increase in the left gaze implicates that either the right inferior oblique or left inferior rectus are involved.

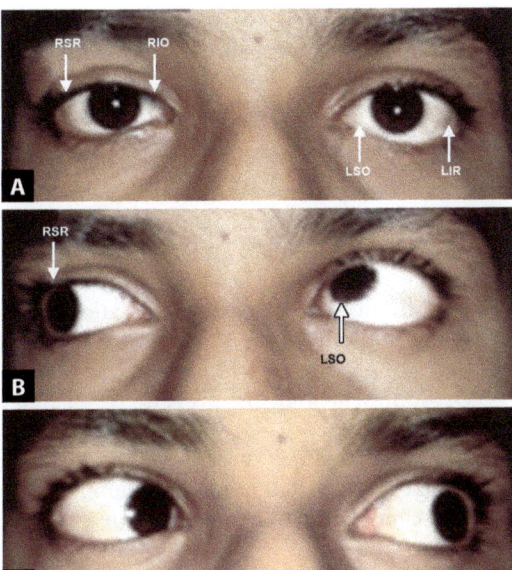

Figs. 1A to C: Left superior oblique palsy: (A) Left hypertropia. Four muscles could be involved; left superior oblique (LSO), left inferior rectus (LIR) or right superior rectus (RSR), right inferior oblique (RIO); (B) Since the hypertropia worsens on right gaze; we have zeroed down to two muscles; RSR or LSO; (C) On head tilt test, the hypertropia worsens on left tilt due to overaction of left superior rectus (LSR) muscle.

In this case, the deviation will be worse in opposite gaze, so now from four muscles we have zeroed down to two muscles left SO or right SR deviation is *worse on opposite gaze (WOOG)*.

Step 3: Also known as *Bielschowsky's head tilt* test is done to assess, in which head tilt direction is the hypertropia worse **(Fig. 1C)**
- For the head tilt test, the patient is asked to fixate at a distant target at 3 m.
- Increase in left hypertropia on left head tilt implies the left SO is involved, and increase in right hypertropia on left head tilt indicates the RSR is involved. Since tilt on left side will cause extorsion in right eye, which needs to compensated by an intorsion of the eye to balance head movement. In addition, since the SO is paralyzed the SR needs to overact to bring about the desired intorsion, which is accompanied by elevation. This increased

elevation is seen as worsening of hypertropia on same side of head tilt.

In fourth nerve palsy, the hypertropia is better on opposite tilt.

Bilateral SO palsy should be excluded in patients with closed head trauma.
- Due to underaction of SO, which is responsible for depression in adduction, in bilateral palsy cases there will be alternate hypertropia that increases on adduction. Hence, on left gaze there will be right hypertropia and on right gaze there will be left hypertropia. Orthophoria may be present in primary position.
- Extorsion of >10° is recorded either by using double Maddox rods or synoptophore.
- Bielschowsky head tilt test is positive on both the sides.

Primary underaction of the SO muscle in fourth nerve palsy results in:
- Overaction of ipsilateral antagonist, inferior oblique
- Overaction of the contralateral yoke muscle (inferior rectus)
- Secondary underaction of antagonist of contralateral yoke (SR)

The combination of these muscle effects is variable and often depends on whether or not the deviation is long-standing.

Hess Charting

On Hess charting, the affected eye shows a smaller constricted field with greatest restriction in the direction of action of paralytic muscle with overaction of the ipsilateral antagonist muscle. Contralateral eye shows overaction of the muscles.

For example, recently acquired left fourth nerve palsy would have following abnormalities:
- Left chart (chart of left eye with right eye fixing) is smaller than the right (chart of right eye with left eye fixing)
- Left chart shows underaction of the SO and overaction of the inferior oblique
- Left chart shows overaction of the inferior rectus and underaction (inhibitional palsy) of the SR

Evaluation of Torsion

Unilateral fourth nerve palsy is characterized by <8° of cyclodeviation while bilateral cases may have >10° of cyclodeviation.

Double Maddox rod test: It includes following steps:
- Red and green Maddox rods, with the cylinders horizontal, are placed one in front of either eye
- Each eye will therefore perceive vertical line of light
- In the presence of cyclodeviation, the line perceived by the paretic eye will be tilted and therefore distinct from that of the other eye
- One Maddox rod is then rotated until both lines become parallel to each other
- The amount of rotation can be measured in degrees and indicates the amount of cyclodeviation

Fundus—Indirect ophthalmoscopy and fundus photography: Useful methods for evaluation of cyclodeviation. Normally the fovea is located between the two horizontal lines, one passing through the center of disc and the other cutting the lower pole of the disc tangentially. The usual location is in the middle of these two horizontal lines, in cases of SOP because of extorsion it is displaced downward.

Field charting: Vertical displacement of blind spot suggests torsion.

Forced duction test: Exaggerated forced duction test was described by Guyton is done to look for laxity on the SO tendon. The globe is grasped with Pierce Hoskins forceps in superotemporal and inferonasal quadrant. The globe is retracted inside the orbit and the eye is elevated and adducted. The globe is rocked in intorsion and extorsion movement. A normal taut SO tendon will cause globe to pop up during this maneuver and a click is felt by the examiner. It is always imperative to compare it with other eye to differentiate between the normal and lax tendon. To test tension in the inferior oblique muscle—the globe is grasped inferotemporal and superonasal quadrant and is then retracted, depressed, and adducted.

Checking fourth CN function in third palsy: Vertical actions cannot be tested, as there is third CN involvement (adduction). To solve this, note a limbal or conjunctival landmark. Ask the patient to look down. The patient will not be able to look down as the eye is abducted and not adducted. However, the eye should intort as the SO works. Check for the conjunctival landmark to see if the eye is intorting.

If the conjunctival landmark is moving the eye is intorting, thus the fourth CN is intact.

■ DIFFERENTIAL DIAGNOSIS

A case of fourth CN palsy has to be differentiated from following:
- Thyroid eye disease
- Ocular surgery
- Orbital fracture
- Neurosurgery
- Childhood strabismus
- Skew deviation
- Third nerve palsy
- Myasthenia gravis
- Decompensated hyperphoria

■ INVESTIGATION

Blood investigations to rule out risk factors, such as diabetes, hypertension, and other cause of microangiopathy should be done. Neuroimaging is required only when it is associated with other neurological signs.

■ MANAGEMENT

Observation

Congenital decompensated and presumed microvascular palsies commonly resolve spontaneously. All patients are seen every 1–2 months while being monitored for stability/recovery. Unilateral cases of vascular origin usually recover within 6 months. Small-unrecovered deviations with vertical/horizontal diplopia can be managed long-term by incorporating prisms into spectacles (Also, see chapter on sixth nerve palsy).

Surgical Management

The choice of surgical options is influenced by various factors:
- Laxity of SO tendon
- Presence of IO overaction
- Amount of deviation in primary position
- Gaze of maximum deviation

Table 1: Management of IV nerve palsy (Von Noorden modification of Knapp's classification): for a case of left superior oblique palsy.

Class	Maximum deviation in gaze	Management
1.	Dextroelevation (L/R maximum in this gaze)	Left inferior oblique recession
2.	Dextrodepression	Left superior oblique tuck or Harada-Ito's procedure ± Right inferior rectus recession
3.	All right gazes	• If hypertropia <25 PD then left inferior oblique recession • If hypertropia >25 then add left superior oblique tuck
4.	All down and right gazes	Treatment plan as in 3 with right inferior rectus recession or left superior rectus recession
5.	All downgazes	Left superior oblique tuck with right inferior rectus recession
6.	Bilateral with a "V" pattern	Bilateral surgery as in class 5
7.	All downgazes, primary gaze, and dextroversion	Explore trochlea

Table 1 shows the algorithm for the management of SO palsy according to Knapp's classification. To correct for torsion Harada-Ito procedure is done. For bilateral acquired cases, perform bilateral Harado-Ito procedure is done to correct torsion.

VIVA QUESTIONS

Q.1. What is the course of fourth nerve?
Ans. The nucleus of fourth nerve is located in the midbrain at the level of inferior colliculi, ventral to the Sylvian aqueduct.

The axons of the fasciculus curve posteriorly around aqueduct; the fourth nerve decussates completely in anterior medullary velum
↓
The trunk leaves the brainstem on the dorsal surface enters the cavernous sinus
↓
Superior orbital fissure
↓
Intraorbital part enters orbit
↓
The intraorbital part innervates the SO muscle

Q.2. What are the causes of isolated fourth nerve palsy?

Ans. Congenital cases are usually idiopathic. However, congenital fourth nerve palsy may remain asymptomatic till vertical fusional ability has reduced, resulting in decompensation.
Trauma frequently causes bilateral fourth nerve palsy.
Microvascular lesions are relatively common.
Aneurysms and tumors are extremely rare.

Q.3. What is relationship of fourth nerve with other structures in cavernous sinus?

Ans. The fourth nerve passes through the lateral wall of cavernous sinus in between third nerve and first division of the fifth nerve. The nerve then passes through the superior orbital fissure outside the annulus of Zinn on its lateral side.

Q.4. Why fourth nerve is so vulnerable to trauma?

Ans. It is the thinnest and longest CN (75 mm). It is the only CN that comes out from the dorsal aspect of the brainstem.

Q.5. How would you differentiate between unilateral and bilateral SOP?

Ans. Refer to **Table 2**.

Q.6. How would you differentiate between congenital and acquired SOP?

Ans. Refer to **Table 3**.

Q.7. How would you differentiate between congenital and ocular torticollis SOP?

Ans. Refer to **Table 4**.

Table 2: Differences between unilateral and bilateral superior oblique palsy.

Investigations	Unilateral	Bilateral
Cover test	Hyperdeviation in 1° position	Slight hyperdeviation in 1° position
Extraocular movements	Hypertropia and diplopia on lateral versions of affected side with slight V pattern	Reversal of hypertropia and diplopia on lateral versions with large V pattern
Abnormal head posture	Chin depression, head tilt and head turn	Chin depression
Torsion	Mild extorsion	Extorsion >10°

Table 3: Differences between congenital and acquired SOP.

Parameters	Congenital	Acquired
History	Long-standing head tilt. No history of trauma	No long-standing head tilt history of acute trauma
Facial asymmetry	Present	Absent
Ocular motility	No diplopia	Diplopia +
Force duction test	Lax superior oblique tendon	No lax superior oblique tendon
Vertical fusional reserve	>40 prism diopters	<20 prism diopters
Torsion (double Maddox rod test)	No extorsion	Extorsion <150

Table 4: Congenital versus ocular torticollis.

Congenital	Acquired
Onset at birth	Rarely before 18 months
Passive straightening of head difficult	Easy passive straightening
Neck muscles firm	Palpation negative
No visual disturbances	Diplopia is frequent
Tilt not affected by occlusion	Generally, straightens on occluding the paralytic eye

Q.8. How would you do Parks–Bielschowsky three-step tests?

Ans. Given in examination.

Q.9. How do you localize the lesion in case of fourth nerve palsy?

Ans. The fourth CN decussates immediately as it originates and lies dorsally making it more susceptible to damage. A damage to the fourth nerve at this point usually results in bilateral palsy. The CN then passes through cavernous sinus and superior orbital fissure where it can be involved. However, in cases with trochlear nerve involvement in cavernous sinus and superior orbital fissure there is usually concurrent involvement of other CNs too (3rd, 5th, and 6th) passing through these structures.

BIBLIOGRAPHY

1. Bagheri A, Fallahi MR, Abrishami M, Salour H, Aletaha M. Clinical features and outcomes of treatment for fourth nerve palsy. J Ophthalmic Vis Res. 2010;5(1):27-31.
2. Borchert MS. Principles and techniques of the examination of ocular motility and alignment. In: Miller NR, Newman NJ (Eds). Clinical Neuro-ophthalmology, 6th edition. Philadelphia: Lippincott Williams & Wilkins; 2005. pp. 887-906.
3. Von Noorden GK, Campos EC. Binocular Vision and Ocular Motility: Theory and Management of Strabismus, 6th edition. St. Louis: Mosby; 2002.

OPTIC NEURITIS

Ritu Nagpal, Adarsh Shashni

INTRODUCTION

Optic neuritis (ON) is the term used for the inflammation of optic nerve. It is also called papillitis (when the head of the optic nerve is involved) and retrobulbar neuritis (when the posterior of the nerve is involved). It is caused by many different conditions, and it may lead to complete or partial loss of vision. The most common cause is acute demyelinating ON often associated with multiple sclerosis (MS).[1-3]

In examinations, ON can be given as both long and short cases.

HISTORY

Chief Complaint

Usual history is a young adult patient, typically <45 years of age, (but may be of any age) presents with unilateral vision loss developing over a period of several hours to few days.

This may be associated with:
- Periocular pain (seen in almost 53%–92% of cases), especially with eye movement that may precede or coincide with visual loss.
- Reduced contrast and color vision—loss of color and contrast at times out of proportion to loss of VA strongly suggests optic nerve pathology. Abnormal color vision by Ishihara plates was found in 88% of involved eyes in the optic neuritis treatment trial (ONTT). Many a times patient may complain of color desaturation refers to a qualitative intereye difference in color perception that can be tested by comparing vision of a red object with each eye. A patient with monocular "red desaturation" may report that the red color appears "washed out," pink, or orange when viewed with the affected eye. It is important to remember that problems of color vision can persist even after complete clinical resolution.

Few symptoms when present strongly points toward an association with multiple sclerosis such as:
- Bright flashes of light with movement of affected eye (phosphenes)
- Flashes of light induced by noise, smell, taste, touch (photism)
- Diplopia, nystagmus, dysarthria, dysphagia
- Electric shock-like sensation on neck movement (*Uhthoff phenomenon*)
- Sudden worsening of vision on exercise or increase in body temperature (*Lhermitte sign*)

- *Pulfrich phenomenon*, in which anomalous perception of the direction of movement of an object occurs due to asymmetry of conduction velocity in the optic nerves
- Weakness and stiffness of lower limbs
- Numbness and paresthesias
- Sphincter disturbances

History of Present Illness

The onset and progression shows a characteristic pattern in a typical case of ON. Visual loss is acute or subacute, varies from mild reduction to no perception of light and progresses over 7–10 days before reaching a nadir. By 2–3 weeks the VA starts improving and almost complete recovery occurs by 4–5 weeks of onset.

The pain is typically dull aching type exacerbated by touching or moving the eye. It reaches maximal severity within 24–36 hours and spontaneously abates within 48–72 hours in few cases it may persist for a long time and atypical causes of ON must be ruled out in such cases.

Past History

Similar episodes in past may be there. In the ONTT, the recurrence rate was 35% within 10 years. Subgroup analysis showed a higher recurrence rate (48%) in patients with MS compared to those without MS (24%).[1,2]

Past Surgical History

History of prior surgery, such as shunt surgery, optic nerve fenestration, and cardiac or any spinal surgery must be recorded carefully.

Past Medical History

A careful systemic history is required to rule out other causes of optic nerve dysfunction such as NAION. Hypertension, DM, hyperlipidemia, collagen vascular disease, antiphospholipid antibody syndrome, erectile dysfunction, hypotension, hyperhomocysteinemia, sleep apnea syndrome, previously diagnosed multiple sclerosis and any previous cerebrovascular accident must be noted carefully. Prior history of peptic ulceration and tuberculosis is important especially when intravenous (IV) steroid therapy is planned.

■ EXAMINATION

Systemic Examination

A complete neurological workup is a must in all cases of ON.

Ocular Examination

Visual Acuity

Uncorrected as well-corrected VA must be recorded in all cases. VA on presentation and VA of the other eye often guides the initial treatment. Serial VA monitoring helps in differentiating typical from atypical form of ON. It must be remembered VA in optic neuropathies, but does not correlate perfectly with the extent of optic nerve dysfunction, so it is a somewhat insensitive measure.

Eyeball

Usually normal; however, nystagmus and ocular motor nerve palsies may be seen in some cases.

Lids, Conjunctiva, and Cornea

Usually normal.

Pupils

Presence of relative afferent pupillary defect (RAPD) is an important sign of optic nerve dysfunction. It must be remembered that RAPD is a nonspecific sign of optic neuropathy. In bilateral cases, or in cases with a preexisting optic neuropathy in the fellow eye, an RAPD may not be apparent.

Anterior Segment/IOP

Usually normal.

Posterior Segment

Slit lamp biomicroscopic examination using a 90D/78D lens and indirect ophthalmoscopy:
- Vitreous—in a typical case of ON vitreous is usually normal
- Optic disc
  - Papillitis with hyperemia and swelling of the disc (**Fig. 1**), blurring of disc margins, and distended veins (**Fig. 2**) is seen in one-third of patients with ON.
  - Two-thirds of these patients have retrobulbar neuritis with a normal funduscopic examination.

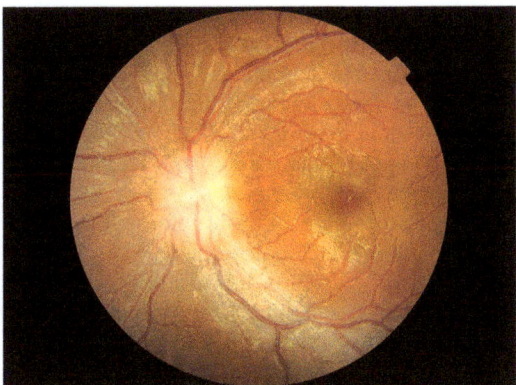

Fig. 1: Papillitis with hyperemia and swelling of the disc.

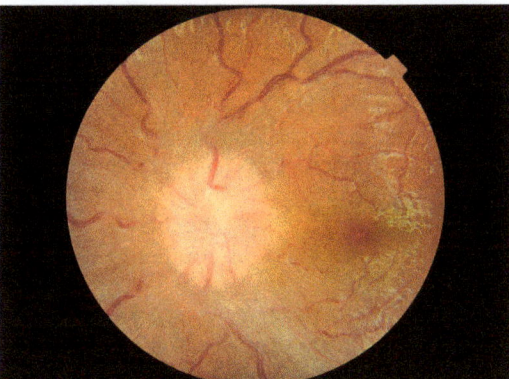

Fig. 2: Papillitis with blurring of disc margins, and distended veins.

- It must be remembered that the disc swelling of demyelinating ON is diffuse and presence of any segmental changes, altitudinal swelling, pallor, arterial attenuation, and splinter hemorrhages suggests some alternate diagnosis.
- Papillitis is more common in children <14 years old and in certain ethnic populations, including black South Africans and Southeast Asians.
- Peripapillary hemorrhages are rare in ON, but are a common accompaniment to papillitis due to anterior ischemic optic neuropathy normal or edematous.
- *Macula:* A typical case on ON may not show any abnormality. Presence edema, exudates, or star formation suggest atypical nature of the disease.

- Perivenous sheathing or periphlebitis retinae can be seen in about 12% of patients with ON and implies *a high risk for MS.*
- Examination of fellow eye is important. Disc pallor [commonly temporal disc pallor which may extend beyond the disc margin into adjacent retinal nerve fiber layer (RNFL)] in the fellow eye suggests previous ON.

■ INVESTIGATIONS

The diagnosis of ON is usually made on clinical grounds.

- *Color vision and contrast sensitivity:*
  - Decreased color vision and contrast sensitivity are highly characteristic of ON.
  - Poor color vision, particularly out of proportion to loss of acuity, is a very sensitive indicator of optic neuropathy.
- *Visual field:* The most common field defect seen in demyelinating ON is diffuse depression of sensitivity in the entire central 30° followed by altitudinal/arcuate defects and focal central/centrocecal scotoma
- *Visual evoked potential (VEP):*
  - Decrease in amplitude and prolongation of latency can be seen. A delay in the P100 of the visual evoked response (VER) is the electrophysiologic manifestation of slowed conduction in the optic nerve as a result of axonal demyelination.
  - This test is not specific for diagnosis of acute optic neuritis (AON).
  - In ONTT 67% cases had fellow eye abnormalities.
- *Magnetic resonance imaging:*
  - MRI of the brain and orbits with gadolinium contrast provides confirmation of the diagnosis of acute demyelinating ON. *MRI with FLAIR (fluid attenuated inversion recovery) sequencing and gadolinium infusion and fat suppression* when available is the preferred modality.
  - Usual finding shows white matter abnormalities characteristic of MS such ovoid periventricular (>3 mm) and corpus callosum plaques with long axis perpendicular to the ventricular margins dark on T2 and hyperintense on T1. The longitudinal extent of nerve involvement as seen on MRI correlates with visual

impairment at presentation and with visual prognosis.
- The reported prevalence of white matter abnormalities varies from 23 to 75%. In the ONTT, almost 40% of patients had MRI lesions.
- It also provides important prognostic information regarding the risk of developing MS. Individuals with white matter abnormalities are at a higher risk of developing MS.
- *Lumbar puncture:*
   - Lumbar puncture is not an essential diagnostic test in ON, but should be considered in atypical cases.
   - Abnormality is seen in >90% cases. It shows leukocytosis, raised IgG levels, raised IgG/albumin index, and oligoclonal IgG bands.
- *Optical coherence tomography (OCT):* OCT shows RNFL thinning in most (85%) of patients with ON. However, it does not have any diagnostic value since these abnormalities are also common in patients with MS who do not have a clinical history of ON.
- *Additional investigations:* To be done in the presence of atypical features
   - Complete hemogram with ESR and CRP
   - Antinuclear antibody, anti-ds-DNA antibody
   - Mantoux test
   - IFN-ψ release assay (Quantiferon TB Gold)
   - Chest X-ray
   - Gallium scan
   - Serum ACE levels
   - Serum and CSF VDRL and FTABs
   - Serum neuromyelitis optica (NMO) IgG levels
   - Spinal MRI
   - Anti-Lyme antibody titer
   - Mitochondrial gene mutation (11778 and 14484).

DIFFERENTIAL DIAGNOSIS

The differential diagnoses for unilateral sudden decrease in vision include following:[1-3]
- *Optic neuritis:*
   - Sudden onset vision loss with subsequent improvement (VA usually between 6/18 and 6/60)
   - Cellular reaction in the vitreous overlying the optic disc and presence of retinal exudates suggestive of papillitis
   - Normal appearing optic disc in retrobulbar neuritis
   - Central visual loss (central scotoma).
- *Ischemic optic neuropathy:*
   - Sudden onset vision loss with no or incomplete improvement
   - Chalky white edematous disc with overlying hemorrhages
   - Sectoral disc edema
   - Nerve fiber bundle-type field defects (originating from and involving the physiologic blind spot) typically respecting the horizontal meridian.
- *Compressive optic neuropathy:*
   - Slowly progressive vision loss
   - Chronic disc edema with optociliary shunt vessels
   - Presence of pseudodrusen
   - Central visual loss (central scotoma)
- *Papillophlebitis:*
   - Mild vision loss (6/12 or better)
   - Slow progression compared to ON or NAION
   - Mild disc swelling
   - Disc surface telangiectasia
   - Spontaneously resolves.
- *Central retinal vein occlusion (CRVO):*
   - Sudden onset of visual blurring with severity depending on the type of CRVO; ischemic or nonischemic
   - Dilated and tortuous vessels with dot/blot and flame hemorrhages in all four quadrants, most numerous in the periphery
   - Cotton wool spots, optic disc and macular edema
   - FFA–delayed A-V transit time, blockage by hemorrhages
   - Disc collaterals, epiretinal gliosis, and pigmentary changes at macula in chronic stage
- *Leber's hereditary optic neuropathy:*
   - Acute or subacute painless loss of central vision
   - Sequential involvement of the fellow eye within weeks or months

- Disc hyperemia with obscured margins
- Dilated and tortuous posterior pole vasculature (telangiectatic microangiopathy)
- Swelling of the peripapillary nerve fiber layer (pseudoedema)
- FFA—absence of dye leak
- Central or centrocecal scotoma
- Usually poor prognosis

■ CLASSIFICATION OF OPTIC NEURITIS

Optic neuritis may be classified either on the basis of ophthalmoscopic findings or on the basis of underlying etiology.

Ophthalmoscopic Classification

- Retrobulbar neuritis—characterized by normally appearing optic nerve head; adults usually present with retrobulbar neuritis associated with multiple sclerosis.
- Papillitis—characterized by hyperemia and edema of the optic disc; peripapillary flame-shaped hemorrhages may or may not be present. Cells can also be present in the posterior vitreous. Papillitis is frequently encountered in children.
- Neuroretinitis—as the name suggests neuroretinitis is associated with papillitis and inflammation of the nerve fiber layer resulting in a macular star development. This is the least common type of ON.

Etiological Classification

- Demyelinating—the most common type
- Parainfectious—usually occurs following a viral infection or immunization
- Infectious—occurs due to sinus infections or in association with cat scratch fever, syphilis, Lyme disease, cryptococcal meningitis in patients with AIDS and herpes zoster
- Noninfectious—occurs in association with systemic causes, such as sarcoidosis, systemic lupus erythematosus, polyarteritis nodosa, and other forms of vasculitis

Depending upon Course of the Disease

For typical and atypical, See **Table 1**

■ TREATMENT

Acute Therapeutic Options for Optic Neuritis

Routine treatment of typical demyelinating ON with corticosteroids is not advised due to lack of long-term benefit and the potential for side

Table 1: Difference between typical and atypical optic neuritis.

Feature	Typical optic neuritis	Atypical optic neuritis
Onset	Acute	Chronic
Age	Young patient (mean age in ONTT was 32 years)	Older patient
Sex	Caucasian female	Male
Laterality	Typically unilateral	Bilateral simultaneous or rapidly sequential
Pain	>90% have pain with eye movements. This helps to differentiate optic neuritis from NAION	Lack of pain or protracted pain
Optic disc	Appears normal in two-thirds of cases	Significant papillitis
Hemorrhage	Usually not seen	Marked hemorrhages
Exudates	Uncommon	Macular star may be seen
Uveitis	Rare	Pars planitis, choroiditis, phlebitis
Course	Vision initially worsens over several days and then spontaneously starts improving. About 75% patients recover visual acuity of 6/9 or better	Lack of improvement or progression

effects.[1-3] There are specific situations where corticosteroids may be offered to shorten the period of functional impairment. Corticosteroids, therefore, are considered for following patients:
- Who require faster recovery, such as occupational requirements
- Patients with severe bilateral visual loss
- Poor vision in the fellow eye

Regimen: IV methyl prednisolone 1 g daily for 3 days followed by oral prednisolone (1 mg/kg/day) for 11 days and then tapered over 3 days. Oral corticosteroids were associated with an increased risk of recurrence of ON in ONTT hence this form of therapy should be avoided.

VIVA QUESTIONS

Q.1. What are the signs of optic nerve dysfunction?

Ans. Signs of optic nerve dysfunction include:
- Reduced VA for distance and near
- Afferent pupillary defect
- Dyschromatopsia mainly affecting red and green
- Diminished light brightness sensitivity
- Diminished contrast sensitivity
- Visual field defects depending on the underlying pathology

Q.2. How do you differentiate typical ON from atypical ON?

Ans. Refer to **Table 1**.

Q.3. What were the results of ONTT?

Ans. The objectives of the study were to evaluate the efficacy of corticosteroid for the treatment of AON and to investigate the relationship between ON and multiple sclerosis.
- *Patients were randomized into three arms:* placebo, oral (low-dose) prednisone (1 mg/kg/day for 14 days) and high-dose IV methyl prednisolone (250 mg four times daily for 3 days), followed by oral prednisone (1 mg/kg/day for 11 days).
- At 6 months, color vision and contrast sensitivity and visual fields were found to be significantly better in the methyl prednisolone arm; however, after 1 year, there was no significant difference between treated and untreated patients in any of the functional outcome.
- IV methyl prednisolone was found to accelerate the rate of visual recovery over the first 15 days. By day 30 nearly complete recovery occurred in all patients.
- No significant difference was found between oral prednisolone and placebo in any of the parameter. At 12 months, all three groups were similar in terms of visual functions.
- In a subsequent analysis, patients randomized to receive treatment with high-dose IV methylprednisolone in conjunction with 11-day low-dose oral prednisone taper exhibited a significantly reduced risk of developing clinically definite multiple sclerosis (CDMS) (defined by the development of new neurologic symptoms attributable to demyelination other than ON in either eye occurring at least 4 weeks after the study entry and lasting >24 hours with abnormality documented on neurological examination) over the subsequent 2 years. Beyond 2 years no significant disease-modifying effects of steroids was seen.

Q.4. What is the overall risk of developing multiple sclerosis in a patient presenting with ON?

Ans. Approximately 15%–20% of MS patients present with ON. In patients with established MS, ON occurs in 50% cases at some point of time. The overall 10 years risk of developing MS following an acute episode of ON with one or more characteristic brain lesions, normal brain MRI is 56% whereas it is 22% if the MRI is normal. At 15 years the risk increases to 25% in patients with normal baseline MRI and 70% in patients with abnormal baseline MRI.[1-3]

Q.5. What is the role of brain MRI?

Ans. The likelihood of progression of ON to MS is best predicted by brain MRI done at the time of diagnosis. In the ONTT baseline, brain MRI was found to be the most powerful predictor of likelihood of CDMS.

Q.6. What are the low risk factors for MS?

Ans. These are lack of pain, severe disc edema, peripapillary hemorrhage, retinal exudates and mild VA loss.

Q.7. What are the diagnostic criteria for diagnosis of MS?

Ans. *McDonald criteria:* Clinical history and presentation in the presence of neuroimaging abnormalities with or without CSF abnormalities or abnormal VEP response. Recurrent ON in the absence of other clinical or laboratory manifestations is not sufficient for diagnosis.

Q.8. What is NMO?

Ans. Neuromyelitis optica or Devic's disease is characterized by necrotizing demyelinating lesions of bilateral optic nerves and spinal cord. The spinal lesions extend contiguously over three of more vertebral segments. Serum antibody, NMO-IgG, which targets the autoantigen aquaporin-4, is a useful marker for diagnosis. Treatment with rituximab has been tried to be beneficial.

Q.9. What are the treatment modalities available for AON apart from corticosteroids?

Ans. Treatment modalities available for acute ON are described below:[4,5]
- *Short-acting agents (for acute exacerbations):* High-dose IV steroids
- *Longer-acting agents (delay the development of CDMS):*
  - *Disease modifying drugs:* Interferon β-1a and 1b, glatiramer acetate
  - *Immunosuppressives:* Mitoxantrone, natalizumab, fingolimod
- *Newer treatment options:*
  - *Intravenous immunoglobulins (IVIg):* have been tried for acute ON but with no long-term effects on visual function or on the latency of VEP responses after AON.
  - *Plasma exchange (PLEX):* PLEX has demonstrated efficacy in the treatment of refractory AON and in AON associated with NMO. The addition of PLEX to IV methylprednisolone in the acute treatment of NMO-associated AON has showed significant improvement in high-contrast acuity, visual fields and temporal RNFL thickness, but not low-contrast letter scores or color vision. The early, first-line use of PLEX in the treatment of AON is yet to be evaluated. PLEX is presumed to mediate a therapeutic effect, at least in part, through the removal of pathogenic humoral and plasma factors.
  - *Erythropoietin:* Systemic infusion of erythropoietin with and without methylprednisolone has demonstrated beneficial effects on retinal ganglion cell (RGC) function and survival in a rat model of experimental autoimmune encephalomyelitis. Erythropoietin administration increases protein levels of various antiapoptotic factors such as phospho-Akt, phospho-MAPK 1 and 2, and Bcl-2 which helps to limit the apoptosis of RGCs after AON. Erythropoietin administration has shown partial recovery of pattern-reversal VEPs and improvement in flash electroretinograms and significant improvement in the thickness of peripapillary RNFL.
- Teriflunomide
- Adrenocorticotropic hormone
- Dimethyl fumarate
- Antibody against LINGO1 (anti-LINGO), a CNS protein that acts as a negative regulator of oligodendrocyte precursor differentiation to promote CNS remyelination phenytoin

Q.10. What are the newer investigative modalities available for the management of AON?

Ans. Various investigative modalities are as follows:
- *OCT and SLP:* To demonstrate RNFL edema which is evident in approximately 80% of the affected optic nerves. On an average, patients with AON lose 22 μm more RNFL in their affected

eye than in their unaffected eye at 3–6 months after the inception of visual symptoms.
- *Diffusion tensor imaging (DTI):* Provides a sensitive modality to complement RNFL structural injury in the evaluation of acute ON injury.
- *Electrophysiology:* Prolongation of the VEP P100 latency is used as a measure of conduction delay through the optic nerve and is a sensitive marker of demyelination. Reduction in the amplitude of VEP serves as a measure of axonal injury. The sensitivity of mfVEP is further enhanced by using low-contrast pattern-reversal stimuli allowing detection of mild residual injury or occult damage in the so-called 'unaffected' eye. The traditional ERG with optical nerve head component (ONHC) waveform—the ONHC waveform represents the transformation of slow membrane conduction to fast salutatory conduction, as axons traverse the lamina cribrosa and become myelinated. After AON, the ONHC waveforms are abolished and later recover, representing the transient effects of conduction block due to reversible demyelination. Eyes with previous ON in patients with MS exhibit changes or loss in the ONHC waveform that correlate with reduction in low-contrast letter acuity, RNFL thickness, visual field depression and amplitude loss and latency delay on mfVEP.
- *Biomarkers:* Serum and plasma neurofilament levels, heavy (NfH) and light (NfL), are elevated in patients with ON, independent of the inflammatory mechanism. The levels of NfH and NfL have been observed to correlate with the extent of vision loss and the loss of retinal nerve fiber thickness following ON.

■ REFERENCES

1. Bowling B. Kanski's Clinical Ophthalmology: A Systematic Approach, 8th edition. Edinburgh: Elsevier; 2015.
2. Albert DM, Miller JW, Azar DT. Albert and Jakobiec's Principles and Practice of Ophthalmology. Philadelphia: Saunders/Elsevier; 2008.
3. Toosy AT, Mason DF, Miller DH. Optic neuritis. Lancet Neurol. 2014;13(1):83-99.
4. Bennett JL, Nickerson M, Costello F, Sergott RC, Calkwood JC, Galetta SL, et al. Re-evaluating the treatment of acute optic neuritis. J Neurol Neurosurg Psychiatry. 2015;86(7):799-808.
5. Petzold A, Wattjes MP, Costello F, et al. The investigation of acute optic neuritis: a review and proposed protocol. Nat Rev Neurol. 2014;10(8):447-58.

ESODEVIATION

Ritika Mukhija, Adarsh Shashni

■ INTRODUCTION

Esodeviations are the most common type of ocular misalignment. It represents 50% of ocular deviations in pediatric age group. In examinations, it is given as long case.

■ HISTORY

Chief Complaint

- Deviation of eyes
- Diminution of vision
- Head posture.

History of Present Illness

- Following points must be recorded in history:
  - Age at onset
  - Constant or intermittent
  - Unilateral or bilateral
  - Progression
  - Abnormal movement of the eyes
  - Preceding history of febrile illness, meningitis, or any neurological events
  - Exacerbating and ameliorating factors
- Patient has history of deviation of eyes that can be present since birth or after some time and can be associated with diminution of vision.

- Onset at 4–6 months of age usually suggests infantile onset esotropia and frequently requires surgical management. However, later onset at 18–36 months is due to accommodative component and can be managed with refractive error correction.
- Patients with freely alternating esotropia have lesser chances of developing amblyopia.
- Family album tomography (FAT) analysis helps in documentation of onset and progression of strabismus.
- History of head posture, chin position, or face turn may be there.

Past History

A detailed ocular history should be elucidated regarding onset, progression, duration of esodeviation, cycloplegic refractive error correction prescribed, compliance with spectacles, and amblyopia therapy. Patient should also be asked about the history of previous surgery, records of previous surgery, and any prism correction. History regarding previous management helps in determining the prognosis and further treatment

Birth History

- Complete birth history should be taken beginning from period of gestation, antenatal complications, type of delivery (normal or forceps), birth weight, delayed cry, milestones, and postnatal trauma or CNS infections. Following factors increases the risk of ET in a child:
- Maternal smoking during pregnancy
- Maternal age (>30 years)
- LBW (low birth weight) baby
- Retinopathy of prematurity and Down's syndrome.

Family History

Note down any history of strabismus in the parents or siblings. There is 73% concordance rate of esotropia in monozygotic twins, as compared to 35% in dizygotic twins.

■ EXAMINATION

General Examination

A careful examination especially focusing on development of the child and the neurological system must be carried out.

Local Examination

Visual Acuity

- Visual acuity chart (for elderly children)
- VER (<6 months).

Fixation preference tests (for young kids):
- Central, steady, and maintained (CSM)
- *Fixation preference:* Alternation
- *Maintenance of fixation:* 15 seconds
- 10 PD BD/BU prism test
- 25 PD BI alternation test
- *Cross fixation:* Tracking past midline.

Measurement of Alignment

Light reflex tests:
- Generally used to assess deviations in small children and in patients who cannot fixate with either or both eyes.
- Require minimal cooperation from the patient
- *Drawback:* Assess only tropias and less accurate than cover testing
- In cases where the goal of surgery is improved appearance and an angle kappa is present, light reflex tests (especially the Krimsky test) are essential as they are likely to be the best choice for determining surgical dosages.

Hirschberg test:
- Patient is asked to fixate at the point source of light shone through pen torch at arm's length.
- The position of light reflex is observed. The reflex is centered in the pupil of the fixating eye, but in a squinting eye the position of reflex will be displaced opposite to that of the deviation.
- Note the distance of the corneal light reflex from the center of the pupil. Each millimeter of light displacement across the cornea is equivalent to 7° of decentration or 14 Δ.
- A light reflection at the pupillary border signifies a 15° or 30 Δ deviation, at the mid-iris a deviation of 30° or 60 Δ, and at the limbus a deviation of 45° or 90 Δ.
- The Hirschberg method relies on a pupil size of 4 mm and performing in a case with dilated pupil is not reliable.
- It provides rough estimate of the angle of strabismus in cases where the patient may not allow prisms to be placed in front of the eyes.

Krimsky test:
- Preferred over the Hirschberg test as it allows a more exact estimate of the alignment.
- However, it requires a cooperative patient.
- Corneal reflex assessment is combined with prisms to measure the angle in a manifest deviation.
- A neutralizing prism is placed (A prism bar starting with a relatively low prism power) over either eye to position the corneal light reflex in its normal position.
- Generally, the prism is placed over the fixing eye to improve visualization of the light reflex in the deviating eye.

Bruckner test:
- Done with a direct ophthalmoscope and the red reflex is watched.
- If the red reflex coming from one eye is different from the other, strabismus is suspected. The deviating eye gives a brighter reflex
- Easy to perform, but it does require some expertise
- Generally used for screening purposes only; it is an excellent test to screen a preverbal child for strabismus, anisometropia or amblyopia.

Cover–uncover test: The gold standard for evaluating strabismus is the cover–uncover test. It can diagnose both the tropia and phoria components. When performed with prisms, it can be quantitative also. It has to be done for both near and distance and with and without refractive correction. The fixation distance should be 33 cm for near and 6 m for distance. For distance fixation target is given of a figure or letter size of 6/9 of Snellen's chart.

Prerequisites:
- Both eyes must be able to fixate the target
- Both eyes must have central fixation
- No severe motility defect

Cover test:
- To start with, cover the apparently fixating eye
- Observe if the apparently deviating eye moves to take up fixation
- If the uncovered eye moves, tropia exists

Uncover test:
- It is done to unmask the phoria.
- After covering the eye fusion breaks and if there is any heterophoria the eye behind the cover deviates. This can be observed with the use of translucent occluder (Spielmann's occluder).
- After removing the cover if it remains deviated, it confirms a latent squint with poor fusion (poor recovery). If it recovers, the examiner observes the speed of recovery, which shows strength of fusion and it is important prognostic sign.

Alternate cover test:
- The purpose of alternate cover test is to break the fusion in order to reveal the total deviation. Alternate cover test is usually performed after the cover–uncover test.
- The occlude is shifted back and forth between the two eyes many times, covering one eye at a time.
- On removing the cover, one should record the speed and ease with which recovery of the eyes occur to the predissociated state.
- A prolonged manifest deviation on removing the cover shows a poor control and has higher chances of developing a manifest squint.

Prism Bar cover test (PBCT):
- The prism cover test gives a qualitative assessment of the angle of deviation in prism diopter for near and distance fixation.
- The procedure of PBCT is similar to the alternate cover test. However, in this test prisms of increasing power are placed in front of one of the eyes till the eye movement stops.
- Prism is placed such that the apex of the prism points toward the direction of the deviation. Thus, the position of prism is base-out for esotropia, base-in for exotropia, and base-down for a hypertropia.
- Speed of the refixation movements gradually reduce on approaching the extent of deviation.
- No refixation movement occurs once the deviation has been neutralized. Further on increasing the prism strength an opposite movement is observed, known as the point of reversal. The prism strength is further reduced again to find the point of neutralization.
- In cases of incomitant strabismus, (paralytic and restrictive strabismus) deviations should be measured with both normal fixing (primary deviation) and affected eye fixing (secondary deviation). The secondary deviation is always larger than the primary deviation.

Accommodative Convergence to Accommodation Ratio

It characterizes the difference in alignment observed between distance and near fixation. A normal accommodative convergence to accommodation ratio (AC/A ratio) allows the eyes to remain aligned and in focus as a target moves closer. Preoperative determination of AC/A ratio may be helpful in predicting the extent to which a patient may respond to plus lenses when a surgical overcorrection is obtained.

The AC/A ratio can be determined by following methods:
- *Gradient method:* Interpupillary distance (IPD) is not needed as vergence is measured at the same distance. At 33 cm with patient wearing his proper refractive correction, deviation is measured with and without +3.0 DS lens (if assessed using distance target −3.0 SD lens is used) placed in front of both the eyes.
  Prolonged monocular occlusion used to break vergence after effect before test.

  AC/A = Deviation without lens − deviation with lens

  Power of the lens is in diopters
- *Heterophoria method:* Deviation measured at distant vision with full optical correction (no accommodation exerted), and at a near distance (e.g., 33 cm)
  AC/A = IPD + ND − DD/AN [IPD = interpupillary distance (cm); ND = near deviation (diopters); DD = Distance deviation (diopters); AN = Accommodation for near (1/3 = 3 diopters)] (*Note:* Esotropia + sign is used and for Exotropia − sign is used for deviation while calculating AC/A ratio).
- Graphic method, fixation disparity method, and haploscopic method are other methods for AC/A ratio.
  Routine AC/A ratio is normally not done clinically; instead, the difference in measurements at distance and near is assessed. Any difference of >10 PD suggests an abnormal AC/A relationship and should be considered into the treatment plan for the patient.

Maddox Wing

- The Maddox wing is a handheld device, used for measuring latent and manifest deviations at near, and cyclophoria.
- The instrument is constructed in such a way that the right eye sees only a white vertical arrow and a red horizontal arrow, whereas the left eye sees only horizontal and vertical rows of numbers.
- Patient is asked the number to which the white arrow points that indicates the horizontal deviation.
- The number intersecting with the red arrow indicated the vertical deviation.
- Patient is asked to move the red arrow such that becomes parallel to the horizontal row numbers, this measures the cyclophoria.

Maddox Rod

- Maddox rod is used to measure horizontal and vertical deviations and is a subjective test for measuring torsion.
- Maddox rod consist of a series of fused cylindrical rods that convert a point source of light to a streak at an angle of 90° with the long axis of the rods. Thus, when the glass rods are held vertically, the streak will be perceived horizontally and vice versa.
- The amount of dissociation is measured by the superimposition of the two images using prisms. The apex of the prism is placed in the direction of the deviation.

Fusional Amplitudes

Fusional amplitudes measure the efficacy of vergence movements. It can be tested with prisms bars or synoptophore. A progressively increasingly strong prism is placed in front of one eye, which will then abduct (base-in prism) or adduct (base-out prism) to maintain bifoveal fixation. Thus for fusional amplitude of convergence base-out prism is used and for divergence base in prism is used. When the power of prism exceeds the fusional amplitude, diplopia is reported or one eye drifts in the opposite direction, indicating the limit of vergence ability. This is known as break point and gradually then decreases the strength of the prism till patient realign his eyes this is the recovery point. This should be checked for both distance and near fixation.

Near Point of Convergence

Near point of convergence (NPC) is the nearest point up to which eyes can maintain binocular fixation. NPC can be measured using Royal Air Force (RAF) ruler. The RAF ruler resets on patient's cheeks and a target is slowly moved along the rule toward the patient's eye. The point at which the patient reports diplopia is the subjective NPC. Objective NPC is the point at which one eye drifts. Normally NPC is <10 cm.

Near Point of Accommodation

Near point of accommodation (NPA) is the nearest point up to which the eyes can see clearly. RAF ruler is used to measure the NPA. Patient is shown a line of print mounted on the scale, which is slowly moved toward the patient. The point at which the print becomes blurred is the NPA. At the age of 20 years, the NPA is 8 cm and by the age of 50 years is approximately 46 cm. NPA is not a fixed value and recedes back with age.

Interpupillary Distance

It is measured with the help of two scales or synoptophore.

Diplopia Charting

Test requires red–green glasses. Diplopia charting is done in all nine gazes with the help of a linear light source.

Tests for Binocular Vision and Sensory Anomalies

Worth Four-dot Test

- Worth four-dot test is used to differentiate suppression, BSV, and ARC.
- Worth four-dot test uses a red–green glass to induce dissociation and can be used for distance and near.
- *Procedure:* For distance worth four-dot test patient is seated at a distance of 6 m. Patient is given a red–green glass. The red lens is placed in front of the right eye and green lens is placed in front of the left eye. The red lens filters out all other except red, and green lens filters out all other except green.
- Patient is asked to view the screen with two green, one red, and one white dots.
- Interpretation
  - If patient can see all four lights, then it suggests BSV
  - If the patient can appreciate all four lights despite the presence of manifest deviation, it suggest harmonious ARC
  - In patients with left eye suppression only two red lights are seen.
  - In patients with right eye suppression only three green lights are seen.
  - If the patient appreciates three green and two red lights then it suggests diplopia.
  - Alternating suppression is suggested by the alternate green and red lights.

Bagolini Striated Glasses

- Bagolini striated glasses are used for detecting suppression, BSV, and ARC.
- *Procedure:* Bagolini glasses have two lenses with fine at 45° and 135°. Patient is asked to fixate on a focal light source. Each eye perceives an oblique line of light, which is perpendicular to that perceived by the fellow eye.
- Interpretation
- If the patient appreciates a cross (X) then it suggests BSV. If the patient appreciates a cross even in the presence of manifest strabismus, it suggests harmonious ARC.
- If the patient sees two lines separately that do not form a cross, suggests diplopia.
- If the patients sees only one streak it suggests suppression.
- Presence of a small gap in the center of cross suggests central suppression scotoma (CSS).

Four Δ Prism Test

- It distinguishes bifoveal fixation (normal BSV) from foveal suppression (also known as a central suppression scotoma) in microtropia.
- *With bifoveal fixation:* The prism is placed base-out (microtropia is commonly esotropic not exotropic) in front of the right eye with deviation of the image away from the fovea

temporally, followed by corrective movement of both eyes to the left (kindly read it once, the message is not clear).
- The left eye then converges to fuse the images
- *In left microtropia:* The patient fixates a distance target with both eyes open and a 4 Δ prism is placed base-out in front of the eye with suspected CSS. The image is moved temporally in the left eye but falls within the CSS and no movement of either eye is observed.
- The prism is then moved to the right eye which, adducts to maintain fixation; the left eye similarly moves to the left consistent with the Hering law of equal innervation, but the second image falls within the CSS of the left eye and so no subsequent refixation movement is seen.

Base-out Prism

This is a simple method used for detecting fusion in children. The test is performed by placing a 20 Δ base-out prism in front of one eye of the patient. The prism displaces the retinal image temporally resulting in diplopia. Most children with good BSV can overcome a 20 Δ prism from the age of 6 months; if not, weaker prisms (16 Δ or 12 Δ) may be tried, but the response is then more difficult to identify.

After Image Testing (with Synaptophore)

It is a dissociative test to know suppression, ARC, or central scotoma.

Stereopsis

Various tests, using differing principles, are employed to assess the stereoacuity. Random dot tests (e.g., TNO, Frisby) provide the most definitive evidence of high-grade BSV. Where this is weak and/or based on ARC, contour-based tests (e.g., titmus) may provide more reliable information.
- *Titmus test:* The titmus test consists of a three-dimensional polarized vectograph comprising two plates in the form of a booklet viewed through polarized spectacles. On the right is a large fly, and on the left is a series of circles and animals. The test should be performed at a distance of 40 cm.
- *Randot test:* It uses Julsez's random dot background to mask the monocular clues. It requires polaroid glasses. Near Randot is done at 40 cm and distance Randot is done at 3 m.
- *TNO test:* The TNO random dot test consists of seven plates of randomly distributed paired red and green dots viewed with red–green spectacles, and measures from 480 down to 15 seconds of arc at 40 cm.
- *Frisby Davis distance test:* This is a real depth test measured at 6, 3, or 1 m and measures stereoacuity from 4 to 200 seconds of arc.
- *Lang's pencil gross stereopsis test:* Pencils held horizontally to avoid patient seeing end on view. We ask the patient to touch the pencil tip held by him to that of the examiner. Simple bedside test works well to demonstrate gross stereopsis (3,000–5,000 seconds of arc).
- *Synoptophore test:* The synoptophore compensates for the angle of squint and allows stimuli to be presented to both eyes simultaneously.
- It can thus be used to investigate the potential for binocular function in the presence of a manifest squint and is of particular value in assessing young children (from age 3 years), who generally find the test process enjoyable. It can also detect suppression and ARC.
- The instrument consists of two cylindrical tubes with a mirrored right-angled bend and a + 6.50 D lens in each eyepiece. This optically sets the testing distance as equivalent to about 6 m.
- The synoptophore can measure horizontal, vertical, and torsional misalignments simultaneously and is valuable in determining surgical approach by assessing the different contributions in the cardinal positions of gaze.
- *Hess/Lees testing:* A Hess chart is plotted to aid in the diagnosis and monitoring of a patient with incomitant strabismus, such as an extraocular muscle palsy (e.g., third, fourth, or sixth nerve paresis) or a mechanical or myopathic limitation (e.g., thyroid ophthalmopathy, blowout fracture or myasthenia gravis). The chart is commonly prepared using either the Lees or Hess screen, which facilitate plotting of the dissociated ocular position as a measure of extraocular muscle action. Information provided by the Hess chart should be regarded in the context of other investigations such as the field of BSV.

Forced Duction Test

The FDT is an attempt by the examiner to move a patient's eye farther in a given direction than the patient can move it. Topical anesthetic is placed on the appropriate limbal location (generally 180° away from the duction limitation) with a small cotton swab and the limbal conjunctiva is grasped firmly with a toothed forceps. The patient is asked to rotate the eye fully in the direction of the limited duction. An attempt is then made by the examiner to rotate the eye beyond the position attained by the patient while avoiding globe retraction. Care must be taken not to abrade the cornea.

Patients who have pure nerve palsy exhibit no restriction to full movement by the examiner; patients who have pure restriction (dysthyroid orbitopathy, entrapment of ocular contents after blowout fracture) exhibit restricted movements (sometimes termed a positive FDT). Some patients initially have pure nerve palsy, but contracture of the antagonist muscle results in secondary mechanical restriction of movement. Suction cup devices have been developed for examiners who are wary of using toothed instruments at the limbus; a cotton swab may be a sufficient tool in some patients. Forced duction testing of oblique muscles may be performed, but two forceps are used and the globe is depressed forcibly into the orbit.

Active Forced Generation Test

Active force generation testing may be used to evaluate the ability of a muscle to move the eye against a resisting force. The forceps is placed at the limbus of the anesthetized globe in the meridian of the muscle whose duction is limited and the patient requested to rotate the eye in the direction of the limited duction; the examiner judges through the forceps the relative amount of force generated. Strain gauges have been devised that enable quantitation of this force. This is done in patients with paralytic squint (for example, in esotropia due to 6th CN palsy).

■ CLASSIFICATION

- *Esophoria:* Latent deviation that is controlled by fusion under binocular conditions
- *Intermittent esotropia:* Deviation that is controlled by fusion sometimes, but manifests in exertion/illness

Table 1: Types of comitant esotropia.

Accommodative	Nonaccommodative
Refractive accommodative	Infantile esotropia
Nonrefractive accommodative	Acute onset
Partially accommodative	Acquired or late onset
Hypoaccommodative	• Microtropia • Cyclic esotropia • Nystagmus blockage syndrome

Table 2: Incomitant esotropia types.

Paralytic	6th CN palsy, divergence palsy, myasthenia
Restrictive	Eso DRS, tumor, postoperative, strabismus fixus, endocrine myopathy
Spastic	

- *Esotropia:* Deviation is constantly manifested right, left or alternating comitant **(Table 1)** versus incomitant **(Table 2)** primary/secondary/consecutive
- *Primary:* No other cause; most of the esotropias are primary.
- *Secondary:* Consequence of loss or impairment of vision
- *Consecutive:* Overcorrection of an initial exotropia

■ MANAGEMENT

In all patients of esotropia should undergo full cycloplegic refraction before measurement of deviation.

Occlusion therapy should be given to those with amblyopia.

It depends upon the type of esotropia:
- For accommodative esotropia—all patient requires is full cycloplegic refraction with or without near add depending upon AC/A ratio for correction of their deviation fully **(Table 3)**.
- For partially accommodative esotropia, the accommodative element requires correction with glasses and for the nonaccommodative element surgery is needed.

Table 3: Classification of accommodative esotropia.

	Refractive normo-accommodative	Refractive hyper-accommodative	Nonrefractive hyper-accommodative	Nonrefractive hypo-accommodative
Refractive error	Hyperopia	Hyperopia	Not significant	Not significant
AC/A ratio	Normal no convergence excess	Increased	Increased	Normal
NPA	–	–	–	Remote
NPC	–	–	–	Remote
N-D deviation (prism Diopter)	<15	>15	>15 No significant esotropia for distance	>15

- For nonaccommodative esotropia surgery is needed. For convergence excess (near >distance by 10 PD) bimedial recession or medial recti recession with posterior fixation is done. For divergence insufficiency (distance >nearby 10 PD) bilateral LR resection is preferred. For basic type (near distance disparity <10 PD) either monocular MR recession and LR resection or bimedial recession is done.

VIVA QUESTIONS

Q.1. What is accommodative esotropia?
Ans. Refer to **Table 1** for types.
- *Refractive accommodative:* (Normal AC/A ratio) esotropia restored to orthotropia at all fixation distances and in all positions of gaze by optical correction of underlying refractive error.
  - Onset between 6 months and 5 years of age
  - Associated hyperopia
  - Insufficient fusional divergence
  - Often hereditary
  - Intermittent at onset—becoming constant
  - *Deviation:* 20–40 Δ
  - Precipitation—trauma, illness
- *Treatment of refractive accommodative esotropia:*
  - Cycloplegic refraction
  - Full cycloplegic correction of hypermetropic refractive error
  - Initial atropinization to relax accommodation
  - 60%–70% of these patients respond well to treatment with glasses; the remaining require surgical treatment
  - It is important to treat the entire accommodation (latent + manifest)
  - Orthoptic treatment to overcome suppression and build fusional divergence.
- *Nonrefractive accommodative:* High AC/A ratio
  - Esotropia N >D
  - Abnormally high AC/A ratio
  - *Normal NPA*
  - *Age:* 2–3 years
  - Usually has hypermetropia (2.25 D) but may have myopia.
  - Accommodative component is present—greater deviation at near
  - Accommodation is not linked to refractive error; there is synkinesis with accommodative convergence.
  - *Costenbader:* Small refractive error, remote NPA, small distance but large near deviation
  - Excessive accommodative effort and a large persistent deviation with the refractive error fully corrected

Management: Treat with bifocals and miotics
- Miotics—echothiophate iodide 0.06% or 0.125%/BE OD for 6 weeks—dose may be reduced subsequently
- Complications—RD, iris cysts, etc.

- Most patients improve with therapy
- *Surgery:* Advocated if nonaccommodative component develops

Partially accommodative esotropia:
- Esotropia having both accommodative and nonaccommodative elements are considered as partially accommodative esotropias.
- *May be:* Decompensated accommodative esotropia
- Esotropia with subsequent development of accommodative component

Treatment:
- Eventually amblyopia therapy with or without surgery is needed.
- Cycloplegic refraction with *bifocals*
- Surgical correction of residual deviation (nonaccommodative part)
- Explaining to parents that children would still require glasses after surgery
- Alignment of the eyes with glasses or surgery alone usually does not make the eyes work together. Vision therapy does.
- Occasionally the deviation may increase after patient gains stereopsis for near; one should repeat refraction at this point.
- Supportive orthoptic treatment to promote fusional divergence.
- *Hypoaccommodative:*
  - Esotropia N >D
  - Unrelated to refractive error
  - Weakness in accommodation (primary or secondary) → excess accommodative effort → excess convergence
  - The NPA is receded.

Q.2. Describe clinical features and management of essential infantile esotropia.

Ans.
- *Essential infantile esotropia:*
  - Manifest esodeviation
  - Onset between birth and 6 months of age
  - Neurologically normal infant prevalence
  - 0.1% of newborns
  - Even with this reduced prevalence, it is the most common form of strabismus
- *Clinical characteristics:*
  - Onset from birth to 6 months
  - Large angle (≥30 Δ)
  - Stable angle
  - Initial alternation with cross fixation
  - No clinically apparent CNS involvement
  - Asymmetrical optokinetic nystagmus—OKN asymmetry is present in all infants but becomes symmetrical by 6 months in the normal. Patients with congenital ET retain OKN asymmetry
  - Temporal to nasal (T/N) OKN—smooth, following and rapid refixation
  - Nasal to temporal (N/T) OKN—jerky inaccurate movements with halting refixation
  - *Incidence:* 1%–2%
- *Variable findings:*[1,2]
  - Amblyopia
  - Apparently defective abduction
  - Apparently excessive adduction
  - Up or down shoot on adduction
  - A or V pattern
  - Inferior oblique over action (68%)
  - DVD/DHD (50%)
  - Manifest latent nystagmus (33%)
  - Manifest nystagmus (rare)
  - Anomalous head posture
  - *Heredity:* Transmission may be irregular autosomal dominant, or recessive. Waardenburg reported concordance in monozygous twins to be 81%, compared with 9% in dizygotic
  - History of strabismus in the parents or siblings—positive
  - *Refractive errors:* Most commonly associated with mild hyperopia, followed by moderate and high hyperopia, and lastly myopia associated with hypermetropia (>85%) rare in myopia (6%–8%).

Ciancia syndrome:
- Essential infantile esotropia
- Latent nystagmus
- Head turn toward adducting eye
- Apparently limited abduction in both eyes

Lang syndrome:
- Esotropia
- DVD
- Excycloduction of the nonfixating eye
- Abnormal head posture

Differential diagnosis:
- *Congenital:*
  - Bilateral abducens paralysis
  - Duane syndrome type 1
  - Mobius syndrome
- *Acquired:*
  - Sensory esotropia
  - Refractive accommodative esotropia
  - Nystagmus blockage syndrome
  - Esotropia in association with CNS problems

Management
- *Goals of treatment:*
  - Restoration of single binocular vision
  - Normal visual acuity
  - Normal stereoacuity
  - Normal retinal correspondence
  - Stable sensory and motor fusion
- *Nonsurgical treatment:* Correct all hypermetropias (full cycloplegic refraction)
- *Amblyopia treatment:*
  - Conventional, full-time occlusion
  - End-point being free alternation of the two eyes which is equally maintained.
  - It should be treated before surgery because:
    - The earlier the treatment betters the results.
    - The diagnosis of amblyopia and monitoring of fixation preference difficult, once eyes aligned.
    - Patient neglects their follow-up appointment for amblyopia.
    - The outcome of surgery is less favorable.
    - The only situation when surgery is indicated in the face of residual amblyopia is a tight MR muscle that causes one eye to be buried in the medial canthus even when the good eye is patched.

Surgical management:
- *Timing of surgery:*
  - Early surgery provides better chances of functional improvement.
  - A secondary change that occurs in extraocular muscles, the conjunctiva, and Tenon's capsules makes a surgical correction at later stages more difficult and less predictable.
  - In some cases of infantile esotropia, persisting deviation warrants early surgery (3–4 months).
  - Treatment of infantile esotropia must be started at an early age frequently at 6 months.
  - *Esotropia:* Surgery done within a year of misalignment yields better stereopsis.
- *Surgical approaches:*
  - Bilateral MR recession
  - MR recession with LR resection
  - *Safe limits lesser in infants MR: 5.5 mm, LR: 6.5 mm for recession.*
  - 3 or 4 muscle surgery has also been advocated.
  - *Inferior oblique overaction:* Muscle weakening procedures
  - *Alignment within 7–8 Δ of orthophoria:* Acceptable. However, orthotropia/small—esotropia—*better in comparison*
  - One must carefully look at the fixation pattern to make sure that there is no amblyopia.
  - Treatment after 2 years reduces prognosis for re-establishment of binocular vision.
  - Older children with infantile isotropic need both surgical intervention if the turn is large and vision therapy.
  - Smaller turns may only require vision therapy.

Botulinum toxin: It is an effective treatment modality for the management of infantile esotropia in infants.

Q.3. What are microtropias? Describe its clinical features and management.

Ans. These are ultrasmall angle esodeviations which may be missed by ordinary methods of examination.
- Can be primary or secondary; latter are residual deviation postsurgery.

- Park monofixation syndrome has macular scotoma with good peripheral fusion and fusional amplitude with gross stereopsis.
- Lang's microtropia—small angle heterotropia (<5°) these have harmonious ARC with mild amblyopia and partial stereopsis. These are of three types—type 1 has central fixation; type 2 has eccentric fixation without identity; type 3 has eccentric fixation with identity (this means that angle of anomaly is same as the eccentricity of fixation).
- *Clinical features:*
  - Amblyopia
  - ARC
  - Relative scotoma at fixation spot
  - Near normal fusional amplitude
  - Defective stereopsis
  - Size of deviation (5°-8°)
  - Foveal or eccentric fixation
  - Presence or absence of anisometropia
- *Test used for diagnosis:*
  - Bagolini's glasses—detects central scotoma
  - 4 prism diopter test—already explained
- *Management:* Primarily involves treatment of amblyopia.

Q.4. What is A and V pattern strabismus?

Ans. AV pattern deviations are horizontally concomitant vertical incommitant squint. They can be:
- A esotropia—the amount of deviation is more in upgaze
- A exotropia—amount of exodeviation is more in downgaze
- V esotropia—amount of deviation is more in downgaze
- V exotropia—amount of deviation is more in upgaze
- Y pattern—where there is exotropia in upgaze only, associated with Brown's syndrome

Q.5. What are the various theories for A and V pattern strabismus?

Ans.
- *Horizontal school of thought:* According to this concept the horizontal muscles (medial and LR) are chiefly responsible for A and V pattern strabismus, where in MR mainly acts in downgaze and LR in upgaze. In V esotropia, there is MR overaction which leads to increased adduction in downgaze. V exotropia can occur due to LR overaction which causes increased abduction in upgaze. Similarly, A exotropia occurs due to MR underaction and A esotropia there is underaction of LR.
- *Vertical school of thought:* This suggests that the vertical recti lead to the patterns. SR in an elevator and adductor. Hence, SR underaction will lead to less adduction in upgaze and V pattern.
- *Oblique school of thought:* This is now the most widely accepted theory for the AV patterns. V pattern occurs due to IO overaction and A pattern occurs due to SO overaction.
- *Anatomical factors:* These occur due to variation in the facial features such as mongoloid slant is associated with A esotropia and V exotropia.

  Variations in the structures of the skull, which alter the position of the trochlea, can lead to patterns. Desagittalization where the oblique tendon becomes more parallel to coronal plane is seen in plagiocephaly and results in weakening of the SO leading to V pattern and in sagittalization, where the SO lies more in the sagittal plane due to hydrocephalus can give A pattern.

Q.6. What special measures will you take while examining the patient with A V patterns?

Ans.
- The patient can have abnormal head posture, chin up head posture can be seen with V pattern strabismus and a chin down can be seen with A pattern. All horizontal deviations must be checked for presence of oblique muscle overactions and presence of patterns. Deviation is measured in upgaze of 25° and downgaze 35°. A difference of 15 PD is significant in V pattern and 10 PD difference is significant in A pattern.

Q.7. How will you manage a patient with A V pattern along with horizontal strabismus?

Ans. Horizontal rectus recession and resection are done for the horizontal deviation:
- If associated with oblique overactions— if the patterns are associated with oblique muscle overactions, then oblique muscle weakening should be done. In case of V patterns, IO weakening procedure can be done. Depending on the amount of overaction, Parks or Fink recession for mild and Elliot and Nankin's recession with anterior positioning can be done for more severe overaction. Posterior tenectomy of the SO is preferred for SO overaction.
- If there is no oblique overaction, then the horizontal recti shifting is done. In V pattern, the MR is shifted down and the LR is shifted up. In A pattern, the MR is shifted up and the LR is shifted down. Slanting recession of the horizontal recti can be done. In V esotropia pattern, MR is recessed more inferiorly and in A esotropia, it is recessed more superiorly.

REFERENCES
1. Costenbader FD. Infantile esotropia. Trans Am Ophthalmol Soc; 1961.
2. Gunter K, von Noorden, Emilio C Campos. Binocular Vision and Ocular Motility: Theory and Management of Strabismus, 6th edition. St. Louis: Mosby; 2002.

EXODEVIATION

Shipra Singhi, Adarsh Shashni

INTRODUCTION

Exotropia (XT) is outward deviation of the eyes. It is less more frequently seen than esotropia (ET). The approximate ratio of XT to ET is 1:3. According to some studies XT is more prevalent in the Middle East, the Orient, and Africa. Most studies report a normal distribution of refractive errors with XT.

In examinations, it can be given as a long case.

HISTORY

Chief Complaint

- Deviation of eyes
- Headaches, eyestrain, blurring of vision (older children and adults)
- Difficulty with prolonged period of reading
- Diplopia, photophobia, image is perceived as becoming smaller and coming closer

History of Present Illness

Patient (parents in case of small children) may complain of headaches, eyestrain, blurring of vision (older children and adults), and difficulty with prolonged period of reading.

- *Deviation of eyes:* Deviation of eyes toward outside which can be intermittent or constant. Deviation may be present since birth or shortly after birth.
- *Diplopia:* Seen in adults with a mature visual system, which can be intermittent. Children with intermittent or constant exotropia are less symptomatic as suppression eliminates diplopia.
- *Photophobia:* Bright light dazzles the retina so that fusional vergence is disrupted, causing manifest deviation. Child closes one eye to avoid confusion and diplopia (this phenomenon is called diplopia—phobia)
- *Micropsia:* Rare, patient uses accommodative convergence to maintain BSV. Image is perceived as becoming smaller and coming closer.
- *Refractive error:* Patient may have uncorrected myopia, high degree of uncorrected hypermetropia, anisomyopia, anisoastigmatism can also be there.

History of past illness: Any history of febrile disease or cerebral palsy must be noted. Patients should also be asked about refractive error, compliance with spectacles, and history of occlusion.

Surgical history: History of previous ocular surgery (buckling surgery), strabismus surgery, and use of prisms in postoperative period.

Birth History

- Children with craniofacial anomalies are more likely to exhibit XT.
- Maternal smoking during pregnancy increases the risk of XT (maternal smoking is more commonly associated with ET and for XT it is controversial).
- LBW baby increase the risk.
- Retinopathy of prematurity and Down's syndrome increases the risk of XT.

Family history: Note down any history of strabismus in the parents or siblings. There is 17-fold increased risk in monozygotic twin.

■ EXAMINATION AND SPECIAL TESTS

For examination please refer to chapter of esotropia.

Classification: Based on difference in measurement of deviation for distance and near, intermittent exotropia can be divided into following types:
- Divergence excess pattern–distance deviation exceeds near deviation by 10 prism diopters
- Convergence insufficiency pattern—near deviation exceed distance deviation by 10 prism diopter
- Basic exodeviation—when distance and near deviation is same or does not exceed 10 prism diopter.
- Simulated or pseudodivergence excess—these are basic deviation but appear as divergence excess exotropia due to either tenacious proximal fusional convergence (TPFC) or due to accommodation as in patients with high AC/A ratio. Following test differentiates the true and pseudodivergence excess.

Occlusion test of Scobee-Burian: Differentiate true and simulated divergence excess due to TPFC.
- Distance and near deviation is measured.
- U/L occlusion of one eye for 24 hours (Scobee)/30-45 minutes (Burian)
- Ensure that patient does not use both eyes simultaneously even momentarily.
- Measurement of deviation for near fixation is repeated.

In simulated divergence excess after patching there is increase in near deviation, so that it equals or exceeds that at distant fixation.

True divergence excess is not influenced by occlusion.

+ 3.0 DS lens test: Differentiate true and simulated divergence excess due to accommodative convergence.
- A +3.0 DS lens is used and deviation for near fixation is repeated.
- A large increase of near deviation indicates a high AC/A ratio.
- These patients are good candidate for over minus therapy, i.e., using more minus for myopic and using less plus for hypermetropic to stimulate accommodation that aids in decreasing or controlling the amount of exodeviation.
- Preoperative determination of AC/A ratio may also be helpful in predicting the extent to which a patient may respond to plus lenses when a surgical overcorrection is obtained.

■ TREATMENT

Optical

- Full cycloplegic refraction to be done
- Over minus therapy as described above can be prescribed specially in patients with high AC/A ratio.

Prisms

- Indicated in overcorrected/undercorrected exotropia
- Base-out prisms to stimulate fusional convergence
- Half and one-third of deviation is corrected in intermittent exotropia.

■ ORTHOPTICS

- Antisuppression exercises—appreciation of diplopia
- Convergence exercise is done with the help of a convergence trainer. These do not affect the basic deviation but decrease the manifestation of tropia to phoria.
- Should be done only after antisuppression exercises in cases of suppression

- Should not be done in intermittent exotropia for distance only in whom surgery is planned as can cause postoperative over convergence
- Exercises on synoptophore should always be supplemented by home exercises.
- Aim is to obtain normal NPC.

Occlusion Therapy

- Useful in small angle exotropia
- Occlusion of the preferred eye for 3–5 hours/day decreases the angle of deviation—evaluate 4 monthly

Surgery

Indications: The indications for surgery in:
- Intermittent exotropia include following:
  - Exotropia >50% of waking hours
  - Newcastle scoring >3 **(Table 1)**
  - Deviation ≥20 D
  - Asthenopic symptoms
  - Increasing basic deviation
  - Secondary convergence insufficiency with asthenopic symptoms
  - Development of suppression
  - Decreasing stereopsis

Table 1: Newcastle scoring for intermittent exotropia.

Home control	Score
X(T) or monocular eye closure—never seen	0
<50% times for distance fixation	1
<50% times for near fixation	2
>50% times for both distance and near fixation	3
Clinic control	
Distance	
Immediate realignment after cover test	0
Realignment after blink or refixation	1
No realignment/manifest spontaneously	2
Near	
Immediate realignment after cover test	0
Realignment after blink or refixation	1
No realignment/manifest spontaneously	2

- *In constant exotropia:* Surgery is almost always indicated with preoperative and postoperative orthoptic treatment.

Timing of surgery: Knapp advocated early surgery to prevent sensory changes especially in patients with infantile exotropia.

The best approach is to assess the timing in each case individually.

Factors to consider before surgery:
- Age
- Type and size
- Comparative deviation at 33 cm, 6 m, and in the far distance (20 m)
- The size of the AC/A ratio and determining whether the patient has a true or simulated divergence excess.
- If there is a change of deviation on lateral versions.
- Lateral gaze inhibition (i.e., decrease in deviation on lateral gaze) If there is a V or A phenomenon with or without associated inferior oblique or SO overaction. These should not be missed especially A pattern as this is a risk factor for postoperative residual exotropia.

Aims

- Phoria for distance and near in primary position.
- In children aim of surgery is to either give optimal correction or slightly under correct (up to 8 PD is desirable) as consecutive esotropia can result in amblyopia.
- In adult surgery can be aimed at slight overcorrection (up to 8 PD) as there is risk of exotropic drift in postoperative period especially in patients with poor vision.
- No suppression
- Stereopsis should be salvaged by performing early surgery especially in very young children with constant deviation.

Types of Surgery

- *True divergence excess type:* Bilateral recession of lateral recti
- *Basic exotropia and stimulated divergence excess:* Unilateral rectus recession and MR resection

- *Convergence insufficiency:* Bilateral resection of medial recti
- *Lateral gaze inhibition:* Bilateral lateral recti recession should be avoided.

VIVA QUESTIONS

Q.1. How will you perform occlusion test of Scobee–Burian?
Ans. This is given in examination section.

Q.2. Differentiate between true and simulated divergence and name the tests used for that.
Ans. This is given in examination section.

Q.3. What is epidemiology of exotropia?
Ans. *Incidence:* Exotropia appears less frequently than esotropia (ET). The approximate ratio of XT to ET is 1:3.

In Costenbader's series of 472 patients with IDS, deviation was present.
- At birth—204
- 6 months—16
- 6-12 months—72
- After 5 years—24
- Sex-women (approximately 60-70%) other associations
- Facial symmetry associated with exodeviations
- Children with craniofacial anomalies more likely to exhibit exotropia
- Maternal smoking during pregnancy
- LBW
- 17-fold increased risk in monozygotic twin.

Q.4. What is constant (early onset) exotropia?
Ans. *Constant (early onset) exotropia has following features:* Presentation is often at birth. Primary constant infantile exotropia is rare.
Signs of infantile exotropia:
- Large angle and constant deviation
- No significant refractive error
- DVD may be present.
- Infantile exotropia is usually associated with neurological deficits and should be investigated for the same.
- Treatment is mainly surgical and consists of LR recession and MR resection.

Table 2: Difference between alternating and unilateral constant exotropia.

Alternating	Unilateral
Visual acuity is almost equal in both eyes	Fixation preference
Angle of deviation is large, nearly equal for distance and near	Deviation is large
Associated commonly with secondary vertical deviation, deviating abducted eye is elevated	Vertical deviations are more common
If there is NRC and bifoveal fusion—suppression of deviating eye	• Marked suppression in the deviating eye • Amblyopia is less severe than esotropia • Treatment is almost always surgical

A complete ocular evaluation should be done to rule out secondary sensory exotropia.

Difference between alternating and unilateral constant exotropia is summarized in **Table 2**.

Q.5. Classify exodeviation.
Ans. *Classification:*
- *Comitant:*
  - *Primary:*
    - Infantile exotropia
    - Intermittent exotropia
  - *Secondary:*
    - Sensory exotropia
    - Consecutive exotropia
- *Incomitant:*
  - Paralytic
  - Restrictive
  - Musculofascial anomalies
  - Dissociated horizontal deviation

On the basis of underlying fusional reserve:
- Exophoria XP
- Intermittent exotropia X(T)
- Manifest exotropia XT

Burian's classification of intermittent exotropia:
- *Basic pattern:* Distance and near deviation is almost equal

- *Convergence insufficiency:* Near deviation is larger than distance deviation by >15 PD
- *Divergence excess:* Distance deviation exceeds near deviation by >15 PD
- *Simulated divergence excess:* Initial distance deviation exceeded the near deviation by >15 PD, but after 1 hour of monocular occlusion 2 measurements showed difference of <15 PD.

Burian classification did not specify the type of convergence that was insufficient (accommodative or fusional) which was included in Kushner classification **(Table 3)**.

Duane's classification:
- Divergence excess pattern
- Convergence insufficiency pattern
- Basic exodeviation
- Simulated or pseudodivergence excess

True divergence excess:
- *Exophoria*—exotropia at distance, normal NPC, adequate prism convergence, intermittency, equal vision, good stereopsis, and ARC when exodeviated
- *Costenbader*—definition of divergence excess
- *Near:* Distance >15 PD
- Associated with a high AC/A ratio in 60% Kushner

Simulated divergence excess:
- Exodeviation distance—near >15 PD
- After breaking fusion, distance—near <10PD
- Due to vergence after effect (tonic and accommodative). Dissipated by prolonged mono-ocular occlusion
- Over 80% of divergence excess type patients

Convergence insufficiency:
- Near deviation—distance >15 PD
- Patients have either a low AC/A ratio or a fusional convergence insufficiency
- Patient usually in teens
- Asthenopic symptoms with intermittent diplopia at near
- No X or X(T) initially at distance or near; seen as disease progresses

Q.6. What are Calhounz's phases of exodeviation?

Ans.
- Intermittent exotropia at distance, orthophoria at near, asymptomatic
- Exotropia **(Fig. 1)** at distance, orthophoria/exophoria at near, symptomatic for distance, no suppression scotoma
- Exotropia at distance, exotropia or intermittent exo at near, binocular vision for near, suppression scotoma develops for distance
- Exotropia for distance and near. Lack of binocularity.

Q.7. What are the causes of pseudoexotropia?

Ans.
- Hypertelorism
- Positive angle kappa
- Large IPD
- Broad nasal bridge
- Narrowing of lateral canthi

Q.8. What are the causes of pseudoesotropia?

Ans.
- Negative angle kappa
- Small interpupillary distance
- Epicanthus

Table 3: Classification intermittent exotropia.

Burian classification	Kushner classification
Divergence excess	High AC/A ratio strong proximal convergence
Simulated divergence excess	Tenacious proximal fusion
Basic pattern	Basic pattern
Convergence insufficiency	• Low AC/A ratio fusional convergence insufficiency • Pseudoconvergence insufficiency

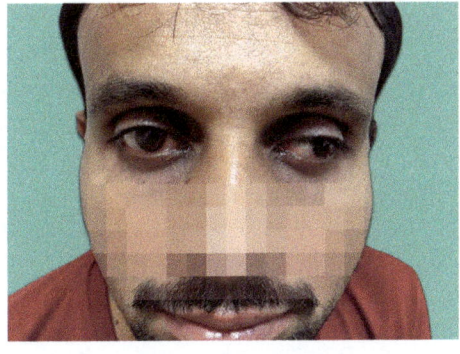

Fig. 1: Left exotropia.

Q.9. What are rules of thumb for prescribing spectacles for young children refractive error without strabismus?

Ans.
- Hyperopia >5 D
- Myopia >3 D
- Astigmatism >2 D if not oblique, >1 D if oblique
- Anisometropia >2 D for myopic, >1 D if hyperopic, >2 D if astigmatic Refractive error with strabismus; treat:
- Hyperopia or hyperopic astigmatism greater than astigmatism >1.25 D (esotropia)
- Myopia >1 D (exotropia) child's age and symptoms as well as other factors must be taken into account.

BIBLIOGRAPHY

1. von Noorden GK, Campos EC. Binocular Vision and Ocular Motility: Theory and Management of Strabismus, 6th edition. St Louis: Mosby; 2002.

SHORT CASES

DUANE RETRACTION SYNDROME

Shipra Singhi, Saranya Devi K

■ INTRODUCTION

Duane retraction syndrome (DRS) falls under the spectrum of congenital cranial dysinnervation disorders (CCDD), resulting from the developmental defects in the innervation of ocular and facial muscles. DRS results from failure of development of sixth nerve nucleus leading to lack of innervation to lateral rectus. Along with this, there is anomalous innervation of the lateral rectus by the third nerve, leading to co-contraction and upshoots during adduction. DRS can be associated with deafness, external ear abnormalities, speech disorder, and skeletal abnormalities. Approximately 10% of DRS cases are familial,[1] and several genetic mutations have been proposed to be associated with DRS.

■ HISTORY

Chief Complaints

Patients present with deviation of either eye, limitation of extraocular movements (EOMs), abnormal movement of eye (upshoot and downshoot), shortening of eye (leash phenomenon), bigger size of eye (retraction of globe), diminution of vision, and abnormal head and face posture.

History of Present Illness

Patients may complain of inward or outward deviation of either eye. Along with that patients have partial or complete limitation of movement on looking laterally (abduction) or medially (adduction). Abnormal movement of eye (upshoot and downshoot) can be there while doing inward movement. Abnormal head posture is adopted in order to maintain binocular single vision, avoiding amblyopia. Narrowing of the palpebral aperture (co-contraction of muscles) can be there. Diminution of vision may be there (anisometropia/amblyopia).

History of Past Illness

History of fever/illness.

Family History

This may be hereditary.

■ EXAMINATION

General Examination/Specific Systemic Examination

Duane retraction syndrome can be associated with:
- *Goldenhar syndrome:* Preauricular tag, hearing limbal dermoid, hemivertebra, and hemifacial hypoplasia
- *Wildervanck syndrome:* Associated with Klippel-Feil anomaly, fused vertebra, low neck hair line, hearing loss
- *Okihiro's syndrome:* Associated with upper limb bony defects (radial ray defects)

Ocular Examination

Abnormal head posture: A face turn is usually present to maintain binocular single vision in primary; usually a face turn to the affected side in types 1 and 3 and to the opposite side in type 2. Long-standing face turn can lead to torticollis and craniofacial asymmetry.

Eyeball: Retraction of the globe on adduction because of co-contraction of the medial and lateral recti with resultant narrowing of the palpebral fissure **(Figs. 1A to C)**.

Extraocular Movement

- There is usually associated complete or partial absence of abduction, with partial deficiency of adduction.
- Severe co-contraction on adduction gives an appearance of pseudoptosis.

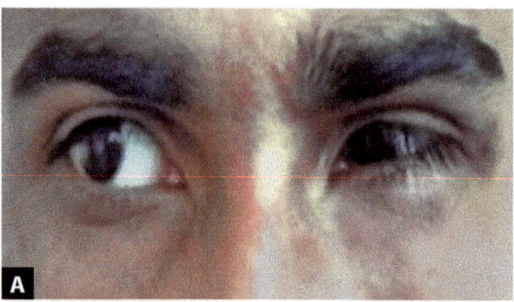
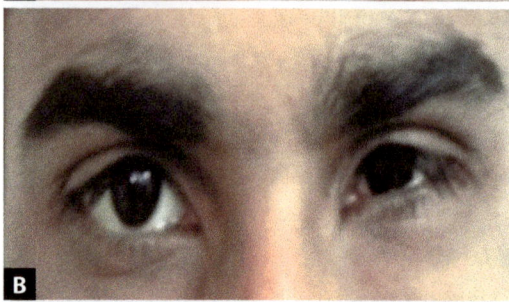
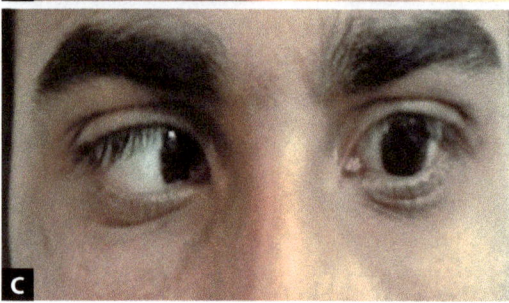

Figs. 1A to C: Left Eso-DRS with left eye limitation of abduction with globe retraction.

- Upshoots and downshoots on adduction result from a tight lateral rectus causing slippage of the globe.
- *Strabismus:* 76% of cases have apparent squint in primary gaze.
- DRS can be associated with hyperopia. Amblyopia (anisometropia) occurs in about 10% of individuals and will respond to standard therapy if detected early.

Special examination for squint: See section on esotropia long case.

Lid: Co-contraction on adduction gives an appearance of pseudoptosis

Conjunctiva: Previous scar of surgery may be there.

Fundus: Disc anomaly may be there (morning glory syndrome).

■ DIFFERENTIAL DIAGNOSIS

It includes:
- *Essential infantile esotropia:* Characterized by large angle esotropia, with onset at 4–6 months; usually have cross fixation and freely alternating esotropia. EOMs are present and can be elicited by doll's eye maneuver.
- *Congenital sixth nerve palsy:* Can be differentiated from DRS by limitation of abduction, but normal adduction and absence of co-contractions
- *Mobius syndrome:* Associated with sixth and seventh nerve palsy

■ MANAGEMENT

Nonsurgical

- Spectacles or contact lenses for refractive error correction
- Prism for correction of small angle deviations and improving the head posture
- Amblyopia therapy
- *Botulinum toxin:* Reduces upshoots and downshoots.

Surgical

Surgery is performed to correct abnormal head posture, manifest strabismus, globe retraction co-contractions, and to improve the binocularity.

Different Scenarios

- *For eso-DRS (type 1):* Recession of medial rectus muscle with horizontal transposition of vertical rectus muscles
- Recession of lateral rectus muscles with Y-splitting of the lateral rectus muscle should be added in patients with severe co-contractions and upshoots
- *For exo-DRS (type 2):* Recession of lateral rectus muscle, with possible Y-splitting in cases with severe upshoots and downshoots
- *Associated V phenomenon with inferior oblique overaction with upshoot:* Horizontal recti plus inferior oblique recession
- *Associated A phenomenon with superior oblique overaction with downshoot:* Ipsilateral horizontal recti recession plus superior oblique weakening
- Recession and retroequatorial myopexy (Faden) of the contralateral synergist can also

be done to correct face turn and may improve the limitation of abduction of the involved eye.
- Y-splitting of lateral recti can be done in upshoot and downshoot.
- In any case, lateral rectus resection should be avoided.

Complications of Surgery
- Undercorrection
- Overcorrection
- Vertical deviations after vertical rectus transposition procedures

VIVA QUESTIONS

Q.1. What is epidemiology of DRS?
Ans. DRS is the most common congenital cranial dysinnervation syndrome with a prevalence of 1/1,000 in general population, accounting for 4% of all strabismus cases. 90% of cases are sporadic. Females (60%) are affected more commonly than males (40%). 80% cases are unilateral. 30% of cases can be associated with other congenital anomalies. DRS can be associated with syndromes such as Goldenhar syndrome, Wildervanck syndrome, Moebius syndrome, and Holt–Oram syndrome

Q.2. Name the systemic syndromes associated with DRS.
Ans. Refer to the discussion part.

Q.3. What is pathogenesis of DRS?
Ans. Various theories are as follows:
- *Myogenic theory:* This theory, suggested by earlier studies, indicates there is fibrosis or inelasticity of the lateral rectus muscles and that the medial rectus muscle inserts abnormally far posteriorly.
- *Neurogenic theory:* There is a disturbance in embryologic development between weeks 4 and 8, which results in an absent abducens nerve with anomalous innervations of the lateral rectus muscle by a branch of the oculomotor nerve. Simultaneous activation of the medial and lateral rectus muscles, as demonstrated by EMG studies, may be the cause of global retraction.

Q.4. Describe surgical management in DRS—indications and procedures.
Ans. Refer to Management.

Q.5. Classify DRS.
Ans. *See* Tables 1 and 2.

Table 1: Classification of Duane retraction syndrome (DRS).

Type 1	Type 2	Type 3	Type 4
Poor abduction, good adduction	Poor adduction, good abduction	Poor adduction, poor abduction	Paradoxical abduction on attempt adduction
6th nerve agenesis abnormal innervation of LR by a branch of 3rd on attempted adduction	6th nerve intact, abnormal branch of 3rd nerve innervates both LR and MR	6th nerve agenesis, 3rd nerve split and equally innervate both LR and MR	6th nerve agenesis, 3rd nerve split abnormally to innervate both LR and MR, with more innervation going towards LR

(LR: lateral rectus; MR: medial rectus)

Table 2: Classification (Huber) of Duane retraction syndrome (DRS).

Type 1	Type 2	Type 3
Most common, characterized by: - Limited or absent abduction - Normal or mildly limited adduction - Esotropia in primary	Least common, characterized by: - Limitation of adduction - Normal or slight limitation of abduction - Exotropia in primary	Characterized by: - Limitation of both adduction and abduction. - Ortho in primary

REFERENCE

1. von Noorden GK, MD, Campos EC. Binocular Vision and Ocular Motility: Theory and Management of Strabismus, 6th edition, by Gunter K. von Noorden, MD, and Emilio C. Campos, MD, St Louis: Mosby; 2002.

OCULAR MYASTHENIA GRAVIS

Shipra Singhi, Adarsh Shashni

INTRODUCTION

Myasthenia gravis (MG) is an autoimmune disease characterized by the formation of antibodies against the postsynaptic acetylcholine receptors, resulting in impaired neuromuscular conduction and weakness of skeletal muscles. This further causes progressive muscle weakness and fatigue with recovery of strength after a period of rest. Weakness is experienced once number of receptors is 30% or less.[1]

HISTORY

Chief Complaint

This includes drooping of eyelid, double vision, limitation of eye movements, abnormal eye movement, difficulty in eye closure, light sensitivity, fatigue of eye muscles, difficulty in swallowing, speech, breathing, muscular weakness, and lack of facial expression.

Past History

This includes previous history of similar complaints or any history of thymoma, thyroid dysfunction, intracranial mass, lung carcinoma.

Past Surgical History

This includes any history of surgery of extraocular muscles or ptosis or thymoma, thyroid dysfunction, intracranial mass, and lung carcinoma.

SYSTEMIC MYASTHENIA GRAVIS

- Symptoms usually appear in the third decade, and present with progressive fatigue that worsen on exercise and improve on taking rest.
- Ptosis and diplopia can be the presenting features.
- Proximal muscles of limbs, muscles of facial expression, and mastication are most commonly involved. Patients can typically complain of difficulty in squatting and combing hair.
- Facial expressions can be absent known as myopathic facies.

There may be several reasons why eye muscles are more frequently involved. However, this is not completely understood.

One hypothesis is that patients may simply notice eye weakness more often than mild weakness in other muscle groups in the body. Another hypothesis is that the eye and eyelid muscles are structurally different from muscles in the trunk and limbs. For example, they have fewer acetylcholine receptors, which is where the defect occurs in autoimmune MG. Eye muscles contract much more rapidly than other muscles and may be more likely to fatigue.

Perhaps the most important difference between eye and eyelid muscles compared with other muscles of the body is that eye muscles respond differently to immune attack. The differences in the response of eye muscles to immune attack may explain why eye muscles are also targeted in other autoimmune conditions, such as autoimmune thyroid disease.

OCULAR MYASTHENIA

Ninety percent of patients can have ocular involvement **(Table 1)** with two-thirds of patients having ptosis and diplopia. <10% of patients have ptosis alone and <30% have diplopia alone.[1]

Ptosis: Ptosis is usually bilateral and asymmetric with diurnal variation that worsens on prolonged upgaze (fatigue test).

Cogan lid twitch: To elicit the sign patient is asked to look down and then to look up, on this saccadic movement there is a brief upshoot of the eyelid. As the patient looks up on manually elevating the eyelid, fine oscillatory movements of the fellow eyelid can be noted.

Table 1: Ocular signs of myasthenia gravis.	
Muscle involved	**Clinical sign**
Levator palpebrae superioris	• Ptosis • Cogan's lid twitch • Lid hopping • Enhanced ptosis
Extraocular movements (EOMs)	• Cranial nerve III, IV, or VI weakness • Gaze palsies • Pseudo-internuclear ophthalmoplegia (unilateral or bilateral) • Complete ophthalmoplegia • Intrasaccadic fatigue • End gaze nystagmus
Orbicularis oculi	• Weakness of forced closure • Peek sign

Diplopia: Diplopia along with ptosis can be the presenting feature of two-thirds of patients. There can be involvement of any extraocular muscle that does not follow any particular cranial nerve. Diplopia can occur on abduction and adduction or on elevation and depression. Patients may acquire a head posture to avoid diplopia. For example, if the patient is not able to look up, patients can tilt their head back to look up.

Nystagmoid movements: Nystagmoid movements, as the name suggests, are nystagmus like movements. Nystagmoid movements result due to involvement of the slow twitch muscle fibers, responsible for gaze holding. This results in fixation drift following saccades.

Ocular flutter and opsoclonus: These entities consist of saccadic oscillations with no inter-saccadic interval; in ocular flutter oscillations are purely horizontal, and in opsoclonus they are multiplanar. Causes include viral encephalitis, myoclonic encephalopathy in infants ('dancing eyes and dancing feet'), as a transient idiopathic occurrence in healthy neonates, or may be drug-induced.

Ocular bobbing: Ocular bobbing movements are characterized by the rapid downward conjugate eye movements followed by a slow drift in the primary position. Besides ocular myasthenia ocular bibbing can be associated with brainstem lesions like pontine and cerebellar hemorrhage, and space-occupying lesions.

Peek sign: The test is used to check the strength orbicularis muscle. Patient is asked to close the eyes tightly, the examiner then tries to open the eyes. Due to weakness of orbicularis one or both eyelids open and it appears that patient is peeking at the examiner, thus known as peek sign.

Forced duction test: Forced duction test is free and helps to differentiate myasthenia from paralytic and restrictive squint.

■ DIAGNOSIS

Investigations

Blood

- AChR-Ab—positive in 80% with generalized MG; positive in only 50% with ocular involvement only also present in 90% of patients with penicillamine-induced MG
- Antistriated muscle Ab
- Antimuscle specific kinase Ab (Anti-MuSK Ab—positive in patients with AChR Ab –ve)
- Thyroid profile
- Erythrocyte sedimentation rate

Imaging

- CXR (chest X-ray)—thymus (anterior mediastinal mass), aspiration pneumonia
- Thoracic imaging (MR, CT, CT/PET) to detect thymoma, present in 10%; imaging may also be used to rule out a lung tumor if Lambert–Eaton syndrome is suspected, or an intracranial mass for ocular myasthenia.

Ice pack test: Ice pack test is a simple bedside test for myasthenia. An ice pack is placed over the ptotic eyelid for not >5 minutes. Ptosis is measured before and after the test. An improvement of >2 mm is considered to be significant. A pre- and post-test picture is taken for the records. The improvement in ptosis is attributed to the fact that lower temperature inhibits the breakdown of acetylcholine by acetylcholinesterase. The test is highly specific and has a sensitivity of 75%.

Sleep test: For sleep test, patient is asked to take rest for 30 minutes in a quiet, darkroom. Pretest and post-test photographs are acquired. An improvement in ptosis and EOMs can be noted after the rest in myasthenia patients.

Patient can also be asked to record his morning and evening pictures, to look for the diurnal variation in ptosis. Similarly old photographs also help to find the underlying cause and increase in ptosis with time.

Fatigue test: Patient is asked to look toward the roof, or toward a target held up. A worsening of ptosis can be noted after a short time.

Acetylcholine receptor (AChR) antibodies: AChR antibodies are present in around only 70% of patients of ocular myasthenia and 90% cases of systemic myasthenia.

MuSK protein antibodies are positive in 50% of those negative for AChR antibodies. The presence of MuSK antibodies usually are associated with systemic myasthenia.

Striational antibodies: Striational antibodies are formed against the contractile elements of striated muscles (like titin). Their presence suggests severe myasthenia and is present in 80-90% patients with thymoma.

Voltage-gated calcium channel antibodies are present in Lambert-Eaton syndrome.

Edrophonium (tensilon) test: The edrophonium (tensilon) test is a first-line diagnostic test for MG. Intially a test dose of 2 mg tensilon is injected intravenously following which 8 mg tensilon is injected. Tensilon is a short-acting reversible acetyl cholinesterase inhibitor, and hence is widely used for the testing. An improvement in the ptosis, extraocular muscle movements, and nystagmoid movements is noted in patients with myasthenia. The test should be done under cardiac monitoring and atropine should be kept ready for reversal in case of bradycardia or asystole.

The test is 85% sensitive in ocular and 95% sensitive in systemic MG. The test aids in diagnosis as well as helps to differentiate cholinergic crisis from myasthenic crisis.

Muscle biopsy reveals neuromuscular junction antibodies and characteristic electron microscopy features, but is not commonly performed.

Thyroid function testing should be performed as autoimmune thyroid disease can be associated with MG.

Electrodiagnostic Studies

- *Repetitive nerve stimulation test* shows a decrease in the compound muscle action potential by 10% in the 4th or 5th response to a train of nerve stimuli.
- *Single fiber nerve electromyography*—evidence of neuromuscular blockade with increased jitter

■ GRADING

Myasthenia Gravis Foundation of America

- Grade 1—affects the ocular muscles only
- Grade 2—mild weakness affecting muscles other than ocular muscles
  - 2A—affects the limb and axial muscles
  - 2B—affects the respiratory and bulbar muscles
- Grade 3—moderate weakness (3A and 3B)
- Grade 4—severe weakness (4A and 4B)
- Grade 5—intubation required

Osserman's Grading

- I—Ocular
- IIA—Mild generalized with slow progression
- IIB—Moderate generalized
- III—Acute fulminant MG
- IV—Late severe MG (takes 2 years to progress from I to II)

■ DIFFERENTIAL DIAGNOSIS

- Fourth nerve palsy
- Third nerve palsy
- Progressive external ophthalmoplegia

■ TREATMENT

Emergencies in crisis (ABC)—treat exacerbating factors, stop medications that can exacerbate, treat fever with antipyretics, treat infections.
- Oral pyridostigmine, neostigmine, steroids, azathioprine, cyclosporine
- Plasmapheresis
- Intravenous immunoglobulin (IVIg)

■ OCULAR MYASTHENIA GRAVIS

People with ocular MG and their caregivers should balance the severity of the symptoms with the risks and benefits of treatment. People who have primarily cosmetic problems due to ptosis or diplopia may consider no pharmacological treatment, such as:
- Wearing dark glasses in bright light, which some patients find helpful.

- Using eyelid tape (a special type of tape used to hold the eyelids open without injuring the eyelids); this can be used for ptosis and may be preferable to drug therapy that alters the immune system using agents such as glucocorticoids (prednisone or similar agents),
- Azathioprine (Imuran), cyclosporine or mycophenolate mofetil (CellCept).
- To avoid diplopia patching, opaque contact lenses, special prism glasses and nonallergic paper tapes can be prescribed.
- For patients presenting with ptosis, crutch glasses, and prism bars can be given. These glasses hold the eyelids open. The crutch wires rest against the socket and holds the eyelid open like a brace or crutch. The gases should be removed regularly to allow blinking. Artificial tears should also be prescribed with the glasses to keep the surface moist.
- Inability to close the eyes due to weakness of orbicularis can result in soap entering the eyes during bathing, and excessive tearing. Swimming goggles can be helpful in such situations.
- Ptosis surgery can be planned in patients not responding to medications and conservative management. Surgery should be considered in patients with stable course.
- When ocular symptoms are severe or disabling, treatment with immune system
- Modulating therapy may be considered.
- Agents that improve neuromuscular transmission, such as *Mestinon* may be helpful for ptosis, but are generally not very useful for diplopia.

■ THYMECTOMY

Thymectomy is usually not considered for people with ocular MG unless thymoma is suspected. Removal of thymus is usually advised for patients with generalized myasthenia.

VIVA QUESTIONS

Q.1. How common is the thymus involved?
Ans. 75% of cases of which 15% are thymomas and 85% are thymic hyperplasia.

Q.2. How common is the thyroid involved?
Ans. Up to 30% of patients with MG have anti-thyroid antibodies.

Q.3. What are the common presentations?
Ans. *Age:* 2 peaks.
- 20–30 years old with female predominance overall; females are more commonly affected in a ratio of 3:2
- >50 years old with male predominance
- Ptosis, diplopia, lagophthalmos
- Extraocular muscles are first affected as they cannot adapt rapidly and even slight weakness can result in diplopia and visual symptoms.
- Dilated and sluggishly reacting pupil can result in photosensitivity.
- Dysarthria, difficulty swallowing (isolated bulbar muscles involvement occurs in 20%)
- Generalized weakness or reduced exercise tolerance
- Respiratory failure in 1%
- Tends to occur extraocular muscles first, then to facial to bulbar and to limbs and truncal

Q.4. What are the complications?
Ans. *Myasthenic crisis:*
- Severe exacerbation of MG
- 10% require intubation
- Treatment complications
- Cholinergic crisis

Q.5. What can exacerbate MG or precipitate crisis?
Ans. *Noncompliance to medications:*
- Infection
- Emotions
- Drugs
- *Antibiotics:* Aminoglycosides, tetracyclines, macrolides and fluoroquinolones
- *CVS:* Beta-blockers, calcium-channel blockers (verapamil)
- *Others:* Chloroquine, quinidine, procainamide, Li, Mg, prednisolone, quinine, penicillamine
- Environmental, emotional, and physical stress can worsen the symptoms.
- Emotional stress, pregnancy, menstruation, bright light, and excessive exercise can also lead to worsening.
- Symptoms worsens toward the end of the day.

Q.6. Ocular involvement is seen in how many patients of MG? What is the most common presenting ocular feature in it?

Ans. 90% of cases have ocular involvement, with two-thirds of patients having both ptosis and diplopia. Less than 10% of patients have ptosis alone and <30% have diplopia alone.

Q.7. Explain the management of myasthenic crisis.

Ans. *See* text.

Q.8. Explain the management of cholinergic crisis.

Ans. *See* text.

REFERENCE

1. Nair AG, Patil-Chhablani P, Venkatramani DV, Gandhi RA. Ocular myasthenia gravis: a review. Indian J Ophthalmol. 2014;62(10):985-91.

MONOCULAR ELEVATION DEFICIT

Gunjan Saluja, Anu Malik

INTRODUCTION

Monocular elevation deficit is characterized by limitation of movements in upgaze both in abduction and adduction. It can be of three types as classified by Ziffer et al. Type 1 results from restriction of inferior rectus; Type 2 results from superior rectus palsy; and Type 3 is caused by supranuclear vertical gaze palsy.

HISTORY

Chief Complaint

Patients present with complains of inability to elevate the affected eye up that is usually associated with drooping of eyelids.

Diplopia can be present in acute onset of elevation deficit.

EXAMINATION

Visual acuity: Visual acuity can be affected in patients with large angle vertical deviation along with severe ptosis and anisometropia.

Abnormal head posture: Patient can have chin-up head posture due to severe ptosis and large vertical deviation. In patients with amblyopia of the affected eye head posture can be absent.

Ptosis/pseudoptosis: Ptosis can be associated with hypotropia because of fascial attachments between the levator palpebrae superioris and superior rectus muscle. Pseudoptosis can be present in primary gaze when fixating with the contralateral eye; however, it improves when the hypotropic eye takes up fixation. Both pseudoptosis and true ptosis can be present in the patient.

Strabismus: There is hypotropia of the affected eye when the unaffected eye is fixing and hypertropia of the contralateral eye when fixating with the affected eye.

Bell's phenomenon: Bell's phenomenon is typically absent in patients of inferior rectus restriction and superior rectus palsy, but is usually present in cases of MED resulting from supranuclear defects. To check Bell's phenomenon patient is asked to gently close the eyes, following which the amount of corneal exposure is seen; Bell's phenomenon can be graded as good, fair, and poor.

Saccades: Upward saccades abruptly stop in cases associated with inferior rectus restriction, are slow in cases of superior rectus palsy, and absent above the midline in supranuclear palsy.

INVESTIGATIONS

Forced Duction Test

Forced duction test is a clinical test to evaluate for restriction. The test is performed under topical or general anesthesia, and patient is asked to look in the direction of restricted gaze. The conjunctiva is held at limbus with forceps and the globe is rotated by the examiner.

Active Force Generation Test

Active force generation test is done under topical anesthesia by asking the patient to look in the direction of the muscle being tested and tug is felt.

Hess charting

See the section on 6th nerve palsy.

Imaging

In patients with acute-onset vertical deviation imaging helps to rule out restriction secondary to muscle entrapment (post-trauma), fibrosis, and inflammation.

■ DIFFERENTIAL DIAGNOSIS

- Brown's syndrome
- Partially recovered third nerve palsy
- Progressive external ophthalmoplegia and congenital fibrosis of extraocular muscles

■ MANAGEMENT

Indications for surgery include:
- Significant vertical deviation in primary gaze
- Significant abnormal head posture
- Deviation-induced amblyopia
- Diplopia in primary gaze
- Restricted binocular fields

Management of MED depends on the forced duction test of inferior rectus. If FDT is tight for inferior rectus, inferior rectus recession is planned.

Knapp's procedure: Knapp's procedure is performed when the forced duction test is free. The medial and lateral rectus muscles are transposed to the insertion of the superior rectus muscle.

Modified Knapp's procedure: Modified Knapp's procedure is planned when there is associated horizontal deviation along with the vertical squint. The horizontal muscle is divided into two halves, where superior halves of the equally divided horizontal muscles are placed near the superior rectus muscle insertion, and correct the vertical deviation, whereas the inferior halves are used for the correction of horizontal deviation.

Augmented Knapp's procedure: Augmented Knapp's procedure utilizes Knapp's procedure combined with posterior fixation sutures on the horizontal recti to increase its effect.

Contralateral eye surgery: To correct residual vertical deviation, contralateral eye superior rectus recession with inferior oblique total anterior positioning should be planned.

VIVA QUESTIONS

Q.1. Explain the vertical gaze pathways.

Ans. The impulse for intentional saccades originates from the contralateral frontal eye field area, whereas the impulse for reflexive saccades originates from the parietal eye field area, located in the posterior parietal cortex. The fibers from the cortex project to the rostral interstitial nucleus of the MLF of Cajal; located in the rostral midbrain. These fibers further project bilaterally to the oculomotor and trochlear nuclei, after passing through the posterior commissure.

Q.2. Classify MED.

Ans. MED has been classified into three types by Ziffer et al.

	MED 1	MED 2	MED 3
Etiology	Inferior rectus restriction	Superior rectus palsy	Supranuclear causes
Extra-ocular movement	Abruptly stops	Saccades slow both above and below midline	Reduced saccadic velocity below midline absent above midline
Bell's	Poor	Poor	Fair to good
Forced duction test	Positive	Negative	Negative

Q.3. What are the secondary causes of MED?

Ans. Acquired caused of MED include trauma, cerebrovascular diseases such as hypertension, thromboembolism, sarcoidosis, and syphilis, or tumors such as pineocytomas, acoustic neuromas and metastases.

Q.4. How will you manage ptosis in a patient with MED?

Ans. MED patients are usually associated with severe complex ptosis, the major hurdle in ptosis correction is poor Bell's. Hence surgery for the improvement of Bell's should be done before ptosis surgery. In patients with large angle vertical deviations not amenable to surgical corrections, crutch glasses can be given.

Q.5. What caution should be taken while planning for inferior rectus recession?

Ans. Inferior rectus is attached to the retractors of lower lid; hence weakening of muscle beyond 5 mm can lead to lower lid retraction and pseudoproptosis.

DISSOCIATED VERTICAL DEVIATION

Gunjan Saluja

■ INTRODUCTION

Dissociated vertical deviation (DVD), also known as alternating hyperphoria/hypertropia, anatopia, double hypertropia, occlusion hypertropia, alternating sursumduction, dissociated double hypertropia, dissociated alternating hyperphoria, and dissociated vertical divergence, is an independent dissociated movement of one eye with respect to another. DVD does not follow Herring's law and can be given in examinations as a short case.

■ COMPLAINT

Patients complain of spontaneous upward deviation of the nonfixing eye.

■ PAST HISTORY

This includes past history of any previous strabismus surgery for esotropia or exotropia.

■ EXAMINATION

Visual acuity: Visual acuity may be reduced due to amblyopia.

Abnormal head posture: Abnormal head posture can be present in the form of chin depression and contralateral head tilt.

Extraocular movements: Inferior oblique overaction is commonly associated with DVD. DVD can also be present in 50% cases of essential infantile esotropia. DVD is bilateral and asymmetric phenomenon. In DVD is elevation along with outward movement and extrusion.

■ MEASUREMENT OF DVD

Dissociated vertical deviation can be comitant or incomitant. In patients of comitant DVD the vertical deviation remains the same in primary gaze, abduction, and adduction, whereas in incomitant DVD the vertical deviation changes in primary, abduction, and adduction.

The variable nature of DVD makes the measurement of the same difficult. Various methods for measurement of DVD are as follows:

Spielmann's translucent occluder: Upward and outward movement of the eye under cover helps in the diagnosis and demonstration of this condition. In the absence of Spielmann's occluder a +4D lens can also be utilized for the same. The purpose is to dissociate the light stimulus reaching both the eyes.

Red filter test: Red image is always lower in the eye occluded by red filter in case of DVD as the eye drifts upwards after dissociation with red filter. This also helps differentiate DVD from hypertropia.

Graded neutral density filter test: Filters of increasing density are held in-front of the fixing eye. This reduces the visual input to the fixating eye which triggers an abnormal innervation to elevators. This further elicits compensatory innervation in depressors in contralateral eye and subsequently shifts downward, sometimes even below the primary position.

Prism bar under cover test: Base-down prisms are held in front of nonfixing eye under occlusion. Alternate occlusion is done till the recovery movement is neutralized. The same procedure is repeated in the other eye as well. In cases with associated inferior oblique overaction, the difference between total upward drift by PBUCT and hypotropic refixation movement by PBCT is contributed by DVD.

Dissociated vertical deviation should be differentiated from inferior oblique overaction and the differentiating points have been highlighted in **Table 1**.

Table 1: Differentiating points between dissociated vertical deviation (DVD) and inferior oblique overaction (IOOA).

	DVD	IOOA
Elevation	Both in abduction and adduction	Overelevation in adduction
V pattern	Often absent	Present
Incycloduction on refixation	Present	Absent
Latent nystagmus	Present	Absent
Saccadic velocity of refixation movement	10–200°/s	200–400°/s
Bielschowsky phenomenon	Present	Absent

■ MANAGEMENT

Nonsurgical management is indicated in patients with latent and small angle DVD with infrequent manifestation and includes refractive correction and correction of associated horizontal deviation.

Surgical Management

Indications:
- Large angle DVD
- Anomalous head posture
- Increasing frequency of manifest phase of DVD in patient with peripheral fusion
- Amblyopia

Superior rectus recession: Superior rectus recession is the most commonly used surgical technique, 7 mm recession of superior rectus is usually performed for the correction of DVD, posterior fixation sutures can further enhance the affect of recession.

Inferior rectus resection/plication: Inferior rectus resection and plication involve the strengthening and shortening of inferior rectus. In inferior rectus plication, the muscle is double-breasted on itself and is not disinserted, thus avoiding the disruption of blood supply to the anterior segment and reducing the risk of anterior segment ischemia.

Inferior oblique total anterior positioning: Inferior oblique total anterior positioning is usually performed in patients of DVD with coexisting inferior oblique overaction. Total anterior positioning involves anterior transposition of inferior oblique near the insertion of inferior rectus. Inferior oblique muscle is converted from an elevator into a depressor after the anterior transposition procedure.

VIVA QUESTIONS

Q.1. What are the various theories of DVD?
Ans. Various theories have been postulated for the pathogenesis of DVD.

Spielmann's theory: DVD results from abnormal persistent immature monocular circuits and an imbalance of binocular stimulation. These can be either visual or vestibular. Vertical pursuit asymmetry can be noted in DVD patients with better pursuits directed when down to up than vice versa. Variability of DVD with postural changes suggests involvement of vestibular or otolithic pathways.

Bielschowsky's theory: According to Bielschowsky, DVD results from alternate and intermittent excitation of subcortical centers governing vertical divergence

Brodsky's theory: Brodsky postulated that DVD results from unequal visual stimulus manifestation of primitive dorsal light reflex. When light stimulus falls from one side of fish, it misregisters it as its subjective vertical meridian with a counterclockwise tilt. As a result, clockwise tilt occurs for equal binocular stimulation. This righting reflex causes vertical divergence of eyes to prevent the corrective body tilt. Therefore, downward movement of ipsilateral eye and upward contralateral eye occurs.

Other theories are manifestation of atavistic oculomotor reflexes present in birds and fishes, elastic preponderance, and paresis of elevators or depressors (bilateral paresis), oblique muscle-induced cycloversion as a nystagmus dampening mechanism, and abnormal visual pathway routing as seen in albinism.

Q.2. How will you evaluate a case of DVD?
Ans. Refer to text.

Q.3. How will you manage a case of DVD?
Ans. Refer to text.

Q.4. What are the possible complications of surgical management of DVD?
Ans. The possible complications include:
- Recurrence of DVD
- Residual DVD
- Large asymmetric SR recessions may lead to vertical imbalance, resulting in hypotropia.
- Upgaze limitation
- Pseudo IO overaction can be seen after SR recession due to fixation duress of contralateral IO.
- *Palpebral fissure changes:* Widening of palpebral fissure is seen in patients with superior rectus recession and narrowing of fissure is seen in patients undergoing inferior rectus resection/plication.

OPTIC DISC EDEMA

Gunjan Saluja, Anu Malik

■ INTRODUCTION

A case of disc edema can be given in examinations as a short/long case. Optic nerve edema can be unilateral or bilateral. Unilateral disc edema usually results from papillitis, neuroretinitis, and ischemic optic neuropathies. The acute stages of Leber's hereditary optic neuropathy (LHON) can present with unilateral disc edema with telangiectasia being the characteristic feature. The common feature in each of these is the sudden-onset profound vision loss, hence the investigations must be advised taking in considerations age, gender, and presenting feature of each of the etiology when suspecting them to be the underlying cause.

On the other hand, bilateral disc edema can be pseudodisc edema or true disc edema. Common causes of pseudopapilledema are optic nerve head drusen and hypermetropia. The differentiating features of true and pseudo disc edema have been summarized in **Table 1**. Papilledema is a specific term used for bilateral disc edema associated with increased intracranial pressure (ICP). The common etiologies are grade 5 hypertensive retinopathy (Keith–Wegner–Beker classification), intracranial space-occupying lesion, spinal cord tumors, and cerebral venous thrombosis. However, if disc edema cannot be explained by the above-mentioned etiology, then diagnosis of idiopathic intracranial hypertension (IIH) should be considered.

Table 1: True and pseudodisc edema.

	True disc edema	Pseudodisc edema
Disc margins	Blurred	Well defined
Disc vasculature	• Obscured • Venous dilation and tortuosity	• Vessels not obscured • Absence of central cup
Surrounding retina	Peripapillary hemorrhages, with cotton-wool spots	Anomalous arterial branching
Fundus fluorescein angiography	Leakage present	No leakage

■ CLINICAL FEATURES

Symptoms: Patients usually present with complaints of headache with no to mild blurring of vision. Some patients may also complain of diplopia in lateral gazes, resulting from sixth nerve palsy.

Signs:
- *Visual acuity:* Visual acuity is usually good in the initial stages of papilledema, until the late stages when optic atrophy ensues in.
- *Pupil:* Relative afferent pupillary defect (RAPD) cannot be elicited in patients with bilateral involvement and will have sluggishly reacting pupil.

- *Extraocular movements:* EOMs must be examined to look for any limitation of abduction and sixth nerve palsy which can result from stretching of nerve due to increased intracranial tension and causes a false localizing sign.
- *Fundus examination:* Fundus examination reveals the presence of an elevated disc with blurred margins and surrounding flame-shaped hemorrhages, exudates, and presence of Paton's lines (Paton's lines result from displacement of retina due to underlying edema; throwing the peripapillary retina into a series of folds running concentrically with the edge of disc).
- Spontaneous venous pulsation (SVP) results from the variation in the pressure gradient along the retinal vein as it traverses the lamina cribrosa. When the ICP rises, the intracranial pulse pressure also rises to equal the intraocular pulse pressure and the SVP ceases.
- *Grading:* Frisen's grading of papilledema helps to determine progression of the papilledema.
    - *Grade 1:* Blurring of nasal disc margin with normal temporal margins
    - *Grade 2:* Blurring of 360° of disc margin with few flame-shaped hemorrhages
    - *Grade 3:* Blurring of disc margin with surrounding hemorrhages and exudates
    - *Grade 4:* Optic atrophy

INVESTIGATIONS

Ultrasonography (USG) B scan: B scan helps to differentiate true and pseudo-disc edema. Optic nerve head drusen can present as a high-amplitude spike due to calcification.

30° test: Increase in the ICP causes an increase in the optic nerve sheath diameter. The difference in the optic nerve sheath diameter (ONSD) in primary position as compared to an eccentric 30° gaze is a useful test to detect papilledema. ONSD can be measured with the help of ultrasound B scan, 3 mm behind the globe from inner edge to inner edge of optic nerve. The site 3 mm behind the globe is recommended as it is believed to be the site with maximum pressure changes along the optic nerve. When the eye rotates to 30° eccentric gaze position, the CSF within the sheath redistributes itself posteriorly, reducing the ONSD. Usually, a reduction of ONSD of >10% from primary position to 30° from fixation is considered positive for fluid in the sheath and a marker of potential increased ICP.

Visual fields: Visual field examination reveals the presence of enlarged blind spot.

Fundus fluorescein angiography: Fundus fluorescein angiography reveals the presence of disc leakage in true optic disc edema as opposed to disc staining without leakage in pseudo-papilledema.

Optical coherence tomography: OCT in papilledema reveals an increase in the RNFL, which eventually normalizes with eventual thinning as the edema resolves. The optic nerve head in papilledema is elevated with smooth internal contour and subretinal hyporeflective space with a recumbent "lazy V" pattern. OCT is also helpful in diagnosis of subtle disc edema.

Magnetic resonance imaging (MRI) brain: MRI brain must be the initial investigation advised (after ruling out pseudopapilledema) to exclude the diagnosis of space-occupying lesion.

Magnetic resonance venography (MRV): MRV helps to rule out cerebral venous thrombosis. Cerebral venous thrombosis can be further attributed to a large number of causes, which include Behçet's disease, septic and tumor emboli, and autoimmune diseases such as systemic lupus erythematosus (SLE) and primary coagulopathy. Hence, once cerebral venous thrombosis is detected on MRV, investigations to diagnose the underlying pathology must be done.

Lumbar puncture: After excluding the space-occupying lesion, lumbar puncture should be done, and increased opening pressure, should warrant further investigation.

MANAGEMENT

Management depends on the underlying cause as mentioned in the following text.

Management of Idiopathic Intracranial Hypertension

Conservative Management

Diet control and weight reduction: The precise relationship between weight gain or obesity and raised ICP is not clear, but the benefits of weight reduction have been demonstrated repeatedly. Studies have demonstrated that loss of approximately 6% of body weight is associated with a reduction in papilledema and discontinuation of systemic treatment.

Medical Management

In a patient with good visual acuity and with primary complaints of headache, medical management is indicated.

Carbonic anhydrase inhibitors (CAIs): CAIs, such as acetazolamide, are the treatment of choice. The Idiopathic Intracranial Hypertension Treatment Trial (IIHTT) is a multicenter, double-blind, placebo-controlled, North American clinical trial that reported the results of use of acetazolamide with a low-sodium weight-reduction diet compared with diet alone. Use of acetazolamide resulted in modest improvement in visual field function in patients with mild visual loss. The trial also reported improved quality of life outcomes at 6 months with acetazolamide.

Mechanism of action: CAIs such as acetazolamide and methazolamide present in the choroid plexus, decrease CSF production, and also act as mild diuretics.

Dose: Acetazolamide in adult patients is usually started at 1 g daily (250 mg QID or 500 mg BID), with a maximum recommended daily dose of 4 g.

Adverse effects: Adverse effects of acetazolamide include paresthesias, lethargy, and altered taste. Hypokalemia is an important adverse effect and hence electrolytes must be monitored.

Topiramate: Topiramate is an antiepileptic drug; it inhibits carbonic anhydrase and can suppress appetite. It has proven to have similar effects such as acetazolamide in terms of papilledema and headache. The dose of topiramate in IIH is from 25 to 50 mg BD. The drug has side effects such as depression, cognitive slowing, and has potential teratogenic risks.

Surgical Management

In acute or rapidly progressive disease, cases of treatment failure are the indications of surgical management.

- *Cerebrospinal fluid diversion procedures:* The commonly performed surgical procedures include CSF diversion using ventriculoperitoneal, ventriculoatrial, or lumboperitoneal shunt. CSF shunting is the most widely performed surgical treatment for IIH. Shunting results in rapid normalization of the ICP, resolution of papilledema, and improvement of vision. All shunt procedures have a high long-term failure rate and often need revision because of obstruction or failure.
- *Optic nerve sheath decompression:* It is an effective treatment in patients with papilledema and severe visual loss but does not improve headache. The procedure rapidly reduces papilledema and bilateral improvement in visual function is seen in many cases. The procedure has little effect on ICP, but symptomatic improvement is due to local reduction in pressure on the nerve by lowering the intrasheath pressure. In long run, it results in fibrous scar formation between the dura and the optic nerve, thus protecting the anterior optic nerve from ICP. Patients with improvement or apparent remission after optic nerve sheath decompression should remain under close follow-up.

VIVA QUESTIONS

Q.1. What are the causes of disc edema?
Ans. Refer to text.

Q.2. How will you differentiate between true and pseudo disc edema?
Ans. *See* **Table 1**.

Q.3. How will you grade disc edema?
Ans. Refer to text.

Q.4. How will you investigate a case of disc edema?
Ans. Refer to text.

Q.5. How do you differentiate between ischemic and nonischemic optic neuropathy?
Ans. *See* **Table 2**.

Q.6. How will you manage a case of IIH?
Ans. Refer to text.

Table 2: Differences between arteritic and nonarteritic ischemic optic neuropathy.

Features	Arteritic	Nonarteritic
Etiology	Giant cell arteritis	Diabetes, hypertension, hypercholestremia, sleep apnea causing obstruction of posterior ciliary artery
Age	>70 years	Middle-aged (40–60)
Symptoms	Sudden onset blurring of vision associated with pain and jaw claudication	Painless sudden onset blurring of vision
Visual acuity	No perception of light to perception of light	6/60 to 6/18
Fundus	Pallid disc edema	Disc edema with small disc
Investigation	Raised ESR and CRP	Raised BP, RBS, cholesterol
Management	Steroids and immunosuppressants	Correction of underlying systemic condition

Q.7. How will you approach a patient with disc edema?
Ans. Management algorithm

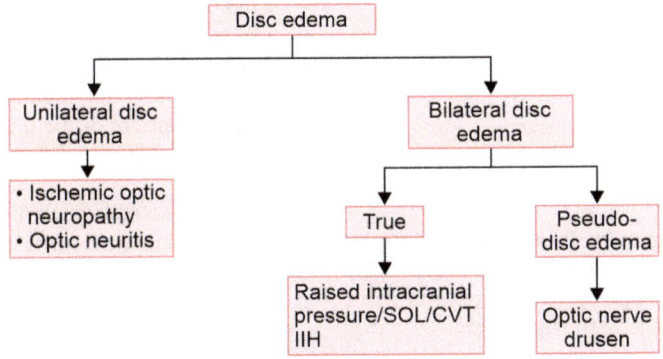

OPTIC ATROPHY

Gunjan Saluja, Anu Malik

■ INTRODUCTION

Optic atrophy is defined as loss of ganglion cells with ensuing pallor of optic disc. Optic atrophy can be given in examinations as a short case.

■ CLINICAL PRESENTATION

Age

Age can help to determine the underlying cause.
Age 0–10 years:
- Cerebral vision impairment
- Trauma shaken baby syndrome
- Secondary to atypical optic neuritis

Adolescents:
- Traumatic optic neuropathy
- Hereditary optic neuropathy

Young adults:
- Post-optic neuritis
- Traumatic optic neuropathy
- Toxic optic neuropathy
- Secondary to IIH

Old age:
- Ischemic optic neuropathy
- Traumatic

Table 1: Differentiation between glaucomatous optic neuropathy and nonglaucomatous optic atrophy.

	Glaucomatous optic atrophy	Nonglaucomatous optic atrophy
Age	Usually in patients >50 years	Young patients
Disc features	• Increased cup disc ratio with loss of neuroretinal rim • Nasalization and bayonetting of vessels with baring of circumpapillary vessels • RNFL loss present	Pallor of neuroretinal rim not correlating with cupping
Visual field	• Follows horizontal midline • Affects periphery first	• Follow vertical midline • Center involving

- Toxic optic neuropathy
- Compressive optic neuropathy secondary to space-occupying lesion

■ EVALUATION

Visual acuity:
- Reduced
- Can range from No perception of light to 6/60 or even better

Anterior segment: Normal

Pupil: RAPD is present.

Fundus:
- *Primary optic atrophy:* Primary optic atrophy occurs without any antecedent edema of optic nerve. Primary optic atrophy results from retrograde damage to the optic nerve.
- *Secondary optic atrophy:*
  - Occurs with antecedent edema of optic nerve
  - Can occur secondary to optic neuritis, ischemic optic neuropathy, and papilledema
  - Disc margins are blurred.
- *Consecutive optic atrophy:* Occurs secondary to retinal pathologies that affect the inner retina and its blood supply. The common etiologies of consecutive optic atrophy are retinitis pigmentosa, pathological myopia, extensive retinochoroiditis, and central retinal artery occlusion. Optic nerve head is waxy pale with a normal cup disc ratio.

Table 1 differentiates glaucomatous and nonglaucomatous optic atrophy.

Kestenbaum index: Kestenbaum capillary index is the number of capillaries visible over the optic disc. The normal number of capillaries visible over the disc is 10. More than 12 suggests hyperemic disc whereas <6 suggests atrophy.

■ INVESTIGATIONS

- *Color vision:* Reduced
- *Contrast sensitivity:* Reduced
- *Visual field:* Visual field defects vary and depends upon the underlying cause. There can be enlargement of the blind spot, paracentral scotoma, altitudinal defects, and bitemporal defects.
- *VEP:* Increased latency of P100
- *OCT:* Thinning of retinal nerve fiber layer

■ IMAGING

Magnetic Resonance Imaging

Magnetic resonance imaging should be ordered to rule out space-occupying lesion. MRI shows thinning of optic nerve with optic nerve sheath distension due to increased amount of CSF.

■ MANAGEMENT

- Management depends on underlying cause and focuses on preventing any further damage.
- Low vision aids should be prescribed after the stabilization of the pathology.

VIVA QUESTIONS

Q.1. Difference between primary and secondary optic atrophy.

Ans.

	Primary	*Secondary*
Etiology	Retrobulbar neuritis, toxic and traumatic optic neuropathy, compressive optic neuropathy	Disc edema, papillitis, ischemic optic neuropathy
Disc margins	Well-defined	Ill-defined
Appearance	Chalky-white	Gray–white
Lamina cribrosa	Visible	Obscured
Retinal vessels	Normal	Peripapillary sheathing

Q.2. What are the types of optic atrophy?

Ans.
- Primary optic atrophy
- Secondary optic atrophy
- Glaucomatous optic atrophy
- Consecutive optic atrophy

Q.3. How will you differentiate between glaucomatous and nonglaucomatous optic atrophy?

Ans. *See* **Table 1**.

Q.4. What is Kestenbaum Index?

Ans. *See* text.

CHAPTER 6

Lens

LONG CASES

ZONULAR CATARACT

Manpreet Kaur, Ashutosh Kumar Gupta, Jeewan S Titiyal

■ INTRODUCTION

Zonular cataract is the most common visually significant variant of pediatric cataract. It may be congenital or occur at a later stage of development and is characterized by an opacity which occupies a discrete zone in the lens. It is usually bilateral and has an autosomal dominant inheritance pattern.

It may be given as a long or short case in postgraduate examination.

■ HISTORY

Chief Complaints

The informants are usually the parents who notice few or all of the following symptoms:
- Child does not recognize objects, toys, or parents (diminution of vision)
- White pupillary reflex (*leukocoria*)
- Involuntary continuous rhythmic movements of the eye (*nystagmus*)
- Deviation of eye (*strabismus*)

History of Present Illness

Etiology and genetics: It is usually hereditary with an autosomal dominant genetic pattern. This type of congenital cataract may be caused by mutations in the heat-shock transcription factor-4 gene (HSF4) located at 16q21-q22.1.

An environmental form of zonular cataract may occur and is associated with vitamin D deficiency. Occasionally, maternal rubella infection contracted between 7th and 8th week of gestation may also cause zonular (lamellar) cataract.

Age at presentation: Patients with zonular cataract usually present in early childhood, though occasionally, they may present soon after birth.

Presenting features: Bilateral involvement is characteristic of zonular cataracts. Since the patients are often in the pre-school age group, a definitive history of diminution of vision may be difficult to elicit. The parents usually notice that the child is unable to see toys placed nearby, stumbles often and does not recognize faces of familiar persons. The parents may notice a white reflex or leukocoria. In cases where there is an asymmetric involvement of both eyes, strabismus may be the presenting complaint. Congenital cases may have associated involuntary ocular movements due to impaired development of fixation.

Antenatal and perinatal history: A history of fever associated with rash may be present in the mother in the antenatal period, which may point toward rubella as the causative etiology. It is essential to rule out maternal malnutrition and history of drug or toxin intake in the antenatal period. Recurrent neonatal infections and malnutrition should be ruled out.

Family history: A positive family history of congenital or developmental cataract is present.

EXAMINATION

General Examination/Specific Systemic Examination

Zonular cataract is familial and usually not associated with any underlying systemic disorder.

However, a detailed examination is essential to rule out systemic disorders that are commonly associated with bilateral congenital cataracts, such as toxoplasmosis, other agents, rubella, cytomegalovirus, and herpes simplex (TORCH) syndrome, galactosemia, and various mutational syndromes. The presence of microcephaly, deafness, cardiac abnormalities, and developmental delay points toward an underlying systemic etiology and warrants a need for further investigations.

Ocular Examination

Visual acuity: Visual acuity may be difficult to establish in very young children. Indirect evidence of diminution of vision includes:
- Child does not follow objects or light.
- Inability to maintain central steady fixation.
- Child resists occlusion of the better eye.
- Strabismus (usually convergent squint)
- Nystagmus

Objective assessment of visual acuity may be made by the following tests:
- *Infants:* Preferential looking tests, Teller acuity cards, Catford drum test, optokinetic nystagmus, and visual-evoked responses
- *1–2 years:* Worth's ivory ball test, Sheridan's ball test, and Boek's Candy test
- *2–5 years:* Dot acuity test, Miniature toy test, Sheridan–Gardiner test (HOTV) test, Tumbling E test, Allen picture cards, Beale-Collins picture chart tests, Kay picture test, Landolt C test, and Snellen's chart

Eyeball: Strabismus may be present, usually convergent squint. Nystagmus is present in cases with congenital onset of cataract.

Eyelids, conjunctiva, cornea, sclera, iris, and pupil: Examination is usually unremarkable. Microcornea may be present in cases with underlying systemic syndrome.

Intraocular pressure is usually normal. If there is associated glaucoma, congenital rubella syndrome must be ruled out.

Lens: Typically, zonular cataract occurs in the zone of fetal nucleus surrounding the embryonic nucleus. The main mass of the lens internal and external to the zone of cataract is clear, except for small linear opacities such as spokes of a wheel (riders), which may be seen toward the equator **(Figs. 1 and 2)**.

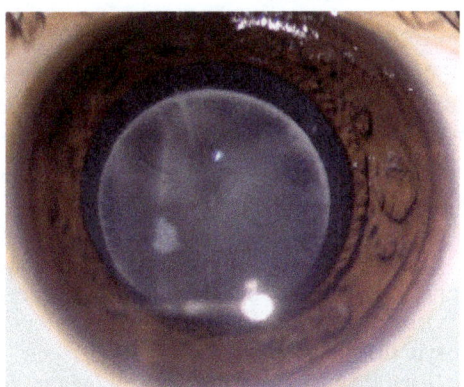

Fig. 1: Zonular cataract with clear periphery and riders.

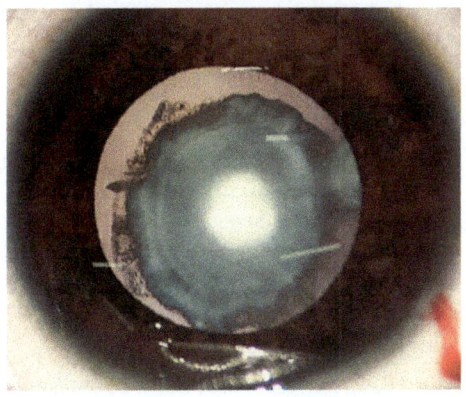

Fig. 2: Zonular cataract retroillumination.

Vitreous and fundus: Examination is usually normal in bilateral zonular cataract. Salt and pepper retinopathy may be present in congenital rubella syndrome. Persistent fetal vasculature (PFV) may be associated, especially in unilateral cases.

■ DIFFERENTIAL DIAGNOSIS

- Persistent fetal vasculature
- Retinoblastoma
- Endophthalmitis
- Retinal detachment
- Toxocariasis
- Coat's disease
- Retinopathy of prematurity
- Astrocytic hamartoma
- Vitreous hemorrhage

■ INVESTIGATIONS

Systemic Investigations

Zonular cataract with positive family history and established hereditary basis for the cataract does not warrant any further investigation.

In other cases with bilateral cataract, the investigations should include the following:
- *Serology for intrauterine infections:* TORCH titers (TORCH = toxoplasmosis, rubella, cytomegalovirus, herpes simplex virus, other viruses such as varicella), VDRL titers for syphilis
- *Urine examination:* Urinalysis for the presence of reducing sugars (galactosemia); urine chromatography for amino acids (Lowe's syndrome)
- Serum electrolytes (serum calcium and phosphorus)
- Fasting blood glucose
- Serum galactokinase
- Thyroid function tests
- Referral to a pediatrician may be warranted for dysmorphic features or suspicion of other systemic diseases. Genetic testing and chromosome analysis may be useful in this context.

Ocular Investigations

- *Visual evoked responses (VER):* To assess visual acuity and estimate visual potential.
- *Biometry:* Axial length and keratometry measurements for intraocular lens (IOL) power calculation
- A-scan ultrasonography to give an estimate of axial length in infants and children uncooperative for biometry.
- *B-scan ultrasonography:* To rule out any posterior segment pathology.

■ MANAGEMENT

Conservative Management

Partial cataracts, cataracts with <3 mm diameter and pericentral cataracts may not immediately require surgery and can be observed. Pupillary dilatation with 2.5% phenylephrine and part-time occlusion of good eye may be tried in unilateral partial cataracts.

Surgical Management

Indications for Treatment

- Cataract >3 mm diameter
- Dense nuclear cataract obstructing view of fundus
- Associated strabismus/nystagmus
- VA <20/80

Time of Surgical Intervention

- Bilateral dense cataracts require early surgery within 6–8 weeks of age to prevent the development of stimulus deprivation amblyopia. In asymmetrical cataract, the eye with the denser cataract should be addressed first.
- Unilateral dense cataract should be operated as soon as possible, ideally before 4–6 weeks of age. Refraction on the first postoperative day with early onset of amblyopia therapy is indispensable. Results are often poor due to dense amblyopia and noncompliance with occlusion therapy.
- Bilateral partial cataracts may not require surgery until later, if at all. In case of doubt, it may be prudent to defer surgery and maintain the level of near vision the patient has, as opposed to diminishing the same by usage of monofocal intraocular lenses. Monitor lens

opacities and visual function and intervene later if vision deteriorates.
- Partial unilateral cataract can usually be observed or treated nonsurgically with mydriasis, and possibly part-time contralateral occlusion to prevent amblyopia.

Biometry and Intraocular Lens Power Calculation

Accurate measurements of axial length and keratometry may be difficult in the preoperative period because of poor patient cooperation and poor fixation. Usually, examination under anesthesia has to be performed to determine axial length and keratometry. Immersion biometry is more predictable than the contact method for IOL power calculation.

An under-correction of the IOL power is usually recommended in cases of pediatric cataract to account for the myopic shift following IOL implantation. Dahan et al. suggest an under-correction of 10% in children between 2 and 8 years and under-correction of 20% in children <2 years of age. They also suggested IOL power selection based on axial length alone (**Table 1**). Indian eyes have been seen to have a lower rate of elongation and change in keratometry, and thus, a smaller under-correction has been seen to suffice.

In cases with unilateral cataract, emmetropia may be aimed for to minimize the risk of amblyopia. Piggyback IOL or IOL exchange may be needed at a later date in such cases.

Surgical Procedure

The primary surgical management consists of *lens aspiration or lensectomy*. Coaxial or bimanual lens aspiration via limbal route is preferred. Pars plana lensectomy may be undertaken in cases where IOL implantation is not planned.

Anterior capsulorhexis may pose a challenge due to the elastic pediatric anterior capsule, which has a propensity to extend. Cohesive ophthalmic viscoelastic device (OVD) such as Healon GV facilitates anterior capsulorhexis as it maintains anterior chamber stability and offsets the vitreous upthrust.

Posterior continuous curvilinear capsulorhexis (PCCC) with limited anterior vitrectomy is

Table 1: Intraocular lens (IOL) power based on axial length (Dahan's formula).

Axial length (mm)	IOL power (D)
17 mm	28 D
18 mm	27 D
19 mm	26 D
20 mm	24 D
21 mm	22 D

recommended for children <5 years of age to minimize the risk of visual axis opacification (VAO) and subsequent additional surgical procedures. In children 8 years and older, lens aspiration with IOL implantation is performed. Between the ages of 5 and 8 years, a posterior capsulorhexis without a limited anterior vitrectomy usually suffices.

Primary IOL implantation is preferred in all unilateral cataract cases as well as bilateral cases when possible. In-the-bag implantation of single-piece hydrophobic IOL is preferred. Multipiece IOL in the sulcus may be implanted when in-the-bag IOL implantation is not possible.

Wound closure by stromal hydration alone may be inadequate because of low scleral rigidity, and sutures are often required to effectively seal the corneal incisions.

Postoperative Visual Rehabilitation

Postoperative occlusion therapy and visual rehabilitation is essential to achieve optimal outcomes, as postoperative amblyopia may limit the visual potential in even a well-done cataract surgery. Optical correction in an aphakic child depends upon the patient's age and laterality of aphakia.
- Aphakic glasses are effective for visual rehabilitation in older children with bilateral aphakia. However, they result in unacceptable anisometropia and aniseikonia in unilateral aphakia. Aphakic glasses are heavy, cosmetically unattractive and result in spherical as well as prismatic aberrations.
- Contact lenses provide a superior optical solution for both unilateral and bilateral aphakia. Tolerance is usually reasonable until the age of about 2 years; problems with

compliance may start after this period as the child becomes more active and independent. Contact lens may become dislodged or lost, leading to periods of visual deprivation with the risk of amblyopia. Maintenance of hygiene may be problematic in young children, leading to a risk of microbial keratitis. The maintenance issues and financial cost limit the widespread usage of contact lenses.
- Intraocular lens implantation is increasingly being performed in young children and even infants and appears to be effective and safe in selected cases. Awareness of the rate of myopic shift, which occurs in the developing eye, combined with accurate biometry, allows the calculation of an IOL power targeted at initial hypermetropia (correctable with spectacles), which will ideally regress toward emmetropia later in life. However, final refraction is variable and emmetropia in adulthood cannot be guaranteed.
- Occlusion therapy to prevent and treat amblyopia is vital in order to achieve optimal outcomes, especially in cases that have undergone unilateral cataract surgery. Atropine penalization may also be considered.

Complications

- *Visual axis opacification (VAO)* is nearly universal if the posterior capsule is retained in a child under the age of 6 years. An intact anterior hyaloid phase provides a scaffold for proliferation of lens epithelial cells and may result in VAO despite posterior capsulorhexis. The incidence of opacification is reduced when posterior capsulorhexis is combined with vitrectomy. Surgical membranectomy via limbal or pars plana route is required for management. Nd:YAG capsulotomy may be tried in cooperative children.
- *Secondary membranes* may form across the pupil, particularly in microphthalmic eyes or those with associated chronic uveitis. A fibrinous postoperative uveitis in an otherwise normal eye, unless vigorously treated, may also result in membrane formation. Thin membranes can be treated with laser capsulotomy, thick membranes may require surgical excision.
- *Secondary glaucoma* may develop in 3–32% of eyes undergoing pediatric cataract surgery. Pupillary block glaucoma may occur in the immediate postoperative period, especially in microphthalmic eyes. Secondary open-angle glaucoma may also develop years after the initial surgery. It is, therefore, important to monitor the intraocular pressure regularly for many years.
- *Retinal detachment* is an uncommon and late complication after cataract surgery. The incidence of retinal detachment following cataract surgery has been reported between 1 and 1.5%.

VIVA QUESTIONS

Q.1. What is the etiology of congenital cataracts?

Ans. *Etiology of bilateral cataracts:*
- Idiopathic
- Familial (hereditary); usually autosomal dominant
- Chromosomal abnormality—Trisomy-21 (Down), Trisomy-18 (Edward), Trisomy-13 (Patau). Other translocations, deletions, and duplications
- *Craniofacial syndromes:* Hallermann-Streiff, Rubinstein-Taybi, Smith-Lemli-Opitz.
- Musculoskeletal—Conradi, Albright, myotonic dystrophy
- Renal—Lowe, Alport
- Metabolic—galactosemia, Fabry, Wilson, mannosidosis, diabetes mellitus
- Maternal infection (TORCH diseases)—rubella, cytomegalovirus, varicella, syphilis, toxoplasmosis
- Ocular anomalies—aniridia, anterior segment dysgenesis syndrome
- Iatrogenic—corticosteroids, radiation (may also be unilateral)

Etiology of unilateral cataracts:
- Idiopathic
- Ocular anomalies—persistent fetal vasculature (PFV), anterior segment dysgenesis, retinal detachment
- Traumatic (rule out child abuse)

Table 2: Morphological variants of pediatric cataract associated with systemic diseases.

Systemic disease	Cataract morphology	Associated findings
Fabry syndrome	Spoke-like	Corneal whorls
Mannosidosis	Spoke-like	Hepatosplenomegaly
Diabetes	Vacuoles	↑Blood glucose level
Hypoparathyroidism	Multicolor flecks	↓Serum calcium
Myotonic dystrophy	Multicolor flecks	Characteristic facial features, tonic "grip"
Wilson disease	Green "sunflower"	Kayser–Fleischer corneal ring
Lowe syndrome	Thin disciform	Hypotonia, glaucoma

Q.2. What are the contraindications for IOL implantation in pediatric cataract?

Ans. *Contraindications of IOL implantation are:*
- Microphthalmos
- Rubella cataract
- Aniridia
- Uveitis

Q.3. What are the surgical challenges faced in pediatric cataracts?

Ans. The intraoperative challenges faced in pediatric cataracts are:
- Difficulty in capsulorhexis formation
- Positive intravitreal pressure
- Intraoperative miosis
- Wound leak

Q.4. What are characteristic morphological variants of pediatric cataracts associated with systemic diseases?

Ans. Refer **Table 2**.

Q.5. Explain IOL power calculations in pediatric patients.

Ans. Refer text.

Q.6. Which is the best IOL power calculation formula for pediatric cataract?

Ans. At present there is no consensus on the best IOL formulae in pediatric cataract. All available IOL power calculation formulae are developed for adults, so they are not perfect in pediatric eyes.

The infant aphakia treatment study, the largest multicentric trial on pediatric cataracts reported Holladay 1 and the SRK/T provides the best outcomes in terms of residual errors.

Q.7. What is the role of artificial intelligence (AI) in the management of pediatric cataracts?

Ans. Artificial intelligence combines large data sets with computer science to make an intelligent computer program that can make predictions or classifications, and take decisions not unlike humans, for problem solving. The diagnosis and management of pediatric cataracts usually necessitate an adequately trained ophthalmologist. As such, patients who do not have access to specialized centers might have a delay in diagnosis, paving the way to stimulus deprivation amblyopia. Today, there are highly accurate AI software capable of diagnosing, grading, and advising appropriate treatment of pediatric cataracts. There are algorithms that can also explore other potentially significant features of pediatric cataract on slit-lamp examination for further research. These have the potential to expand the reach of healthcare facilities to areas lacking the same.

■ BIBLIOGRAPHY

1. Bradford GM, Keech RV, Scott WE. Factors affecting visual outcome after surgery for bilateral congenital cataracts. Am J Ophthalmol. 1994;117:58-64.
2. Kaur S, Sukhija J, Ram J. Intraocular lens power calculation formula in congenital cataracts: are we using the correct formula for pediatric eyes? Indian J Ophthalmol. 2021;69(12):3442-5.

3. Kugelberg M, Zetterström C. Pediatric cataract surgery with or without anterior vitrectomy. J Cataract Refract Surg. 2002;28(10): 1770-3.
4. Lambert SR, Drack AV. Infantile cataracts. Surv Ophthalmol. 1996;40:427-58.
5. Medsinge A, Nischal KK. Pediatric cataract: challenges and future directions. Clinical Ophthalmology (Auckland, NZ). 2015;9:77-90.
6. Ram J, Brar GS, Kaushik S, Gupta A. Role of posterior capsulotomy with vitrectomy and intraocular lens design and material in reducing posterior capsule opacification after pediatric cataract surgery. J Cataract Refract Surg. 2003;29:1579-84.
7. Vanderveen DK, Trivedi RH, Nizam A, Lynn MJ, Lambert SR. Infant Aphakia Treatment Study Group. Predictability of intraocular lens power calculation formulae in infantile eyes with unilateral congenital cataract: results from the infant aphakia treatment study. Am J Ophthalmol. 2013;156:1252-60.e2.

ECTOPIA LENTIS

Prafulla Kumar Maharana, Ananya PR, Ruchita Falera, Manpreet Kaur

■ INTRODUCTION

Ectopia lentis (subluxation of lens) is characterized by partial displacement of the lens from the patellar fossa. The first case of lens dislocation was reported by Berryat in 1749 and the term *ectopia lentis* was coined by Stellwag in 1856. The terms *ectopia lentis* and *subluxated lens* have been used interchangeably in literature, it is, however, preferable to use ectopia lentis in cases of subluxation secondary to inheritable causes. Lens subluxation may be heritable without associated systemic syndrome, heritable with associated systemic syndrome, in association with ocular comorbidities or because of trauma **(Box 1)**.

The most common cause of lens subluxation is trauma, which accounts for nearly 50% of all cases. Marfan's syndrome is the most common heritable cause of ectopia lentis. Disruption or dysfunction of the zonular fibers of the lens is the underlying pathophysiology of ectopia lentis, regardless of cause (trauma or heritable condition). The degree of zonular impairment determines the degree of lens displacement.

It is given as a long or short case in postgraduate/DNB/diploma examination.

■ HISTORY

Epidemiology

Ectopia lentis can occur at any age. It may be present at birth, or it may manifest late in life. A male preponderance is reported, as males appear more prone to ocular trauma than females. Isolated ectopia lentis and Marfan's syndrome have an autosomal dominant mode of inheritance.

Box 1: Etiology of subluxated lens.
- Traumatic subluxation of lens
- *Hereditary causes without systemic associations:*
    - Isolated ectopia lentis (autosomal recessive isolated ectopia lentis-2 is caused by ADAMTSL4 mutation)
    - Ectopia lentis et pupillae (due to homozygous or compound heterozygous mutation in the ADAMTSL4 gene on Chromosome 1q21)
- *Hereditary causes with systemic associations:*
    - Marfan's syndrome
    - Homocystinuria
    - Weill–Marchesani syndrome
    - Hyperlysinemia
    - Sulfite oxide deficiency
    - Ehlers–Danlos syndrome
    - Crouzon's syndrome
    - Oxycephaly
- *Associated with other ocular diseases:*
    - Mature or hypermature cataract
    - Buphthalmos
    - High myopia
    - Megalocornea
    - Pseudoexfoliation
    - Retinitis pigmentosa
    - Eales disease
    - Retinal detachment

Chief complaints: The patients may present with the following symptoms:
- Decreased or fluctuating vision
- Photophobia
- Glare
- Monocular diplopia
- Suboptimal correction with spectacles.

History of present illness: Heritable ectopia lentis is bilateral, symmetric, and stable from early childhood. Time of onset of disease, its progression and its effect on visual function should be noted. There is frequent change in glasses with a progressive increase in the power of glasses. Subluxation of lens associated with trauma can present with sudden diminution of vision or other symptoms such as photophobia and monocular diplopia.

Past medical history: Ectopia lentis may be associated with underlying systemic disorders and a careful history must be elicited regarding the following:
- Any history of previous cardiac illness must be taken. Cardiovascular manifestations of Marfan's syndrome include aortic and pulmonary artery dilatation, mitral and tricuspid valve prolapse with or without regurgitation. Dilatation of the sinus of Valsalva is found in 60–80% of adult and mitral valve prolapse (MVP) is present in 80% patients.
- Homocystinuria is a recessively inherited disorder caused by deficiency of cystathionine synthase leading to accumulation of homocysteine and methionine. Affected persons have tall, thin habitus similar to Marfan's syndrome patients but infrequent arachnodactyly. Any history of developmental delay or mental retardation should be elicited as homocystinuria is associated with subnormal intelligence.
- History of recurrent fractures, hip dislocation or any musculoskeletal abnormalities should be asked to rule out presence of any connective tissue diseases such as Ehlers–Danlos syndrome.

Family History

A three-generation pedigree chart must be prepared. History of similar complaints in siblings and parents should be specifically asked.

EXAMINATION

Systemic Examination

A careful systemic examination must be carried out and the findings suggestive of underlying systemic disorders must be noted.

Marfan's syndrome may present with the following systemic signs:
- Long thin limbs
- Arachnodactyly-long spider like fingers
- *Arm span:* Height ratio >1.05
- Upper segment of body (head to pubic bone): Lower segment ratio <0.86
- Scoliosis
- Chest wall deformities (pectus excavatum/pectus carinatum)
- Thumb sign (the thumb sign is positive when the entire distal phalanx of the adducted thumb extends beyond the ulnar border of the palm)
- Wrist sign (the wrist sign is positive when the tip of the thumb covers the entire fingernail of the fifth finger when wrapped around the contralateral wrist)
- High-arched palate

Musculoskeletal anomalies are also present in homocystinuria, Weill–Marchesani syndrome and connective tissue disorders.

Cardiovascular examination should be performed to rule out underlying valvular heart defects in Marfan's syndrome.

Homocystinuria may have associated mental retardation and may necessitate IQ testing and evaluation of higher mental functions.

Ocular Examination

Visual acuity: Visual acuity should be carefully assessed considering the following points:
- Uncorrected visual acuity and best-corrected visual acuity (BCVA) must be assessed in all cases.
- Near vision should be documented.
- Refraction should be carried out through phakic and aphakic zones **(Fig. 1)**.

Eyeballs: Strabismus may be associated with Marfan's syndrome, and if uncorrected in children can result into amblyopia. It may be a presenting sign of the disorder. Delayed and inadequate correction of refractive errors as well as deficient fibrillin in extraocular muscle pulleys causing their instability may explain the high incidence of strabismus in Marfan's patients.

Conjunctiva is usually normal.

Cornea: Patients with Marfan's syndrome can present with flat cornea (cornea plana) or steep cornea. Associated keratoconus may be present. Ectopia lentis et pupillae is associated with increased corneal diameters.

Sclera: Thinning of sclera may be present, giving it a *bluish hue* in Marfan's disease as well as in cases of connective tissue disorders such as osteogenesis imperfecta and Ehler–Danlos syndrome.

Anterior chamber and angle:
- Ectopia lentis is usually associated with a deep anterior chamber, however, it may be irregular.
- Gonioscopy must be done in all cases to rule out angle recession (in post-traumatic subluxation of lens) and enlarged iris processes (in ectopia lentis et pupillae).

Iris:
- Thinning and flattening of iris with loss of iris crypts may be seen in ectopia lentis et pupillae.
- Post-traumatic cases may show iridodialysis.

Pupil:
- The pupil may be eccentrically placed as in cases of ectopia lentis *et pupillae* where the pupil is displaced opposite to the direction of subluxation.
- The pupil may be poorly dilating on account of hypoplastic dilator muscles.
- Persistent pupillary membrane may also be seen in some cases.
- Relation of the lens with respect to the undilated pupil should be noted.

Lens:
- Any evidence of phacodonesis should be documented.
- Evidence of cataract, if any, should be documented. Early onset of cataractous changes in ectopia lentis has been well documented.
- Extent of subluxation should be noted in clock hours.
- Direction of subluxation **(Fig. 2)** must be noted.
- *Zonules:* Condition of the zonules should be documented as they may be stretched in cases of Marfan's disease **(Fig. 3)** or broken in

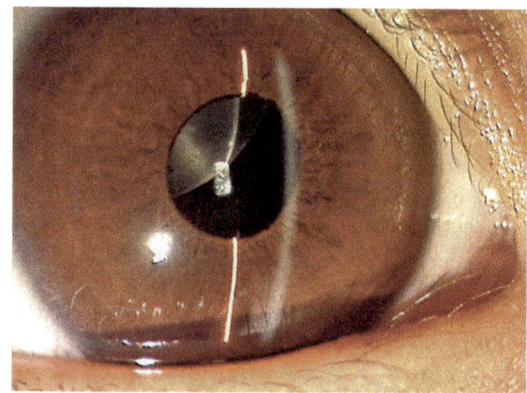

Fig. 2: Superotemporal displacement.

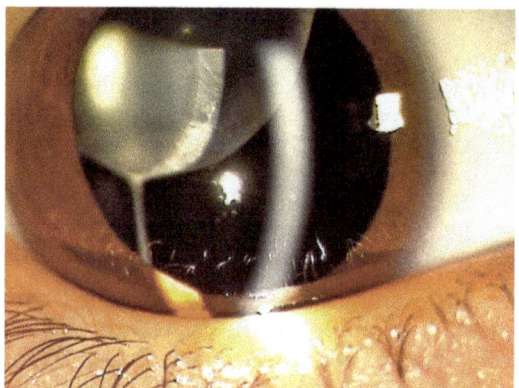

Fig. 1: Phakic and aphakic zones in ectopia lentis.

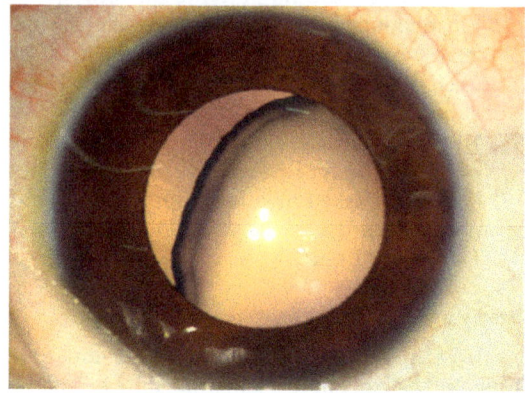

Fig. 3: Stretched zonules in cases of Marfan's disease.

case of homocystinuria. Some cases may be associated with absence of zonular fibers.

The subluxation of the lens is generally superotemporal in cases of Marfan's syndrome. Preferential focusing of ultraviolet B light on the inferonasal quadrant of the crystalline lens is hypothesized to explain the predominantly superotemporal dislocation **(Fig. 2)** of the lens in Marfan syndrome, while it is inferonasal in cases of homocystinuria. However, the direction of subluxation is not pathognomonic, and it may occur in any direction. Premature cataracts and other lens and capsule opacities are commonly found in Marfan's syndrome with presentation at a younger age (30–50s) compared to the general population.

In some cases, the patients may be aphakic with posterior dislocation of the lens into the vitreous cavity.

Intraocular pressure: Intraocular pressure should be documented in all cases. Primary open-angle glaucoma is most common, but glaucoma can be secondary to anterior lens dislocation or anterior chamber angle abnormalities.

Fundus examination:
- *Distant direct ophthalmoscopy examination:* A crescent-shaped reflex seen on distant direct ophthalmoscope is pathognomonic of subluxated lens.
- Detailed fundus examination is mandatory in all cases. Retinal detachment may occur in 5–11% of patients with Marfan's syndrome, and its incidence increases to 8–38% in the presence of ectopia lentis. Unstable subluxated or dislocated lens capsule exerts traction on the vitreous base, leading to small tears or holes in the retinal periphery. Axial myopia presents in Marfan's syndrome predisposes to early vitreous liquefaction and posterior vitreous detachment, retinal thinning, lattice degeneration, and peripheral breaks.

■ DIFFERENTIAL DIAGNOSIS

Ectopia lentis is diagnosed clinically on the basis of slit-lamp examination. Various etiologies responsible for ectopia lentis are tabulated in **Box 1**. Marfan's syndrome and homocystinuria are common heritable systemic disorders associated with ectopia lentis and their differentiating features are summarized in **Table 1**.

■ INVESTIGATIONS

Systemic Investigations

A case of ectopia lentis must be managed with a multidisciplinary approach along with a pediatrician, cardiologist, and orthopedician. It should be evaluated for underlying systemic abnormalities.
- X-ray chest/ECG (electrocardiogram)/2D Echo (two-dimensional echocardiography) should be done in all cases to rule out cardiac abnormalities in Marfan's syndrome.
- Sodium nitroprusside test (in urine) must be done to rule out homocystinuria.
- X-rays of spine and extremities are undertaken to evaluate the skeletal deformities.

Ocular Investigations

- *Biometry* should be done to calculate IOL power.

Table 1: Differentiating features of Marfan's disease and homocystinuria.

Clinical features	Marfan's disease	Homocystinuria
Etiology	Fibrillin-1 (FBN1) gene mutation on chromosome 15	Deficiency of cystathionine synthase leading to accumulation of homocysteine and methionine
Mode of inheritance	Autosomal dominant	Autosomal recessive
Mental retardation	Absent	Present
Direction of subluxation	Superotemporal subluxation of lens	Inferonasal subluxation of lens
Condition of zonules	Primarily present with stretched zonules	Absent and broken zonules

- *B-scan ultrasonography:* In cases of mature cataract where the fundal view is obscured, an ultrasonography (USG) must be done to rule out retinal detachment or any posterior segment pathology.

MANAGEMENT

Conservative Management

- A complete refraction considering the undilated central pupillary position, size of the phakic and aphakic zones and preferred visual axis needs to be done.
- Appropriate spectacle correction, aphakic glasses, or contact lens can be given.
- Other methods such as miotics to minimize diplopia or mydriatics to enlarge the aphakic zone are rarely used these days.

Surgical Management

Indications for Surgery

- Subluxated lens bisects the pupil leading to a phakic and aphakic zone in an undilated pupillary axis.
- Cataractous lens
- Associated complications such as glaucoma or pupillary block
- Presence of lenticular astigmatism
- Anteriorly or posteriorly dislocated lens surgical management of subluxated lens depends on the degree of subluxation. The following are the modalities of management mainly for secondary causes of lens subluxation.
- *Subluxation <3 clock hours:* In cases of lens subluxation of <3 clock hours, slow motion phacoemulsification with posterior chamber intraocular lens (PCIOL) implantation in the bag can be attempted. Slow motion phacoemulsification includes phacoemulsification at low flow rate, low vacuum, and low infusion bottle height in order to minimize stress on the zonules.
- *Subluxation of 3–5 clock hours:* In case of lens subluxation of 3–5 clock hours, slow motion phacoemulsification can be done. Insertion of capsular tension ring (CTR) or capsule tension segments (CTS) may be needed to support the bag. With the use of CTR, any force that is transmitted to the capsule does not directly impact the adjacent zonules but is rather distributed to the entire zonular apparatus.
- *Subluxation of 5–7 clock hours:* Slow motion phacoemulsification with the use of Cionni ring or a CTS with CTR with PCIOL implantation can be attempted in cases of severe or progressive zonular weakness. Cionni ring has a hook, which needs to be kept opposite to the direction of decentration. A transscleral suture applied to it allows it to be pulled peripherally thereby counteracting the capsular bag decentration.
- *Subluxation of >7 clock hours:* Intracapsular cataract extraction (ICCE) with intrascleral haptic fixation or sclera fixated IOL (SFIOL), iris fixated IOL or ACIOL implantation can be done in cases with extensively subluxated cataractous lens.
- In cases with significant posterior subluxation of lens, pars plana lensectomy (PPL) with pars plana vitrectomy (PPV) can be done, followed by IOL implantation in the anterior chamber or sulcus-fixated IOL.

The use of capsular support devices is not preferred in cases of progressive zonular weakness. These are of particular importance in secondary causes of subluxation such as post-traumatic subluxation of lens and pseudoexfoliation where the basic zonular anatomy is not compromised.

In heritable ectopia lentis with or without underlying systemic disorders, intralenticular lens aspiration (ILLA) (**Figs. 4A to D**) is the preferred technique, which is described as follows:

- In this technique, two openings are made in the lens capsule with a microvitreoretinal (MVR) blade and the lens matter is aspirated using a bimanual irrigation and aspiration system.
- The capsular bag is then cut and aspirated using a vitrectomy probe.

This technique has several advantages such as:

- The lens can be stabilized with the irrigation cannula, the area to be aspirated can be brought into focus, and a complete lens aspiration can be easily performed.
- Additionally, the irrigation cannula hydrates the cortical matter, enabling complete aspiration.
- Furthermore, creating two small capsular openings in the midperiphery of the lens

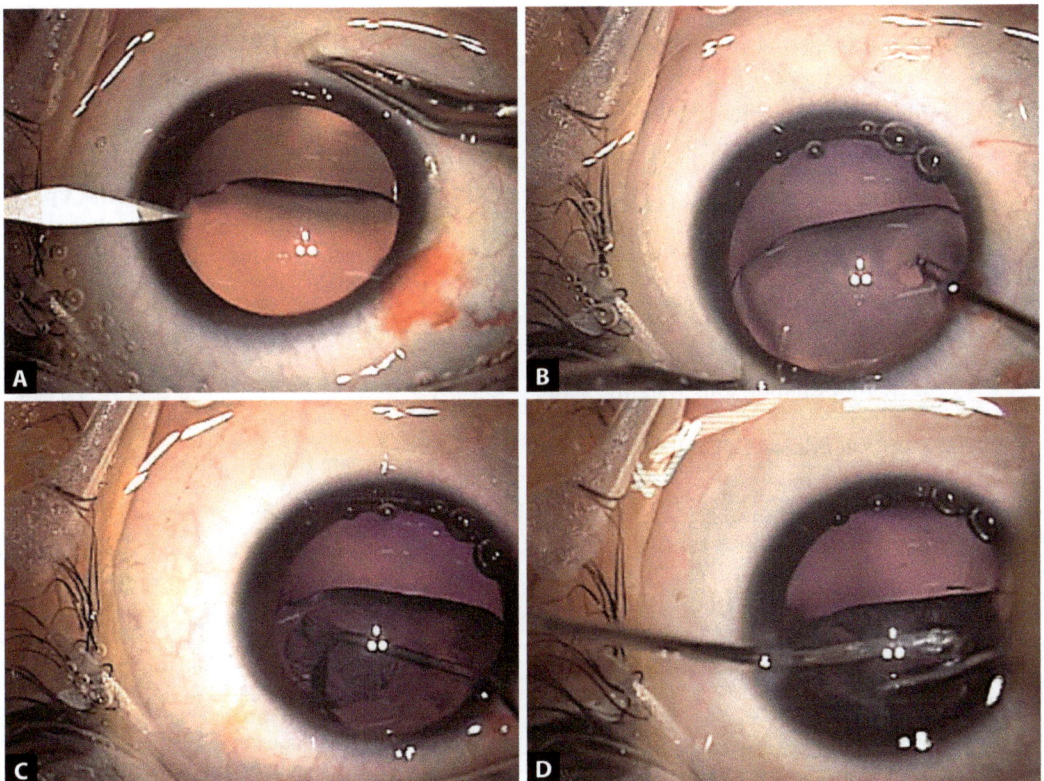

Figs. 4A to D: Intralenticular lens aspiration.

that are directly visible often eliminates the problem of poor visibility.
- There is less chance of vitreous becoming hydrated and lens matter falling into the vitreous cavity, as aspiration is intralenticular.
- Another added advantage is that the capsular rim is left intact. This may allow IOL implantation in the sulcus once the capsular rim fibroses, thus avoiding the complications and difficulties associated with anterior chamber and sulcus-fixated IOLs.

VIVA QUESTIONS

Q.1. What is the etiopathogenesis of Marfan's disease?
Ans. Marfan's syndrome is an autosomal dominant disorder with near complete penetrance and variable expression. There is a mutation in the fibrillin locus (FBN1), which lies on the long arm of chromosome 15 (15q21). This results in abnormal biosynthesis of fibrillin, a 350 kD *cysteine-rich glycoprotein which is a major constituent of microfibrils present in connective tissue of suspensory ligaments of crystalline lens.*

Q.2. What are the differences between Homocystinuria and Marfan's disease?
Ans. Refer **Table 1**.

Q.3. Type of astigmatism seen in subluxation of lens.
Ans. Irregular/compound myopic astigmatism is seen due to following mechanism:
- Weak zonules lead to relaxation of lens capsule (which is normally in a state of stretch by zonules) making the lens more spherical along the axis with increased lens power and consequent myopia.

- Area where zonules are still intact, the lens remains as such or may slightly bulge.
- Therefore, there is more myopia in one axis while less myopia in other axis.

Q.4. What are the diagnostic criteria for Marfan's syndrome?

Ans. Marfan's disease is diagnosed according to modified Ghent's criteria.

In absence of family history:
- Aortic root dilation (Z score >2) and ectopia lentis
- Aortic root dilation and FBN1 mutation
- Aortic root dilation and systemic score >7 points
- Ectopia lentis and FBN1 with known aortic root dilation

In presence of family history:
- Ectopia lentis and family history: Marfan's syndrome
- Systemic score (>7 points, table) and family history of Marfan's syndrome
- Aortic dilation and family history of Marfan's syndrome

Systemic feature	Score
Wrist and thumb sign (either of the above: 1)	3
Pectus carinatum deformity (pectus excavatum or chest asymmetry: 1)	2
Hind foot deformity (plain pes planus 1)	2
Pneumothorax	2
Dural ectasia	2
Protrusio acetabuli	2
Reduced US/LS and increased arm/height and no severe scoliosis	1
Scoliosis or thoracolumbar kyphosis	1
Reduced elbow extension	1
Facial features (3/5): (dolichocephaly, enophthalmos, down-slanting palpebral fissures, malar hypoplasia, and retrognathia)	1
Skin striae	1
Myopia >3 diopters	1
Mitral valve prolapse (all types)	1

Maximum total: **20 points; score ≥7 indicates systemic involvement.**

Q.5. What are the different techniques of sclera fixated IOL (SFIOL)?

Ans. The different techniques of SFIOL differ primarily in terms of use of sutures, creation of scleral flap, and creation of scleral tunnel. Most techniques use polymethylmethacrylate (PMMA) IOLs with eyelets (sutured) or a three-piece IOL (optic acrylic, haptic prolene/polypropylene).

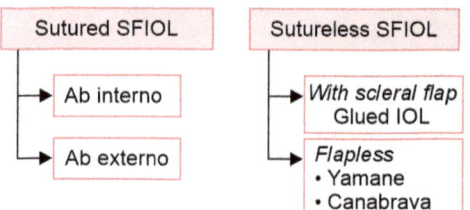

The popular techniques of SFIOL are described below in the table.

Technique	Principle
Sutured SFIOL	• Ab externo technique—needle from scleral flap into eye • Ab interno technique—needle through corneoscleral tunnel, brought out through the scleral flap
Glued IOL	• Two partial-thickness scleral flaps are created 180° apart at 3 and 9 o'clock positions • Sclerotomies made under the scleral flaps 1.5–1.75 mm from the limbus • Scleral tunnels are made at the edge of the scleral flap with the help of a 26 G bent needle or an MVR knife • Haptics are externalized by micro forceps/SFIOL forceps using a handshake technique
Yamane technique	• Two angled sclerotomies are made, 180° apart, through the conjunctiva 2 mm from the limbus using a 30-gauge needle • The haptics are exteriorized by threading them into the lumen of a 30 G needle • The ends of the haptics are cauterized to make a flange • The flange of the haptics is pushed back and fixed into the scleral tunnels

Contd...

Contd...

Technique	Principle
Canabrava technique	• 5–0 polypropylene sutures are inserted through eyelets of the haptics of a single-piece non-foldable IOL • Using ophthalmic cautery flanges are created at the ends of the suture at the eyelets and the externalized end

BIBLIOGRAPHY

1. Anteby I, Isaac M, BenEzra D. Hereditary subluxated lenses: Visual performances and long-term follow-up after surgery. Ophthalmology. 2003;110:1344-8.
2. Goel S, Sahay P, Singhal D, Maharana PK, Titiyal JS, Sharma N. Intraoperative optical coherence tomography-guided release of lenticulo-corneal adhesion and lens aspiration in anterior dislocation of lens with corneal edema. Indian J Ophthalmol. 2020;68(3):510-2.
3. Kumar B, Muni I. Scleral Fixation of Intraocular Lenses. In: StatPearls. Treasure Island (FL): StatPearls Publishing; 2023.
4. Loeys BL, Dietz HC, Braverman AC, Callewaert BL, De Backer J, Devereux RB, et al. Revised Ghent criteria for the diagnosis of Marfan syndrome (MFS) and related conditions. J Med Genet. 2010;47:476-85.
5. Maharana PK, Sahay P, Mandal S, Lakshmi CC, Goel S, Nagpal R, et al. Outcomes of surgical intervention in cases of ectopia lentis. Indian J Ophthalmol. 2022;70(7):2432-8.
6. Nelson LB, Maumenee IH. Ectopia lentis. Surv Ophthalmol. 1982;27:143-60.
7. Nemet AY, Assia EI, Apple DJ, Barequet IS. Current concepts of ocular manifestations in Marfan syndrome. Surv Ophthalmol. 2006; 51:561-75.
8. Rubin SE, Nelson LB. Ocular manifestations of autosomal dominant systemic conditions. Duane's Clinical Ophthalmology on CD-ROM. Vol. 3. Ch. 58. Philadelphia: Lippincott Williams & Wilkins, 2006.
9. Sahay P, Maharana PK, Shaikh N, Goel S, Sinha R, Agarwal T, et al. Intra-lenticular lens aspiration in paediatric cases with anterior dislocation of lens. Eye (Lond). 2019;33(9): 1411-7.
10. Sinha R, Sharma N, Vajpayee RB. Intralenticular bimanual irrigation: aspiration for subluxated lens in Marfan's syndrome. J Cataract Refract Surg. 2005;31(7):1283-6.

SHORT CASES

LENTICONUS

Manpreet Kaur, Prafulla Kumar Maharana, Jeewan S Titiyal

■ INTRODUCTION

A localized conical protrusion of the anterior or posterior capsule of the lens, along with the underlying cortex, is referred to as a lenticonus. The anomaly is mostly restricted to the axial area and can reach a diameter of 2–7 mm. Posterior lenticonus is more common than anterior lenticonus and is usually unilateral and axial in location. Anterior lenticonus is bilateral and usually associated with Alport syndrome.

It is given as short case in postgraduate examination.

■ HISTORY

Chief Complaints

- Decrease in visual acuity
- Minimal improvement with spectacle or contact lenses.

History of Present Illness

Epidemiology: Alport syndrome, a hereditary systemic disease with a prevalence of 1/5,000 in a normal population, is associated with bilateral anterior lenticonus. Alport syndrome is inherited in an X-linked fashion in 85%, autosomal recessive pattern in 10%, and least commonly, autosomal dominant.

Posterior lenticonus is a unilateral congenital defect that usually occurs in a sporadic manner, with a prevalence of 1–4 per 100,000 children. It has no predilection for either sex. It may also occur in association with Lowe syndrome (oculocerebrorenal syndrome).

Age at presentation: Anterior lenticonus manifests before the age of 30 years, most commonly in the second decade. Posterior lenticonus is a congenital anomaly and the age at diagnosis lies between 3 and 7 years.

Presenting features: Patients with anterior lenticonus present with gradual progressive diminution of vision in both eyes. It is not amenable to correction by either spectacles or contact lenses.

Posterior lenticonus is unilateral, and amblyopia is the most significant visual problem associated with it. Amblyopia may be a result of the optical distortion induced by the conical protrusion of the lens surface, anisometropia or by visual deprivation due to cataract.

Alport syndrome may present with pain, watering, diminution of vision and photophobia due to corneal erosions.

Progressive vision loss may occur if associated with posterior polymorphous dystrophy.

Associated ocular features: Anterior lenticonus may be associated with the following ocular anomalies:
- Dot-and-fleck retinopathy
- Posterior polymorphous corneal dystrophy
- Temporal macular thinning
- Subcapsular and cortical cataract
- Arcus juvenilis.

Posterior lenticonus may be associated with the following ocular manifestations:
- Amblyopia
- Subcapsular and cortical cataract
- Strabismus
- Glaucoma (in Lowe syndrome).

Family history: Autosomal dominant inheritance has been described, in bilateral cases. Male patients with anterior lenticonus may have a positive family history of hearing loss of early onset, hematuria and renal insufficiency, suggestive of Alport syndrome.

■ EXAMINATION

Systemic Examination

Alport syndrome is characterized by progressive renal failure and sensorineural deafness in addition to anterior lenticonus. Defective Type 4 collagen (found in the glomerular basement membrane, lens capsule, stria vascularis of the cochlea, internal limiting membrane, Bruch's membrane of the retina, Bowman's and Descemet membrane of the cornea) is implicated. The earliest and most common manifestation of Alport syndrome is hematuria, which may be gross or microscopic; the latter present in all males and 95% of females. Males with X-linked Alport syndrome and both sexes with autosomal recessive Alport syndrome develop proteinuria. Proteinuria of nephrotic range may occur in as many as 30% of patients and worsen with age. Hypertension is usually present in males with X-linked Alport syndrome and in both sexes with autosomal recessive Alport syndrome. Incidence and severity increase with age and degree of renal failure.

Bilateral, high-frequency sensorineural hearing loss begins by late childhood and is present in approximately 50% of male patients with X-linked disease by the age of 25 years, and about 90% are deaf by the age of 40 years.

Posterior lenticonus may be associated with Lowe syndrome (oculocerebrorenal syndrome). It is a rare X-linked recessive disorder characterized by congenital cataracts, hypotonia and areflexia, intellectual disability, proximal tubular acidosis, aminoaciduria, phosphaturia, and low-molecular-weight proteinuria. Nonsyndromic cases have been hypothesized to occur due to the traction exerted by the hyaloid artery remnants on the capsule, vitritis, or overgrowth of posterior lens fibers.

Ocular Examination

Eyeball: Strabismus may be present in cases with posterior lenticonus. Eyeball shape and movements are normal.

Lid: Eyelids are normal.

Conjunctiva: Conjunctival examination is normal.

Cornea: Posterior polymorphous corneal dystrophy may be observed in cases with anterior lenticonus, characterized by endothelial vesicles. Posterior lenticonus may be associated with microcornea.

Sclera: Scleral examination is normal.

Iris: Iris examination is normal.

Pupil: Pupils are normal.

Intraocular pressure: Glaucoma may be present in 50% of cases with Lowe syndrome.

Lens: A localized, sharply defined, transparent, conical projection of the lens capsule and cortex, generally axial in location (**Fig. 1**). There is an increase in lens thickness.

"Oil-droplet" reflex is observed on retroillumination (**Fig. 2**).

Associated subcapsular and cortical opacities appear in advanced stages of lenticonus.

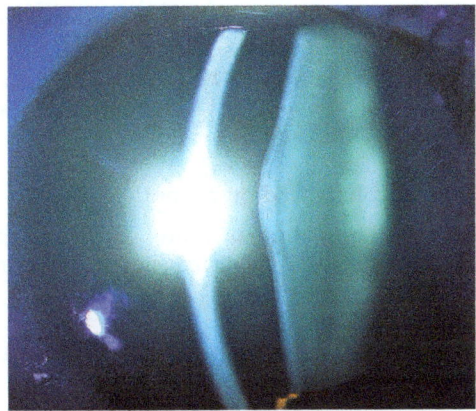

Fig. 1: Transparent, localized, axial, sharply demarcated conical projection of the lens capsule and cortex in anterior lenticonus. There is an increase in lens thickness.

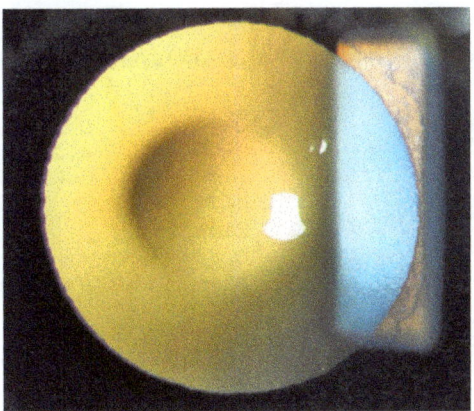

Fig. 2: Oil-droplet reflex observed on retroillumination in a case of anterior lenticonus.

Vitreous: Posterior lenticonus may be associated with persistent fetal vasculature, as mentioned above.

Fundus: A dot-and-fleck retinopathy may be observed in cases with anterior lenticonus. Temporal macular thinning may also be observed in cases with anterior lenticonus.

Retinoscopy: Scissoring reflexes are observed on retinoscopy.

■ DIFFERENTIAL DIAGNOSIS

The diagnosis of lenticonus is clinical in nature and is easily confirmed on a slit-lamp examination. The differences between anterior and posterior lenticonus are highlighted in **Table 1**.

Anterior lenticonus is rare and bilateral, and may be associated with the following syndromes:
- Alport syndrome (most common association with anterior lenticonus)
- Waardenburg syndrome (rare).

Posterior lenticonus is more common and unilateral. It may be associated with the following conditions:
- Sporadic (most common)
- Associated with persistent hyperplastic primary vitreous
- Associated with hyaloid artery remnant
- Familial posterior lenticonus and microcornea
- Lowe syndrome (oculocerebrorenal syndrome)
- Trauma

■ INVESTIGATIONS

Systemic investigations should be undertaken to evaluate associated syndromes.
- Renal function tests
- *Urine examination:* Hematuria and proteinuria
- *Audiometry:* Evaluate sensorineural hearing loss
- *Renal biopsy* to assess glomerular damage and ultrastructure of the glomerular basement membrane.

Ocular Investigations

- An increase in lens thickness may be seen on A-scan ultrasonography.
- B-scan ultrasonography may reveal herniated lenticular material on the posterior aspect of the lens.
- Aberrometry reveals lenticular astigmatism and aberrations.
- Biometry to calculate intraocular lens power.

Table 1: Differentiating features of anterior and posterior lenticonus.

Clinical features	Anterior lenticonus	Posterior lenticonus
Laterality	Bilateral	Unilateral
Age at presentation	Second decade	3–7 years
Etiology	Associated with Alport syndrome	• Usually sporadic • May be associated with Lowe syndrome
Sex	M > F	M = F
Associated ocular features	• Posterior polymorphous corneal dystrophy • Cataract • Dot-and-fleck retinopathy • Temporal macular thinning	• Amblyopia • Strabismus • Cataract • Glaucoma (in Lowe syndrome)
Associated systemic features	• Renal dysfunction • Sensorineural hearing loss	• Usually none • Renal and cerebral manifestations in Lowe syndrome
Management	Lens aspiration with IOL implantation	• Lens aspiration with IOL implantation • Amblyopia therapy

MANAGEMENT

- Patients with good visual acuity can be managed initially with spectacles or contact lenses.
- Lens aspiration with *in-the-bag* intraocular lens implantation is the treatment of choice in patients with poor vision and amblyopia.
- Amblyopia management with occlusion therapy is mandatory in cases with unilateral posterior lenticonus to achieve optimal visual outcomes.
- Screening of family members of X-linked Alport syndrome is imperative.
- Multispecialty care of syndromic cases (for management of proteinuria, hypertension, and sensorineural hearing loss in Alport syndrome and neuropsychiatric manifestations of Lowe syndrome).

VIVA QUESTIONS

Q.1. Describe the pathogenesis of anterior lenticonus associated with Alport syndrome.

Ans. Alport syndrome is caused by mutations affecting the gene that encodes for type IV collagen. Type IV collagen is present in the basement membranes of the glomerulus, cochlea, lens capsule, and cornea. Histopathologic examination of the anterior lens capsule shows thinning and vertical dehiscences. Initially, an increase of the lens thickness is observed with thin anterior capsule in the central area, followed by progressive central protrusion of the capsule-cortex complex and development of anterior lenticonus.

Q.2. Describe the pathogenesis of posterior lenticonus.

Ans. The pathogenesis of posterior lenticonus is obscure; remnants of the hyaloid arterial system applying traction on the posterior lens capsule as well as a disturbance in the tunica vasculosa have been suggested as possible mechanisms. Vitritis or an overgrowth of posterior lens fibers that produce a phakoma of the lens have also been suggested as possible pathophysiologic mechanisms. In bilateral cases, a genetically determined congenital weakness of the posterior lens capsule may be the causative factor.

BIBLIOGRAPHY

1. Colville DJ, Savige J. Alport syndrome: a review of the ocular manifestations. Ophthalmic Genetics. 1997;18:161-73.
2. Jacobs K, Meire FM. Lenticonus. Bull Soc Belge Ophthalmol. 2000;(277):65-70.

POSTERIOR POLAR CATARACT

Manpreet Kaur, Ananya PR, Jeewan S Titiyal, Sandeep Gupta

INTRODUCTION

Posterior polar cataract is an uncommon form of congenital cataract, with an incidence of about 3-5 in 1,000. It is bilateral in 65-80% of the cases. It poses a surgical challenge due to its fragile posterior capsule and an increased risk of posterior capsule rupture with vitreous loss.

It is given as short case in postgraduate/DNB/diploma examination.

HISTORY

Chief complaints: The patient presents with the following complaints:

- Diminution of vision for distance and near
- Glare, especially during night driving
- Intolerance to bright light.

History of Present Illness

Epidemiology and genetics: Posterior polar cataract has an autosomal dominant inheritance pattern, although it may occasionally be sporadic. Positive family history may be present in 40-55% of the patients. There is no gender predilection and the disease is usually bilateral in nature.

Presenting features: Early cases may present with complaints of glare and reduced vision in bright light. There is a difficulty in near work and intolerance to bright light. The cause of glare, reduced contrast sensitivity and decreased visual acuity is forward light scattering (light scattering toward the retina). The diminution of vision is progressive in nature.

Patient profession must be noted carefully, since it may influence decision making before cataract surgery.

EXAMINATION

General Examination/Specific Systemic Examination

Posterior polar cataract may be associated with number of systemic diseases such as:
- Psychosomatic disorders
- Ectodermal dysplasia
- Rothmund syndrome
- Scleroderma
- Congenital dyskeratosis
- Incontinentia pigmenti (Bloch–Sulzberger syndrome)
- Congenital ichthyosis

Ocular Examination

- *Eyeballs:* Microphthalmia may be an associated feature.
- *Eyelids* are usually normal.
- *Conjunctiva* is usually normal.
- *Cornea:* Microcornea may be present.
- *Sclera, iris, and pupil* are usually normal.
- *Intraocular pressure* is normal.

Lens: A dense, circular plaque in the axial, posterior aspect of the lens giving rise to the classic Bull's eye appearance is seen. Concentric rings of opacity are present around the central opacity (onion peel pattern) **(Fig. 1)**. Vacuoles and smaller areas of degenerated lens material may also be seen surrounding this area.

Coexistent nuclear sclerosis may be present in advanced cases.

In cases where the other eye has already undergone cataract surgery, it is important to examine the posterior capsule status of the fellow eye carefully. This is especially important where the cataract is in an advanced stage and it is difficult to rule out posterior polar cataract. In presence of any sign of posterior capsule rent in the operated eye (such as posterior capsular rupture, decentered IOL, vitreous strands, pupillary peaking, IOL in sulcus, etc.), the cataract in the other eye must be suspected as posterior polar cataract and all precautions during surgery must be taken.

Vitreous: Oil-like droplets or particles, if visualized in the anterior vitreous, should raise the possibility of a preexisting capsular rent **(Fig. 2)**. This is also known as "fishtailing."

Fundus: Examination is usually normal; signs of incontinentia pigmenti may be present, if associated.

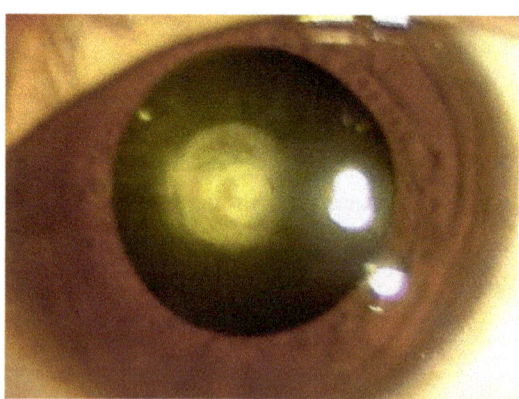

Fig. 1: Posterior polar cataract with concentric rings of opacity (onion-peeling or Bull's eye appearance).

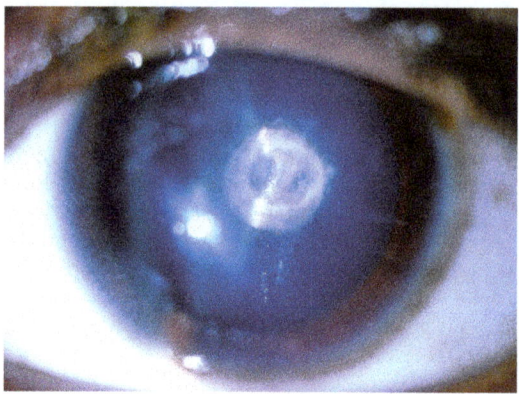

Fig. 2: Preexisting posterior capsular defect in a case of posterior polar cataract with whitish particles in anterior vitreous.

DIFFERENTIAL DIAGNOSIS

- *Posterior subcapsular cataract:* There is generally a clear space between the posterior subcapsular cataract and the posterior capsule.
- *Posterior lenticonus:* There is a conical protrusion of the posterior capsule and underlying cortex, which may or may not be associated with cataract.

CLASSIFICATION

Three different classification systems have been described as:

Duke Elder Classification

- *Stationary form (most common—accounts for 65% of cases):* A round, clearly delineated opacity over the central posterior capsule, with surrounding concentric thickened rings (Bull's eye pattern). Smaller satellite rosette lesions may be present around the central opacity. Nuclear sclerosis may camouflage the opacity.
- *Progressive form:* Whitish opacification in the form of a radiating rider occurs in the posterior cortex. It has feathery and scalloped edges and does not extend as far anteriorly as the original opacity. The nucleus remains uninvolved.

Singh Classification

- *Type 1:* Posterior polar opacity is associated with posterior subcapsular cataract.
- *Type 2:* Sharply defined round or oval opacity with ringed appearance such as an onion with or without grayish spots at the edge.
- *Type 3:* Sharply defined round or oval white opacity with dense white spots at the edge often associated with thin or absent posterior capsule. These dense white spots are a diagnostic sign (Daljit Singh sign) of posterior capsule leakage with or without repair and extreme fragility.
- *Type 4:* Combination of the above three types with nuclear sclerosis.

Schroeder Classification

Based on the effect of opacity on pupillary obstruction in the red reflex testing in pediatric patients, and its importance lies in the early recognition of amblyopia, and recognition of cases in which surgical management can be deferred.

- *Grade 1:* Small opacity not hampering the optical quality of the clear segment of the lens **(Fig. 3)**.
- *Grade 2:* Obstruction of two-thirds of the red reflex but without any optical distortion.
- *Grade 3:* Disc-like opacity surrounded by an area of further optical distortion; clear red reflex surrounding this zone is seen only after dilation of the pupil.
- *Grade 4:* Opacity completely occluding the reflex; with no sufficient red reflex even after pupillary dilation.

Vasavada's Classification

Vasavada divided posterior polar cataract (PPC) based on the status of posterior capsule:
- PPC with impending posterior capsular dehiscence
- Pre-existing capsular dehiscence with PPC
- Spontaneous dislocation of PPC.

INVESTIGATIONS

Preoperative anterior segment optical coherence tomography can be performed to recognize a deficient posterior capsule and counsel the patient in advance.

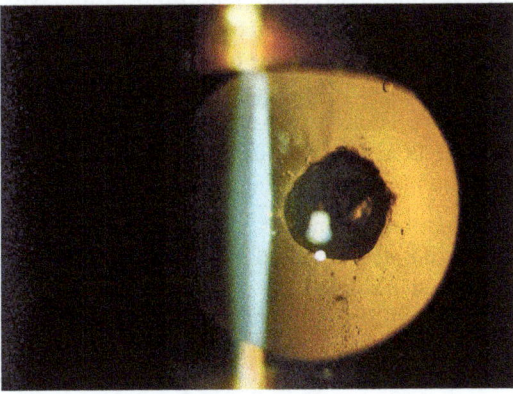

Fig. 3: Disc-like opacity in the posterior capsule on retroillumination.

Intraoperative microscope-integrated optical coherence tomography (MiOCT): Three morphological variants of PPC have been described based on MiOCT findings by Titiyal et al.
1. Type I, with intact PC and a clear area between the posterior capsule and the opacity.
2. Type II having shadowing and inability to delineate PC in the center but with intact PC in the periphery of the opacity.
3. Type III with dense opacity, extensive shadowing, and inability to delineate PC.

■ MANAGEMENT

Preoperative counseling: It is essential to inform the patient of the possibility of a posterior capsular rent, a relatively long duration of surgery, need for posterior segment intervention, and a prolonged visual recovery time. Additionally, the prospect of leaving the patient aphakic and future interventions for the same should be explained. The need for Nd:YAG capsulotomy for residual plaque should be discussed.

Surgery in posterior polar cataract: Posterior polar cataract poses a unique surgical challenge, with a high incidence of posterior capsular rupture ranging from 8 to 36%. Various techniques have been described to avoid intraoperative complications in posterior polar cataract, such as inside-out phacoemulsification, slow motion phacoemulsification, bimanual microphacoemulsification, viscodissection, pre-surround division technique and layer-by-layer phacoemulsification, etc. The basic surgical principle governing these techniques is avoidance of hydrodissection and attempting to create a cushion of cortical matter with careful hydrodelineation. The aim is to avoid stress on the compromised posterior capsule during surgery.

Capsulorhexis: Aim is to keep an adequate sulcus (approximately around 5 mm) so that the IOL can be placed in sulcus in case of PCR.

Hydrodissection should be avoided since it may result in the rupture of the thinned posterior capsule or widen any congenital capsular opening. Gentle hydrodissection with minimal fluid in multiple quadrants, without a fluid wave passing across the weak posterior capsule, may be attempted if necessary.

Hydrodelineation should be done carefully with minimal fluid (not >0.2 cc) to achieve multiple planes of separation (seen as multiple golden rings in coaxial illumination) so that the nucleus can be aspirated *layer-by-layer*.

Phacoemulsification parameters: Slow phacoemulsification with low parameters, with the power being not >60%, bottle height 55–70 cm, vacuum 30–100 mm Hg and aspiration rate of 15–25 mL/minute. These parameters prevent sudden shallowing of the anterior chamber.

Nucleus emulsification: A fine chopper should be used, and the endonuclease incised in perpendicular meridians without countertraction, followed by emulsification of the quadrants. Nuclear rotation should be avoided.

Epinucleus removal: Viscodissection may be employed to remove the epinucleus. Ophthalmic viscosurgical device (OVD) is injected under the rim of the capsulorhexis in one quadrant to elevate the epinucleus, which can then be aspirated using irrigation/aspiration (I/A) handpiece, in a centripetal fashion (peripheral epinucleus aspirated before central).

Adequate anterior chamber stability: It is provided by the low-infusion and low-vacuum system. Biaxial microincisional phacoemulsification may be used to enhance safety and reduce risk of complications. Anterior chamber should not be allowed to collapse at any step during surgery.

Residual plaque: Occasionally, the opacity may dislodge spontaneously due to infusion pressure during cortex removal. However, if a part of the opacity is firmly adherent to the capsule and does not separate, it can be left *in situ* and later, an Nd:YAG capsulotomy may be performed to clear it out.

Management of posterior capsular defect (pre-existing/iatrogenic): If a defect is present in the posterior capsule, a dispersive OVD such as Viscoat should be injected over the area of defect before withdrawing the phaco or I/A probe from the eye. The defect may be converted into a posterior capsulorhexis, after which an anterior vitrectomy may be performed, if needed. The IOL can be placed in the bag in cases with a small PCR. If in-the-bag IOL implantation is not possible, sulcus implantation of a multipiece IOL may be done followed by optic capture in the bag, if needed.

VIVA QUESTIONS

Q.1. Describe the pathogenesis of posterior polar cataract.

Ans. The developing lens obtains its nutrition through the tunica vasculosa lentis (TVL), a transitory vascular network, supplied by the hyaloid artery posteriorly, which forms an anastomosis with the anterior pupillary membrane via the capsulopupillary vessels. Posterior polar cataracts are hypothesized to be caused by the persistence of the hyaloid artery, or alternatively, by the invasion of the lens by mesoblastic tissue. A genetic mutation causing lens fibers to develop abnormally and form an opacity close to or adherent to the posterior capsule is also suspected. Even though they form during embryonic life or in early infancy, posterior polar cataracts usually become symptomatic 30–50 years later.

Q.2. What is the inheritance pattern of posterior polar cataract?

Ans. Refer text.

Q.3. Classify posterior polar cataract.

Ans. Refer text.

■ BIBLIOGRAPHY

1. Duke-Elder S. Congenital deformities. Part 2. Normal and Abnormal Development. System of Ophthalmology; Vol. III. St. Louis: CV Mosby; 1964.
2. Kalantan H. Posterior polar cataract: a review. Saudi J Ophthalmol. 2012;26(1):41-9.
3. Lee MW, Lee YC. Phacoemulsification of posterior polar cataracts: a surgical challenge. Br J Ophthalmol. 2003;87:1426-7.

MICROSPHEROPHAKIA

Manpreet Kaur, Devika S Joshi, Prafulla Kumar Maharana

■ INTRODUCTION

Microspherophakia is a developmental abnormality and is characterized by a crystalline lens, which has a small diameter and spherical shape due to weak zonules exerting inadequate tension at the equator. The entire lens diameter can be characteristically visualized during slit-lamp examination with a fully dilated pupil.

It is given as short case in postgraduate/DNB/Diploma examination.

■ HISTORY

Chief complaint: The patient with microspherophakia presents with the following features:
- Diminution of vision
- Acute painful red eye with diminution of vision (*acute angle-closure episode*).

History of Present Illness

Genetics: Isolated spherophakia is an autosomal recessive disorder resulting from homozygous mutations in LTBP2 (13q24.1-q32.12). Parental consanguinity was present in reported families.

Microspherophakia is a clinically and genetically heterogeneous disorder and usually found in association with Weill–Marchesani syndrome. Other syndromes that may be associated include Marfan's syndrome, Peter's anomaly, Alport syndrome, Lowe syndrome, homocystinuria, mandibulofacial dysostosis, and Klinefelter's syndrome.

Etiopathogenesis: Microspherophakia is a result of the faulty development of the secondary lens fibers during embryogenesis. The underdeveloped zonules of Zinn are unable to exert enough force on the lens to make it form the usual oval shape.

Presenting features: The disease is bilateral in nature. The patient presents in childhood with diminution of vision and the use of high minus lenses as a result of the lenticular myopia. The lens may subluxate into the vitreous cavity in advanced cases. Secondary angle-closure glaucoma may occur because of pupillary block induced by the spherical lens. The pupillary block manifests as an acute onset diminution of vision associated with pain and circumciliary congestion.

EXAMINATION

General Examination/Specific Systemic Examination

Systemic examination should be undertaken to evaluate the manifestations of the associated syndromes.

Features of *Weill–Marchesani syndrome* include short fingers (i.e., brachydactyly) and muscular hypertrophy. *Marfan's syndrome* is associated with arachnodactyly, tall stature, high-arched palate and cardiac valvular anomalies.

Homocystinuria, mandibulofacial dysostosis, Alport's syndrome, and Klinefelter's syndrome may also rarely be associated with microspherophakia.

Ocular Examination

The *eyeballs and eyelids* are usually normal.

Conjunctiva: Circumciliary congestion may be present in cases presenting with acute angle-closure episode.

Cornea: It is usually normal. Corneal opacity is usually present in Peter's anomaly.

Sclera: Scleral thinning and posterior staphyloma may be present in Marfan's syndrome.

Anterior chamber is shallow.

Iris and pupil: Sphincter dysplasia may be present, and pupils may be ectopic.

Intraocular pressure: IOP is raised in cases of pupillary block.

Inverse pupillary block: Forward movement of spherical lens or anterior subluxation of lens due to weak and long zonules, causing crowding of AC angle, which in longstanding cases may lead to peripheral anterior synechiae formation.

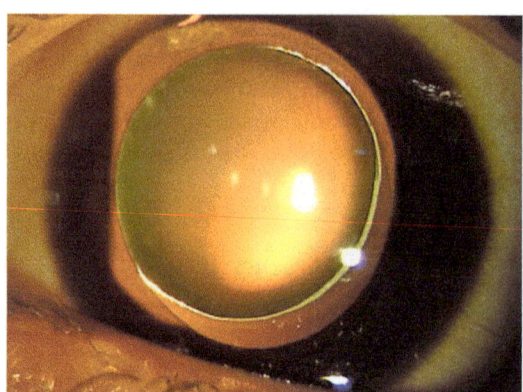

Fig. 1: Whole lens is visible with full mydriasis in a case of microspherophakia.

Miotics are contraindicated due to risk of promoting pupillary block.

Lens: There is a decrease in the equatorial lens diameter and the whole lens is visible with full mydriasis **(Fig. 1)**. The anteroposterior lens diameter is increased and the lens assumes a relatively spherical shape. The lens may move with changes in posture and may dislocate or subluxate into the anterior chamber or vitreous.

Vitreous: Posteriorly dislocated lens may be visible in the vitreous cavity in advanced cases.

Fundus: Glaucomatous optic nerve head cupping may be visible in cases with coexistent secondary glaucoma. Posterior staphyloma, myopic crescent and retinal detachment may be present.

Refraction: High myopia is present without an increase in axial length.

DIFFERENTIAL DIAGNOSIS

The lens findings on slit-lamp examination are pathognomonic and characteristic of microspherophakia. The differential diagnoses for the etiology of microspherophakia are described in **Table 1**.

INVESTIGATIONS

Systemic Investigations

Systemic investigations are directed toward the underlying syndrome, and may include X-rays of

Table 1: Differential diagnoses for the etiology of microspherophakia.

Features	Familial microspherophakia	Weill–Marchesani syndrome	Marfan's syndrome	Peter's anomaly	Klinefelter's syndrome	Alport's syndrome	Lowe syndrome
Inheritance	Autosomal recessive	Autosomal recessive, rare autosomal dominant	Autosomal dominant	Autosomal dominant, autosomal recessive	X-linked (aneuploidy)	X-linked	X-linked recessive
Other ocular features (in addition to microspherophakia)	Ectopia lentis, lenticular myopia, posterior staphyloma, ectopic pupil, retinal detachment, glaucoma	Ectopia lentis (displaces inferiorly), posterior synechiae, glaucoma	Ectopia lentis, glaucoma, axial myopia, retinal detachment, blue sclera, iris hypoplasia	Anterior segment dysgenesis (corneal opacity, glaucoma, sclerocornea, corectopia, iris hypoplasia, cataract)	Microphthalmia, colobomas of the iris, choroid and optic nerve, strabismus	Lenticonus, posterior polymorphous corneal dystrophy, dot-and-fleck retinopathy, temporal macular thinning	Congenital cataract, glaucoma
Systemic features	None	Short stubby fingers (brachydactyly), short stature, broad hands, joint stiffness	Cardiac and musculoskeletal anomalies	Developmental delay, dysmorphic facial features, cardiac, genitourinary, and central nervous system malformation	Tall stature, gynecomastia, small testes, and infertility	Renal dysfunction, sensorineural hearing loss	Central nervous system and renal anomalies, hypotonia

spine and extremities, cardiac echocardiogram and genetic testing as needed.

Ocular Investigations

Specular microscopy: For endothelial cell count, especially in cases with coexistent glaucoma.

Perimetry: To evaluate visual fields in cases with secondary glaucoma.

Biometry: Axial length and keratometry for IOL power calculations.

B-scan ultrasonography: To evaluate cases with posterior staphyloma or posteriorly dislocated lens.

■ MANAGEMENT

Management of Lens

Clear lens extraction, with or without goniosynaechiolysis, is the treatment of choice for myopia and glaucoma in microspherophakia.

Indications for Lens Extraction

- Cataract
- Corneolenticular touch
- High myopia
- Intermittent pupillary block
- Secondary glaucoma.

Surgical Approach

- Lens aspiration via limbal route
- Pars-plana lensectomy.

Surgical Challenges

Capsulorhexis: Iris hooks may be needed to stabilize the lens.

Intraocular Lens Implantation

- Successful in-the-bag implantation of acrylic single piece hydrophobic lens has been described; however, phacodonesis persists in the postoperative period.
- Capsular support using a modified capsular tension ring (M-CTR) and capsular tension segment (CTS) sutured to the sclera along with implantation of a foldable intraocular lens inside the bag may be tried.
- Scleral fixated IOL in the same sitting or a second sitting can be done in cases without capsular bag support.
- Aphakic glasses or contact lens may be prescribed in cases where IOL is not implanted.

Management of Glaucoma

The pupillary-block glaucoma associated with microspherophakia is also known as *inverse glaucoma* as miotics aggravate the condition by stimulating ciliary muscle contraction, thereby loosening the zonules and further increasing anterior lens displacement. Mydriatic-cycloplegics tighten the zonules and are the preferred treatment.

Nd:YAG laser peripheral iridotomy is useful in relieving angle-closure glaucoma and should be done prophylactically in all cases of microspherophakia.

Raised IOP may be managed with topical and oral anti-glaucoma medications; trabeculectomy or tube shunt surgeries may be required in chronic cases refractory to conservative medical therapy.

VIVA QUESTIONS

Q.1. Describe the pathogenesis of microspherophakia.

Ans. An arrest of development of the secondary lens fibers or the insertion of abnormally thin secondary fibers are said to be responsible for the development of microspherophakia. Both may be secondary to a nutritional deficiency from defects in the tunica vasculosa lentis and occur at the 5–6 months of embryonic life when the lens is normally spherical.

An alternative theory suggests that microspherophakia is caused by a lack of tension in the rudimentary zonular fibers of the lens, which arrests development so that the lens remains spherical.

Q.2. What is inverse pupillary block glaucoma?

Ans. Refer text.

Q.3. What are the syndromes associated with microspherophakia?

Ans. Refer **Table 1**.

■ BIBLIOGRAPHY

1. Bhattacharjee H, Bhattacharjee K, Medhi J, DasGupta S. Clear lens extraction and intraocular lens implantation in a case of microspherophakia with secondary angle-closure glaucoma. Indian J Ophthalmol. 2010;58(1):67-70.
2. Chan RT, Collin HB. Microspherophakia. Clin Exp Optom. 2002;85(5):294-9.
3. Willoughby CE, Wishart PK. Lensectomy in the management of glaucoma in spherophakia. J Cataract Refract Surg. 2002;28:1061-4.

POSTERIOR CAPSULAR OPACIFICATION

Prafulla Kumar Maharana, Manpreet Kaur

■ INTRODUCTION

Posterior capsular opacification (PCO) or after-cataract is the most common complication of cataract surgery, with an incidence of 2–63%, 3 years after phacoemulsification. It is a major cause of diminution of vision in the postoperative period after an uneventful extracapsular cataract surgery.

It may be given as a short case in postgraduate/DNB/diploma examination.

■ HISTORY

Chief complaint: The patient presents with the following complaints:
- Diminution of vision
- Glare.

History of Present Illness

The patient presents few months to few years after undergoing an extracapsular cataract extraction. The interval between surgery and PCO ranges from 3 months to 4 years after the surgery. There is an inverse correlation with age and young age is a significant risk factor for PCO. There is a history of good gain in visual acuity following cataract surgery, following which there is a gradual, painless, progressive diminution of vision. In early cases, the best corrected visual acuity may be optimal but the patient may complain of glare.

■ EXAMINATION

General Examination/Specific Systemic Examination

Systemic examination is usually unremarkable.

Ocular Examination

Visual acuity: There is a decrease in the uncorrected as well as best spectacle corrected visual acuity (BSCVA), both for distance and near. Refraction must be done in all cases to find out the BSCVA.

The *eyeballs and eyelids* are usually normal.

Conjunctiva is usually normal. Conjunctival scars may be present in cases that have undergone ECCE or SICS.

Cornea: Scars of previous cataract surgery may be present. Sutures or suture marks may be present.

Sclera: Scleral incision may be visible in cases that have undergone SICS.

Iris: Usually normal; however, in complicated cases iris atrophy, chafing, peripheral anterior synechiae or capsuloiridic adhesion must be noted carefully.

Pupil: Usually normal; however, in complicated cases abnormality in shape and size may be there. In cases with dense PCO, pupillary reflexes must be noted carefully to rule out relative afferent pupillary defect (RAPD) to determine the visual prognosis.

Intraocular pressure is usually normal: Following Nd:YAG laser capsulotomy, a transient rise in IOP often occurs. So, any raised IOP or glaucoma must be controlled with medication, most commonly an alpha agonist such as apraclonidine/brimonidine, before proceeding for capsulotomy.

Lens: Intraocular lens is present in the bag, or rarely in the sulcus. Any IOL decentration, adhesion between anterior capsular margin and posterior capsule or between iris and posterior capsule must

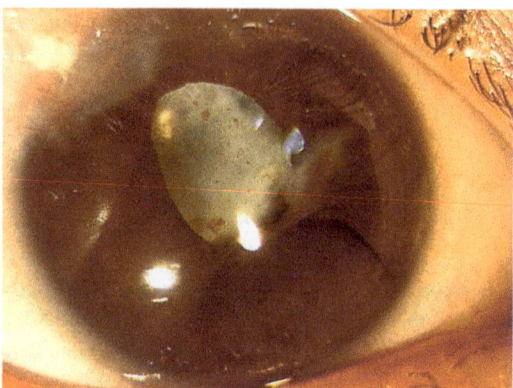

Fig. 1: Posterior capsular opacification, fibrotic type.

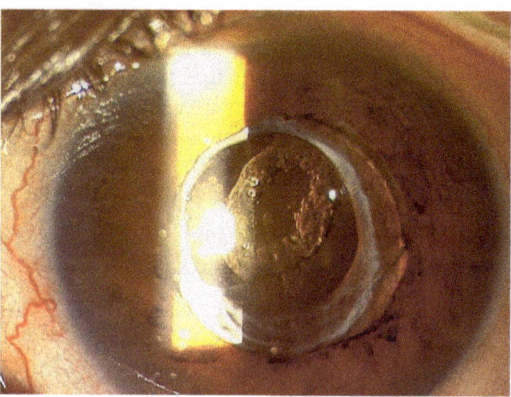

Fig. 2: Soemmering's ring.

be noted carefully as these clinical conditions increase the risk of early PCO formation.

Posterior capsular opacification is visible behind the lens. Different morphological variants of PCO may be observed, such as fibrotic type **(Fig. 1)**, Elschnig pearls and Soemmering's ring **(Fig. 2)**.

Vitreous: Usually normal; may not be clearly visible as a result of media haze induced by PCO.

Fundus: A thorough fundus examination is essential to rule out any retinal tear/hole/traction since Nd:YAG laser capsulotomy increases the risk of retinal detachment. Cystoid macular edema must be ruled out as the inflammation induced by laser capsulotomy predisposes toward the development of macular edema. Indirect ophthalmoscopy must be done in all cases.

■ DIFFERENTIAL DIAGNOSIS

Localized Endophthalmitis

Propionibacterium acnes may induce a chronic endophthalmitis with low-grade inflammation that may mimic a PCO. The bacteria are sequestered within the capsular bag and form whitish precipitates and plaques. Laser capsulotomy is contraindicated in such cases to avoid dispersion of the infective material into the vitreous cavity.

Cell Precipitates and Membranes

Breakdown of the blood-aqueous barrier as a result of cataract surgery may lead to inflammation and the aqueous dispersion of erythrocytes, chronic inflammatory cells such as macrophages and giant cells as well as protein, pigments, and fibrin. They may form thin, translucent diffuse or punctate opacities that may mimic PCO. Increased frequency of topical steroid instillation may help resolve such inflammatory membranes.

Capsular Bag Distention Syndrome

Capsular bag distention syndrome (CBDS) is a complication of continuous curvilinear capsulorhexis done in phacoemulsification and in the bag IOL implantation. It usually presents in the immediate postoperative period, with shallowing of the anterior chamber, unexpected myopic refraction, and accumulation of liquefied substance between the implanted lens and posterior capsule with forward protrusion of the intraocular lens. It may rarely present many years after surgery with reduced vision but no significant refractive change. The management consists of Nd:YAG capsulotomy or capsular bag lavage.

■ INVESTIGATIONS

- *B-scan ultrasonography:* To rule out any posterior segment complications. Presence of PVD is a good sign before proceeding for laser capsulotomy since risk of traction and subsequent retinal detachment is less. A posterior segment ultrasonographic examination also helps to rule out low-grade endophthalmitis, especially *Propionibacterium acnes* (*P. acnes*) endophthalmitis.

- *Pentacam:* Not done routinely. Scheimpflug imaging may be useful to document a distended capsular bag with fluid accumulation behind the lens in CBDS.

CLASSIFICATION
- Clinically, PCO can be divided into two types:
  1. *Regeneratory PCO:* Regeneratory PCO is a result of migration of lens epithelial cells along the posterior capsule, behind the IOL. These cells (also known as bladder cells due to their appearance) proliferate to form layers of lens material and *Elschnig pearls*, leading to opacification. When arranged in a form of ring (between anterior capsular rim and posterior capsule), it is called *Soemmerring's ring* (**Fig. 2**). It is more common and is one of the important causes of a decrease in visual function after cataract surgery.
  2. *Fibrotic PCO:* In fibrotic PCO, lens epithelial cells of the anterior capsule undergo transformation to myofibroblasts, causing fibrosis and contraction of the capsule bag. This can lead to decentration of the IOL and hinder visualization of the peripheral retina.
- Sellman and Lindstrom have described four grades of posterior capsule opacification (**Table 1**).
- Tetz et al. described a morphological scoring system of PCO by obtaining standardized retroillumination photographs of the pseudophakic anterior segments using a photo slit lamp, grading the density of the opacification from 0 to 4 and multiplying it by the fraction of capsule area involved behind the IOL optic.

MANAGEMENT

Conservative Management
Cases with mild PCO that achieve optimal visual acuity with refraction may be observed and kept on regular follow-up. Refraction with prescription of glasses may be adequate in such cases.

Nd: YAG Laser Capsulotomy
- *Indications*
  - Interference with daily activities
  - Decreased vision
  - Increased glare
  - Difficulty visualizing the fundus
- *Preoperative preparation:* Before beginning the capsulotomy, informed consent should be obtained. 1 hour before the laser capsulotomy, a drop of a pressure-lowering drug such as apraclonidine may be administered along with a mydriatic to dilate the pupil. Topical anesthesia drops are administered.
- *Procedure/laser parameters:* An Abraham YAG capsulotomy lens is used in conjunction with a coupling agent, such as 2% hydroxypropyl methylcellulose. Laser spots are applied in a cruciate, circular, inverted U or "Christmas-tree" pattern. Cruciate pattern is most commonly used. The capsulotomy should be centered on the visual axis with diameter slightly larger than the mesopic pupil size. Laser energy is set at 1–3 mJ and posterior offset of laser beam is set at 125–150 μm to avoid hitting the lens.
- *Post-laser medication:* After the procedure, topical anti-glaucoma medications may be prescribed for a week along with topical steroids to reduce inflammation.

Membranectomy
Surgical membranectomy may be indicated in the following situations:
- Pediatric patients
- Uncooperative or mentally challenged patients
- Dense fibrotic PCO.

Table 1: Sellman and Lindstrom posterior capsule opacification (PCO) grades.

Grade	Definition
1	No or slight PCO without reduced red reflex, also no pearls at all or pearls not to the IOL edge
2	Mild PCO reducing the red reflex, Elschnig pearls to the IOL edge
3	Moderate fibrosis or Elschnig pearls inside IOL edge but with a clear visual axis
4	Severe fibrosis or Elschnig pearls covering the visual axis and severely reducing the red reflex

Surgical Approach
- Limbal route—with anterior vitrectomy cutter
- *Pars-plana route:* Especially, in dense fibrotic PCO with *in-the-bag* IOL, where it may be difficult to access the posterior capsule via limbal route.

VIVA QUESTIONS

Q.1. Describe the prevention of PCO.

Ans. Following factors may help to minimize the incidence of PCO:

Surgical techniques to prevent PCO formation:
- Cortical cleaving hydrodissection and cortical clean-up
- In-the-bag IOL fixation
- Optic capture within posterior capsulorhexis
- Optimally sized continuous curvilinear capsulorhexis with 360° IOL coverage
- Capsular devices such as E-ring (equator ring)

IOL-related factors ("Ideal" IOL):
- Biocompatible IOL material to reduce stimulation of cellular proliferation
- Hydrophobic IOLs have lower rates of PCO formation.
- Maximal IOL optic—posterior capsule contact, angulated haptic, "adhesive" biomaterial to create a "shrink wrap"
- IOL optic geometry—square, truncated edge (according to the Sandwich theory, which states that PCO development is reduced when there is maximum contact between the IOL and the posterior capsular bag).

Q.2. Describe the pathogenesis of PCO.

Ans. The development of PCO is a very dynamic process, and involves three basic phenomena—proliferation, migration, and differentiation of residual lens epithelial cells (LECs). LECs left behind in the capsular bag after cataract surgery convert from epithelial to mesenchymal cells, deposit collagen and generate lens fibers (being fibroblastic in morphology), leading to PCO development. Equatorial differentiation of cells to fiber-like structures leads to Soemmerring's ring formation. Near the rhexis, cell swelling forms globular Elschnig's pearls. Several cytokines and growth factors play a major role in the pathogenesis of PCO, such as interleukins, transforming growth factor β (TGF-β) and fibroblast growth factor 2 (FGF-2), which stimulate myofibroblastic differentiation and attachment of LECs to the underlying posterior capsule. Cytokine production may be initiated by the surgically induced break in the blood-aqueous barrier and subsequent leakage of plasma protein into the aqueous humor.

Younger patients, diabetics, and patients with preexisting ocular pathologies like uveitis are predisposed to early development of PCO.

Q.3. What do you mean by "A" and "E" cells?

Ans. The anterior-central zone (corresponding to the zone of the anterior lens capsule) consists of a monolayer of flat cuboidal, epithelial cells with minimal mitotic activity. In response to a variety of stimuli, these anterior epithelial cells (*"A" cells*) proliferate and undergo fibrous metaplasia. Continuation of anterior lens cells around the equator form the equatorial lens bow (*"E" cells*). Unlike within the A-cell layer, cell mitoses, division, and multiplication are quite active in this region, and new lens fibers are continuously produced in this zone throughout life.

Q.4. Describe the Soemmering's ring and Elschnig pearls.

Ans. Elschnig pearls consist of clusters of swollen, opacified epithelial "pearls" or clusters of posteriorly migrated equatorial epithelial (E) cells (Bladder or Wedl cells).

The Soemmering's ring **(Fig. 3)** is a dumbbell or donut-shaped lesion that often forms following any type of ECCE (manual or phacoemulsification). Equatorial cells (E-cells) are responsible for formation of a Soemmering's ring. The pathogenetic basis of a Soemmering's ring is rupture of the anterior lens capsule with extrusion of nuclear and some central lens material.

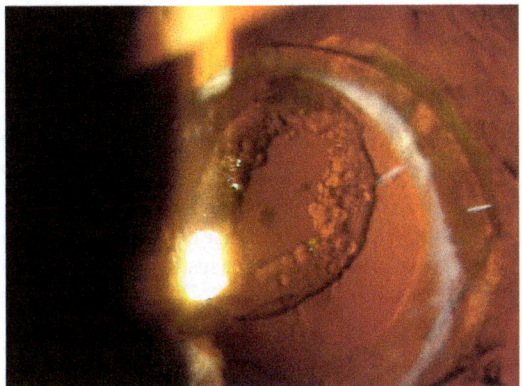

Fig. 3: Soemmering's ring with bladder cells.

Soemmering's ring is a direct precursor to PCO.

Q.5. What are the drugs/agents used intraoperatively to reduce PCO?

Ans. Intraocular application of pharmacologic agents has been investigated to prevent PCO. The basic principle is to selectively destroy the LECs and avoid toxic side effects on other intraocular tissues such as corneal endothelium. Pharmacologic agents being investigated include antimetabolites (such as methotrexate, mitomycin, daunomycin, 5-FU, colchicine, and daunorubicin), proteases (dispase), anti-inflammatory substances, hypo-osmolar drugs, and immunological agents. Sealed capsular irrigation (SCI) device has been developed to precisely deliver the pharmacological agents within the capsular bag, while minimizing the potential for collateral ocular damage. Implantation of intracapsular ring may prevent central PCO after cataract surgery by mechanically blocking migration of lens epithelial cells toward the central visual axis.

BIBLIOGRAPHY

1. Pandey SK, Apple DJ, Werner L, Maloof AJ, Milverton EJ. Posterior capsule opacification: a review of the aetiopathogenesis, experimental and clinical studies and factors for prevention. Indian J Ophthalmol. 2004;52:99-112.
2. Raj SM, Vasavada AR, Johar SRK, Vasavada VA. Postoperative capsular opacification: A review. Int J Biomed Sci. 2007;3(4):237-50.
3. Tami R, Sellman TR, Lindstrom RL. Effect of a plano-convex posterior chamber lens on capsular opacification from Elschnig pearl formation. J Cataract Refract Surg. 1988;14(1):68-72.

TRAUMATIC CATARACT

Deepali Singhal, Ruchita Falera, Manpreet Kaur

INTRODUCTION

Cataract formation is a well-known complication of blunt and penetrating trauma. It results from direct lens trauma or concussion effect on the lens and is often associated with trauma to cornea, iris, angle, and posterior segment.

It is given as short case in postgraduate/DNB/diploma examination.

HISTORY

Chief complaint: Presenting complaints depend on the type of injury.

Blunt trauma
- Progressive diminution of vision
- Whitish opacity
- Monocular diplopia, if associated with subluxation

Penetrating trauma
- Sudden diminution of vision
- Whitish opacity.

History of present illness: Onset, duration, and mode of trauma should be recorded.
- Onset and duration of diminution of vision and whitish opacity should also be noted.
- Any history of deviation of eye or limitation of motility should be noted.
- It is important to note if there is any medico-legal case associated with trauma.

Past history: Any history of ocular surgery or glaucoma should be enquired.

EXAMINATION

Systemic Examination

A complete systemic examination should be done including cranial nerves examination, especially in cases associated with acute onset diplopia. It is important to remember the ABC (airway, breathing, circulation) in a case of acute trauma with involvement of multiple systems.

Ocular Examination

Visual acuity: Uncorrected and best-corrected visual acuity (BCVA) helps in planning the treatment, especially in early cataract. It is important to note projection of rays since it can suggest presence of posterior segment complications of blunt trauma such as retinal detachment (RD). Assessment of near vision should not be missed.

Eyeball: Ocular deviation and extraocular movements, both uniocular and binocular, should be tested.

Eyelid: Laceration or scarring may be seen. Assessment of lid margin abnormalities occurring secondary to scarring, such as ectropion, or entropion or trichiatic lashes is also important.

Conjunctiva: Subconjunctival hemorrhage, chemosis, or scar may be present.

Cornea: On slit-lamp biomicroscopy, following signs must be noted.
- Corneal clouding/edema
- Corneal perforation
- Corneal opacities of any depth, namely nebular/macular/leucomatous
- Sutures may be seen in repaired perforations
- Intrastromal foreign body may be present.

Sclera: Repaired scleral perforation or scar should be looked for.

Anterior chamber: Anterior chamber (AC) cells, flare, hyphema, vitreous, or lens matter must be looked for.

Iris: Iridodonesis/iridodialysis/posterior synechiae/iris atrophy may be present.

Pupil: Sphincter tear, eccentric pupil/traumatic mydriasis **(Fig. 2)**, oval/peaking pupil/irregular/vitreous entangling pupillary area should be ruled out. Direct and consensual light reactions of both eyes should be recorded. Presence of relative afferent pathway defect (RAPD) suggests posterior segment complications such as RD or traumatic optic neuropathy.

IOP: IOP may be raised due to angle recession/subluxation or trabecular damage.

IOP may also be low in case of globe perforation or vitreous loss. In acute cases of trauma, IOP is low due to ciliary shock.

Gonioscopy: Angle recession, pigmentation, PAS, cyclodialysis, zonular dialysis, and trabecular meshwork splitting may be seen.

Lens: Lens examination should include:
- Determination of type and extent of cataract
- Intumescent or normal thickness lens
- Associated intact or ruptured anterior capsule
- Status of the zonules.

In majority of young patients, the opacity is localized and stationary, which starts in subcapsular zone and eventually lies deeply due to the formation of new lens fibers.

Whereas older age group is associated with more diffuse and progressive cataract due to activation of degenerative process of senile cataract.

Morphological classification of traumatic cataract due to blunt trauma is as follows:

Vossius Ring

Vossius ring is the epicapsular deposition of iris pigment. It is a reddish-brown ring corresponding to the pupillary aperture, about 1 mm in breadth formed due to extreme miosis at the time of trauma. It is usually segmented due to constrictions on the posterior surface of iris. At times, a double ring can be seen due to immediate pupillary constriction followed by dilatation.

Localized Subcapsular Opacities

- *Disseminated subepithelial opacity:* Small, discrete/flake like anterior subcapsular opacities, which are commonly stationary. This can also present as a large, round, discrete-layered opacity called as *Cataracta Nodiformis*.[1]

- *Cobweb opacity:* It presents as a subcapsular and a more diffuse filmy structure supporting fine dust-like opacities commonly in young patients. This can be seen in both blunt and penetrating trauma. It is permanent, occurs in the absence of capsular rupture and may be due to mechanical damage to the epithelium.[1]
- *Zonular (Lamellar) opacity:* It is the result of disseminated opacities occurring extensively over the lens or rosette opacity. This is a rare presentation as a unilateral zonular cataract, seen in young patients. The density may vary while the outline is irregular and typical riders may be evident.
- *Rosette cataract:* Early/late.
  Early rosette cataract:
  - It is recognized shortly after trauma, few hours to few weeks.
  - It may be seen in anterior subcapsular area in concussive injuries or in posterior subcapsular area in penetrating injuries.
  - Initially seen as fine-fluid droplets formed between the radiating lens fibers, which then form feathery parallel rays radiating from the dark suture lines **(Fig. 1)**.
  - In mild injuries, these are translucent and may disappear within a few days.
  - More commonly, they are permanent, stationary, and cause vision impairment. It is gradually buried deeply in cortex due to formation of new lens fibers.

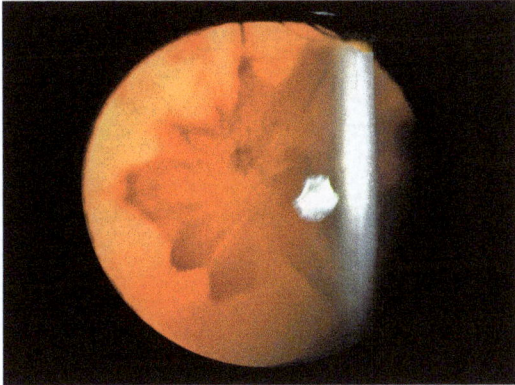

Fig. 1: Rosette cataract.

  Late rosette cataract:
  - Seen few years after trauma.
  - It is located deep in the cortex or nucleus and is due to minimal degree of damage to subcapsular fibers.
  - In early rosette, the sutures run up to the center of petals and the rays run from them as a midriff whereas, in late rosette, the sutures run between the petals which are formed by the outcrop of rays from two neighboring sutures. It can also extend much further in the periphery and may turn backwards to form a second posterior rosette.
- *Post-traumatic atrophy of the lens:* It may be seen few years after a severe blunt trauma where lens capsule is intact. It is characterized with thinning of the lens substance and associated with shrinkage of the nuclear and cortical matter, which can be symmetrical or asymmetrical leading to deformation of whole architecture. Anterior capsule seems to be flatter without folds, which are present in penetrating trauma.
- *Presenile and senile changes:* These can be observed in the form of coronary cataract, water clefts, punctate cortical opacities, and sclerotic nuclear opacities. There is rapid and premature progression of such changes as compared to senile cataract.

Diffuse concussion cataract: It is rare and is usually associated with capsular tear. It is due to rapid imbibition of aqueous by the lens matter leading to opacification. In case of a large tear, the swollen lens fibers may herniate into anterior chamber and vitreous, and later become granular and necrotic. In young patients, slow and total absorption of cataract may occur, whereas, in the old, iritis and secondary glaucoma may occur.

Vitreous: Vitreous hemorrhage may be present or vitreous base avulsion with a bucket handle appearance may be seen.

Fundus: Retinal dialysis, giant retinal tear with retinal detachment, and macular hole can occur due to trauma. Indirect ophthalmoscopy with indentation of periphery is a must in all cases of trauma. Other features include commotio retinae, traumatic optic neuropathy, or disc avulsion.

■ DIFFERENTIAL DIAGNOSIS

- Uveitic cataract
- Developmental cataract (unilateral)
- Glaucomafleckens.

■ INVESTIGATIONS

- *Biometry:* Axial length and keratometry
- *Visual potential assessment:* Laser Interferometry or VER
- *Ultrasonography:* For posterior segment evaluation
- *NCCT head and orbit/X-ray orbit:* To look for IOFB and orbital injuries.
- *UBM:* To identify occult zonular damage and posterior capsular rupture.

■ MANAGEMENT

Standard recommendation in acute-onset traumatic cataract with penetrating/perforating injuries is primary globe closure followed by a secondary lens aspiration with IOL placement. This is because the degree and visual significance of cataract may not be apparent in the acute setting and a small opacity may become visually insignificant later. Moreover, IOL power calculation and decision about the type of lens and positioning may be compromised in acute setting and surgery may be difficult due to hazy media.[1,2]

Indications of Surgery

- Anterior capsular rupture with swollen lens or lens matter in AC require primary lens aspiration.
- Lens-induced glaucoma or inflammation
- Visually significant cataract causing diminution of vision
- Poor visualization of posterior segment, which impedes management of posterior segment injuries.

Primary cataract removal helps control inflammation and allows early direct visualization of posterior segment. In children, cataract surgery should be performed within 1 year of ocular trauma to reduce the risk of amblyopia. In the acute setting, accurate IOL calculations may be difficult to obtain so data from the other eye can also be taken.

Surgical Management

The surgical approach depends upon the capsular and zonular status and degree of lens injury **(Fig. 2)**. There can be four different scenarios such as:
1. Non-dislocated cataract with intact capsule
2. Anterior capsular rupture with cataract
3. Posterior capsular rupture with cataract
4. Subluxated lens with cataract **(Fig. 3)**.

Nondislocated Cataract with Intact Capsule

Standard phacoemulsification technique can be used with associated glaucoma and iris injuries taken into consideration. Adequate size capsulorhexis should be made with capsular staining which will help in better visibility. Anterior

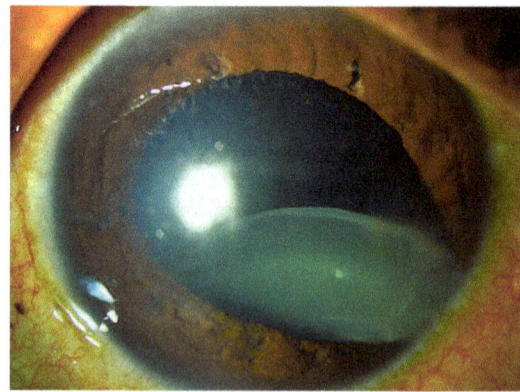

Fig. 2: Subluxated lens.

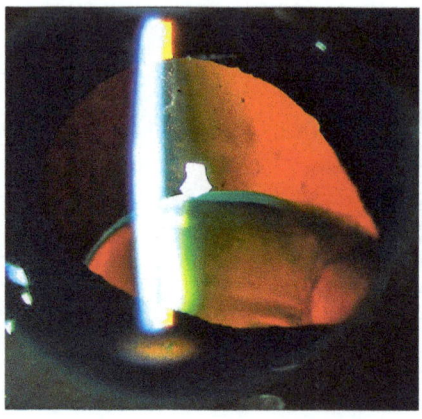

Fig. 3: Subluxated cataract.

capsular staining can be performed with trypan blue 0.06%. Generous hydrodissection should be done with low flow phacoemulsification to avoid stress on the zonules.[2]

Anterior Capsular Rupture with Cataract

Primary lens aspiration should be performed in these cases to decrease the chances of inflammation and secondary glaucoma. After the initial incision, viscoelastic should be injected and the extent of anterior capsular rupture along with the presence of vitreous prolapse should be determined. Vitrectomy cutter should be used in cut/IA mode to remove the vitreous and cortical matter from AC. Then, the anterior capsulorhexis can be completed and lens aspiration is done. In cases of thick fibrotic capsule, Vannas scissors can be used to complete the capsulorhexis. Femtosecond laser-assisted anterior capsulorhexis can also be performed to minimize zonular stress.[1,2]

Posterior Capsular Rupture with Cataract

The management depends upon the type and the size of tear. In type I tears the margins are *thickened and fibrosed*, so there are less chances of extension with irrigation. Type 2 tears are present in early surgeries, and they have *thin, transparent* margins, which may rapidly enlarge during irrigation. Tears larger than 6 mm are unable to support in the bag IOL. When using an anterior approach, further hydration of vitreous and extension of tear should be avoided by using dry aspiration techniques and meticulous control of infusion and anterior vitrectomy. Phacoemulsification with low-flow settings should be used. Posterior pars plana approach is used in cases of posterior dislocation, and if there is associated retinal pathology.[2]

VIVA QUESTIONS

Q.1. Describe the pathophysiology of cataract in trauma.

Ans. Several mechanisms have been described for cataract formation after ocular trauma, which includes coup injury, contrecoup, and equatorial expansion. Coup injury is the direct trauma to the lens epithelium and capsule leading to imbibition of aqueous and cataract formation. Contrecoup refers to damage occurring at a distal site due to shock waves, which can disrupt the capsule and the lens fibers. Blunt trauma causes anteroposterior compression and equatorial expansion of the globe, which results in transmission of shock waves. This may result in damage to capsule causing necrosis and increased permeability, or damage to lens fibers, or zonular dehiscence. Damage to lens fibers can also result from the impact of aqueous and iris or lens rebound mechanism.

Q.2. Discuss the seven rings of trauma.

Ans. *See* section of traumatic RD.

■ REFERENCES

1. MacFaul PA, Duke-Elder SS. Concussion and contusion. In: System of Ophthalmology, volume. XIV, part I, 1972. Henry Kimpton.
2. Mian SI, Azar DT, Colby K. Management of traumatic cataracts. Int Ophthalmol Clin. 2002; 42(3):23-31.

CHAPTER 7

Instruments

OPHTHALMIC INSTRUMENTS

Pranita Sahay, Devesh Kumawat

The ophthalmic instruments can be classified into the following.

■ LID SPECULUM

It is used to keep the lids open during any ocular surgery. The two commonly used lid speculums are described below.

Universal Metallic Eye Speculum

As the name suggests, the same speculum can be used for either eye (right or left), but the disadvantages are that it is heavy in weight and cannot keep the eyelashes away from the operating field **(Fig. 1)**.

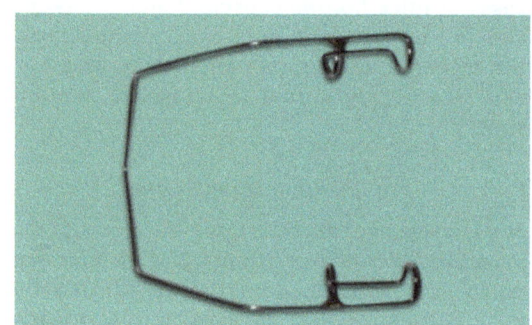

Fig. 1: Universal metallic eye speculum.

Self-retaining Barraquer Eye Speculum

This lid speculum has a screw that helps in giving desired exposure of the surgical site which can be changed as per the surgery or surgeon's choice.

The disadvantage is that the screw increases pressure over the eyeball and thereby increases the intraocular pressure. Hence, it is not advisable in perforated cases **(Fig. 2)**.

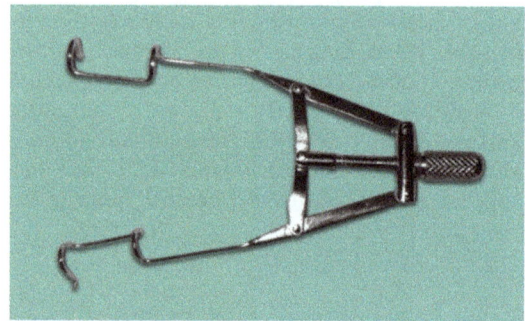

Fig. 2: Self-retaining Barraquer eye speculum.

Uses

- All intraocular surgeries such as cataract surgery, glaucoma surgery, keratoplasty, buckling, and other vitreoretinal surgery
- Removal of conjunctival and corneal foreign body
- Examination of children and patients with severe blepharospasm.

■ FORCEPS

Forceps of different design are available for different purposes.

Plain Forceps

It is a blunt forceps without any tooth.

Its tip has serrations (either horizontal or vertical) for holding tissue **(Fig. 3)**.

Uses

- For holding conjunctiva, scleral flap, or skin
- For holding the sutures while tying.

Globe Fixation Forceps

The tip of this forceps is toothed for better grip while holding the tissue.

It is used to hold the conjunctiva and episcleral tissue near the limbus **(Fig. 4)**.

Uses

- For fixing the eyeball during surgery
- For holding the eyeball during forced duction test.

Superior Rectus-holding Forceps

It is a toothed forceps with "S" shaped curve specially designed to fit into the orbit while trying to grasp the muscle belly **(Fig. 5)**.

Colibri Forceps

It is a fine-toothed forceps for holding flaps of cornea or sclera and rarely the iris **(Fig. 6)**.

Lim Forceps

It is also a toothed forceps for holding the cornea or sclera and rarely the iris **(Figs. 7A and B)**.

Iris Forceps

These are toothed forceps especially designed for holding the iris for the purpose of iridectomy.

Epilation Forceps

It is a small stout forceps with blunt and flat ends **(Fig. 8)**.

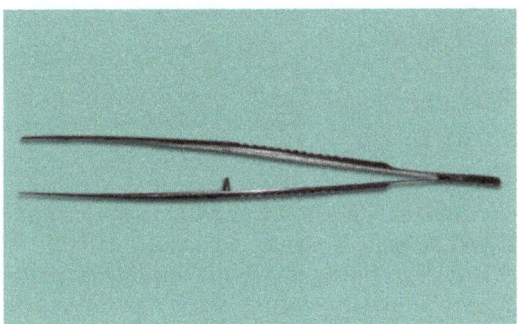

Fig. 3: Plain forceps.

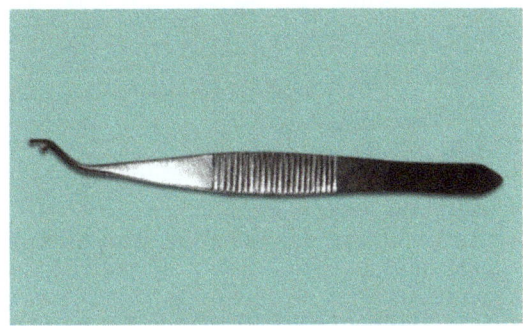

Fig. 5: Superior rectus-holding forceps.

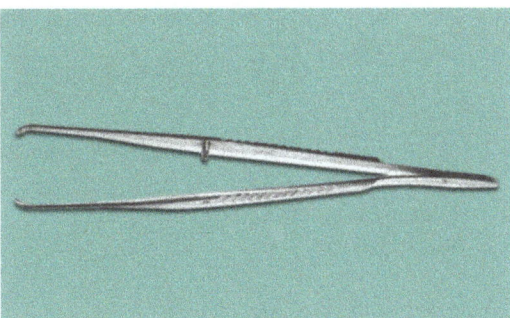

Fig. 4: Globe fixation forceps.

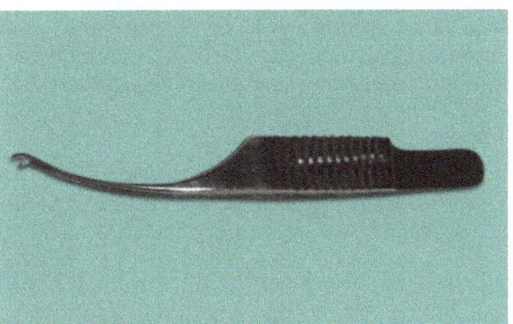

Fig. 6: Colibri forceps.

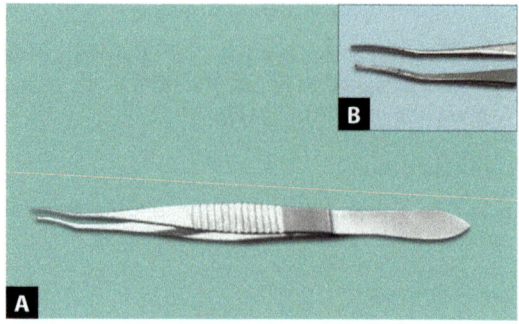

Figs. 7A and B: (A) Lim forceps; (B) Magnified view of tip showing toothed end.

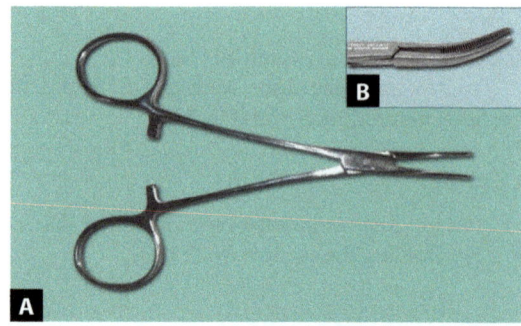

Figs. 9A and B: Artery (hemostatic) forceps: (A) Plain; (B) Curved (Inset).

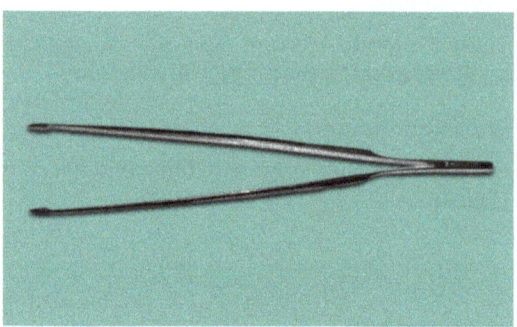

Fig. 8: Epilation forceps

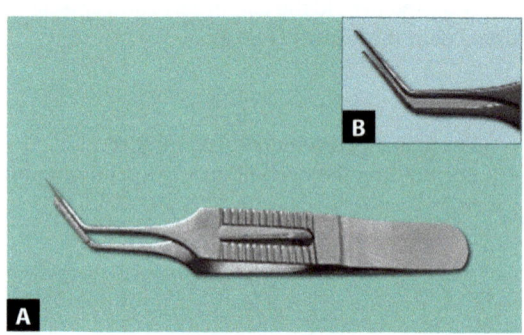

Figs. 10A and B: (A) Utrata capsulorhexis forceps; (B) Magnified view of its tip.

Uses

- Epilation of cilia in trichiasis and stye
- Removal of cilia after electrolysis and cryotherapy.

Artery (Hemostatic) Forceps

It is a blunt-tipped forceps with multiple serrations near the tip and a locking mechanism near the other end. It is available in various sizes small, medium, and large. The small-sized forceps are called mosquito forceps and are the most commonly used variety in ophthalmic surgeries **(Figs. 9A and B)**.

Uses

- Holding the bleeders during surgery
- To crush the muscle before cutting in squint surgery.

Utrata Capsulorhexis Forceps

This forceps has a fine titanium tip with a sharp point that enables to initiate the capsular tear then securely grasp the capsule to perform the capsulorhexis. It has an "iris stop platform" at 8.5 mm from the tip to stop the shaft of the forceps from completely closing when tips are closed **(Figs. 10A and B)**.

McPherson Forceps

It is a fine sharp tipped non-toothed forceps with angulation **(Fig. 11)**.

Uses

- Holding the intraocular lens (IOL) while implanting it
- Holding the suture while tying the knot
- Suture removal.

Pierse Hoskins Forceps

It is a fine-toothed tissue holding forceps **(Fig. 12)**.

Instruments

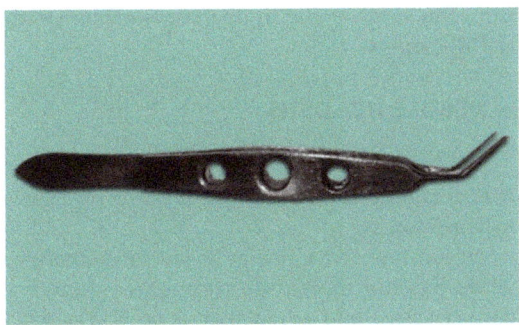

Fig. 11: McPherson's forceps.

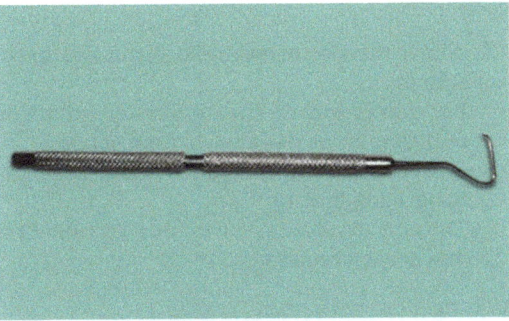

Fig. 14: Green hook.

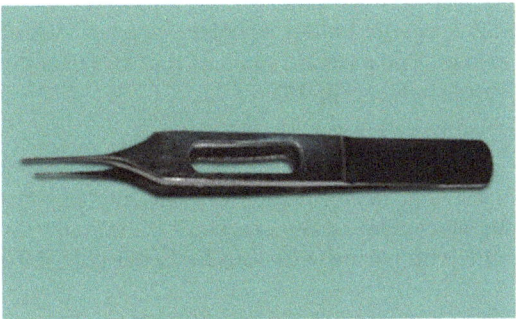

Fig. 12: Pierse Hoskins forceps.

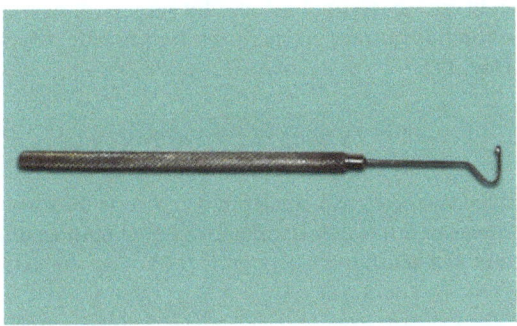

Fig. 15: Jameson hook.

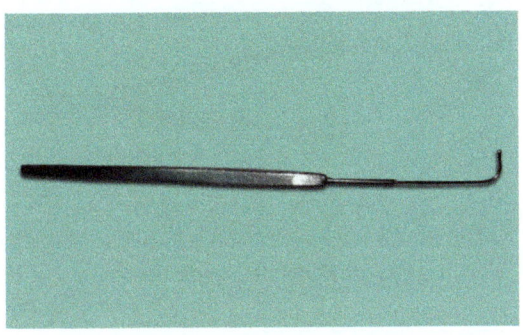

Fig. 13: Lens hook/Von Graefe retractor.

Uses

- Holding the corneal tissue firmly
- For suture tying
- For forced duction test.

■ HOOKS AND RETRACTORS

Lens Hook/Von Graefe Retractor

It has a flat metal handle which is curved at its end and has a knob **(Fig. 13)**.

Uses

- For applying pressure on the limbus at 6 o'clock position during delivery of lens in intracapsular cataract extraction as well as extracapsular cataract extraction
- It can be used as an alternative to muscle hook in squint surgery.

Green Hook

It has a straight shaft with flat-ended hooked tip. It is used for hooking the muscle during squint or enucleation surgery **(Fig. 14)**.

Jameson Hook

It has a straight shaft with flat-hooked end and paddle-shaped tip. It is used for retrieving the rectus muscles at their insertion site during squint or enucleation surgery **(Fig. 15)**.

Desmarres Lid Retractor

It is a saddle-shaped instrument available in two sizes—small and large **(Fig. 16)**.

Uses

For double eversion of the eyelid and evaluation of superior fornix
- For retraction of the upper eyelid while removing corneal sutures or foreign body
- For retraction of the conjunctiva after peritomy in buckling surgery.

The only disadvantage with this instrument is that it is not self-retaining.

Cat's Paw Lacrimal Wound Retractor

It is used to retract the soft tissue from the operative field during lacrimal sac and lid surgery. It has an added advantage of having a hemostatic effect (**Fig. 17**).

Müller's Self-retaining Adjustable Hemostatic Retractor

It has two limbs with three pins in each. As the name suggests, it has the advantage of being hemostatic and self-retaining along with retracting the skin from the surgical site in dacryocystorhinostomy (DCR) surgery.

■ NEEDLE HOLDERS

Barraquer Needle Holder

It is available in two designs with or without a locking system.

It has fine serrations at its jaw for better grip while passing the suture through conjunctiva, cornea, sclera, and extraocular muscles (**Fig. 18**).

Castroviejo Needle Holder

It is a needle holder with an S-shaped locking system. The uses are same as that of Barraquer needle holder (**Fig. 19**).

Arruga Needle Holder

It is a large needle holder with one end being flat for placement of the surgeon's thumb and the other end having serrations for better grip of the

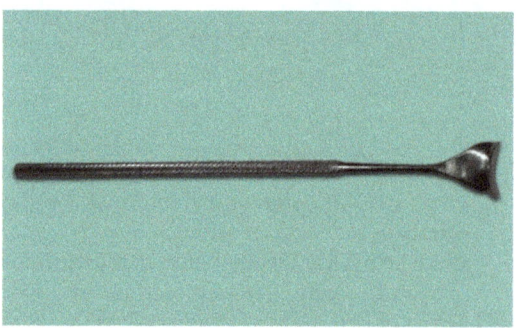

Fig. 16: Desmarres Lid retractor.

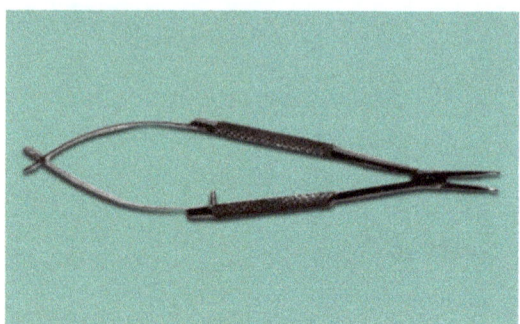

Fig. 18: Barraquer needle holder.

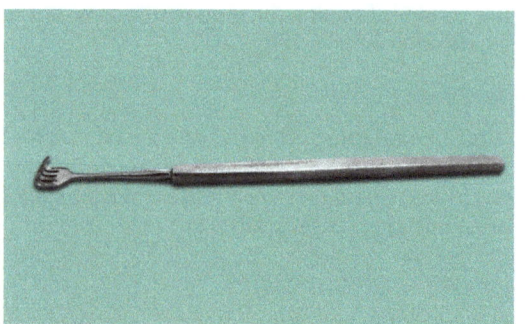

Fig. 17: Cat's paw lacrimal wound retractor.

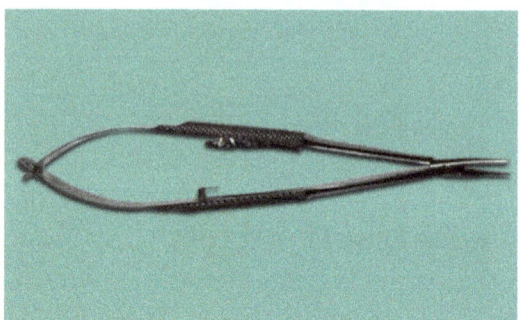

Fig. 19: Castroviejo needle holder.

suture. It is available in two designs—with and without a locking system **(Fig. 20)**.

Uses

- In eyelid surgery
- For passing superior rectus bridle suture

■ CASTROVIEJO CALIPER

It is a divider-like instrument with a graduated scale at one end (marking in millimeters) and the other arm moves by a screw over the scale **(Fig. 21)**.

Uses

- Measuring the diameters of host or donor cornea
- Marking the site for muscle insertion in recession surgery
- Marking the site for pars plana entry for either surgery or intravitreal injection

■ KNIVES

Von Graefe Knife

It is a long, narrow, thin blade with a sharp tip with cutting edge on one side. It was used for making the corneoscleral entry in cataract surgery.

Keratome

It is a thin blade with a diamond-shaped apex and cutting edge on both sides. It is available in both straight and curved design as well as in various sizes (2.8 mm, 3 mm, 3.5 mm, and 5.5 mm). It is used for making self-sealing corneal incisions in cataract surgery, iridectomy, and keratoplasty **(Fig. 22)**.

Micro Vitreo Retinal (MVR) Blade

It is a fine straight instrument with triangular knife at its distal end having cutting edge on both the sides. The instrument is predominantly used for making side port entry during cataract and other anterior segment surgical procedures. The 'V' lance design of MVR blade is used for creating watertight ports during posterior segment surgeries. **(Fig. 23)**.

Crescent Knife

It is blunt-tipped instrument with bevel side of the knife up and having cut-splitting action on both the sides **(Fig. 24)**.

Uses

- For dissection in pterygium surgery
- For dissection of the scleral flap in trabeculectomy/small incision cataract surgery

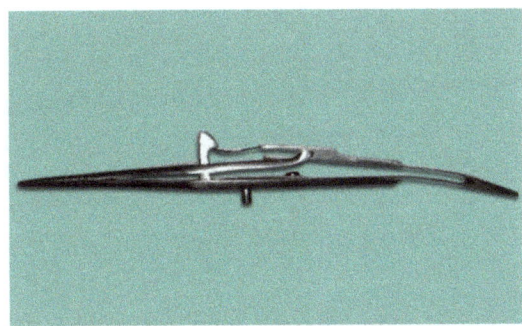

Fig. 20: Arruga needle holder.

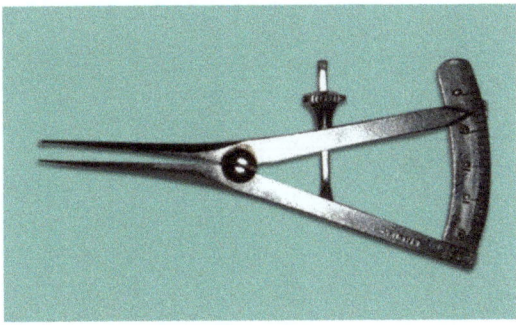

Fig. 21: Castroviejo caliper.

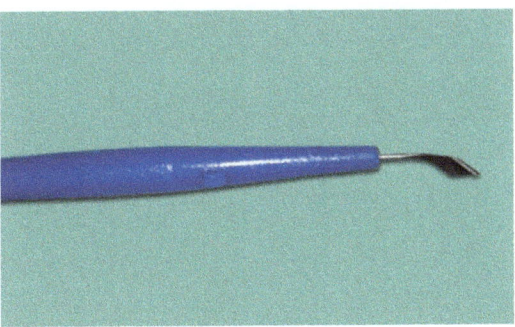

Fig. 22: Keratomes.

(SICS)/Descemet's stripping automated endothelial keratoplasty (DSAEK)
- For corneal dissection in anterior lamellar keratoplasty.

■ SCISSORS

Steven Tenotomy Scissors

It is a plain scissor with blunt ends. It comes in two designs—straight and curved **(Fig. 25)**.

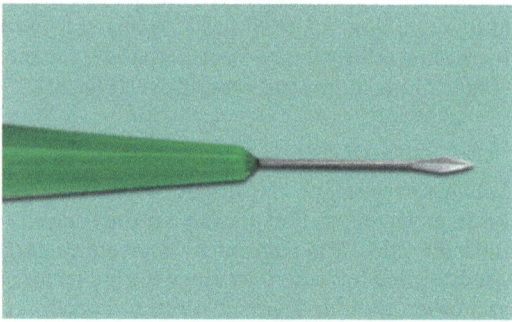

Fig. 23: Micro Vitreo Retinal (MVR) blade.

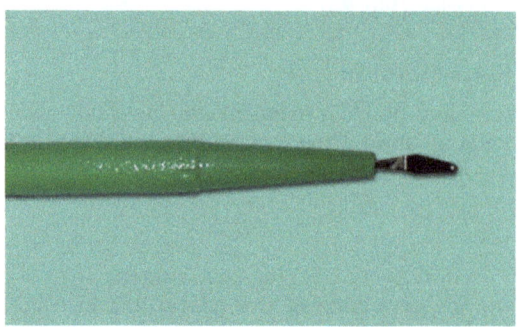

Fig. 24: Crescent knife.

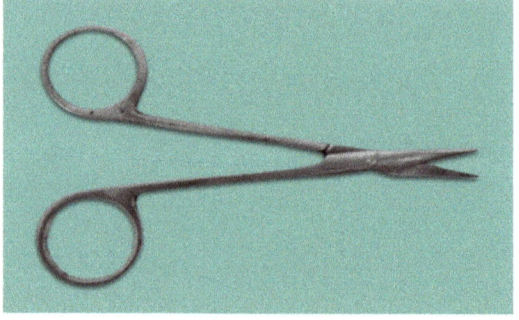

Fig. 25: Steven tenotomy scissors.

Uses
- For cutting the muscle
- For blunt dissection of the soft tissue in squint and oculoplasty procedures.

Castroviejo Corneoscleral Scissors

It is a fine-curved scissor that works on spring action **(Fig. 26)**.

Uses
- To enlarge the corneal or corneoscleral incision for intracapsular cataract extraction (ICCE)/extracapsular cataract extraction (ECCE)
- To enlarge corneal incision in keratoplasty
- To cut the scleral tissue flap.

DeWecker Scissors

It is a fine scissor with small blades at right angle to the arm that works on spring action **(Fig. 27)**.

Uses
- For performing iridectomy

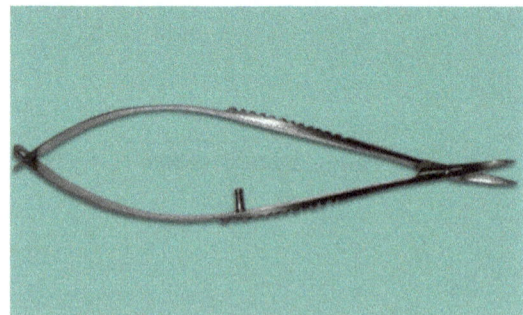

Fig. 26: Castroviejo corneoscleral scissors.

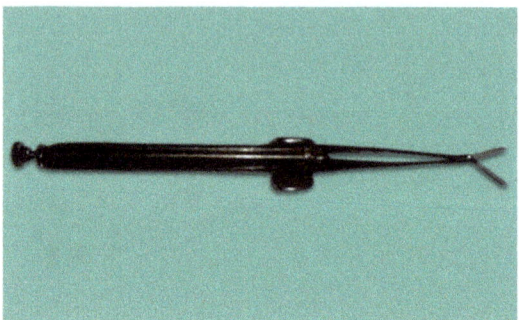

Fig. 27: DeWecker scissors.

- For cutting the vitreous strands prolapsing from the wound.

Westcott's Scissors

It is a stout scissor with straight or curved blades that work on spring action.

It is used for conjunctival dissection **(Fig. 28)**.

Vannas Scissors

It is a fine scissor that works on spring action. It has two wings to operate—one sharp and one blunt **(Fig. 29)**.

Uses

- For cutting sutures
- For anterior capsulotomy in ECCE
- For cutting the vitreous strand while performing anterior vitrectomy.

Enucleation Scissors

It is a thick-curved scissor with blunt tip used for cutting the optic nerve in enucleation surgery **(Fig. 30)**.

■ OTHER INSTRUMENTS

Cataract Surgery

Lens Spatula

It has a metallic handle with spoon-shaped end which is used to apply pressure at 12 o'clock position for expression of nucleus in Smith's technique in extracapsular cataract extraction **(Fig. 31)**.

Wire Vectis

It is a wire loop attached to metallic handle **(Fig. 32)**.

Uses: It is used to remove subluxated lens in ICCE as well as nucleus in ECCE.

Irrigating Wire Vectis

It is a modification of the wire vectis. It has a hollow rim with a 0.3-mm opening at the anterior end and a hollow handle at the posterior end which is attached to a hub similar to that of a hypodermic

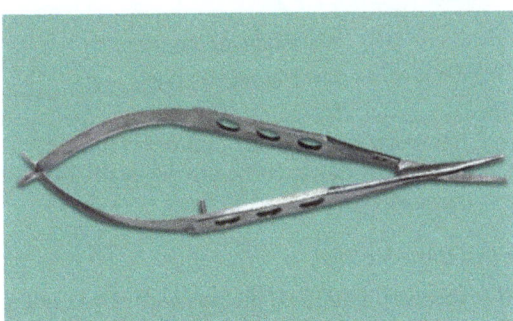

Fig. 28: Westcott scissors.

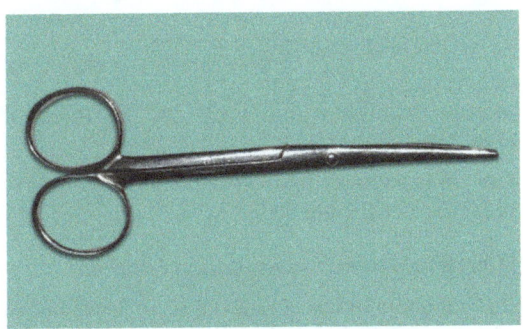

Fig. 30: Enucleation scissors.

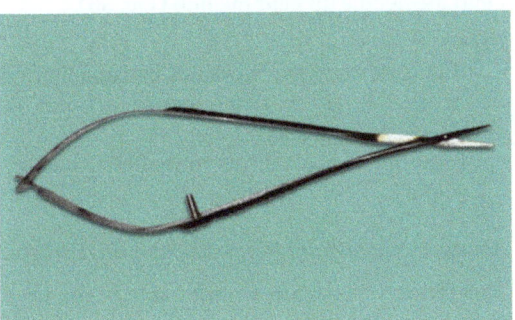

Fig. 29: Vannas scissors.

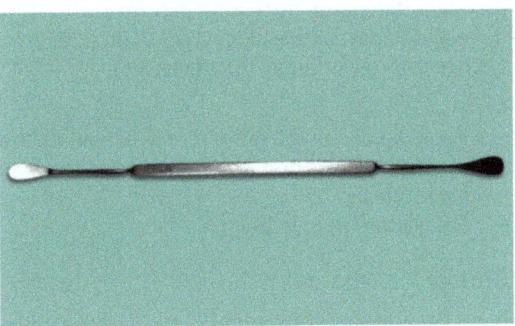

Fig. 31: Lens spatula.

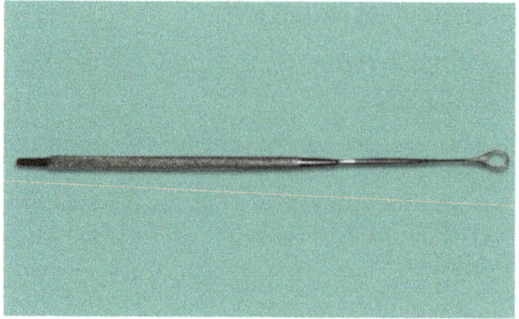

Fig. 32: Wire Vectis.

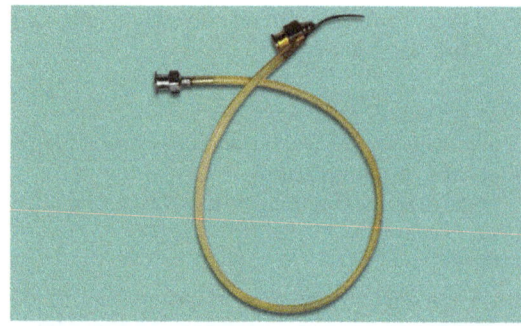

Fig. 34: Simcoe irrigation and aspiration cannula.

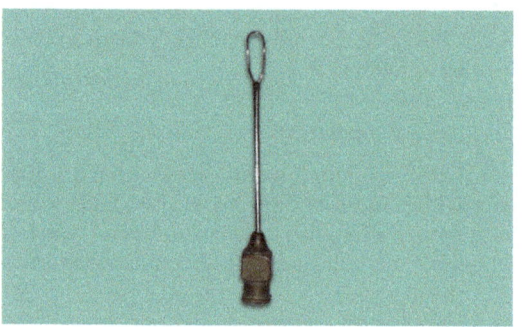

Fig. 33: Irrigating wire Vectis.

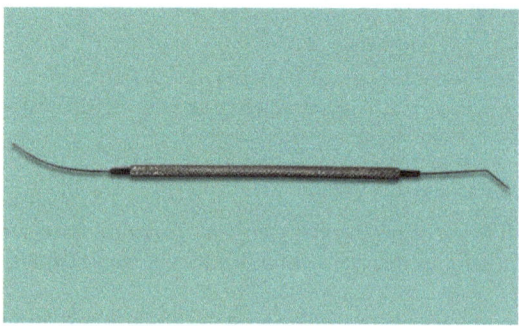

Fig. 35: Dastoor iris repositor.

needle through which fluid can be injected **(Fig. 33)**.

Uses: It is used for hydro/viscoexpression of the nucleus in ECCE and SICS.

Simcoe Irrigation and Aspiration Cannula

It is available in the classical and reverse design with both right-handed and left-handed models available in each design. It has an irrigation system through the main port and aspiration system through the port on the side which is attached to a syringe through a silicon tube **(Fig. 34)**.

Uses
- For irrigation and aspiration of cortical matter in ECCE and open sky cataract surgery in keratoplasty
- For aspiration of hyphema.

Dastoor Iris Repositor

It is a flat and straight/bent blade with blunt edges **(Fig. 35)**.

Uses
- To reposit the iris in the anterior chamber
- To tuck the donor cornea underneath the host cornea in keratoplasty surgery.

Cystotome Needle

It is prepared with a 26-gauge needle by bending the needle tip down while holding the bevel up. Then, while maintaining this needle orientation, bend the needle up near the hub **(Fig. 36)**.

Uses
- It is used to make the anterior capsulotomy in ECCE as well as capsulorhexis in phacoemulsification.
- Posterior capsulorhexis in pediatric cataract surgery.

Arruga Intracapsular (Capsule Holding) Forceps

This forceps has a cup at inner side of the tip of each limb. The edges of the cup are smooth and atraumatic to the lens capsule **(Fig. 37)**.

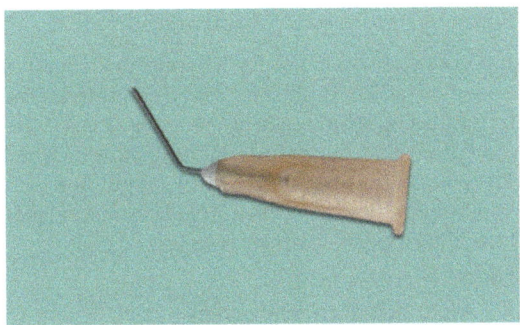

Fig. 36: Cystotome needle.

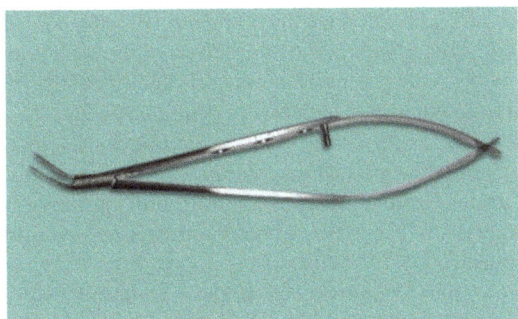

Fig. 38: Intraocular lens (IOL)-holding forceps.

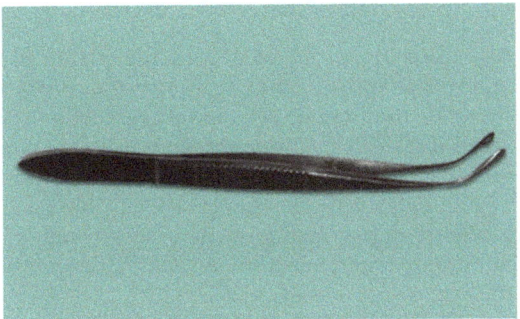

Fig. 37: Arruga intracapsular (capsule holding) forceps.

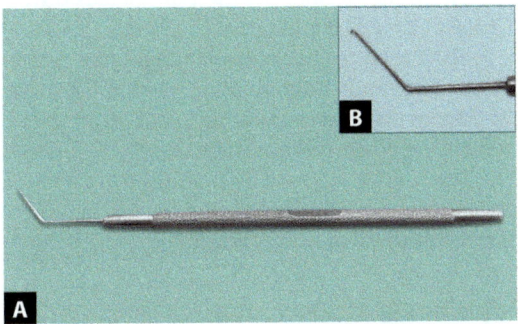

Figs. 39A and B: (A) Sinskey hook or intraocular lens (IOL) dialer; (B) Magnified view of its blunt tip.

Uses
- For removal of the lens during forceps method of intracapsular cataract extraction
- For removal of the lens capsule remnant after accidental extracapsular cataract extraction.

Intraocular Lens-holding Forceps

It is a spring action forceps with short, blunt, and curved blades smooth edges and tips. It is used to hold the optic of non-foldable polymethylmethacrylate (PMMA) intraocular (IOL) during implantation **(Fig. 38)**.

Sinskey Hook or Intraocular Lens Dialer

It is a fine instrument with a bent tip. The tip can engage the dialing holes of the IOL **(Figs. 39A and B)**.

Uses
- Dialing of the non-foldable PMMA IOL for proper positioning in the capsular bag or sulcus

- For nucleus manipulation in phacoemulsification.

Chopper

It is similar in appearance to the Sinskey hook, but the difference lies in the tip which is sharp with cutting edges in a chopper. It is used to split or chop the nucleus into smaller pieces during phacoemulsification **(Figs. 40A to C)**. Sharp tip choppers are useful in hard cataract and vertical chopping technique. Choppers can also have a blunt/knobbed tip which is useful in soft cataract and horizontal chopping technique.

Phaco Needle Tip

It is made of titanium with a distal opening 0.9 mm in diameter with a silicon sleeve which has two openings on the side 180° apart, through which the irrigation fluid flows. The phaco needle threads directly onto the phaco handpiece **(Figs. 41A to C)**.

The tip can have bevel with 0°, 15°, 30°, 45°, or 60°. The greater is the angulation of the bevel tip, better is the sculpting effect and visibility of the tip but leads to poor occlusion. The 30° bevel offers the best compromise and leads to better sculpting, visibility as well as occlusion. The silicon sleeve acts as an insulator and the fluid flowing through the sleeve keeps the tip cool and prevents wound burn.

The Kelman tip has a 22° angulation of the shaft 3.5 mm from the tip. This enhances the emulsification as well as allows the surgeon to use the phaco tip for manipulation of nucleus during surgery **(Figs. 41B and C)**.

The flared tip has an outer diameter greater at the distal end of the tip than 1–2 mm behind it. This helps to enhance the emulsification effect and reduce the postocclusion surge.

The Cobra tip is a bell-shaped tip, which increases the surface producing the ultrasound to reduce the level of energy required.

Bimanual Irrigation and Aspiration

It consists of two cannulas wherein the irrigation and aspiration functions are decoupled. The irrigation cannula which is connected with irrigation port maintains the anterior chamber. The aspiration cannula is used to aspiration port and helps in removing cortical matter/viscoelastic from the anterior chamber **(Fig. 42)**.

Uses
- Aspiration of cortical matter
- Viscoelastic washout.

Intraocular Lens Injector

It is used for insertion of foldable IOL in the anterior chamber. It has a plunger that pushes the IOL loaded in IOL cartridge through a small incision. The plungers are available two designs—push insertion and screwed insertion of IOL **(Fig. 43)**. Currently, a lot of IOLs are available in pre-loaded form as well which do not require such injectors for IOL placement in the eye.

Nuijts–Lane Toric Bubble Marker

It is used for toric IOL/phakic IOL implantation **(Fig. 44)**. Preoperative three reference points are marked at the limbus with the help of this instrument at 0, 90 and, 180 degrees. This marking is done with a patient in upright posture to avoid the effect of cyclotorsion in supine posture. At the time of marking the bubble position should be central to avoid tilting of the instrument. The marked reference points are used to guide intraoperative accurate placement of Mendez toric marker gauge which provides

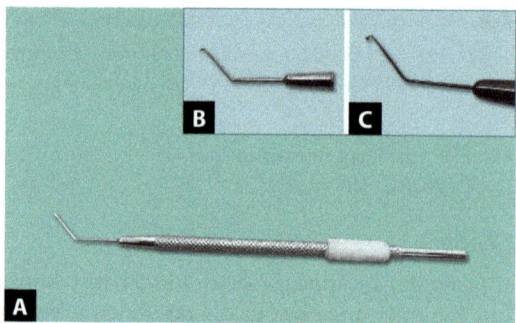

Figs. 40A to C: (A) Chopper; (B) Magnified image of sharp tip chopper; (C) Magnified image of blunt tip chopper.

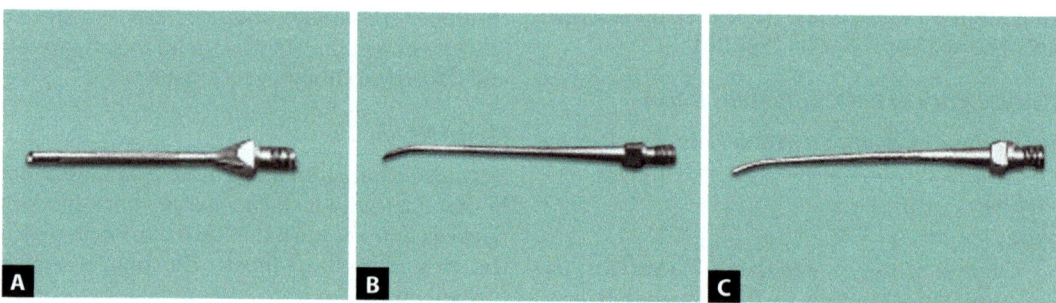

Figs. 41A to C: Phaco needle tip; (A) Straight tip; (B) Kelman tip with 30° bevel; (C) Kelman tip with 45° bevel.

Instruments

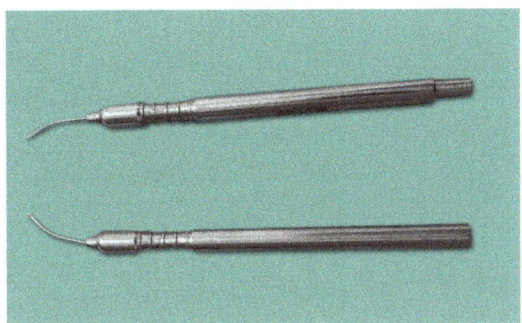

Fig. 42: Bimanual irrigation and aspiration.

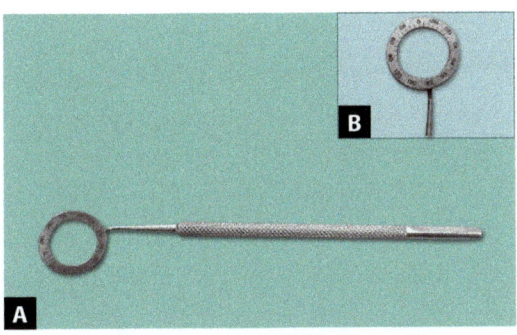

Figs. 45A and B: Mendez toric degree gauge ring marker.

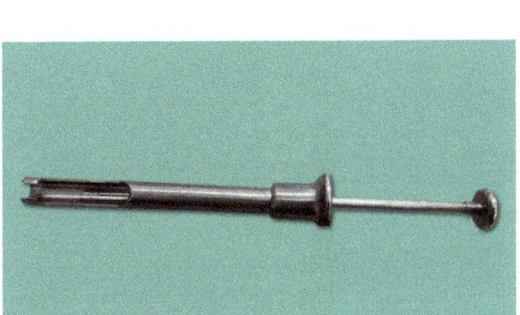

Fig. 43: Intraocular lens (IOL) injector.

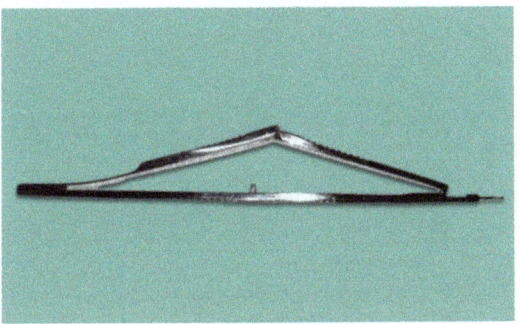

Fig. 46: Kelley's punch.

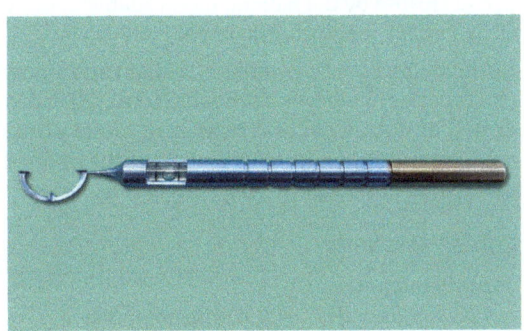

Fig. 44: Nuijts–Lane toric bubble marker.

the final guide for marking the implantation axis of toric IOL. The bubble marker has marking on both sides; hence can be used for both left and right eye.

Uses
- Placement of corneal incision
- Toric IOL/phakic IOL placement
- Arcuate keratotomy placement.

Mendez Toric Degree Gauge Ring Marker

After the preoperative marking of reference points, the intraoperative marking of implantation axis is done with the help of Mendez toric degree gauge ring marker. It has an angulation for easy placement of marker on cornea in supine position. The ring has marking from 0 to 180°. Different models are available with 10° and 5° steps **(Figs. 45A and B)**.

Glaucoma Surgery

Kelley's Punch

It is used to perform punch sclerostomy in trabeculectomy surgery **(Fig. 46)**. The instrument creates hemi-oval punches of size 0.5–0.75 mm.

Harms Trabeculotome

Harms trabeculotome is used for performing trabeculotomy surgery in cases of congenital glaucoma. It consists of a curved approximately 9-mm long tip that is introduced externally into the Schlemm canal and is used to break the inner wall

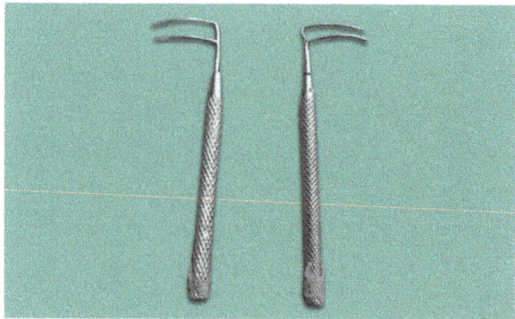

Fig. 47: Harms trabeculotome.

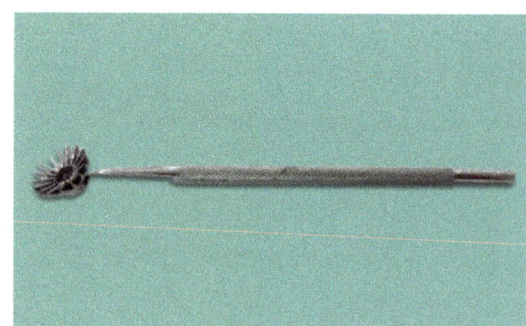

Fig. 49: Radial keratotomy (RK) marker.

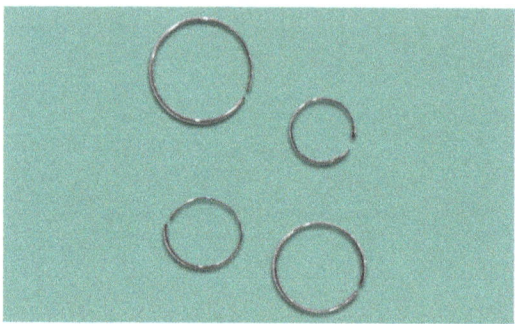

Fig. 48: Flieringa ring.

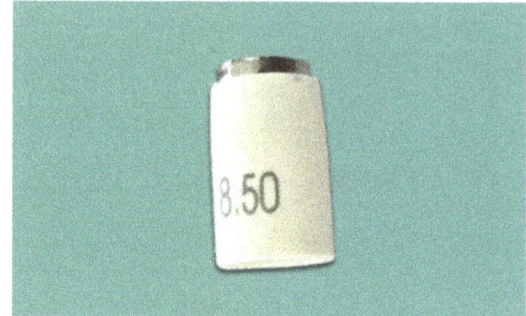

Fig. 50: Disposable handheld trephine.

of Schlemm canal to allow outflow of aqueous. It is available in two curves designed for left-sided and right-sided entry in the Schlemm canal (**Fig. 47**).

Keratoplasty

Globe Fixation Rings

Flieringa ring: It is made of stainless steel and is useful for maintaining the architecture of the globe once the host corneal button has been removed. They are available in 11 sizes from 12 to 22 mm (**Fig. 48**).

Uses: Keratoplasty in aphakic eyes especially where vitrectomy has been performed. Keratoplasty in pseudophakic eyes and pediatric eyes as the eyeball has a tendency to collapse in these cases after trephination.

Disadvantage is that it can distort the shape of the eyeball and cause an oval cut during trephination and subsequent high astigmatism.

McNeill–Goldman ring: It provides support at four strategically placed sutures. The ring has medial and temporal openings for greater access to the surgical field and two lid retractors to prevent eyelid closure by the patient. It is available in three sizes—small, medium, and large.

Corneal marking instruments: Radial keratotomy (RK) marker, Vajpayee corneal marker (20 radial arms), and Anis corneal marker (8 radial arms) are the various instruments that guide the optimal placement of sutures in keratoplasty (**Fig. 49**).

Corneal Trephines

Types of trephines
- *Conventional circular cutting trephines*
  - Handheld
    - Ranging from 3 to 17 mm in diameter. In some trephines, there is a central obturator, which can be adjusted to select the depth of the corneal cut and hence an inadvertent entry into the anterior chamber (**Figs. 50 and 51**).
    - However, the obturator obscures the view of central cornea which may result in inaccurate centration during trephination of the recipient's cornea.

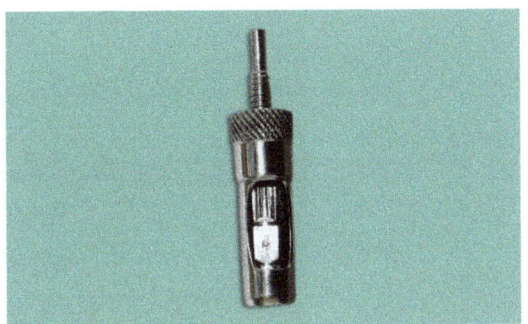

Fig. 51: Handheld trephine with obturator.

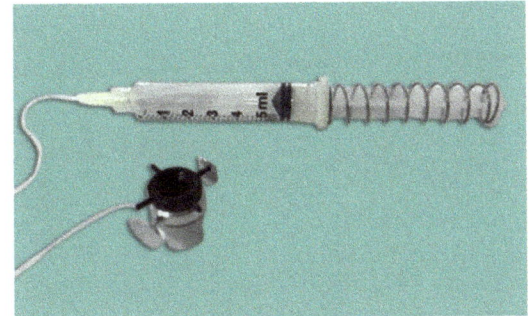

Fig. 52: Hessburg–Barron trephine.

- The examples of hand-held trephines with obturator are the Castroviejo trephine and the Grieshaber-Franceschetti trephine.
- *Mechanized*: The disadvantages associated with motor driven trephines include corkscrew edge effect on the corneal stroma.
- *Suction-fixation type*
    - It is devised to obtain a perpendicular cut in the recipient cornea. These trephine systems essentially consist of an outer corneal suction ring for fixation and an inner circular cutting blade.
    - Hessburg-Barron trephine has a crosshair device for improved centration and an outer ring of corneal marks at equal intervals to assist in suture placement. It is available in diameters.
    - 6.0–9.0 in 0.5 mm increments as well as diameter of 7.75 mm. For each spoke (90°) turned, the blade is lowered or raised approximately 0.06 mm **(Fig. 52)**.
    - The Barron vacuum punch features a solid stainless-steel blade which is permanently mounted in a nylon housing. Four steel guideposts align with four corresponding holes in the cutting block base, automatically centering the blade over the donor cornea.

Special-purpose type
- The Olson calibrated cornea trephine system used to trephinate both the donor and recipient corneas. The system consists of the anterior chamber maintainer, the reusable blade holder (with micrometer setting), and the suction ring. One revolution of the micrometer is equivalent to 500 μm.
- *Skin biopsy punches:* The skin biopsy punches, which have been used in dermatological practice, are especially useful in harvesting of small patch grafts used for tectonic purposes in cases of impending/frank perforation.
- *Single point cutting trephines:* The single point cutter trephines were designed to decrease corneal torsion, e.g., Leiberman single point cutter.
- *Combination trephines:* Hanna trephine system has got a circular razor-cutting blade and incorporates many of the salient features of single point cutting trephines.
- *Noncontact trephines (lasers):* Laser noncontact trephination eliminates corneal topography distortion, provides the visualization of the entire cornea, and enhances centration.

Graft Holder (Paton Spatula)

Graft is placed over viscoelastic and is kept covered till the recipient dissection is complete **(Fig. 53)**.

Cutting Block

The various cutting blocks available for corneal grafting are paraffin block, Teflon block, and polycarbonate and nylon blocks **(Fig. 54)**.

The Kaufmann corneal cutting block is the simplest design which consists of a Teflon block with a metal cover.

The Brightbill corneal cutting block made up of teflon is the modern, compound curved block

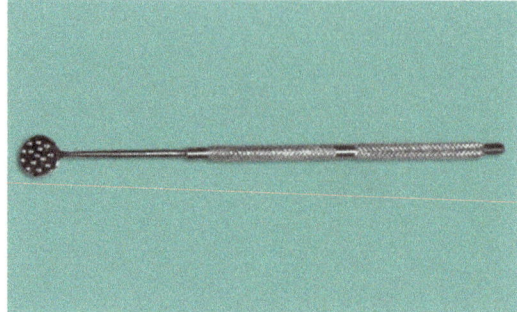

Fig. 53: Paton spatula.

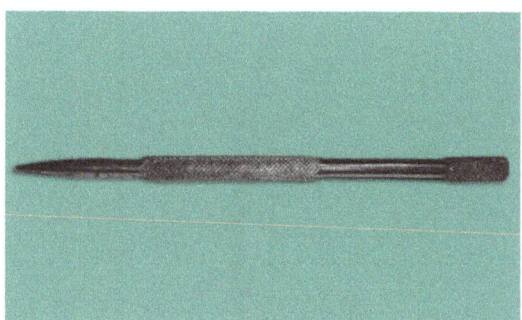

Fig. 55: Blade breaker.

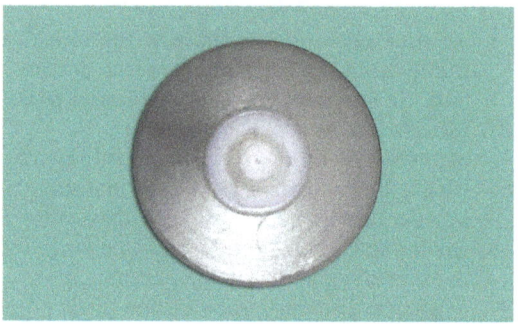

Fig. 54: Teflon block.

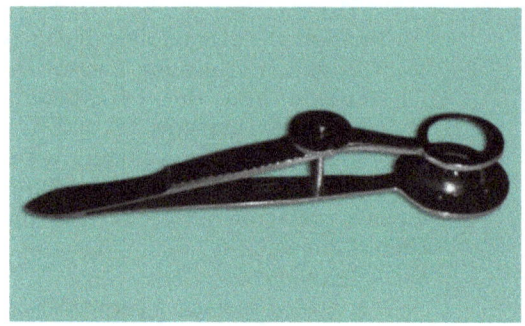

Fig. 56: King's clamp.

which approximates the central, midperipheral and peripheral curvature of the donor tissue.

Corneal Endothelial Punches

To cut a donor button from endothelial side corneal punches are also available which use disposable trephine blades. The advantage of corneal punch is that they yield sharp vertical cuts without beveling, e.g., Cottingham corneal punch, Troutman corneal punch, IOWA PK press corneal punch, Lieberman gravity-action punch, Rothman–Gilbard corneal punch.

Cutting Instruments

Blade breaker: A disposable razor blade is broken and mounted on the tip of a metallic pencil handle. It is used for a controlled entry into the anterior chamber **(Fig. 55)**.

Diamond knife: This is the sharpest cutting instrument and is available in various sizes and shapes. It is the most durable and useful instrument for stab incisions as well as to complete the trephine cuts.

Forceps with special functions
- *Double corneal forceps, colibri style:* It has two 2.75-mm long tips separated 1 mm with 1 × 2 teeth. It is 72-mm long and has a serrated handle.
- *Colibri-style Polack double corneal forceps:* It is used for the first corneal suture. The cut edge of the graft is gently grasped at the junction of the epithelium and stroma with fine-toothed forceps.

Instruments for donor cornea dissection in lamellar keratoplasty
- *Barron's artificial anterior chamber and clamp:* The chamber is used to mount the donor tissue and maintain adequate pressure while lamellar dissection or full thickness trephination is being performed. It is designed in a bright blue color to provide a high contrast background for visualizing the cornea and aiding in the lamellar dissection of the cornea.
- King's clamp **(Fig. 56)**.

Lamellar Dissectors

Tooke knife: The pocket for the initiation of the lamellar dissection may be performed with a Tooke's knife. It has a smooth blade at one end, which can be inserted intralamellarly to create a pocket.

Paufique knife: It has a double-edged sharp angled blade that helps in outlining the graft, making the pocket, and in dissecting the lamellar plane.

Desmarres lamellar dissector: It is used in the open type of dissection, which has a curve in its vertical meridian, and it is used to sweep across the fibers in a cutting and teasing motion. A duckbill shape lamellar dissector is used for closed type of dissection, which is curved in the horizontal dimension.

Gill's lamellar dissector: It has a 3-mm wide blade which can be either straight or curved.

Guarded diamond knife: It is a micrometer adjusted guarded diamond knife, useful for obtaining irregular shaped lamellar grafts.

Crescent knife: This is another useful instrument for the lamellar dissection. It has a 2.0 mm blade.

Automated Lamellar Therapeutic Keratoplasty Machine

The Moria automated lamellar therapeutic keratectomy (ALTK) microkeratome system utilizes the CBm microkeratome and an artificial chamber which is manually driven by the surgeon. Multiple microkeratome heads may be used to achieve dissection of various thicknesses ranging from 130 to 350 (130, 150, 250, 300, and 350 μm). The Moria ALTK artificial anterior chamber requires a donor scleral rim that is symmetrically >16 mm (maximum 19 mm) in diameter to provide proper vacuum during the microkeratome pass. The surgical time is greatly reduced as compared to manual dissection technique **(Figs. 57 and 58)**.

Descemet's Stripping Automated Endothelial Keratoplasty Spatula (Stripper)

It is designed to strip the recipient's Descemet's membrane during the DSAEK procedure. The DSAEK strippers, made of surgical steel, are available in 45° and 90°-angled models, in both

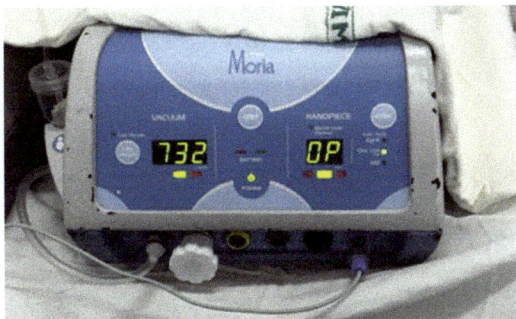

Fig. 57: Moria automated lamellar therapeutic keratectomy microkeratome system.

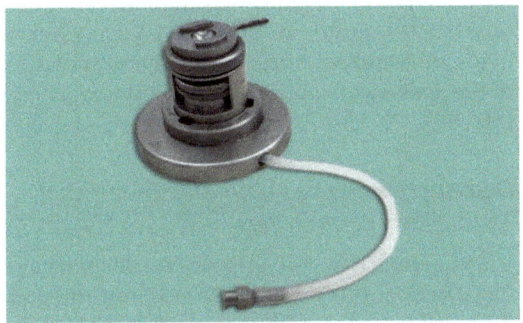

Fig. 58: Moria artificial chamber maintainer.

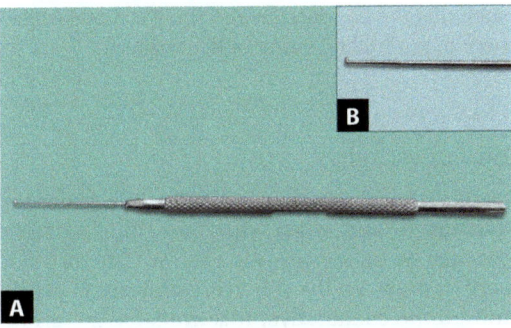

Figs. 59A and B: Descemet's stripping automated endothelial keratoplasty (DSAEK) spatula (Stripper).

irrigating and non-irrigating versions. The angled tips facilitate the efficient dissection and removal of Descemet's membrane without inadvertent damage to the stroma **(Figs. 59A and B)**.

Busin Glide

It allows insertion of the taco by pull-through technique through 3.2-mm incision. It facilitates

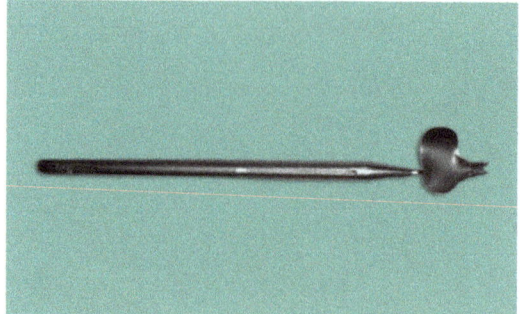

Fig. 60: Busin glide.

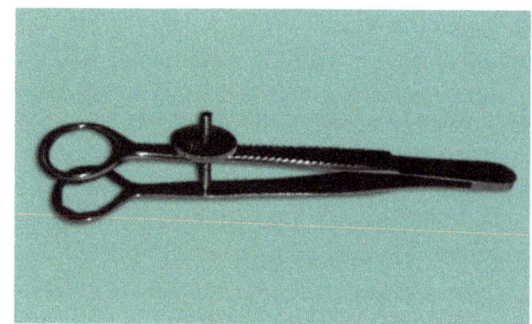

Fig. 61: Chalazion clamp.

the unfolding of the graft and simplifies centration of the donor button in the anterior chamber. It helps to minimize intraoperative manipulation of the graft and the possibility of endothelial loss **(Fig. 60)**.

Descemet's Stripping Automated Endothelial Keratoplasty Busin Forceps

It is a microincision forceps with 20G diameter and distal action. It is designed to position the graft in the glide and to pull it from the glide into the anterior chamber. Its tips have been specifically designed to contact the periphery of the graft such that the endothelial and the stromal surfaces remain untouched in the optical zone.

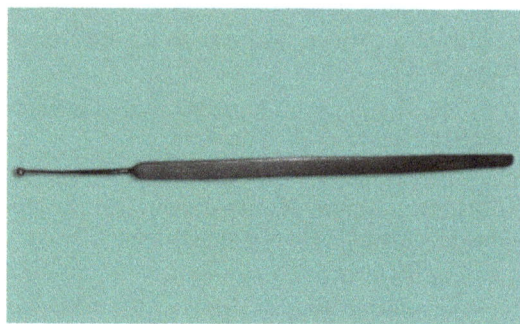

Fig. 62: Chalazion scoop.

Lid Surgery

Chalazion Clamp

It consists of a circular disc attached a circular rim attached to each other with the help of a handle that can be tightened with a screw. The disc side is placed toward the skin while the rim is placed toward the conjunctiva. It is available in various sizes from 10 to 21 mm. It is used to stabilize the lid and chalazion, and also provides hemostasis while performing incision and curettage of the chalazion **(Fig. 61)**.

Chalazion Scoop

It has a small cup with sharp margins attached to a narrow handle. It is used to scoop out the contents of chalazion during incision and curettage **(Fig. 62)**.

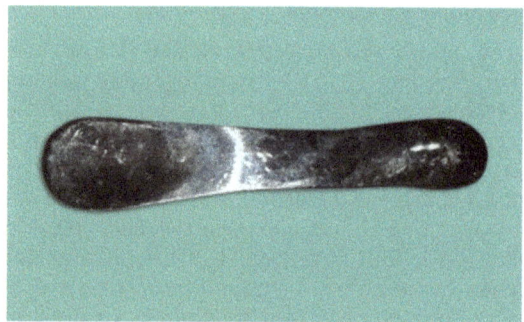

Fig. 63: Jaeger's lid spatula.

Jaeger Lid Spatula

It is a simple metal plate having a slightly convex surface on both ends. It is used to support the lid, as well as protect the globe during lid surgeries such as entropion, ectropion, ptosis, etc. **(Fig. 63)**.

Lid Clamp or Snellen's Entropion Clamp

It has a D-shaped plate attached to a U-shaped rim which when tightened with the help of a

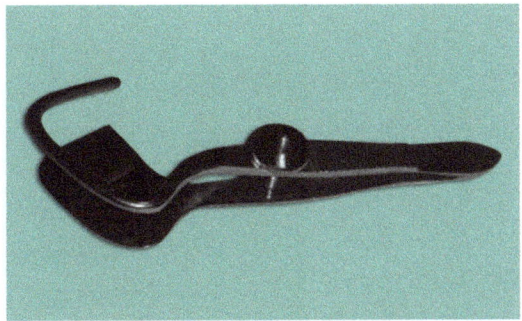

Fig. 64: Lid clamp or Snellen's entropion clamp.

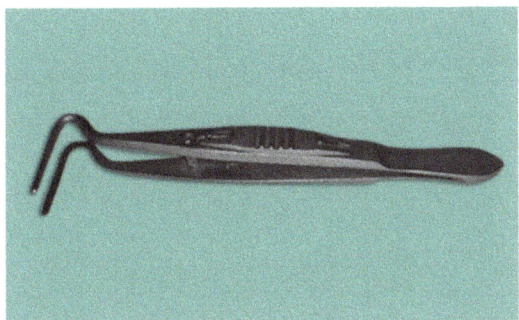

Fig. 65: Berke's ptosis clamp.

screw clamps the tissue and provides hemostasis. There are separate clamps for the right and left eye. The plate is placed on the conjunctival side while the rim is placed on the skin side and the handle is always directed temporally **(Fig. 64)**.

It offers the advantage of being self-sustaining and providing hemostasis. The disadvantage is that it reduces the surgical field and can cause pressure necrosis of the tissue, if applied too tightly. It is used in lid surgeries such as ectropion and entropion to stabilize the lid, protect the eyeball, and provide hemostasis.

Berke's Ptosis Clamp

It is a clamp with J-shaped end with internal serrations. It has a locking mechanism as well. It is used to hold the levator palpebral superioris muscle during ptosis surgery **(Fig. 65)**.

Crawford's Fascia Lata Stripper

It is used in ptosis surgery for harvesting the fascia lata. It has a proximal slot for holding the fascia lata and has the advantage of harvesting the tissue through a small incision.

Lacrimal Sac Surgery

Nettleship Punctum Dilator

It has a conical pointed tip and is used to dilate the puncta prior to probing or syringing. It is available in multiple sizes corresponding to the probe sizes **(Fig. 66)**.

Bowman Lacrimal Probe

It is available in sizes ranging from #0000 (0.5 mm diameter) to #4 (1.4 mm diameter) **(Fig. 67)**.

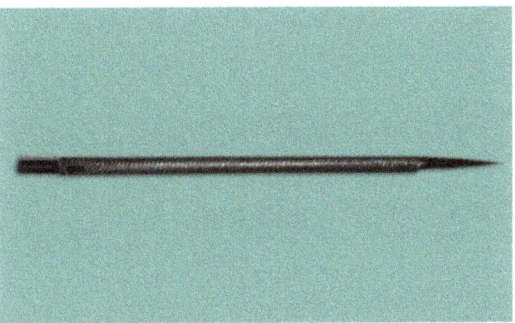

Fig. 66: Nettleship's punctum dilator.

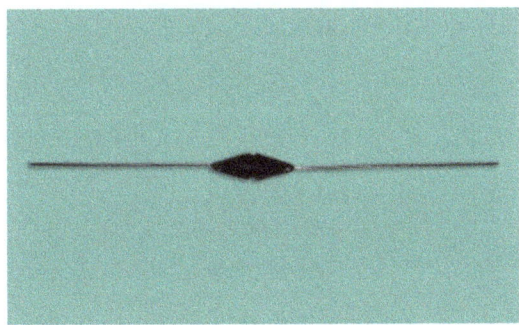

Fig. 67: Bowman lacrimal probe.

Uses
- Probing the lacrimal canaliculi and nasolacrimal duct to find the location of block
- DCR surgery
- Therapeutic probing in children.

Freer Periosteal Elevator

It is a double ended instrument with two tear-drop shaped tips, often is used to lift the periosteum and lacrimal sac from underlying fossa **(Figs. 68 and 69)**.

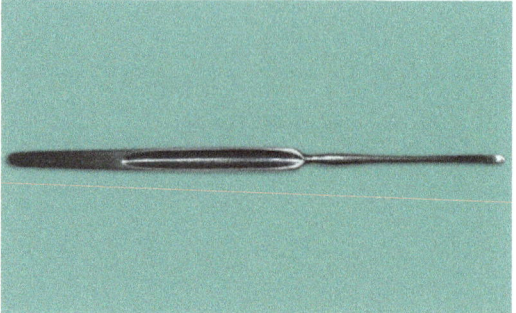

Fig. 68: Freer periosteal elevator.

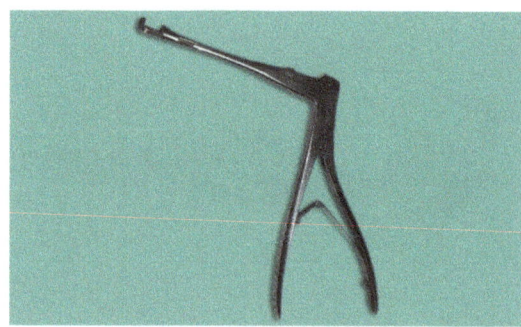

Fig. 71: Kerrison bone punch.

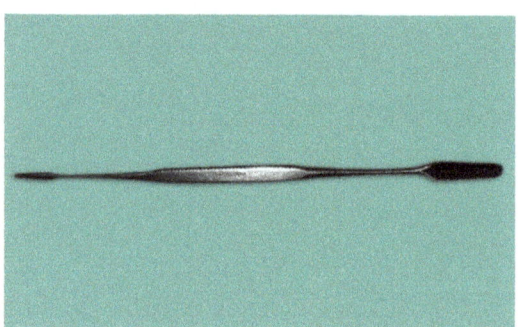

Fig. 69: Lacrimal sac dissector and curette.

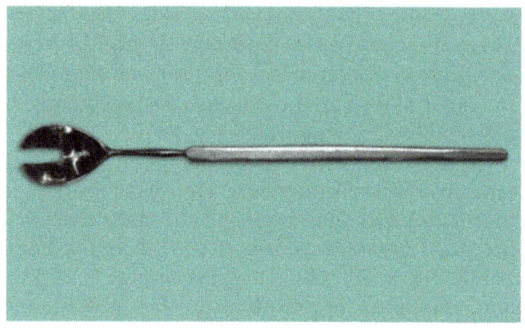

Fig. 72: Wells enucleation spoon.

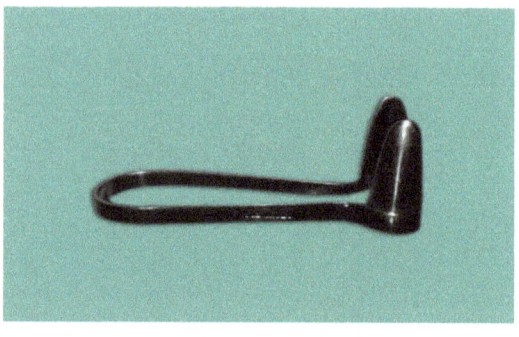

Fig. 70: Thudichum nasal speculum.

Thudichum Nasal Speculum

It is used for anterior rhinoscopy **(Fig. 70)**.

Kerrison Bone Punch

It is available in various sizes ranging from size 0 = 1 mm to size 4 = 5 mm. It has a cutting end up or down design. It is predominantly used to create an ostium in DCR surgeries **(Fig. 71)**.

Enucleation and Evisceration Surgery

Wells Enucleation Spoon

It is a spoon-shaped instrument with a central cleavage to engage the optic nerve during enucleation procedure so that it can be easily cut with an enucleation scissor **(Fig. 72)**.

Mule Evisceration Spatula

It consists of a handle with small but stout rectangular blade with convex surface and blunt edges at its distal end. It is used to separate the uveal tissue from sclera in evisceration surgery **(Fig. 73)**.

Evisceration Curette

It consists of a round cup with blunt margins attached to a handle. It is used to curette out the intraocular contents during evisceration surgery.

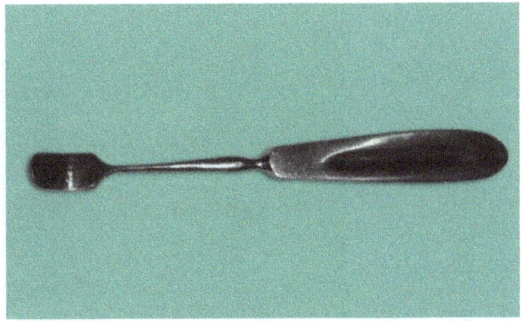

Fig. 73: Mule evisceration spatula.

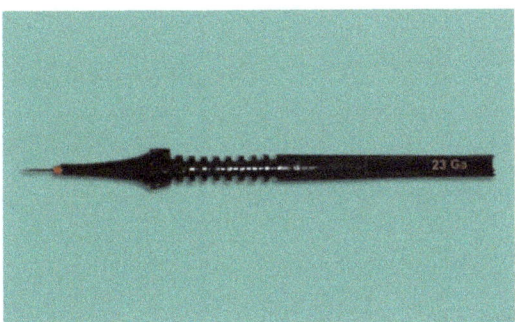

Fig. 74: Trocar.

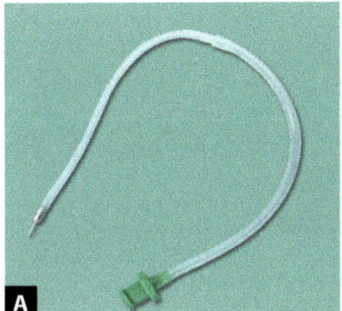
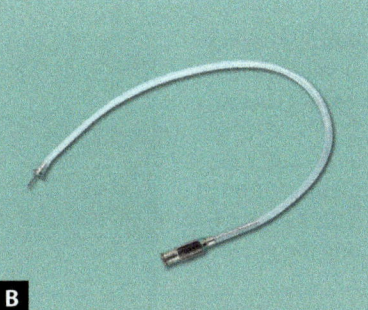
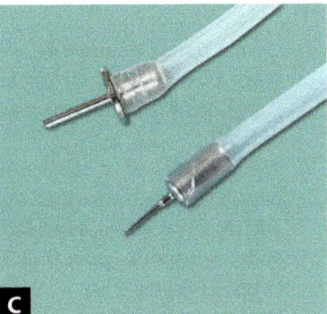

Figs. 75A to C: Infusion cannula. (A) 4-mm long tip canula; (B) 6-mm long tip canula; (C) Magnified image to compare the size of tips.

Vitreoretinal Surgery

Trocar and Cannula

Trocars are used to make pars plana sclerotomy entries. Trocar needle can be 20G/23G/25G/27G.

Microcannulas made up of polyimide, are preloaded on the needle trocars. Microcannula can be valved or nonvalved. Valved cannulas eliminate the need for plug placement while exchanging instruments or removing it.

Combined components of the trocar needle, microcannula, and trocar handle are referred to as the trocar-cannula assembly. This system maintains the alignment between the entry holes in conjunctiva and sclera, as well as provides unobstructed instrument access **(Fig. 74)**.

Infusion Cannula

Self-retaining infusion cannulas of different sizes according to microcannula (20G/23G/25G/27G) are used to introduce irrigating solution into the vitreous cavity **(Figs. 75A to C)**. The commonly used infusion cannula has a tip length of 4 mm. Infusion cannula with 6-mm long tip is used in cases with choroidal detachment or edema wherein the 4-mm tip may not be long enough to enter the vitreous cavity. 6-mm long canula is wider in diameter and is suture fixed to 20G sclerotomy incision without the microcannula.

Vitrectomy Cutter

Vitreous cutters utilize suction and inclusive shearing force to cut vitreous.

These can be of two broad types:
1. *Electrodynamic cutters:* It is heavy, becomes hot causing fatigue and exacerbates tremors.
2. *Pneumatic cutters:* It is light, so cause fewer tremors and are cheap.

Vitrectomy cutters are of three types based on the cutting mechanism:
1. *Cutters using rotating mechanism:* There is risk of vitreous spooling and traction on retina.

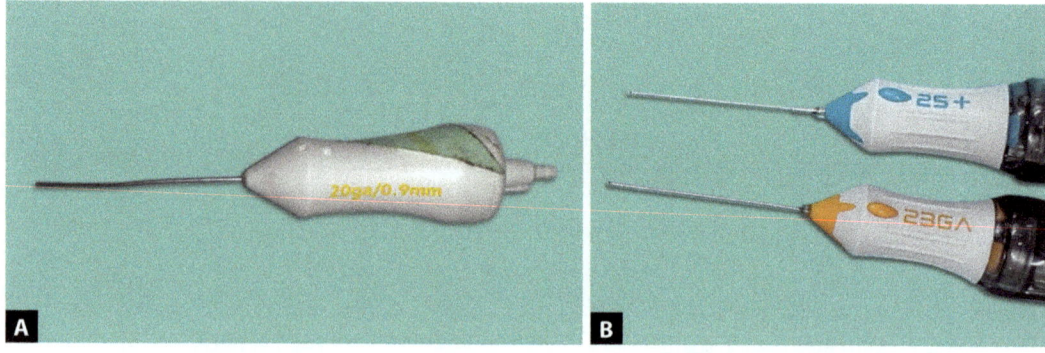

Figs. 76A and B: Vitrectomy cutters. (A) 20G cutter; (B) Micro-incisional vitrectomy system cutters—23G and 25G.

2. *Cutter using oscillating mechanism/Peyman type:* This type of cutter is considered to be superior to the first one as it has less shearing effect.
3. *The guillotine type cutters:* It has an outer tube which is fixed and has an opening through which vitreous is aspirated. The inner tube slides across the port thus cutting the vitreous **(Figs. 76A and B)**.

While the conventional vitrectomy system used 20G cutters, the micro-incisional vitrectomy systems use 23G, 25G, or 27G cutters **(Figs. 76A and B)**.

End-grasping Forceps

These forceps have jaws at the tip to hold tissues at the edge only. The tips are fine and allow visualization of the tissue while grasping. These are used for epiretinal membrane peeling **(Fig. 77)**.

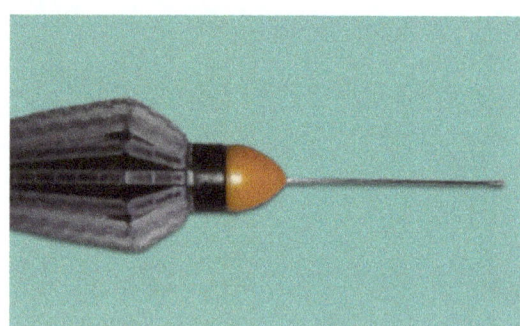

Fig. 77: End-grasping forceps.

Internal Limiting Membrane Forceps

These have fine tips with smaller jaws which help in picking up of delicate tissues such as internal limiting membrane (ILM). These are used for internal limiting membrane peeling in macular hole surgery **(Fig. 78)**.

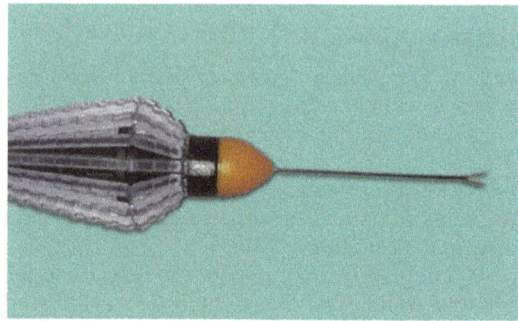

Fig. 78: Internal limiting membrane (ILM) forceps.

Serrated Forceps

These have large flat grasping blades without jaws, which help to attain strong grip over tissues while managing proliferative vitreoretinopathy. These are used in tough epiretinal membrane peeling and retinal pucker release.

Foreign Body Forceps

These are large gauge forceps with serrated or diamond-dusted tips for removal of intraocular foreign bodies. These have stout jaws which help in firm holding of the foreign bodies **(Fig. 79)**.

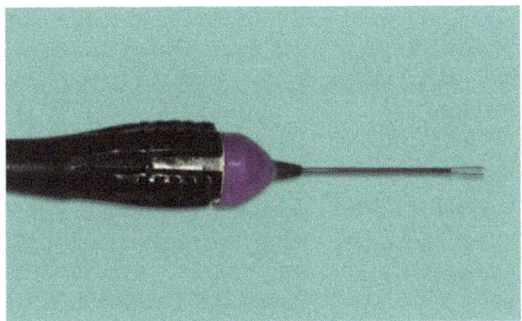

Fig. 79: Foreign body forceps.

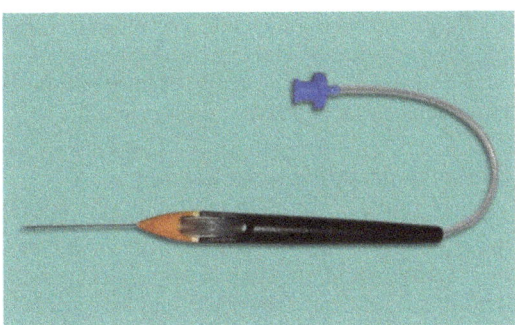

Fig. 81: Back flush.

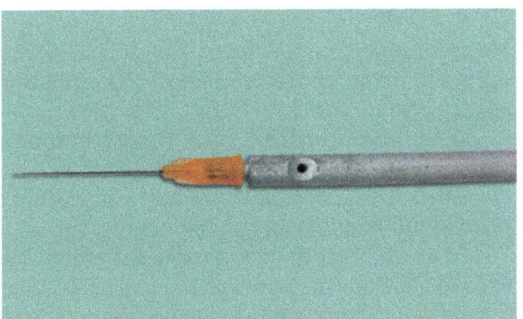

Fig. 80: Charles flute needle.

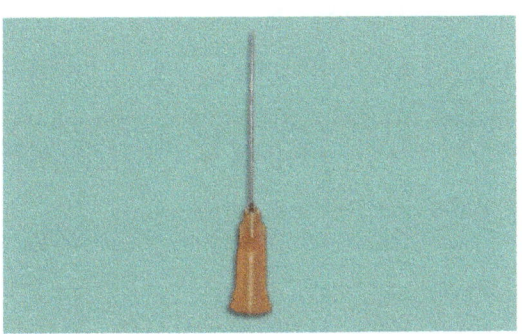

Fig. 82: Soft silicone tip cannula.

Extrusion Instruments

Charles flute needle: It consists of a blunt needle attached to a detachable handle. It is used for controlled passive extrusion of fluid during internal drainage of subretinal fluid, removal of preretinal blood, and fluid-air exchange. Internal channel leads to an exit port on the side of handle.

Egress of fluid occurs when cannula tip is in fluid and exit port is open, driven by infusion pressure which is above the atmospheric pressure. The blunt tip can be replaced with a soft silicone tip needle as well which decreases the risk of iatrogenic retinal damage **(Fig. 80)**.

Backflush is a modified flute handle with large silicone reservoir. Pressure on this reservoir leads to retrograde flushing of the fluid or accidentally aspirated/incarcerated tissues. It can also be used to disperse sedimented preretinal bleed. It can be used with either blunt or soft tip needle **(Fig. 81)**.

Cannula

Cannula tips can be of several types:
- *Silicone brush tip cannula:* The soft silicone brush tip allows gentle brushing and manipulation of the retina. These are excellent for manipulation and removal of blood from the retina surface.
- *Diamond-dusted soft silicone tip cannula:* These are used for triamcinolone removal.
- *Charles flute cannula:* This helps to aspirate blood and debris from the posterior segment. Smooth, finished tip provides atraumatic entry and reduces risk of trauma to surrounding tissue.
- *Soft silicone tip cannula:* The soft flexible tip on the cannula provides atraumatic entry through retinal or macular tears or holes. These are used for fluid-fluid or fluid-air exchange in vitrectomy surgery **(Fig. 82)**.
- *Dual bore cannula:* Simultaneous infusion of heavy liquids and aspiration of intraocular

fluids with dual bore cannula helps to control constant intraocular pressure during injection.

Cannula can be connected to flute handle or backflush handle or active extrusion handle.

Diamond-dusted Membrane Scraper

Tano diamond-dusted membrane scraper (DDMS) helps to find the edge of the epiretinal membranes. It is made of tongue-shaped soft silicone with inert diamond dust. Perfectly suited for both ILM and epiretinal membrane (ERM) removal, the diamond dusted, soft silicone tip helps in finding and grasping the edge of the membrane quickly and easily **(Fig. 83)**.

Retinal Pick

Retinal pick has a straight shaft with 0.5 mm angled tip **(Figs. 84A and B)**. This can be used for induction of posterior vitreous detachment, internal limiting membrane peeling initiation, and for engaging and lifting proliferative epiretinal membranes.

Finesse Loop

Finesse flex loop is used for scarping and initiating the ILM peeling. The surgeon-adjustable retractable nitinol loop has tines that allow no >85% penetration into the ILM. It has a concave shape to impede penetration with increasing force **(Figs. 85A and B)**.

Vitreoretinal Scissors

Horizontal scissors are used for delamination during epiretinal membrane removal. Their cutting edge moves conformal to the retinal surface.

Their blades can have a gentle curve or can be straight, with angle of 30 or 45° to the shaft.

Vertical scissors have vertical blades with pointed tips that move along the axis of shaft.

Proximal blade moves down toward the fixed distal blade to cut the tissue vertically. These are used for epiretinal membrane segmentation **(Fig. 86)**.

Viewing Lenses

Wide-angle viewing lenses: These lenses provide a wider view of the fundus during vitrectomy surgery and allow peripheral shave vitrectomy. These could be contact or noncontact in nature. Contact wide-angle lenses come in pediatric and

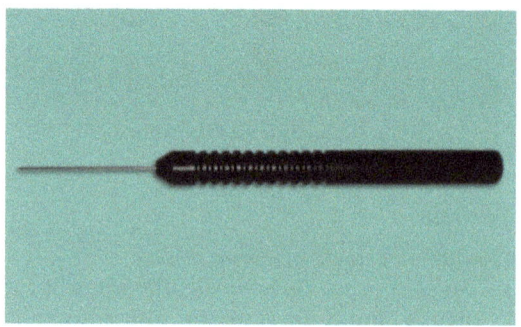

Fig. 83: Diamond-dusted membrane scraper.

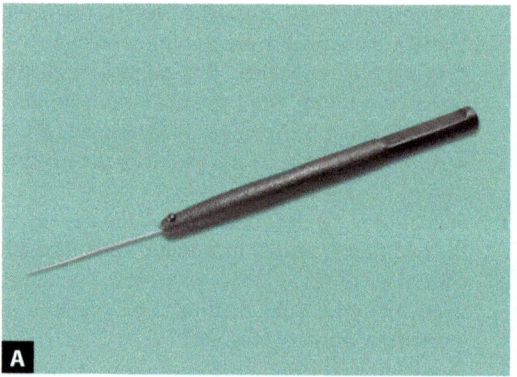
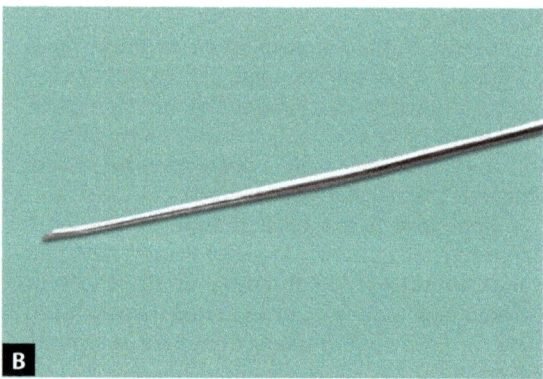

Figs. 84A and B: (A) Retinal pick; (B) Magnified image of the angled tip.

Instruments

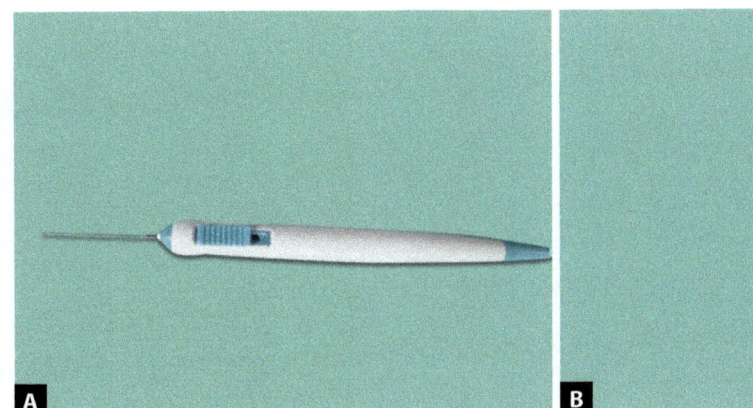

Figs. 85A and B: (A) Finesse flex loop; (B) High magnification image of the adjustable nitinol loop at the tip.

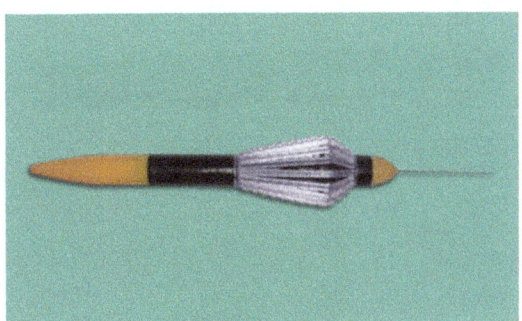

Fig. 86: Vitreoretinal scissors.

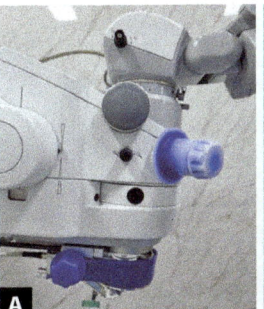 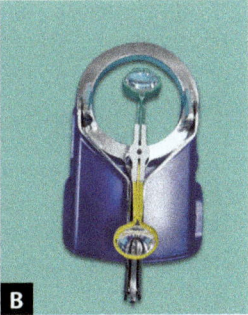

Figs. 88A and B: ReSight noncontact viewing system. (A) In attached state to the microscope; (B) Assembly of lenses (yellow lens for wide-angle viewing and green for posterior pole viewing) and holder.

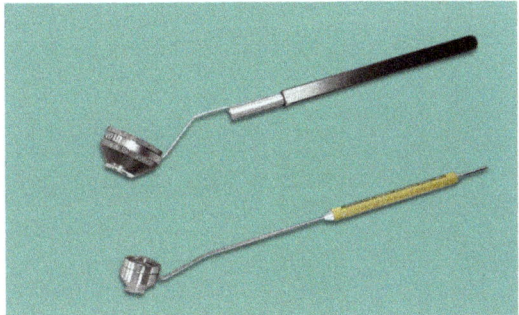

Fig. 87: Pediatric and adult size contact wide angle lenses.

adult sizes **(Fig. 87)**. The noncontact systems do not require an assistant to hold the lens handle **(Figs. 88A and B)**. Resight (Carl Zeiss Meditec AG, Jena, Germany) and Binocular Indirect Ophthalmo Microscope (BIOM; Oculus, Wetzlar, Germany) are the common noncontact viewing systems.

Macular lenses: Like the wide-angle viewing lenses, these could be contact or noncontact in nature. Contact lenses include plano-concave irrigating lens and self-retaining Chalam lens **(Figs. 89A and B)**. Noncontact systems also have a macular lens for a magnified view.

Gass Retinal Detachment Hook

Used for localization of retinal breaks onto the sclera in retinal detachment surgery **(Fig. 90)**.

Magnets

These are used to remove magnetic intraocular foreign bodies. Electromagnets are more powerful

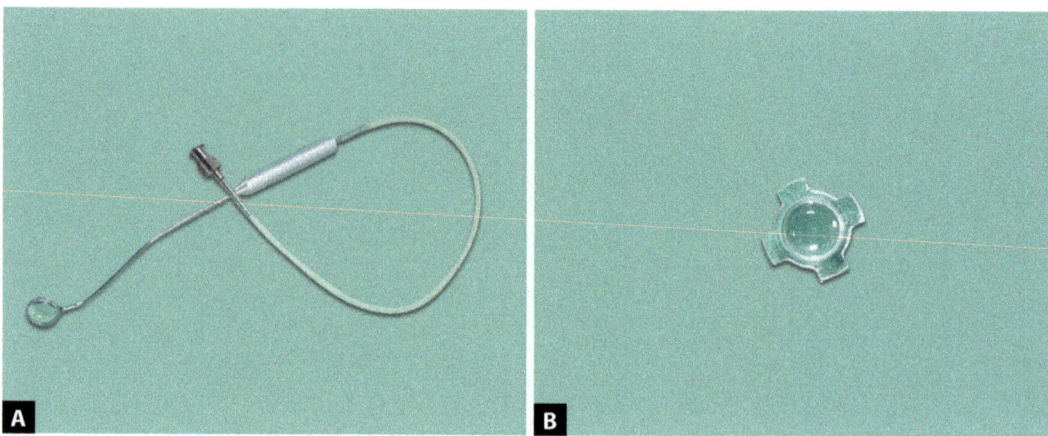

Figs. 89A and B: Contact lenses. (A) Irrigating hand-held plano-concave lens; (B) Self-retaining Chalam lens with flanges.

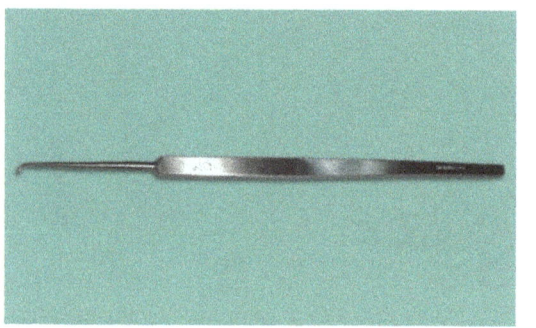

Fig. 90: Gass retinal detachment hook.

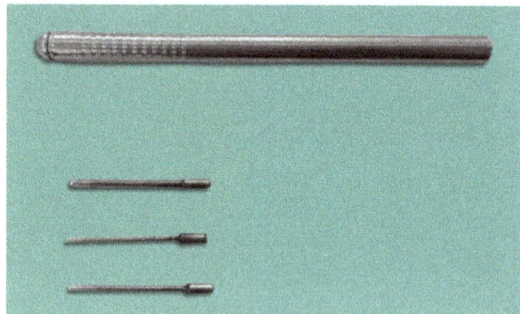

Fig. 91: Magnets.

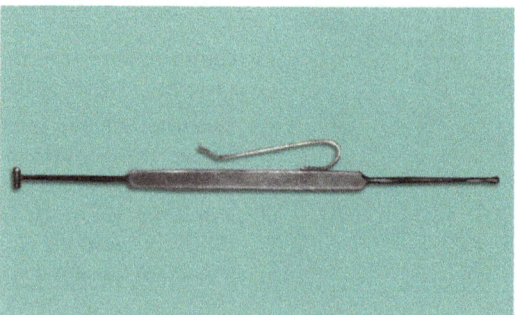

Fig. 92: Schocket scleral depressor.

than rare earth magnets (REM) and their magnetic force can be varied but they are used only as external magnets. Rare earth magnets are available for both intraocular and extraocular use **(Fig. 91)**.

Schocket Scleral Depressor

It has a rounded end designed for depressing the sclera, and a curved marking end for reaching behind the globe **(Fig. 92)**.

CHAPTER 8

Supplementary Chapter of Glaucoma

LONG CASES

PRIMARY OPEN ANGLE GLAUCOMA

Dewang Angmo, Vaishali Ghanshyam Rai, Ritika Mukhija

■ INTRODUCTION

Glaucoma is a chronic, degenerative optic neuropathy which may or may not be associated with raised intraocular pressure (IOP). The glaucomas are classified by the appearance of the iridocorneal angle into two broad categories open angle **(Fig. 1)** and closed angle. In open-angle glaucoma (OAG) the iridocorneal angle is open (unobstructed) and normal in appearance but aqueous outflow is diminished.[1] It may be of primary or secondary type. Primary (no other associated disease) open-angle glaucoma (POAG) includes both adult-onset disease (occurring after 40 years of age) and juvenile-onset disease (occurring between the ages of 3 and 40 years of age). Secondary (secondary to some other disease in eye) OAG include those associated with pseudoexfoliation or pigment dispersion syndrome.[1] Primary open angle glaucoma case is commonly kept in practical examination as long case.[2]

■ HISTORY

Epidemiology

Primary open angle glaucoma primarily affects persons >40 years of age, which is the second leading cause of blindness in the United States and the leading cause of blindness among black Americans. In India, it accounts for almost half of the cases (5.8% of blindness in India is attributable to glaucoma). Gender predilection is controversial, most study reports no predilection.[1,2]

Chief complaints: POAG can present in the following ways:
- Commonly an incidental finding on ocular examination.

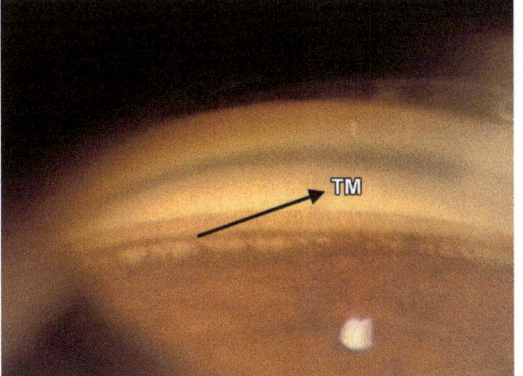

Fig. 1: Open angles on gonioscopy.
(TM: trabecular meshwork)

- POAG has no associated symptoms or other warning signs before the development of advanced visual field loss.
- Patient may present with eye pain and redness and gradually diminishing vision for distance.
- Other complaints can be blurred vision with or without color halos, frequent change of glasses or early morning or afternoon blurred vision with or without heaviness in eyes depending on IOP peak.

History of Present Illness

History must include the onset and progression of vision loss. In addition, following points must be noted:
- Brief history of patient's previous records to get baseline IOP.
- Patient who is already on treatment for glaucoma, it is important to know how many medications he/she is using and whether this treatment has sufficiently controlled IOP and visual field loss.
- Must also check for compliance of medications
- Patient's previous visual fields record should be checked to know the progression of glaucoma.
- Any other record such as OCT, GDx.

History of Past Illness

Past history of ocular trauma is important to rule angle recession glaucoma.

Surgical History

History of previous ocular surgery like cataract surgery, retinal surgery, trabeculectomy, penetrating keratoplasty or any laser procedure such as peripheral iridotomy (PI) must be recorded.

History of Systemic Illness

- Hypertensive, thyroid diseases and diabetic patients are at increased risk of developing POAG.
- *Cardiovascular disease:* Systemic hypertension (HTN) has weak association with glaucoma. Beta-blockers given for systemic HTN can reduce IOP and so a patient who is on systemic beta-blockers, topical ones should be avoided as the first-line therapy. Thyroid diseases and diabetic patients usually show more association with POAG.
- *Vasospastic diseases:* Migraine, Raynaud's syndrome may be associated with increased incidence of glaucoma.
- *Hemodynamic crisis*: Acute blood loss (postpartum hemorrhage, ruptured abdominal aneurysm, severe trauma, stroke) can cause severe systemic hypotension, destabilizing the ocular blood flow and increase the optic nerve damage.
- *Endocrine*: Diabetes and thyroid may have an increased risk of glaucoma. Cushing's syndrome cause endogenous release of corticosteroids.
- It is very important to ask about cardiovascular disease, renal diseases and bronchial asthma before deciding on antiglaucoma treatment.
- History of disorders which cause endogenous release of corticosteroids, e.g., Cushing's syndrome must be enquired.

Drug History

- History of use of ocular and systemic medications, especially if patient is already on systemic beta-blockers (topical beta-blockers would work suboptimally) must be enquired.
- Known local or systemic intolerance to ocular or systemic medications.
- History of long-term use of corticosteroid in any form like eye drop, nasal spray (example for allergic rhinitis), systemic (example for asthma) is important to rule out steroid-induced glaucoma.
- Long-term systemic use of steroids following any major organ transplantation surgery, e.g., liver or kidney transplant surgery.
- Long-term topical use of steroids following keratoplasty or chronic allergic keratitis, e.g., vernal keratoconjunctivitis.
- History of systemic use of topiramate needs to rule out.
- Any hypersensitivity reaction to antiglaucoma medications both topical and sulpha allergy.

Family History

Relatives of POAG patients are at higher risk for developing glaucoma. The severity and outcome of glaucoma in family members, including history of visual loss from glaucoma is also important.

Personal History

Alcohol, smoking (as both can have toxic effects on optic nerve which is already compromised due to glaucoma), excessive weightlifting, trumpet blowing or yoga postures or exercises involving Valsalva maneuver.

■ EXAMINATION

General Examination/Specific Systemic Examination

Detailed systemic examination to rule out neurofibromatosis, Sturge-Weber syndrome, carotid-cavernous fistula, thyrotoxicosis exophthalmos which cause elevated episcleral venous pressure and secondary open angle glaucoma must be done.

Ocular Examination

Eyeball: Usually looks normal.

Lids: Usually normal. In patient who is already on antiglaucoma medications like prostaglandin analogs look for hyperpigmentation of lid margin and long eyelashes.

Conjunctiva: All antiglaucoma medications can cause some form of conjunctival toxicity so always look for conjunctival congestion. This congestion is more in inferior quadrant.

Cornea: The cornea is typically normal in POAG. Ocular hypertension has a higher incidence of increased central corneal thickness (CCT) hence CCT measurement is important. Thinner CCT corneas are at higher risk for POAG. IOP is also affected by CCT. Fluorescein (Na fluorescein 1%) staining with cobalt blue light examination of cornea is advisable to look for corneal surface toxicity caused by some antiglaucoma medications.

Pupils: The pupils are examined for direct and consensual light reflex. Relative afferent pupillary defect indicates advanced glaucoma.

Anterior segment: A slit-lamp biomicroscopic examination of the anterior segment can provide evidence of physical findings associated with narrow angles, corneal pathology, or a secondary mechanism for elevated IOP such as pseudoexfoliation, pigment dispersion, iris and angle neovascularization, or inflammation.

IOP: IOP is measured in each eye, preferably using a Goldmann applanation tonometer before gonioscopy or dilation of the pupil. Time of day should be recorded because of diurnal variation.

Points to be noted for IOP:
- Done by NCT/GAT
- Time of procedure
- CCT
- On what antiglaucoma drugs—number and timings
- Compliance of patient
- Baseline IOP

Gonioscopy: The diagnosis of POAG requires careful evaluation of the anterior-chamber angle to exclude angle closure or secondary causes of IOP elevation, such as angle recession, pigment dispersion, peripheral anterior synechiae, angle neovascularization **(Fig. 1)**.

Optic disc and retinal nerve fiber layer: It is best done using +90D or +78D lens with slit-lamp under dilated pupils. Following points must be remembered **(Table 1)**:
- Early findings include enlargement of the optic disc cup, deep cup, thinning or saucerizing of the neural rim **(Fig. 2)**, disc hemorrhages, and peripapillary atrophy (common at beta zone) **(Fig. 3)**.
- The diagnosis of glaucoma should be strongly considered if vertical CD ratio ≥0.7 or asymmetric cupping between two eyes is >0.2.
- Changes at lamina cribrosa—laminar dot sign.
- Changes at neuroretinal rim—look for focal or diffuse defect in neuroretinal rim which does not obey ISNT rule.
- For glaucoma superior and inferior loss occurs.
- For neuro-ophthalmic cause temporal and nasal loss of NRR occurs.
- Vascular changes—nasalization of retinal vessels, bayoneting of vessels, baring of circumlinear vessels.
- Changes in retinal nerve fiber layer (RNFL)—look for focal or diffuse defect in RNFL using red-free illumination (green filter).

Table 1: Commonly used antiglaucoma medications.

Class	Mechanism	Drugs	Dose	Ocular side effects	Systemic side effects
Prostaglandin analogs (prostamide)	Increase in uveoscleral outflow of aqueous humor	Latanoprost (Xalatan)—0.005%, travoprost (Travatan)—0.004%, tafluprost (Zioptan)—0.0015%, bimatoprost (Lumigan)—0.01%, 0.03% Unoprostone (Rescula)—0.15%	HS	Conjunctival hyperemia, lengthening and darkening of eyelashes, brown discoloration of the iris, uveitis, macular edema	Minimal; may be related to headaches
β-adrenergic blockers	Reduction of aqueous humor production	Timolol (0.5/0.25%), levobunolol, carteolol, metipranolol, betaxolol	OD or BD	Irritation and dry eyes	Contraindicated in patients with asthma, chronic pulmonary obstructive disease, and cardiac failure, bradycardia
α-adrenergic agonists	Initial reduction of aqueous humor with subsequent effect of increase in outflow	Brimonidine (0.1/0.15%), apraclonidine	TID sometimes BD	Irritation, dry eyes, allergic reaction	CNS effects and respiratory arrest in young children (contraindicated <2 years); caution in patients with cerebral or coronary insufficiency, postural hypotension, renal or hepatic failure
Carbonic anhydrase inhibitors	Reduction of aqueous humor production	Dorzolamide (2%), brinzolamide (1%), acetazolamide (oral)	TID sometimes BD	Irritation, dry eyes, burning sensation with topical agents	Oral form may be associated with paresthesia, nausea, diarrhea, loss of appetite and taste, lassitude, or renal stones
Cholinergic agonists	Increase in aqueous humor outflow	Pilocarpine (0.5/1.0/2.0%), carbachol	Usually QID, but may vary	Irritation, induced myopia and decreased vision due to ciliary spasm	Ciliary spasm leading to headaches in young patients
ROCK inhibitors (Rho kinase inhibitors)	Relaxation of smooth muscle cells in trabecular meshwork thus decreasing outflow resistance	Ripasudil (0.4%), netarsudil (0.02%)	Ripasudil BD, Netarsudil OD	Conjunctival hyperemia, subconjunctival Hemorrhage, corneal verticillata	Minimal

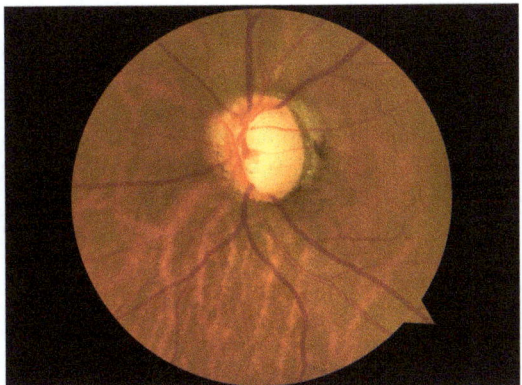

Fig. 2: Enlargement of the optic disc cup, thinning or saucerizing of the neural rim and peripapillary atrophy.

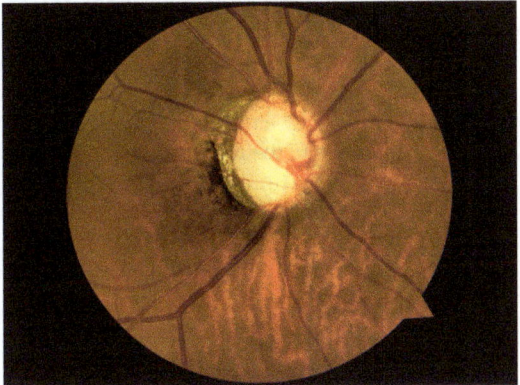

Fig. 3: Advanced glaucoma with near total cupping, thinned neural rim and peripapillary atrophy.

Look for other abnormalities of fundus that might account for visual field defects, e.g., optic nerve pallor, tilted disc, disc drusen, optic disc pits, optic nerve hypoplasia, neurological disease, macular degeneration, and other retinal disease.

■ DIFFERENTIAL DIAGNOSIS

Ocular hypertension—Following points help in differentiation:
- High IOP > 21 mm Hg on two consecutive occasions with applanation tonometry
- Normal optic disc and neuroretinal rim (NRR)
- Normal visual field
- Open angles on gonioscopy
- Absence of any other ocular disease causing raised IOP.

Pigmentary glaucoma: following points help in differentiation:
- Younger age group 20–30 years
- Pigments dispersion on corneal endothelium, lens surface
- Midperipheral iris transillumination defect
- Wide open angles with dark broad pigmentation of trabecular meshwork on gonioscopy.

Pseudoexfoliation glaucoma—following points help in differentiation:
- Higher IOP and greater 24 hours IOP fluctuation
- Exfoliation material deposits on corneal endothelium, at pupillary margin, on lens surface, upon trabecular meshwork on gonioscopy.
- Diffuse loss of NRR
- Greater visual field loss

Steroid-induced glaucoma—following points help in differentiation:
- History of corticosteroid intake in any form
- History of endogenous disease causing increased blood corticosteroid levels
- Usually bilateral but can be unilateral also
- Other ocular side effects due to steroid use, e.g., posterior subcapsular cataract.

Angle recession glaucoma—Following points help in differentiation:
- Past history of ocular trauma
- Angle recession on gonioscopy
- Other signs may be seen as phacodonesis, iridodonesis, traumatic cataract or retinal tear
- Usually unilateral.

Normal Tension Glaucoma

- Glaucomatous optic disc cupping
- IOP in statistically normal range
- Usually hypertensive and cardiac patients
- Usually associated with optic disc hemorrhage

■ INVESTIGATIONS

Following investigations are done in a case of POAG:

Diurnal variation in IOP: IOP needs to be recorded every 3 hourly for 24 hours, important for
- Diagnose early cases of glaucoma
- Assess pretreatment baseline IOP (highest recorded IOP before the diagnosis of glaucoma without any medication)

- Pick-up nocturnal rise of IOP
- Helpful in timing of antiglaucoma medications
- Assess maximum-minimum variation of IOP—IOP difference of 8 mm Hg or more between any two readings is significant.

Pachymetry: To estimate central corneal thickness and correction of IOP accordingly.

Perimetry: Usually automated perimetry to document visual field loss.

Retinal nerve fiber layer thickness: Retinal nerve fiber layer (RNFL) assessment by optical coherence tomography (OCT), GDx and Heidelberg retinal tomogram (HRT).

Fundus photography: For documentation of optic nerve head changes.

MANAGEMENT

- *Patient counselling and lifestyle modifications:*
  - Lifelong therapy and follow-up is essential
  - Aim is to preserve vision with medications not gain vision
  - Vision once lost will not come back
  - Regular aerobic exercise
  - Quit smoking, alcohol
  - Meditation and breathing exercises have shown to decrease IOP
  - Avoid head down yoga postures
  - Control hypertension and diabetes
- *Medical treatment:*
  - Target IOP: In every diagnosed case of glaucoma, target IOP should be calculated to halt or prevent further glaucomatous damage to optic nerve and visual field loss progression.
  - Start with one or two medication based on target IOP (*See* viva section). Beta-blockers and prostaglandin (PG) analogs are often the first choice (*See* **Table 1**).[2]
  - Adjuvant treatment with neuroprotectives like N-methyl D-aspartate (NMDA) receptors like memantine; alpha 2 adrenergic agonists-like brimonidine; Calcium channel blocking agents, e.g., flunarizine, nimodipine, antioxidants or nitric oxide synthetase inhibitors can be considered.
  - Follow every 3 months in mild to moderate visual field loss cases and 1 monthly in advanced cases. Every patient should be checked for compliance and tolerance to antiglaucoma medications. IOP with Goldmann applanation tonometry should be recorded at each follow-up to monitor IOP control and target IOP with medication.
  - Visual fields with standard automated perimetry should be done every year in ocular hypertension with high-risk cases, every 6 monthly in mild to moderate cases while every 3 monthly in advanced cases to monitor progression of disease and modification in treatment accordingly.
- *Laser trabeculoplasty:* The indications of laser trabeculoplasty include—
  - In patients who cannot or will not use medications reliably due to cost, memory problems, difficulty with instillation, or intolerance to the medication.
  - To reduce the number of glaucoma drops
  - Failure of medical therapy as a less invasive alternative therapy compared to surgery
  - The available methods of laser trabeculoplasty are:
    - Argon laser trabeculoplasty (ALT)—more than 75% of unoperated eyes have a good reduction of IOP initially. Within 5 years, 30% to >50% eyes need additional surgical management. Repeat ALT usually (90%) fails to control IOP by 2 years.
- *SLT (Selective laser trabeculoplasty):* It uses Q-switched frequency doubled Nd:YAG. The efficacy of SLT is similar to ALT.
- Micropulse laser trabeculoplasty
- *Filtration surgery—Trabeculectomy:* Indications:
  - Patients from rural areas where follow-up is likely to be difficult
  - Patients with baseline IOP of more than 40 mm Hg where even maximal medical therapy will be unsuccessful
  - Patients who have lost one eye due to glaucoma at presentation
  - Failure to control IOP after maximal tolerated medical therapy

- Patient develops side-effects of antiglaucoma treatment
- IOP not at target on three topical medications or progression of visual fields despite maximum medical therapy
- Poor compliance to medical therapy.
- *Glaucoma drainage devices:*
  Indications:
  - Patients who have failed filtering surgery with antimetabolites
  - Patients whose conjunctiva is so scarred from previous surgery that filtering surgery with antimetabolites is at high risk for failure.
- *Nonpenetrating glaucoma surgery:*
  - Viscocanalostomy
  - Nonpenetrating deep sclerectomy
  - Sinusotomy
  - Canaloplasty.
- *Minimally invasive glaucoma surgeries:*
  Indication: Mild/moderate glaucoma
  Types of implants: (They help improve outflow)
  - Trabecular—iStent, Hydrus
  - Suprachoroidal stents—iStent supra, Gold Micro-shunt, MINIject
  - Subconjunctival implants—XEN, PreserFlo, Express shunt

  Excisional MIGS:
  - BANG—Bent Ab interno needle goniectomy
  - Kahook blade

  Endoscopic cyclophotocoagulation (ECP): Decreases inflow

VIVA QUESTIONS

Q.1. What are the most important parameters on clinical examination that lead you to investigate the patient for open angle glaucoma?

Ans.
- Raised intraocular pressure (IOP)
  - Optic disc cupping:
    - Retinal edema
    - A suspicious disc with increased vertical cup-to-disc (CD) ratio more than or equal to 0.7
    - Asymmetric cupping between two eyes >0.2
    - A diffuse or focal thinning of the neuroretinal rim which does not obey the ISNT rule (normally the inferior rim is thickest followed by superior, nasal and temporal), and a retinal nerve fiber layer defect in red free light.
- Field changes suggestive of glaucoma
- Additional risk factors, e.g., age, myope, diabetes mellitus, hypertension, thyroid disease, family history of glaucoma.

Q.2. What is the importance of DVT in POAG management?

Ans. Diurnal variation is very important in a glaucoma patient both for—
- Diagnosis—to establish baseline IOP, determine magnitude of IOP fluctuation and the timing of peak IOP.
- Management—to establish diurnal control with ocular hypotensive drugs and maintain IOP below target with a fluctuation of less than 5 mm Hg, instill medicines at a time to cover peak IOP spikes.

Q.3. Define target IOP and how you will calculate target IOP?

Ans. Target IOP may be defined as a pressure, rather a range of intraocular pressure levels within which the progression of glaucoma and visual field loss will be delayed or halted. It is calculated depending on severity of glaucomatous optic damage. The severity of glaucoma damage can be estimated using the following scales:
- *Mild*: Characteristic optic nerve abnormalities consistent with glaucoma and a normal visual field as tested with standard automated perimetry.
- *Moderate*: Characteristic optic nerve abnormalities consistent with glaucoma and visual field abnormalities in one hemifield and not within 5° of fixation.
- *Severe*: Characteristic optic nerve abnormalities consistent with glaucoma and visual field abnormalities in both hemifields and loss within 5° of fixation in at least one hemifield.

Depending on severity of glaucomatous optic disc damage, American Academy of

Ophthalmology has given guidelines to estimate target IOP as follow:
- In mild damage cases—30% reduction of IOP from baseline IOP
- In advanced damage cases—40% reduction of IOP from baseline IOP
- In ocular hypertension cases—20% reduction of IOP from baseline IOP
- In normal tension glaucoma (NTG) cases—30% reduction of IOP from baseline IOP.

Q.4. What are the qualitative evaluation and quantitative evaluation of optic nerve head in case of glaucoma?

Ans. *Qualitative evaluation:*
- Contour of the neuroretinal rim
- Optic disc hemorrhage
- Parapapillary atrophy
- Bared circumciliary vessels
- Appearance of retinal nerve fiber layer.

Quantitative evaluation:
- Optic disc size (vertical disc diameter)
- Cup disc ratio
- Rim disc ratio.

Q.5. Which cup disc ratio is important horizontal or vertical and why?

Ans. The vertical cup disc ratio is more important since early neuroretinal rim loss occurs preferentially in upper and lower poles of disc.

Q.6. Why Goldmann's applanation tonometry should be done before gonioscopy and before dilatation of pupils?

Ans.
- During gonioscopy angle of anterior chamber opens up due to pressure over cornea, which results in reduction of IOP and applanation tonometry performed after gonioscopy gives low IOP than correct IOP.
- By dilatation of pupil there is transient rise in IOP 4–5 mm Hg that also gives high IOP than actual IOP on applanation tonometry if performed on dilated pupils.

Q.7. Which are preperimetric diagnostic tools of glaucoma?

Ans. Preperimetric diagnostic tools can defect early glaucomatous damage in RNFL even before that damage can be located on perimetry. These are GDxVCC, HRT, OCT and SWAP.

Q.8. What is the pathogenesis of primary open angle glaucoma?

Ans.
- *Genetics:*
  - *MYOC*: Myocilin (GLYC1A, chromosome 1), associated with juvenile open angle glaucoma and ≈4% of adults with POAG
  - *OPTN*: Optineurin (GLYC1E, chromosome 10)
  - *Other loci*: GLYC1B, GLYC1C
- *Pressure-dependent (mechanical factors):*
  - Increased IOP® compression and backward bowing of lamina cribrosa
    - Obstruction of axoplasmic transport
    - Ganglion cell death
- *Ischemic factors/pressure independent (esp significant for NTG):*
  - Vascular perfusion compromise (DM, HTN, migraine, Raynaud's phenomenon
  - Abnormal coagulability
  - Nocturnal hypertension, significant blood loss
- *Neurodegenerative factors:*
  - Primary ON damage leads to glutamate release, which interacts with cell receptors that leads to an increase in intracellular calcium levels
  - This triggers cell death via apoptosis and leads to further release of glutamate and a vicious cycle occurs.

Q.9. What is the role of central corneal thickness (CCT) in ocular hypertension (OHT)/open angle glaucoma (OAG)?

Ans. CCT measurement is important before diagnosing glaucoma and deciding the management, while it is not helpful in predicting risk of progression of existing glaucoma. CCT influences IOP measurement by applanation tonometry and therefore it is important to note CCT in every patient being evaluated for glaucoma. CCT can be broadly categorised as: Thin (<500 μm), Normal and Thick (>570 μm).

Refractive surgeries reduce the CCT and therefore the IOP measurements in such patients would be falsely low.

Q.10. Classify antiglaucoma drugs, their common side effects.

Ans. Refer to any Standard Textbook (*See* Table 1).

Q.11. Recent advances in pharmacotherapy in glaucoma.

Ans.
- Rocklatan – Fixed drug combination of Netarsudil + Latanoprost.
- Latanoprostene bunod (0.024%)—nitric oxide donar. Approved by FDA in 2017.
- Trabodenoson—Adenosine receptor agonist

Q.12. Newer drug delivery systems in glaucoma.

Ans.
- Durysta—Bimatoprost intracameral implant (10 mcg)
- iDose-Travoprost intracameral implant—In trials
- Contact lens-based drug delivery—silicon hydrogel soft contact lens with nanoparticles. In trials currently.
- Timoptic-XE 0.25%—Nanoparticles-based technology. Ph sensitive hydrogel formulation turns from solution to gel after coming in contact with tear film, thereby enhancing drug delivery.

Q.13. What is PAP in glaucoma?

Ans. Prostaglandin-associated periorbitopathy is a term to describe the eyelid and orbital changes that occur due to use of topical prostaglandin eye drops. It includes upper lid ptosis, deepening of upper lid sulcus, involution of dermatochalasis, periorbital fat atrophy, mild enophthalmos and inferior scleral show.

Q.14. What are the risk factors for progression of glaucoma?

Ans. Family history of glaucoma, low socioeconomic status, old age and young age, cardiovascular diseases, migraine, thin cornea and disc hemorrhage.

■ REFERENCES

1. Kwon YH, Fingert JH, Kuehn MH, Alward WL. Primary open-angle glaucoma. N Engl J Med. 2009;360(11):1113-24.
2. Weinreb RN, Aung T, Medeiros FA. The pathophysiology and treatment of glaucoma: a review. JAMA. 2014;311(18):1901-11.

Index

Page numbers followed by *b* refer to box, *f* refer to figure, *fc* refer to flowchart, and *t* refer to table

A

Abadie's sign 5, 37
Abduction, limitation of 376
Aberrant regeneration 371
Abetalipoproteinemia 252
Acanthamoeba 90, 91, 93*f*
   cysts 101
   keratitis 96
      antimicrobials for 108
Accommodation, near point of 398
Accommodative esotropia 401
   classification of 401*t*
Acetazolamide 187, 316
   mechanism of action of 317
Acetylcholine receptor antibody 416
   test 22
Acquired immunodeficiency
      syndrome 76
Acral lentiginous melanoma 14
Active force generation test 371, 378,
      400, 418
Acute corneal graft rejection 140,
      142, 142*f*, 143*f*
   differential diagnosis of 143*t*
   risk factors for 145
Acyclovir, topical 105
Adduction 369*f*
   limitation of 377*f*
Adenocarcinoma
   pleomorphic 49
   primary 48
Adenoid cystic carcinoma 4, 44*f*, 46,
      47, 49, 50
   prognosis of 50
Adenoma
   pleomorphic 46, 47, 49, 50
   sebaceous 70
Adnexa 343, 348
   ocular 231
Adrenergic blocking agents, topical 41
Aflibercept 227, 291
Age-related eye disease study
      classification 289*t*
Age-related macular degeneration
      187, 214, 267, 280, 283,
      284*f*, 287, 290, 357
   classification of 288*t*
   management of 290*t*
   treatment of 290

Aicardi syndrome 332
Air-assisted deep anterior lamellar
      keratoplasty 117, 131
Allen picture cards 429
Allergic eye disorders 91
Allergic reactions 51
Alpha-adrenergic agonists 490
Alport's syndrome 442, 445, 449, 450
Alstrom syndrome 254
Alternaria 94
Alternate cover test 396
Amblyopia 175, 220, 330, 400, 411,
      412, 435, 442
   management of 177
   treatment 403
Amelanotic melanoma 314
Amikacin 103
Amniotic membrane
      grafting 149, 163
      pterygium excision with 149
      transplantation 160
Amorphous hyaline 126
Amphotericin B 103
Amsler charting 261
Amsler grid 287, 290
   testing 232
Amsler-Dubois chart,
      modified 270, 271*f*
Amsler–Krumeich classification
      113*t*, 120
Amyloidosis 211, 217, 296
Anemia 216, 243, 246
Anesthesia
   infraorbital 4
   supraorbital 4
Aneurysm 368, 373
Angiography, wide-field 233
Angioma, retinal 214
Angiotensin-converting enzyme 160
   inhibitor, use of 243
Angle closure glaucoma 491
   classification of 186*t*
   management of 186*t*
   mechanisms of 188
Angle recession
   glaucoma 202, 203
   mechanism of 205
Angle, neovascularization of 199*f*, 202
Aniridia 110, 169, 196, 351
Anisometropia 220, 411, 412

Anophthalmia, bilateral 28*f*
Anophthalmos 175
Anterior chamber 31, 96, 135, 142,
      152, 183, 191, 215, 224,
      231, 281, 295, 318, 335,
      343, 348, 352, 362, 436,
      450, 458
   angle of 206
   cells, grading of 295*f*
   paracentesis 101
Anterior segment 340, 489
   dysgenesis 172, 196
   ischemia 379, 421
   optical coherence tomography
      101, 114, 125, 148, 176
   surgeon 354
Antiangiogenic drugs 200
Antibiotics 417
Anticholinergic agents 183
Anticorticosteroid therapy 316
Antifungals 103*t*
   topical 103
Antiglaucoma
   drugs 197, 199, 495
   medications 490*f*
Anti-inflammatory drugs 200
Antineutrophil cytoplasmic
      autoantibodies 232
Antinuclear antibodies 232
Antioxidant supplementation 289
Antiphospholipid antibody
      syndrome 388
Anti-vascular endothelial growth
      factors 150, 239*t*, 291
   agents 199, 227, 291, 323
   injections 219
Antivirals
   agents 76
   oral 105
Aphakia 351
   bilateral 431
Aphakic bullous keratopathy 135
Arden's ratio 360
Argon laser trabeculoplasty 492
Arruga intracapsular forceps 470, 471*f*
Arruga needle holder 466, 467*f*
Arsenic exposure 10
Arteriovenous malformations 85
Arteritic ischemic optic
      neuropathy 425*t*

Index

Artery
  forceps 464, 464f
  posterior communicating 373
Artificial intelligence, role of 433
Artificial tears 41
Aspiration 472, 473f
  cannula 470, 470f
Aspirin 79, 316
Asteroid hyalosis 217
Asthma, atopy-bronchial 110
Astigmatism 1
  type of 439
Asymmetric bow tie 120
Atrophy, macular 357f
Audiometry 444
Auscultation 6, 82
Autofluorescence 357
Autograft
  damage 150
  reversal of 150
Autoimmune disease 414
Automated lamellar therapeutic
  keratoplasty machine 477
Avastin 291
Avellino corneal dystrophy 125f
Axenfeld–Rieger syndrome 169
Azathioprine 145, 417
Azoles 102

B

Backflush 483, 483f
Bacteria, atypical 96
Bacterial keratitis 96, 103t
  management of 101
Bagolini striated glasses 370, 398
Ballett's sign 5, 37
Bandage contact lens 104
Band-shaped keratopathy 158, 160f
  associations of 159t
  histopathology of 161
  pathogenesis of 161
Bardet–Biedl syndrome 254
Bard-Parker blade 106
Bare sclera technique 149
Barkan's membrane 194
Barraquer eye speculum, self-
  retaining 462, 462f
Barraquer needle holder 466, 466f
Barron's artificial anterior chamber
  and clamp 476
Basal cell carcinoma 9, 11, 12, 68
  different histological types of 13
  lids manifestation of 14t
  pigmented 10f
Basal cell nevus syndrome 332
Basal hole diameter 261
Bassen–Kornzweig syndrome 252

Batten–Mayou syndrome 311
Beale–Collins picture chart tests 429
Beaten-bronze appearance 357
Beck's sign 5, 37
Becker and Armaly studies 208t
Beer belly appearance 158
Belin ABCD grading system 114t
Bell's palsy 76
  ocular
    manifestations of 75t
    signs of 75
    symptoms of 75
Bell's phenomenon 17, 20, 60, 418
  inverse 18
Berger's space 216
Berke's criteria 53t
Berke's method 17
Berke's ptosis clamp 479, 479f
Best corrected distance
  visual acuity 113
Beta-blockers 417
Beta-adrenergic blockers 490
BETT classification 365
Bevacizumab 291
Bielschowsky's head tilt test 383
Bielschowsky's phenomenon 421
Bielschowsky's theory 421
Bifoveal fixation 398
Big bubble deep anterior lamellar
  keratoplasty 117, 131
BIGH3 gene 129
Biguanide 108
Bimanual irrigation 472, 473f
Binocular function 370, 377
Binocular vision, tests for 398
Biogenic implants 29
Biointegrated implants 29
Biometry 430, 431, 437, 452, 460
Bionic eye, significance of 257
Biopsy 85
  corneal 101, 126
  excision 8, 11
Birth
  injury, forceps-related 195
  trauma 53, 171, 172, 195, 195t
Bladder cells 457f
Blade breaker 476f
Bleeding disorder 214
Blepharitis 68
  chronic marginal 152
Blepharochalasis 54
Blepharoconjunctivitis 68
Blepharokymographic analysis 73
Blepharophimosis 53, 63, 65, 66f
  epicanthus inversus ptosis
    syndrome 20, 64f, 66
  syndrome 53, 54, 58

Blepharoptosis 64
Blood
  disorders 221
  retinal barrier 234
  sugar 7, 73
    postprandial 230
Blowout fracture 30, 33, 371, 399
  etiopathogenesis of 33
Blunt tip chopper 472f
Blunt trauma 205, 363
Boek's Candy test 429
Bone, metastatic carcinoma to 159
Bony spicules 253f, 257
Boston's sign 5, 37
Botulinum toxin 372, 403, 412
  injection 41, 379
  role of 62
Bowman's lacrimal probe 479, 479f
Bowman's layer 156
Bowman's membrane 120
Brachydactyly 450
Bradycardia 30
Brain, magnetic resonance imaging
  of 191, 392, 423
Brainstem auditory evoked
  response 73
Branch retinal artery occlusion 197
Branch retinal vein occlusion 197,
  229, 232
  causes of 234
  classification of 235
  pathogenesis of 235
  risk factors for 230t
Brimonidine tartrate 197
Brodsky's theory 421
Brow suspension ptosis repair 20, 53
Bruckner test 396
Bruch's theory 33
B-scan ultrasonography 344, 348,
  430, 438, 452, 454
Buckling theory 33
Bull's eye
  appearance 446f
  maculopathy 357
    differential diagnosis of 358
Bullae formation 134f
Bullous keratopathy 91
Buphthalmos 165, 193, 195, 197, 434
  bilateral 193f
  differential diagnosis of 195
Burian's classification 408, 409
Busin glide 477, 478f
Byron Smith classification 26

C

Calcium-channel blockers 417
Cannula 481, 483
  tips 483

Capsular bag distention
        syndrome 454
Capsular support devices, use of 438
Capsule
    holding forceps 471*f*
    tension segments 438
Capsulorhexis 448
    anterior 431
Carbon monoxide 311
Carbonic anhydrase
        inhibitors 424, 490
Carcinoma 46
    lung 414
    metastatic 2
    mucoepidermoid 48
    sebaceous 70
Carcinosarcoma 48
Cardiovascular disease 174, 222, 488
Cardiovascular system 309
Carotid angiography 8
Carotid artery disease 201
Carotid cavernous fistula 9, 38, 201
Carotid ischemic diseases 197
Castroviejo caliper 467, 467*f*
Castroviejo corneoscleral scissors
        468, 468*f*
Castroviejo needle holder 466, 466*f*
Cat's eye syndrome 332
Cat's paw lacrimal wound retractor
        466, 466*f*
Cataract 149, 173, 297, 298, 328, 330,
        343, 430, 461
    bilateral 432
    congenital 432
    cortical 442
    development of 345
    diffuse concussion 459
    extraction 256
    formation 457
        pathomechanism of 345
    hypermature 434
    mature 434
    nondislocated 460
    partial 430
    pathophysiology of 461
    pediatric 433*t*
    snowflake 318
    subcapsular 442, 447
    subluxated 460*f*
    surgery 137, 211, 212*t*,
        214, 345, 469
    traumatic 457
    type of 345
    unilateral 432
    zonular 428-430
Cataracta nodiformis 458
Cataractous lens 438

Cavernous hemangioma 83, 84, 84*t*
    course of 83
    management of 83
Cavernous sinus 380
    structures in 386
Ceftazidime 103
Cellulitis, orbital 2
Central areolar choroidal
        dystrophy 357
Central corneal
    guttae 134, 134*f*
    lesions 163
    opacity 173
    thickness 110, 113, 157, 169,
        489, 494
    ulcer 93*f*
Central herpetic disciform
        keratitis 135
Central nervous system 190, 340
Central retinal
    artery occlusion 197, 310*f*, 311
    vein occlusion 197, 222, 225*f*,
        226*f*, 390
        pathogenesis of 227
        risk factors for 227
        types of 223*t*, 228
Central serous chorioretinopathy
        312, 314*f*, 315
    pathogenesis of 317
    risk factors with 317*t*
Cerebrospinal fluid 379
    diversion procedures 424
Cerebrovascular accident 239
Ceroid lipofuscinosis 357
Chalazion 68
    clamp 478, 478*f*
    scoop 478, 478*f*
Chandler's syndrome 135, 168, 170
Charge syndrome 332
Charles flute
    cannula 483
    needle 483, 483*f*
Charleux sign 112
Chelation 160
Chemosis, conjunctival 150
Chemotherapy 12
    systemic 69, 306
Cherry-red spot 309, 310, 310*f*
    bilateral 310
    causes of 310
    differential diagnosis of 310, 311*b*
    pathophysiology of 311
    unilateral 310
Chest compression 215
Chloroquine 254, 417
    retinal toxicity 357
Cholinergic agonists 490

Chopper 471, 472*f*
Chorioretinal venous
        anastomosis 227
Chorioretinopathy, chronic central
        serous 313
Choristoma 80
Choroidal coloboma 330, 332
    pathophysiology of 331
Choroidal excavation 304, 329*f*
Choroidal mass 268
Choroidal melanoma 299, 300, 301*t*,
        303*t*, 305-307
    diagnosis of 304, 306
    pigmented 303*f*
    prognostic factors of 307
    risk factors for 306
Choroidal neovascular membrane
        220, 325, 357
    classification of 288
Choroidal neovascularization 262,
        283, 287, 289, 290, 330
    membrane 286*f*
    progression of 292
Choroidal nevus 303*t*
Choroidal pathologies 301*t*
Choroidal rupture 363
Choroideremia 254
Choroiditis, ultrawide-field
        pseudocolor of 268*f*
Ciancia syndrome 402
Cicatricial ectropion 56, 57*f*
    generalized 58
    management of 58
    severe 58
Cicatricial entropion 61
    causes of 61
Ciliary body band, widening of 204*f*
Clinical activity score 39
Coat's disease 201, 246
Cobweb opacity 459
Cogan twitch sign 21
Cogan–Reese syndrome 168, 169
Colibri forceps 463, 463*f*
Colibri-style polack double corneal
        forceps 476
Collaborative ocular melanoma 307
        study 303*t*
Collagen cross-linking 104, 154
    role of 158
Collagen vascular disease 388
Coloboma 327, 329*f*, 331, 333
    atypical 331
    choroidal excavation of 329*f*
    histopathology of 331
    isolated 87
    macular 329
    posterior segment 331

simple 87
types of 331, 334
typical 331
zonular 329*f*
Color haloes 121
Color vision 389, 426
Comitant esotropia, types of 400*t*
Complete blood count 7, 341, 372
Compressive optic neuropathy 390
Computed tomography 11, 52, 80, 84
high-resolution 45
scan 7, 31, 32*f*, 38, 78
Cone-rod dystrophy 110, 254, 357
Confocal microscopy 101, 125, 136, 143, 169
Congenital corneal opacity 172*b*
causes of 171*t*
differential diagnosis of 172*t*
Congenital cranial dysinnervation disorders 411
Congenital glaucoma 153, 165, 171, 172, 192, 192*t*, 193*f*, 195, 195*t*
classification of 196
management of 196
Congenital hereditary endothelial dystrophy 135, 136, 159, 160*f*, 164, 164*f*, 165, 165*f*, 166, 166*f*, 166*t*, 172
complications of 167
Congenital hereditary stromal dystrophy 165, 172
Congenital ptosis 18-20, 51, 54
causes of 53
Conjunctiva 6, 31, 36, 45, 55, 64, 68, 71, 72, 87, 90, 92, 110, 123, 134, 141, 147, 152, 155, 159, 162, 164, 183, 191, 198, 203, 206, 209, 215, 224, 231, 244, 252, 281, 295, 300, 318, 326, 335, 352, 361, 370, 382, 388, 412, 429, 436, 443, 446, 450, 453, 458, 489
bulbar 11
palpebral 11
Conjunctival autograft
edema 150
pterygium excision with 149
Conjunctival closure, primary 149
Conjunctival dermoid 80*t*
cyst 79, 80
Conjunctival flaps 104, 106
Conjunctival intraepithelial neoplasia 148
Connective tissue disorders 91, 152
noninflammatory 110

Conservative therapy 354
Contact lens 92, 115, 153, 431, 486*f*
wear 109
Contraceptives, oral 233
Contracted socket 24, 27, 28*f*
causes of 27
mechanism of 28
mild 26
moderate-to-severe 26
morphological classification of 26*t*
Contusion, orbital 311
Convergence, near point of 398
Cool compresses 41
Cornea 7, 11, 18, 31, 45, 55, 64, 68, 72, 90, 93, 94, 123, 134, 141, 147, 152, 155, 159, 162, 164, 168, 171, 173, 183, 191, 193, 198, 203, 206, 209, 215, 224, 231, 237, 244, 252, 281, 300, 318, 328, 335, 343, 348, 352, 362, 370, 377, 383, 388, 429, 436, 443, 446, 450, 453, 458, 489
anterior 123
ectatic protrusion of 111*f*
normal 120
plana 436
posterior surface of 168*f*
Corneal biopsy 101, 126
indications of 106
Corneal blood staining 172
Corneal choristoma classification 178
Corneal collagen cross-linking, role of 154
Corneal Dellen 150
Corneal diameter, normal 152*f*, 195
Corneal disorders 169
Corneal dystrophy 110
classification of 126
macular 121, 128, 129, 132
posterior polymorphous 110, 135, 136, 138, 152, 166, 166*t*, 171, 172
Corneal endothelial
punches 476
reflex, increased intensity of 112
Corneal erosion, recurrent 121, 122, 128, 137
Corneal exposure
medical treatment for 74
supportive care for 74
syndromes 159
Corneal graft rejection 140
Corneal guttae, causes of 138
Corneal nerves, prominent 112
Corneal opacification, neonatal 172

Corneal opacity 122, 173
congenital 172*b*
treatment of 172
Corneal pachymetry 136
Corneal perforation 94, 150
Corneal protrusion 155
Corneal scar 111, 111*f*, 150, 175
Corneal sensations 94, 125
Corneal stromal dystrophy 121
differential diagnosis of 127*t*
Corneal stromal edema, stage of 134
Corneal thickness 125, 165*f*
Corneal thinning 94, 111, 150, 155
Corneal tomography 148, 153, 156
Corneal transplantation 116
Corneal trephines 474
Corneal ulcer 90, 91*t*, 94*f*, 95*f*, 106, 107
differential diagnosis of 98*t*
etiological diagnosis of 106
grading of 97*t*, 107
Corneoscleral laceration 172
Coronary artery disease 368
Corticosteroids 41, 349
intralesional 71
topical 71, 105
Corynebacterium diphtheriae 91, 92
Cotton-wool spots 223, 245, 246*f*
severe 247*f*
Cover test 377, 383
Cover-uncover test 396
Cowen's sign 5, 37
Cox's postulates 364
Cranial nerve 4
Craniofacial syndromes 432
Craniosynostosis 180
lymphomas 2
Crawford's fascia lata stripper 479
C-reactive protein 217, 372, 379
Crescent knife 467, 468*f*, 477
Crescentic lamellar keratoplasty 157
Crinkled cellophane maculopathy 325
Cryoglobulinemia 311
Cryopexy, anterior retinal 199
Cryosurgery 12
contraindications of 12
Cryotherapy, anterior retinal 219
Cryptophthalmos 89
Curvature 113
Curvularia 94
Cuticular drusen 284
Cyanoacrylates 106
Cycloablative procedures 194
Cyclodestructive procedure 201, 202
Cyclodialysis 205
Cyclophotocoagulation 192
Cycloplegics 349
refraction 175

Cyclosporine 144, 417
Cyclotropia, subjective 377
Cyst 78
    anterior 81, 81t
    gross examination of 340
    intracorneal 172
    intravitreal 340f
    subretinal 340
Cystadenolymphoma 46
Cystadenoma 47
Cysteine-rich glycoprotein 439
Cysticercosis 342
    intraocular 342
    life cycle of 341
    posterior segment 339
Cysticercus cellulosae 339
Cystoid
    macular edema 251, 253f, 259, 287, 296f, 297, 325
    retinal spaces 288f
Cystotome needle 470, 471f

D

Dahan's formula 431t
Dalrymple's sign 5, 37
Dapsone toxicity 311
Dastoor iris repositor 470, 470f
Decompression, orbital 42
Deep anterior lamellar keratoplasty 116, 117t, 129t
    diamond-knife-assisted 118, 131
    different techniques of 130
Deep dermoid 77, 78, 81
    cyst 80, 81t
Deep stromal lesions 128
Deep vein thrombosis 493
Degeneration 129, 130t
Delleman syndrome 86
Dellen formation 175
Deoxyribonucleic acid 108, 239
Depression 369f
    scleral 329
Dermoid 171, 172, 176
    cyst 2, 77
        epidermal 80
    differential diagnosis of 176t
    epidemiology of 80, 178
    grading of 178
    medial anterior 78
    ocular 179
    recurrent 175
    superficial 77
Dermolipoma 175
Descemet's folds 156
Descemet's membrane 138, 171, 176, 193
    tears in 171

Descemet's stripping automated endothelial keratoplasty 137-139, 139t, 165, 166f
    busin forceps 478
    spatula 477, 477f
Descemetocele 94f
Descemetorhexis 137
Desmarres lamellar dissector 477
Desmarres lid retractor 465, 466f
Developmental glaucoma, Hoskin's anatomic classification of 196t, 197
Devic's disease 393
Dewecker scissors 468, 468f
Dexamethasone 208
    implant 323t
Diabetes mellitus 91, 206, 222, 317, 433
Diabetic macular edema 267, 317, 319f-321t
    pathogenesis of 322
Diabetic papillopathy 245, 250
Diabetic retinopathy 197, 216, 236, 241, 245t, 246
    study
        epidemiology of 413
        pathogenesis of 413
Diameter hole index 262
Diamidine 108
Diamond knife 476
Diamond-dusted
    membrane scraper 484, 484f
    soft silicone tip cannula 483
Diffusion tensor imaging 394
Digital eversion test 60
Diplopia 150, 367, 376, 382, 387, 405, 415
    acute onset of 367
    charting 31, 371, 377, 380, 398
    management of 380
    persistent 34
    vertical 382
Disc
    collaterals 225
    coloboma 332
    edema 425
        causes of 424
    margins, blurring of 389f
    neovascularization 216, 238f
    opacity 447f
    sparing of 329f
    swelling of 389f
Disciform scar 284f, 285f, 288f
Dislocation, late 355
Disposable handheld trephine 474f
Disseminated subepithelial opacity 458

Dissociated vertical deviation 420, 421t
    measurement of 420
    theories of 421
Distant direct ophthalmoscopy examination 353, 437
Dot acuity test 429
Dot-blot hemorrhage, pathophysiology of 248
Double corneal forceps 476
Down syndrome 110
Doyne honeycomb retinal dystrophy 284
Droplets, coalescence of 162f
Drusen 281, 292
    high-risk characteristics of 281
Dry age-related macular degeneration 281
    management of 289
Dry eye 159
Dry socket 25
    treatment of 27
Dual bore cannula 483
Duane's classification 409
Duane's retraction syndrome 86, 175, 378, 411
    classification of 413t
    management in 413
Dubowitz syndrome 65
Duke elder classification 447
Dumbbell dermoids 81
Dysarthria 387
Dysostosis
    craniofacial 180
    multiplex 309
Dysphagia 387
Dysthyroid orbitopathy 371
Dystopia, inferior 36f
Dystrophic calcification 281
Dystrophy 127, 129, 130, 130t, 132, 360
    endothelial 126, 171
    epithelial 126
    macular 124f, 127, 132, 138, 357f, 358, 358t
    pattern 284

E

Eales' disease 201, 217, 219, 220, 434
    central 217f
Ear
    abnormalities 63
    anomalies 180f
E-cells 456
Echinocandins 102
Ectasia, corneal 111, 156f
Ectopia lentis 434, 436, 436f, 437

Ectopic lacrimal gland 175
Ectropion 55, 57, 58
　acquired 56
　congenital 56, 58, 196
　extreme 57
　grades of 57
　involutional 56, 61
　mechanical 56
　moderate 57
　paralytic 56, 57f
　surgical management of 57
　tests for 55
　uvea 237, 244
Edema 31, 142f
　angioneurotic 110
　corneal 136, 168, 168f, 277
　　epithelial 134
　macular 224f, 225f, 226, 317
Edrophonium chloride test 21, 416
Ehlers-Danlos syndrome 110, 152, 435
Electrolytes, serum 430
Electromyography 73
Electroneurography 73
Electrophysiology 358
Electroretinogram 226
Electroretinography, multifocal 321
Elschnig's operation 58
Elschnig's pearls 455, 456
Emphysema, subcutaneous 30
Encephalotrigeminal
　　angiomatosis 190
End-grasping forceps 482, 482f
Endocrine 2
Endophthalmitis 264, 296
　endogenous 341
　infectious 143
　localized 454
Endoscopic cyclophotocoagulation 493
Endothelial cell count, normal 138
Endotheliitis 105
Endothelium 142
Enophthalmos 34, 51
Enroth's sign 5, 37
Entis et pupillae 436
Entropion 25, 59, 60f
　acute spastic 61
　common types of 61
　congenital 60-62, 62t
　correction, spacer graft for 62
　management of 62
　spastic 61
Enucleation
　scissors 469, 469f
　surgery 480
Enzyme-linked immunosorbent
　　assay 73, 230

Epiblepharon 61, 62, 62t
Epibulbar dermoid 175
Epicanthus
　fold 66
　inversus syndrome 53, 63-65, 66f
Epidermal appendages 174f
Epidermal dermoid 80, 80t
　cyst 80
Epikeratophakia 118
Epilation forceps 463, 464f
Epiphora 63
Epiretinal membrane 234, 251,
　　267, 297, 298, 323, 325,
　　326f, 327
Epiretinal proliferation 325
Episcleral plaque brachytherapy 306
Episcleral scarring 343, 348
Epithelial defect, corneal
　　persistent 150
Epithelial stromal TGFBI
　　dystrophies 126
Epithelioid cell melanoma 307
Epitheliomas, sebaceous 70
Epithelium 123
Erectile dysfunction 388
Erythrocyte sedimentation rate 7,
　　217, 372, 379
Erythropoietin 393
Escherichia coli 100
Esodeviation 394
Esophoria 400
Esotropia 400, 410
　accommodative 401
　essential infantile 402, 412
　infantile 378
　intermittent 400
　partially accommodative 402
Ethylenediaminetetraacetic acid 160
Evisceration surgery 480
Excimer laser phototherapeutic
　　keratectomy 119, 163
Exodeviation 405, 408
　Calhounz's phases of 409
Exophoria 409
Exophthalmometry 6
Exotropia 371, 405, 407, 408,
　　408t, 409f
　basic 407
　epidemiology of 408
Extensive periorbital involvement 10f
External beam radiotherapy 49, 306
Extraocular diseases 201
Extraocular movement 86, 175, 411,
　　415, 419, 420, 423
Extraocular muscle
　disinsertion 150
　majority of 367

Exudative retinal detachment,
　　inferior 268f
Eyeball 3, 45, 64, 72, 77, 86, 92, 123,
　　134, 141, 147, 152, 155,
　　159, 162, 164, 171, 175,
　　183, 191, 193, 203, 206,
　　209, 215, 224, 237, 244,
　　252, 281, 295, 300, 318,
　　328, 335, 343, 348, 352,
　　361, 368, 388, 411, 429,
　　435, 443, 446, 450, 453,
　　458, 489
Eyebrow 86, 281
Eyelashes 36
Eyelids 4, 10, 16, 25, 31, 36, 55, 64,
　　67, 71, 76, 78, 86, 110, 134,
　　141, 147, 152, 155, 159,
　　162, 164, 191, 206, 209,
　　318, 414, 429, 446, 450,
　　453, 458
　anatomy of 75
　coloboma 85, 88
　　surgical 87f
　defects, reconstruction of 13
　drooping of 51, 63
　dysplastic 64
　ecchymosis 30
　Moll gland of 67
　squamous cell carcinoma of 10f
　tape 417
Eyes
　buphthalmos 194f
　deviation of 405, 428
　high-risk 338
　muscles, fatigue of 414
　normal 377
　protrusion of 3
　surgery, contralateral 419
　wall 365
Eylea 291

F

Fabry syndrome 433
Face 368
Facial
　angiomatosis, bilateral 190f
　appearance 110
　asymmetry 174, 368, 382
　defects 86
　nerve, anatomy of 75
　symmetry 16
Fairly reliable diagnostic sign 357
Fallen over retina 336f
Fanconi's disease 159
Fanconi's syndrome 159
Fasanella-Servat operation 20, 52
Fascicular cavernous sinus
　　portion 374

Fatigability 21
Fatigue test 416
Fellow eye 97, 217, 225, 352
   examination of 125
   management of 338
   role of 221
Femtosecond laser 117
Femtosecond-assisted deep anterior lamellar keratoplasty 118, 131
Fetal fissure 328
Fibroblast growth factor 151
Fibroepithelioma 14
Fibrotic posterior capsular opacification 455
Fibrovascular proliferation 238*f*
Field defect 269
Filtration surgery 194, 201, 204, 349
Fine-needle aspiration
   biopsy 8
   cytology 11, 68
Finesse flex loop 484, 485*f*
Fishman classification 359, 359*t*
Fixation disparity method 397
Fixation preference tests 395
Fleck lesions 359
Fleischer ring 111
Flieringa ring 474, 474*f*
Floaters, significance of 273
Floor repair surgery, complications of 34
Floppy eyelid syndrome 72, 110
Fluconazole 103
Fluocinolone acetonide 323*t*
Fluorescein
   angiogram 255, 297, 319
   angiography 238*f*, 233, 262*f*, 285, 304, 320*f*, 325
   late 233*f*
   staining 60
Fluorinated pyrimidines 102
Fluorometholone 101, 102, 102*t*, 208
Follicular cysts, multiple 70
Foos classification 326
Force duction test 31, 87, 371, 378, 379, 384, 400, 415, 418
Force generation test 31, 379
Forceps 462
   injury 165
Foreign body
   forceps 482, 483*f*
   sensation 121, 158
Forme fruste keratoconus 120
Fortified eye drops 102*t*
Four delta prism test 398
Fourth nerve palsy 381, 387
   isolated 386
   management of 385*t*

Foveal drusen 261
Foville syndrome 381
Fracture, orbital 385
Fraser syndrome 86, 87, 89
Freer periosteal elevator 479, 480*f*
Freidreich-like ataxia 252
Fresh retinal detachment 277*t*
Frisby Favis distance test 399
Frontalis
   flap 53
   overaction 16
Fuchs' endothelial corneal dystrophy 110, 133, 136, 138, 165, 166, 166*t*, 169
   differential diagnosis of 136*t*
   early-onset 138, 138*t*
   late-onset 138, 138*t*
Fuchs' keratopathy 209
Fundal coloboma 327, 329*f*, 334
   classification of 332
Fundus 7, 18, 31, 64, 78, 87, 135, 152, 163, 191, 199, 204, 206, 210, 216, 238, 252, 281, 296, 300, 324, 336, 353, 370, 377, 412, 426, 430, 444, 446, 450, 454, 459
   autofluorescence 288, 304
   coloboma 333*t*
   examination 112, 185, 270, 329, 423, 437
   flavimaculatus 356, 359
   fluorescein angiography 218, 226, 282*f*, 314, 357, 423
Fungal keratitis 96
   management of 102, 104, 104*fc*
Fungus 103

G

Galactosemia 429
Gass clinical grading system 326
Gass retinal detachment hook 485, 486*f*
Gatifloxacin 101
Gaucher's disease 311
Gene therapy 256
Genital anomalies 89
Geographic atrophy 281, 282*f*
Giant cell arteritis 201
Giant retinal dialysis 336, 337
Giant retinal tear 272, 335, 337, 338
   classification of 336, 339*t*
   etiology of 339*t*
   surgery, complications of 338*t*
Gifford's sign 5, 37
Gill's lamellar dissector 477
Glare 121

Glaucoma 182, 192, 192*t*, 214, 224, 231, 256, 277, 297, 348*f*, 442, 487, 494, 495
   advanced 491
   causes of 192, 350
   congenital 153, 165, 171, 172, 192, 192*t*, 193*f*, 195, 195*t*
   developmental 196*t*, 197
   drainage device 349, 493
   inverse 452
   long-standing 159
   low-potency steroid and risk of 208
   mechanism of 205, 256
   newer drug delivery systems in 495
   pathomechanism of 350
   pigmentary 211
   preperimetric diagnostic tools of 494
   progression of 495
   secondary 432
   steroid-induced 206-208, 491
   surgery 192, 214, 473
   treatment of 173
   uveitic 206, 211
Glaucomatocyclitic crisis 206
Glaucomatous optic
   atrophy 427
   neuropathy 186, 426*t*
Glaukomflecken 184*f*
Globe fixation
   forceps 463, 463*f*
   rings 474
Globular corneal protrusion 151*f*, 152*f*
Globus 112
Glomerulonephritis, membranoproliferative 284
Glycosaminoglycan 126
Gold weight implantation 74
Goldberg's disease 311
Goldenhar syndrome 87, 89, 179*t*, 180, 180*f*, 411, 413
Goldmann applanation tonometry 194, 492, 494
Goldmann gonioprisms 189
Goldmann mirror 189
Goldzieher's sign 5, 37
Goltz syndrome 332
Gonioscopy 169, 171, 175, 185, 185*f*, 189, 191, 194, 202, 204, 206, 210, 216, 224, 281, 336, 352, 362, 458, 487*f*, 494, 489
   examination 204

Goniotomy 191, 194
Gopal Krishna classification 26
Gout 159
Graded neutral density filter test 420
Graft
    displacement 150
    failure, late 143
    holder 475
    host junction 145
    rejection 146, 173
        manifestations of 146
Gram stain 99
Granular dystrophy 121, 123, 123f, 124, 127, 128, 132
    early 123f
Granuloma 54
    foreign body 175
    pyogenic 70, 71f
Graphic method 397
Graves' disease 1, 36
Graves' orbitopathy 35, 40, 378
Gravitational tracts 313
Green hook 465, 465f
Griffith's sign 5, 37
Ground-glass appearance 124f
Guarded diamond knife 477
Guillain-Barré syndrome 23, 72
Gunderson's flap 104

H

Haab's striae 165, 171, 195
Haemophilus keratoconjunctivitis 92
Hallervorden-Spatz syndrome 311
Hallucinogenic drugs 257
Hamartoma 80
Handheld trephine 475f
Hanging drop sign 31
Hangliosidosis 311
Haploscopic method 397
Harada's disease 300, 314
Harboyan syndrome 167
Hard drusens 281f
Harms trabeculotome 473, 474f
Hassall-Henle bodies 135
Head
    computed tomography of 191
    posture 63, 368, 376
        abnormal 368
Healing corneal ulcer, signs of 106
Hearing loss 174
Heart failure, congenital 239
Hemangioma 2, 84, 214
    capillary 83, 83f, 84, 84t
    cavernous 83, 84, 84t
    choroidal 192
    location of 84
    orbital 82, 83

Hemangiopericytoma 84
Hematoma 31
    periorbital 30
Hemifacial microsomia 180
Hemifield diabetic macular edema 320f
Hemodynamic crisis 488
Hemorrhage 216, 246f, 248, 233
    flame-shaped 248
    intraoperative 150
    intraretinal 340
    macular 232f
    retinal 223, 246f
    scattered 232f
    subcapsular 150
Hemostatic forceps 464, 464f
Herpes simplex 93
    virus 107, 151, 171
Herpetic eye disease study 107
Herpetic keratitis, recurrent 143
Herring's law 420
Hertel exophthalmometer 31
Hertoghe's sign 5, 37
Hess chart 371, 377, 384, 419
Hess screen 31
Hessburg-Barron trephine 475f
Heterophoria method 397
Higher order aberrations 147
Hip dysplasia, congenital 110
Hirschberg test 395
Histochemical stains, types of 128
Hole closure, types of 265
Holt-Oram syndrome 413
Homocystinuria 434, 437t, 449, 450
Hormone, parathyroid 160
Horner syndrome, congenital 23
Hoskin's classification 197
Host cornea, vascularization of 145
Hotz procedure 61
Human immunodeficiency virus 73, 76
Human papillomavirus 10, 151
    keratitis 145
Hundred-day glaucoma 202
Hurler's syndrome 311
Hybrid contact lenses 116
Hydraulic theory 33
Hydrocortisone 208
Hydrodelamination 118, 131
Hydrodelineation 448
Hydrops, corneal 112f
Hyopia, high 378, 434
Hyperbaric oxygen therapy 256
Hypercalcemia 159
Hyperemia 389f
Hyperesthesia, corneal 112
Hyperglycemia 243

Hyperhomocysteinemia 388
Hyperlipidemia 243
Hyperoleon 348f
Hyperopia 412
Hyperopic correction 313
Hyperparathyroidism 159
Hypertension 243, 300, 309
    idiopathic intracranial 422
    systemic 488
Hypertonic saline solutions, topical 136
Hypertropia 383, 396
Hypoparathyroidism 433
Hypophosphatasia 159
Hypoplastic dilator muscles 436
Hypopyon 96f
    characteristics of 96t
    role of 106
Hypotension 388
Hypoxia 249
    retinal 202

I

Ibuprofen 79
Ice cell 170
Ice pack test 21, 415
Ichthyosis 159
Ideal orbital implant, characteristics of 29
Idiopathic giant retinal tear, pathogenesis of 339
Idiopathic intracranial hypertension 422
    management of 423
Iliff test 17, 52
Immunoglobulins, intravenous 393
Immunohistochemistry 46
Immunosuppressive therapy 144
Implantable miniature telescope 292
Incision biopsy 8, 11
Incomitant esotropia 400t
Incomitant strabismus 396
Indocyanine green 218, 283
    angiography 283, 304, 315
Infantile esotropia 378
    signs of 408
Infections 28, 174, 175
    maternal 432
Inferior oblique overaction 403, 421t
Inferior rectus
    palsy 371
    resection 421
Inflammation 2
    periorbital 4
    suture-related 150
Inflammatory disease 326
Infusion cannula 481, 481f

Inhibitional palsy 384
Injury, orbital 30
Inoculation 99
Insulin use 243
Intercalary membrane 332
Intermediate uveitis 293, 298
    causes of 294*fc*, 298
    differential diagnosis of 298
Intermittent esotropia 400
    Burian's classification of 408
    classification of 409*t*
    newcastle scoring for 407*t*
Internal limiting membrane
    forceps 482, 482*f*
    peeling 263
International Vitreomacular
        Traction Study 326
Interpupillary distance 64, 398
Intracorneal ring segment insert
    116, 118
Intracranial pressure 422
Intralenticular lens aspiration 439*f*
Intraocular lens 263, 430, 431*t*, 471*f*
    choice of 137
    contraindications of 433
    dialer 471
    dislocation 354
    holding forceps 471, 471*f*
    implantation 432, 452
        primary 431
    injector 472, 473*f*
    power calculation 431
    removal 355
Intraocular pressure 7, 78, 95, 97,
    152, 169, 182, 184, 186,
    191, 202, 208, 208*t*, 216,
    237, 252, 270, 272, 281,
    295, 300, 310, 318, 328,
    335, 352, 362, 383, 429,
    437, 443, 446, 450
    elevation 208*t*
    reduction of 136
Intraocular silicone oil 159
Intrastromal corneal lenticule 116
Intrauterine infections, serology
    for 430
Intravitreal triamcinolone 256
    acetonide 206
Inverse pupillary block 450
    glaucoma 452
Involutional ectropion 56, 61
    pathogenesis of 58
Iodine, radioactive 43
Iridectomy, peripheral 349, 350
Iridocorneal endothelial dystrophy
    135, 136, 165, 166, 168*f*
    clinical variants of 170

Iridoschisis 110
Iridotrabecular dysgenesis 172
Iris 7, 31, 64, 87, 97, 135, 152, 160,
    168, 171, 184, 194, 198,
    203, 209, 215, 237, 244,
    252, 281, 300, 328, 335,
    352, 362, 370, 377, 383,
    429, 436, 443, 446, 450,
    453, 458
    adhesion 145
    atrophy 168*f*
        progressive 168
        segmental 184*f*
    coloboma 329*f*, 332
        complete 331
        incomplete 331
    disorders 169
    forceps 463
    melanosis 169
    neovascularization of 198*f*,
        202, 318
    nevus syndrome 170
    nodules 168
    root, retrodisplacement of 204*f*
    vessels, normal 199, 201
Irrigating wire vectis 469, 470*f*
Irvine-Gass syndrome 318
Ischemia
    macular 238*f*
    ocular 201
    orbital 311
    severe
        peripheral 238*f*
        retinal 226*f*
Ischemic central retinal vein
        occlusion 224*f*
Ischemic index 228

J

Jaeger's lid spatula 478, 478*f*
Jameson hook 465, 465*f*
Jellinek's sign 5, 37
Jendrassik's sign 5, 37
Joffroy's sign 5, 37
Jones criteria 101, 106
Joubert syndrome 254
Julsez's random dot 399

K

KANSL1-related intellectual
        disability syndrome 65
Kaposi sarcoma 71
Kasabach-Merritt syndrome 84
Kay picture test 429
Kaye's dots 142
Kearns-Sayre syndrome 15, 54, 252

Kelley's punch 473, 473*f*
Keloids, corneal 176
Keratectomy
    photorefractive 119, 160
    superficial 160, 163
Keratitis 107
    bacterial 96, 103*t*
    epithelial 105
    fungal 96
    healing 94*f*
    infectious 97
    infective 108
    interstitial 138, 159
    specific 96*t*
    type of 105
    viral 93, 96
Keratoacanthoma 70
Keratoconjunctivitis, superior
        limbic 68
Keratoconus 109, 112, 113, 119, 120,
    132, 153, 157, 158
    Amsler-Krumeich classification
        of 113*t*
    anterior segment optical
        coherence tomography
        classification of 114*t*
    differential diagnosis of 113*t*
    percentage index 120
    posterior 120, 171
    refractive surgery in 119
    treatment of 115
Keratoglobus 113, 151, 151*f*, 152-
    154, 154*t*, 157
    acquired 154
    associations of 152*t*
    congenital 154
Kerato-irido-lenticular
        dysgenesis 172
Keratomalacia 172
Keratome 467, 467*f*
Keratometry 110, 114, 125, 148
Keratopathy 54, 59*f*, 60*f*
    band-shaped 158, 160*f*
    congenital band 159
Keratoplasty 474
    endothelial 137, 146, 195
    penetrating 106, 116, 117*t*, 129*t*,
        130, 137, 138, 139*t*, 142*f*,
        154, 158, 166*f*, 194
Keratoprosthesis 159
Kerrison bone punch 480, 480*f*
Kestenbaum capillary index 426, 427
Ketoconazole 104
Keyhole pupil 329*f*
Khodadoust line 142*f*
King's clamp 476, 476*f*
Kinyoun stain 107

Kissing doves appearance 158
Klinefelter's syndrome 450
Knapp's classification 385*t*
Knapp's procedure 54, 419
  modified 419
Knies' sign 5, 37
Kocher's sign 5, 37
Krachmer's line 142
Krause-Kivlin syndrome 173
Krimsky test 396
Krukenberg spindle 183, 184
Kushner classification 409

L

Laceration 365
Lacrimal fossa mass, differential diagnosis of 50
Lacrimal gland 43
  adenoid cystic carcinoma of 44*f*
  mass 78
    differential diagnosis of 46*t*
  tumors 43, 50
    major 47*t*
Lacrimal nerve 4
Lacrimal puncta, position of 56
Lacrimal sac 92
  dissector and curette 480*f*
  surgery 479
Lacrimal system 86, 175
  patency assessment 60
Lactosyl ceramidosis 310
Lagophthalmos 17, 55, 71, 72*f*
  causes of 75*t*
  etiology of 75
Lambert-Eaton syndrome 416
Lamellar keratectomy, anterior 104, 160
Lamellar keratoplasty 154, 157, 476
  advantages of 130
Lamellar laceration 365
Lamellar macular holes 261
Landolt C test 429
Lang's microtropia 404
Lang's pencil gross stereopsis test 399
Lang's syndrome 403
Laser 291, 475
  aiming-beam test 261
  capsulotomy 344*f*
  epithelial keratomileusis 119
  in situ keratomileusis 110
  parameters 455
  peripheral iridotomy 186-188
    procedure 189
  photocoagulation 219, 316
  trabeculoplasty 204, 207, 492
    selective 349

Lateral canthal
  laxity test 60
  resuspension 58
  tendon laxity 56, 57
Lateral tarsal strip procedure 57, 57*f*
Lattice corneal dystrophy 110, 124*f*, 127, 128, 132
Laurence-Moon-Bardet-Biedl syndrome 252
Leash phenomenon 411
Leber's congenital amaurosis 110, 152, 254, 311
Leber's hereditary optic neuropathy 390, 422
Lee screen tests 31
Left superior oblique palsy 383*f*, 385*t*
Lens 7, 31, 64, 87, 97, 135, 152, 160, 163, 171, 184, 194, 199, 204, 206, 210, 216, 224, 231, 237, 244, 252, 259, 281, 295, 300, 318, 328, 336, 343, 348, 352, 362, 370, 383, 428, 429, 436, 443, 446, 450, 453, 458
  absorptive 293
  aspiration 431
  capsule 443*f*
  coloboma 331
  extraction 452
  fibers 459
  hook 465, 465*f*
  macular 485
  posterior dislocated 351
  post-traumatic atrophy of 459
  removal of 354
  spatula 469, 469*f*
  subluxation of 434, 438, 439, 460*f*
  zonular fibers 214
Lensectomy 431
  role of 337
Lenticonus 442
  anterior 443*f*, 444*t*
  diagnosis of 444
  posterior 442, 444, 444*t*, 447
Lenticular astigmatism, presence of 438
Lenticular refractive surgery 116
Lentigo malignant melanoma 14
Leprosy 72
Lesions, types of 47, 48
Leukemia 2, 7, 52, 220, 246, 296, 314
  malignant 2
Leukemic vitreous infiltration 217
Leukocoria 428
Leukodystrophy, metachromatic 311
Levator
  function 52, 53

  muscle, ipsilateral 53
  palpebrae superioris 15, 19, 53, 367, 415
  recession 74
  resection 20, 53, 53*t*
    amount of 53
  subnucleus 375
Lhermitte sign 387
Lids 45, 72, 92, 123, 183, 198, 203, 215, 224, 244, 252, 281, 295, 300, 328, 335, 343, 348, 352, 361, 370, 377, 382, 388, 412, 443, 489
  asymmetry 54
  clamp 478, 479*f*
  closure 72*f*
  coloboma 87, 331
  defect, size of 14
  excursion 17
  fatigue 370
  laxity 59
    generalized 58
    horizontal 58
    inferior 56
  malignancy 13
    signs of 13
  margin 59
    examination 56, 60
  opening, normal 72*f*
  reconstruction, full-thickness 14*t*
  resection procedures, disadvantages of 58
  retraction 38*f*
  signs 5*t*, 37*t*
  speculum 462
  surgery 478
  tumors 9
Light reflex tests 395
Lim forceps 463
Limbal dermoid 87, 171, 172, 174, 174*f*, 175, 175*f*, 180*f*
Limbus 193
Limbus-to-limbus corneal thinning 152*f*
Lincoff rules 274
Lingam Gopal classification 333*t*
Lipodermoid 78
Lithium 159
Locus minoris resistentiae 332
Loewi's sign 5, 37
Low vision
  aids 293
    provision of 290
  causes of 333
Lowe syndrome 433, 442, 443, 449
Lower eyelid
  coloboma 86, 88, 89, 89*t*, 175
  retraction 38

Lucentis 291
Luedde's exophthalmometer 6
Lumbar puncture 390, 423
Lutein 290
Lymph nodes 11
　enlarged 68
　regional 4
Lymphangioma, medial orbital 3*f*
Lymphatic metastasis 69
Lymphoma 2, 7, 46, 52, 175, 217, 296
　malignant 2

M

Macroaneurysm 220
　retinal 216
　rupture 318
Macugen 291
Macula 45, 238, 389
　redness of 310
　sparing of 329*f*
Macular edema 224*f*, 225*f*, 226, 317
　clinically significant 245
　development 454
　　pathophysiology of 248
Macular hole 258, 264, 325
　chronic 357
　controversies of 264
　formation 265
　full-thickness 267, 325
　index 262
　management of 262*t*
　prognosis factor for 264
　repair 266
　surgery for 262
Macular ischemia 238*f*
　fluorescein angiography of 320*f*
　managing 322
Maculopathy, ischemic 319
Maculorhexis 265
Maddox rod 397
　test, double 370
Maddox wing 397
Maffucci syndrome 84
Magnetic resonance
　imaging 8, 52, 78, 80, 84, 175
　venography 423
Malignant melanoma 9, 201
　lids manifestation of 14, 14*t*
Malnutrition 91
Mandibulofacial dysostosis 450
Mann's scheme 178
Mann's sign 5, 37
Mannosidosis 433
Map biopsy 13, 68
Marcus Gunn jaw-winking
　　syndrome 21, 23, 53
Marcus Gunn ptosis 54

Marden-Walker syndrome 65
Marfan's disease 436, 436*f*, 437*t*, 439
　etiopathogenesis of 439
Marfan's syndrome 110, 152, 434-
　　436, 439, 440, 449, 450
Margin crease distance 17
Margin limbal distance 17
Margin reflex distance 16, 17, 19
Mass 77, 174
　around eyeball 4
　intracranial 414
　mushroom-shaped 304*f*
　reducibility of 4
Material over lens capsule 210*f*
Matrix metalloproteinase 151
McDonald criteria 393
McNeill-Goldman ring 474
McPherson's forceps 464, 465*f*
Means' sign 5, 37
Measles 91
Mechanical ectropion 56
　management of 58
Meckel-Gruber syndrome 332
Medial canthal laxity 56
　test 60
Medial rectus, palsy of 368
Medial wall fracture, features of 34
Megalocornea 153
Meibomian glands 67
Melanoma 214, 306
　choroidal 299, 300, 301*t*, 303*t*,
　　305-307
　malignant 9, 201
　superficial spreading 14
　types of 307
Membranectomy 455
Mendez toric degree gauge ring
　　marker 473, 473*f*
Mercury fumes 159
Meretoja's syndrome 132
Mestinon 417
Metabolic disorders 310
Metamorphopsia 232
Metastasis 69, 300
Metastatic disease 314
Methanol 311
Michels syndrome 65
Micro aneurysm development,
　　pathophysiology of 248
Micro vitreo retinal blade 467, 468*f*
Micro-incisional vitrectomy system
　　cutters 482*f*
Microphthalmia, unilateral 28*f*
Microphthalmos 175
Micropsia 405
Microspherophakia 449, 450*f*, 453
　etiology of 451*t*
　pathogenesis of 452

Microsporidiosis 96
Microtropia 399
Microvascular disease 373
Milk alkali syndrome 159
Millard-Gubler syndrome 381
Miniature toy test 429
Minimally invasive glaucoma
　　surgeries 493
Minimum inhibitory
　　concentration 103
Mitomycin C 68, 149, 150, 200
Mitral valve prolapse 110, 435
Moebius' syndrome 412, 413
Moebius's sign 5, 37
Mohs' micrographic
　surgery 11
　technique 68
Moist socket, treatment of 27
Monocular elevation deficit 418
　causes of 419
　management of 419
Mononeuropathy, ischemic 373
Monotherapy 102
Monster vessels 194
Mooren's ulcer 93, 156
Moria artificial chamber
　　maintainer 477*f*
Moria automated lamellar
　　therapeutic keratectomy
　　microkeratome
　　system 477*f*
Motility 268, 328
　restriction 40
Movement's cap phenomenon 5, 37
Moxifloxacin 101
Mucocele 2
Mucolipidoses 171
Mucopolysaccharidoses 165, 171,
　　172, 311
Muir-Torre syndrome 70
Mule evisceration spatula 480, 481*f*
Müller's muscle 15
Müller's self-retaining adjustable
　　hemostatic retractor 466
Multifocal posterior pigment
　　epitheliopathy 313
Multilayered amniotic membrane
　　graft 106
Multiple anterior stromal
　　white dots 124*f*
Multiple sclerosis 392
　risk factors for 393
Multisystem disorder 236
Munson's sign 110, 119
Muscle
　biopsy 416
　proximal 414

Index

Musculoskeletal system 340
Musk protein antibodies 416
Myasthenia
    gravis 15, 54, 378, 399, 414
        ocular signs of 415t
        systemic 414
        ocular 414
Mycobacterium tuberculosis 93
Mycophenolate mofetil 144, 417
Mydriasis 450f
Myeloma, multiple 159
Myocardial infarction 239
Myoepithelioma 46
Myogenic theory 413
Myopia 410
    signs of 274
Myositis 2
    orbital 38
Myotonic dystrophy 54, 433

N

Naffziger method 3
Nankin's recession 405
Nanophthalmos 196
Natamycin 103, 104
Naugle exophthalmometer 6
Near reflex, spasm of 378
Necrotizing stromal herpetic stromal
    keratitis 105
Neodymium:yttrium-aluminum-
    garnet 201
    laser capsulotomy 455
Neoplasia 2
Neoplasms
    ocular 201
    orbital 2
Neovascular glaucoma 185, 197
    causes of 201
    management of 242
    stages of 202, 200t
Neovascularization 201, 216
    surgery influence occurrence
        of 202
Nephropathy 243
Nettleship's punctum dilator 479, 479f
Neurocysticercosis 341
Neurogenic theory 413
Neurological system 309
Neuromyelitis optica 393
Neuronal ceroid lipofuscinosis 254
Neuro-ophthalmology 367
Neuroparalytic disease 141
Neuroretinitis 391
Neurosensory retina 258
Niemann–Pick diseas 311
    infantile 311
N-methyl D-aspartate 492

Nodular melanoma 14
Nodular sebaceous carcinoma 68
Nodules, corneal 162f
Nonarteritic ischemic optic
    neuropathy 425t
Noncontact trephines 475
Nonhealing corneal ulcer,
    signs of 106
Non-necrotizing stromal herpetic
    stromal keratitis 105
Non-nutrient agar 100
Nonpenetrating glaucoma
    surgery 493
Nonproliferative diabetic retinopathy
    242, 246f, 247f
    mild 246f
    mild to moderate 248
    moderate 246f
    severe 246f
    signs of 319f
Nonspecific orbital inflammatory
    disease 38
Nonsteroidal anti-inflammatory
    drugs, role of 250
Noonan syndrome 65
Normal tension glaucoma 491
Norrie disease 159, 201
Nuclear sclerosis 329f
Nuclear sclerotic cataracts 263
Nucleus drop, prevention of 355
Nucleus emulsification 448
Nuijts–Lane toric bubble marker 472
Nystagmoid movements 415
Nystagmus 164, 387, 428

O

Occlusion therapy 407
Ochre membrane 217
Ocular adnexal skin 231
Ocular anomalies 173, 432
Ocular coherence tomography 326f
Ocular disorders
    acquired 152
    hereditary 152
Ocular epibulbar dermoids,
    involvement of 179
Ocular examination 63, 86, 77, 92,
    123, 133, 159, 193, 215,
    237, 259, 313
Ocular flutter 415
Ocular hypertension 491, 494
Ocular inflammatory
    diseases 174, 201
Ocular injury, classification of 365fc
Ocular irritation, chronic 151
Ocular motility 4, 31, 376
Ocular myasthenia 414
    gravis 414, 416

Ocular response analyzer 115
Ocular side effects 299
Ocular surface
    disease 91
    squamous neoplasia 148
Oculo-auriculo-vertebral
    spectrum 180
Oculocardiac reflex 30
Oculodigital sign 254
Oculomotor abnormalities 54
Oculomotor synkinesis 371
Oculoplasty 1
Ohdo blepharophimosis
    syndrome 65
Ointments 136
Okihiro's syndrome 411
Olivopontocerebellar atrophy 357
Oncocytoma 47
Onion-peeling appearance 446f
Opacity
    concentric rings of 446f
    pleomorphic 124f
Open globe injury 364
Open-angle glaucoma 222, 349,
    493, 494
    stage 202
Ophthalmic instruments 462
Ophthalmopathy
    thyroid-associated 35
    treatment of 41
Ophthalmoplegia
    chronic progressive external 38
    external 65
Ophthalmoscopic classification 391
Ophthalmoscopy, indirect 384
Opsoclonus 415
Optic atrophy 425
    consecutive 426
    nonglaucomatous 426t, 427
    primary 426
    secondary 426
    types of 427
Optic disc 45, 220, 223, 489
    cup, enlargement of 391f
    edema 422
    involvement, types of 333t
    pit 314
Optic nerve
    coloboma 331
    compression 1
    disease 215
    dysfunction, signs of 392
    glioma 2, 3f, 201
    head 199, 494
    sheath
        decompression 424
        diameter 423
        meningiomas 2

Index

Optic neuritis 387, 390, 391
  acute 393
  atypical 391, 391*t*
  classification of 391
  treatment trial 387
  typical 391, 391*t*
Optic neuropathy
  ischemic 390, 424
  nonischemic 424
  traumatic 363
Optical coherence tomography 160, 226, 233, 261, 286*f*, 287, 287*f*, 304, 315, 320*f*, 354, 390, 423
  angiography 315
Optociliary shunt vessels 225
Ora serrata 273
Orbicularis
  muscle weakness 56
  muscular tone 60
Orbicularis oculi 415
Orbit 16, 31, 110
  blowout fracture of 30, 33
  computed tomography of 68
  dimensions 9
  metastatic tumor of 2
  pseudotumor of 54
  syndrome 33
  vascular malformations of 84
Orbital disease 69
Orbital floor
  boundaries of 34
  fracture of 30*f*, 32*f*
  repair 33*t*
Orbital implants, types of 29
Orbital inflammation, idiopathic 152
Orbital pulsation 4
Orbital rim 4
Orbital thrill 4
Orbital venography 8
Orbital wall fractures 51
Orbito-lid apposition, grade of 57
Orbitopathy, specific inflammatory 38
Orbscan 114
Orthoptics 406
Osserman's grading 416
Osteogenesis imperfecta 110, 152
Osteoma 2
  episcleral 175
Osteoporosis 159
Ozurdex 227

P

Pachymetry 115, 143, 165, 169, 348, 492
Paget disease 159
Pain 2, 90, 141, 367
  acute 236
  onset of 147
Painful blind eye, treatment for 202
Palpation 82
Palpebral aperture 17
Palpebral fissure
  asymmetry 368
  changes 422
Palsy, partial 379
Pannus 148
Panretinal photocoagulation 199, 240
Panuveitis 296
Papilledema, Frisen's grading of 423
Papillitis 389, 389*f*, 391
Papillopathy, diabetic 245, 250
Papillophlebitis 390
Paralytic ectropion 56, 57*f*
  management of 58
Paralytic squint, stages of 371
Paresis 379
Paresthesia 31
Parks–Bielschowsky three-step tests 383, 387
Pars plana
  route 456
  vitrectomy 227, 322
Patch graft 104, 106
Patchy iris stromal atrophy 184*f*
Paton spatula 475, 476*f*
Pattern-scanning retinal laser 241
Paufique knife 477
Payne sign 5, 37
Pediatric cataract 433*t*
  management of 433
Peek sign 415
Pegaptanib 291
Pellucid marginal corneal degeneration 113, 120, 155, 156, 156*f*, 158
  differential diagnosis of 156*t*, 157*t*
  signs of 158
Penicillamine 417
Pentacam 114, 455
Pentoxifylline, oral 227
Perfluorocarbon liquid, role of 354, 337
Perimetry 492
Peripapillary atrophy 491, 491*f*
Peripheral anterior chamber depth 187
  synechia 169, 186, 200
Peripheral iridotomy 488
Peters' anomaly 165, 170-173, 176, 449
Peters' plus syndrome 171, 173
Phaces syndrome 84
Phaco needle tip 471, 472*f*
Phacoemulsification parameters 448
Phacofragmentation 354
Phenothiazine 254
Phenylephrine test 21
Phlebitis, retinal 217
Phosphate 159
Photodynamic therapy 290, 291, 306, 316
Photophobia 91, 121, 127, 158, 405
Photopsia 269
Phthisis bulbi 159
Pierse Hoskins forceps 464, 465*f*
Piggyback systems 115
Pigment dispersion syndrome 213
Pigment epithelial
  abnormalities 281
  derived growth 291
  detachment 282*f*, 283, 286*f*, 287, 287*f*
Pigment production 94*f*
Pigmentary glaucoma 491
Pilocarpine, topical 187
Pinch and Peel technique 263
Pinch test 55, 59
Pinguecula 148
Pisciform 357
Placental growth factor 239
Plain forceps 463, 463*f*
Plasma exchange 393
Plateau iris syndrome 185
Pneumatic retinopexy 276
  principles of 277
  role of 338
Pochin's sign 5, 37
Polar cataract, posterior 355, 445, 446*f*, 449
Polyenes 102
Polymerase chain reaction 101
Polypoidal choroidal vasculopathy 314
Polypoidal choroidopathy, idiopathic 284
Poor vision, management of 292
Portwine stain 192
Positive angle kappa sign 304
Positron emission tomography 11, 68
Postenucleation socket syndrome 29
Posterior amorphous corneal dystrophy, classification of 184*fc*
Posterior capsular
  defect, management of 448
  opacification 453, 454*f*
    pathogenesis of 456
    prevention of 456
    reduce 457
    regeneratory 455
    rupture with cataract 461

Posterior continuous curvilinear
    capsulorhexis 431
Posterior lenticonus 442, 444,
    444t, 447
    pathogenesis of 445
Posterior polar cataract 355, 445,
    446f, 449
    surgery in 448
Posterior vitreous
    detachment 324, 337
Post-laser medication 455
Post-penetrating keratoplasty
    herpetic keratitis 107
Post-vitrectomized eyes 350
Potassium hydroxide 99
    wet preparation 99
Potato dextrose agar 108
Prednisolone 208, 417
Prematurity, retinopathy of 216, 270
Pre-perimetric test 191
Previtelliform 360
Primary angle closure 182, 184,
    186, 187
    disease 184
    glaucoma 182, 184, 186, 202
Primary open-angle glaucoma 206,
    212t, 487
    management? 493
    pathogenesis of 494
    pre-existing concomitant 202
Prism
    bar cover test 396, 420
    permanent 372
Procainamide 417
Proliferative diabetic retinopathy
    218f, 219, 236
    high-risk 240
    nonhigh-risk 239
Prophylactic laser photocoagulation,
    role of 334
Propionibacterium acnes 454
Propranolol, perioperative oral 192
Proptosis 1, 5t, 37t, 81
    bilateral 2t
    causes of 2t, 9
    direction of 3
    disproportionate 36f
    severe bilateral 36f
Prostaglandin analogs 490
Prostamide 490
Proteinuria 443
Pseudo disc edema 424
Pseudo-cherry-red spot 310
Pseudoesotropia, causes of 409
Pseudoexfoliation 213
    glaucoma 204, 209, 212t, 491
Pseudoexfoliative syndrome 209
    peripheral zone of 210f

Pseudoguttae 135
Pseudohole 325
Pseudohypopyon 360
Pseudomacular holes 261
Pseudomembrane formation 92
Pseudomonas
    aeruginosa 90
    keratitis 96
Pseudophakic bullous
    keratopathy 135
Pseudophakic macular edema 322
Pseudoproptosis 8
Pseudopterygium 148, 148t
Pseudoptosis 16, 51, 54, 418
    appearance of 411
Pseudoretinitis pigmentosa 254
Pseudotumor 2, 8
    cerebri 215
    idiopathic inflammatory 2
Psoralen plus ultraviolet A 10
Psychosomatic disorders 446
Pterygium 147, 148, 148t, 149,
    149t, 150
    atypical 175
    extent of 147
    grading of 147
    inflamed 151
    parts of 148f
    pathogenesis of 150
    recurrence 150
    recurrent 150
    surgery 149, 150
Pterygoid muscle, external 53
Ptosis 15, 20, 21, 23f, 51, 53, 54, 63, 65,
    66, 66f, 81, 370, 414, 418
    acquired 18, 19, 19t, 20
        myogenic 22
        neurogenic 23
    classification of 19t, 20
    congenital 18-20, 51, 54
        myogenic 22
        neurogenic 23
        simple 65
    degree of 53
    hereditary congenital 65
    lower eyelid reverse 23
    management of complicated 54
    mechanical 24
    myogenic 22
    neurogenic 23
    postsurgical 22
    severe complicated 23f
    simple severe congenital 16f, 51f
    surgery 66, 417
    traumatic 22
Pulfrich phenomenon 388
Pulsatile proptosis, causes of 9

Pulseless disease 201
Pupil 7, 18, 31, 45, 73, 97, 135, 152,
    199, 203, 206, 209, 210,
    215, 223, 224, 231, 237,
    244, 252, 281, 295, 300,
    328, 335, 343, 352, 370,
    377, 383, 388, 422, 429,
    436, 443, 446, 450, 453,
    458, 489
    reaction 270
    sparing nerve palsy 373
Putterman's criteria 53t
Putterman's method 17
Pythium 108
    insidiosum 108
    keratitis 96
        specific features of 108

Q

Quadrant retinal hemorrhages 224f
Quinidine 417
Quinine 254, 311, 417

R

Radial keratotomy 110
    marker 474f
Radial optic neurotomy 227
Radial ray defects 411
Radiation
    ionizing 10
    retinopathy 319
    therapy 42
Radiotherapy 28
Raised intracranial
    pressure 183, 487, 493
    tension 370
Random blood sugar 230
Randot test 399
Ranibizumab 234, 291
Recent anterior segment surgery 145
Recombinant tissue plasminogen
    activator 227
Red filter test 420
Refractive accommodative 401
    esotropia, treatment of 401
Refractive error 149, 402, 405, 410
Refractive lens exchange 119
Refractory diabetic macular
    edema 322
Refsum disease 252
Relief classification 39
Renal biopsy 444
Renal failure 159
    degree of 443
Renal function test 230, 444
Repetitive nerve stimulation test 416

Index

ReSight noncontact viewing system 485*f*
Respiratory system 309
Retina 214, 272
Retina
   gyrate atrophy of 254
   vascular abnormalities 217
Retinal angiomatous proliferation 284
Retinal breaks 268, 273
   pattern of 333
   peripheral 264
Retinal change, sign of 249
Retinal detachment 218*f*, 267, 270, 270*b*, 272, 277, 298, 328, 330, 332, 340, 363, 432, 434
   mechanism of 364
   prophylactic management of 278
   surgery for 272*t*
   traumatic 361, 362*f*, 364
   types of 268*t*
Retinal dialysis 363
Retinal diseases 201
Retinal distortion, signs of 324*f*
Retinal laser 243
Retinal nerve fiber layer 191, 489
   thickness 492
Retinal photocoagulation, sectoral 234
Retinal pick 484, 484*f*
Retinal pigment
   epithelial tear 283
   epitheliopathy, diffuse 313
   epithelium 287, 289, 303
      disturbances 340
Retinal prosthesis 256
Retinal tears 363
Retinal vascular
   anomalies 220
   occlusion 215
   occlusive diseases 201
Retinal vein occlusion 222, 229, 318
Retinal vessels, minimal distortion of 324*f*
Retinitis
   pigmentosa 110, 251, 252, 253*f*, 256, 434
      atypical 253
      inversus 254
      paravenous 254
      pericentric 254
      sectoral 253
      sine pigmento 253
      syndromic 252*t*, 254
      unilateral 254
   punctata albescens 253
   sclopetaria 363

Retinoblastoma 201, 214, 272
Retinochoroidal coloboma 333, 334
Retinopathy 216, 247*f*, 249
   in diabetes, prevalence of 241
   hypertensive 246, 319
Retinoschisis 273
Retinoscopy 444
Retinovascular disease 245
Retrobulbar neuritis 391
Retrohyaloid space 216
Retroillumination 447*f*
Retropulsion theory 4, 33
Rhabdomyosarcoma 2, 52
Rhegmatogenous retinal detachment 268*f*, 272
   management of 271
Rho kinase inhibitors 490
Ribonucleic acid 239
Rieseman's sign 5, 37
Rigid gas-permeable lenses 110, 115
Rituximab 42
Rizzuti's phenomena 112
Rizzuti's sign 119
ROCK inhibitors 490
Rosacea 110
Rose K lenses 116
Rosenbach's sign 5, 37
Rosette cataract 459, 459*f*
Rothmund syndrome 446
Rubella, congenital 165
Rubeosis iridis 202
Rubinstein–Taybi syndrome 152, 332
Rule out myasthenic ptosis 21
Rundle's curve 43

S

Saccades 418
Saiton's sign 5, 37
Salmon patch 45
   lesion 50
Sampaolesi line 211
Sandhoff's disease 311, 312
Sarcoidosis 2, 159
Sarcomas 2
Scars
   postinfectious 172
   stage of 134
   steroid-induced 156
Scheimpflug camera 114
Schirmer's strips 93
Schirmer's test 55, 60, 72
Schnyder's crystalline dystrophy 121
Schocket scleral depressor 486, 486*f*
Schroeder classification 447
Schwalbe's line 211
Schwartz–Jampel syndrome 65
Schwartz–Matsuo syndrome 274

Scissors 468
Sclera 7, 64, 87, 95, 135, 152, 193, 203, 206, 215, 224, 252, 281, 295, 300, 331, 335, 352, 361, 370, 377, 383, 429, 436, 443, 446, 450, 453, 458
   fixated intraocular lens, techniques of 440
Scleral buckling 276
   prophylactic 338
   surgery 275
Scleral lenses 116
Scleral necrosis 149, 150
Scleral scarring 343, 348
Scleritis, posterior 314
Sclerocornea 172, 176
Sclerosis 159
   multiple 392
Sclerotic lens 353*f*
Scobee–Burian occlusion test 406, 408
Scotoma, central 214
Scott classification 336*t*
Scott procedure 372
Sea blue histiocyte syndrome 310
Sebaceous cell carcinoma 11
Sebaceous gland carcinoma 9, 10*f*, 67, 67*f*
Sellman and Lindstrom posterior capsule opacification grades 455*t*
Semi-integrated implants 29
Senile
   ectropion 56*f*, 61
   furrow degeneration 156
Sensory anomalies 398
Sensory loss 31
Sentinel lymph node biopsy 13
Serum angiotensin-converting enzyme 232
Shaken baby syndrome 214, 216
Sharp tip chopper 472*f*
Sheridan–Gardiner test 429
Sialidosis 311
Sickle cell disease 220
Silicone
   brush tip cannula 483
   oil
      bubbles of 348*f*
      disadvantages of 277
      filled eyes 343, 346, 350
      induced secondary glaucoma 347
      injection 350
      removal 349
      role of 265, 337
      tamponade 330

Simcoe irrigation 470, 470*f*
Single fiber nerve electromyography 22, 416
Single photon emission computed tomography 11
Sinskey hook 471, 471*f*
Sixth nerve palsy 375, 376*f*, 377*f*, 379*t*, 381*t*
    causes of 380, 380*t*
    congenital 412
    differential diagnosis of 378*t*
    nuclear 380
Sjögren's syndrome 2, 91
Skewed radial axes 120
Skin biopsy punches 475
Sleep apnea syndrome 388
Sling surgery
    bilateral 66*f*
    complications of 54
Slit-lamp 187
    biomicroscopic examination 45, 60
Smith–Lemli–Opitz syndrome 65
Snail-track degeneration 273
Snap-back test 55, 60
Snellen's chart 429
Snellen's entropion clamp 478, 479*f*
Snellen-Rieseman's sign 5, 37
Socket
    area of 25
    assessment of 25
Soemmering's ring 454, 454*f*, 455, 457*f*
Soft drusens 281*f*
Soft silicone tip cannula 483, 483*f*
Solid agar media 99
Spastic entropion 61
    causes of 62
Spectacles 115, 157
Specular biomicroscopy 169
Specular microscopy 125, 135, 143, 452
Spheroidal degeneration 161, 162*f*, 163
    histopathology of 163
Spheroidal keratopathy 159
Spielmann's occluder 420
Spielmann's theory 421
Spindle cell melanoma 307
Spranger's disease 311
Squamous cell carcinoma 9, 11, 68, 70
Squint
    paralytic 371, 372
    special tests for 370, 383, 412
Staphylococcus aureus 90, 92, 93
Staphyloma 171
Stargardt disease 356, 357, 359, 359*t*
    Fishman classification of 359
    pathophysiology of 359, 359*fc*

Stargardt dominant macular dystrophy 358
Stargardt scheme 178
Stellwag's sign 5, 37
Stem cell transplant 257
Stereopsis 399
Stereoscopic fluorescein angiography 285
Steroid-induced glaucoma 206-208
    mechanism of 207
    risk factors for 206
Steroids 144, 208
    administration 207, 208*t*
    implants 298
    side effects of 299
    sparing immunosuppressive drugs 42
    topical 144
    type of 208, 208*t*
Steven tenotomy scissors 468, 468*f*
Stevens–Johnson syndrome 91, 141
Still's disease 159
Still's syndrome 160
Strabismus 40, 150, 175, 367, 410, 412, 418, 428, 429, 442
    A and V pattern 404
    childhood 385
    coexist 20
    paralytic 396
    restrictive 396
Stress, emotional 417
Striational antibodies 416
Stromal dystrophy 126
    congenital 171
    genetics of 132
Stromal edema, progressive 134*f*
Sturge–Weber syndrome 190, 192*t*
Subcapsular opacities, localized 458
Subclinical retinal detachment 278
Subepithelial dystrophies 126
Subepithelial fibrillary lines 112
Subfoveal choroidal neovascularization 319
Subluxated lens, etiology of 434*b*
Subretinal choroidal neovascularization 314
Subretinal fluid 268, 286*f*, 303*f*, 304*f*, 315*f*
    drainage 276
    advantages of 276
    complications of 276
    methods of 276
Suker's sign 5, 37
Sulfamethoxazole 103
Sunglasses 41
Superior oblique paresis
    acquired 386*t*
    congenital 386*t*

Superior rectus
    holding forceps 463, 463*f*
    muscle 419
    recession 421
Superotemporal displacement 436*f*
Supportive therapy 144
Supramaxial resection 53
Surgery 379
    complications of 178
    indications of 354
    ocular 110, 201, 385
    refractive 110
    retinal 326
    timing of 52, 403
Swelling around eyeball 4
Swiss cheese appearance 46
Symblepharon variant, congenital 87
Synaptophore 399
Syndactyly 89
Synoptophore 371
    test 399
Systemic carbonic anhydrase inhibitors 256
Systemic disorders, hereditary 270
Systemic lupus erythematosus 222
Systemic nonsteroidal anti-inflammatory drug therapy 79
Systemic steroid 144
    therapy 79
Systemic therapy, indications of 107

T

Tacrolimus 145
Taenia solium 341
Target sign, peripheral ring of 210*f*
Tarsorrhaphy 74
    permanent 74
    temporary 74
Tay–Sachs disease 311
Tearing 158
Tectonic patch graft 106
Teflon block 476*f*
Telecanthus 66
Tellas's sign 5, 37
Tendon sparing 38
Tenon's cyst 150
Tenon's patch graft 106
Tensilon 416
    test 21, 416
Terrien's marginal degeneration 113, 153, 156
Terson's syndrome 216
Tetrahydrotriamcinolone 208
Thiazides 159
Thick mature epiretinal membrane 324*f*

Thioridazine streaks 254
Third nerve palsy 367, 369f, 370
   causes of 373t, 375
   isolated 373
   localization of 373t
   recurrent isolated 373
Thirteen Q deletion syndrome 332
Thirty degree test 423
Thrombophilia 226
Thudichum nasal speculum 480, 480f
Thymectomy 417
Thymoma 414
Thymus 417
Thyroid 417
   dysfunction 43, 414
   eye disease 6, 36f, 38f, 385
   function test 7, 73, 416
   gland dysfunction, treatment of 41
   ophthalmopathy 2, 399
   orbitopathy 2
   stimulating hormone 38
Thyroid-associated
            ophthalmopathy 35
   classification of 39t
   natural course of 43
   risk factors for 42
Thyrotropin receptor antibodies 38
Thyroxine 43
Tissue
   adhesives 106
   diagnosis 305
Titmus test 399
TNO test 399
Tobramycin 101
Tonometry 78, 125, 175
Tooke knife 477
Topiramate 424
Topolanski's sign 5, 37
TORCH
   diseases 432
   syndrome 429
Torsion, evaluation of 384
Torticollis
   congenital 386t
   ocular 386t
Trabecular meshwork 487
Trabeculectomy 191, 194, 207, 492
Trachoma 159
Traction retinal detachment 267, 269f
Transforming growth factor 151
Transient ischemic attacks 239
Transillumination 6
Transmission theory 33
Transpupillary thermotherapy 291,
         306, 316
Transscleral panretinal
            cryotherapy 199

Trauma 28, 51, 110, 174, 175, 373
   penetrating 172
   posterior segment signs of 363t
   seven rings of 205, 364, 461
   signs of 364
Traumatic hole 260
Traumatic hyphema 205
   sources of 205
Treacher Collins syndrome 86, 89,
         89t, 180
Trephines 475
   types of 474
Triamcinolone acetonide 263
Trifluorothymidine 104
Tri-iodothyronine levels 43
Trimethoprim 103
Trisomy 332
Trocar 481, 481f
Trousseau sign 5, 37
Tube surgery 195
Tumbling e test 429
Tumor
   benign 45
   epithelial 47
   infiltrative 2
   malignant 45
         mixed 48-50
   metastatic 50
   necrosis factor 202
   orbital 38
   periorbital 53
   risk of 308
Tunnel vision, differential diagnosis
         of 256
Tyrosine kinase-based therapies 322
Tyrosinosis 171

U

Uberculoma 300
Uhthoff phenomenon 387
Ulcer 93, 171
   corneal 90, 91t, 94f, 95f, 106, 107
   margins of 93
   ring-shaped 93
Ultrasonic pachymetry 153
Ultrasonography 7, 79, 101, 136, 143,
         165, 226
Ultrasound biomicroscopy 176,
         197, 296
Uncover test 396
Universal metallic eye speculum
         462, 462f
Upper eyelid 67
   coloboma 88, 89, 89t, 175
   mechanical ptosis 18f
   normal position of 20
   retraction 38, 74
Uremia 159

Urine examination 430, 444
Usher syndrome 252
Utrata capsulorhexis forceps 464, 464f
Uveal melanoma 299
   development of 300
Uveitis 220, 269
   chronic 159
   intermediate 293, 298
   management for intermediate 298
   nomenclature 295t

V

Valsalva maneuver 214, 216
Van Herick technique 183
Vancomycin 103
Vannas scissors 469, 469f
Varicella-zoster virus 375
Vasavada's classification 447
Vascular attenuation, severe 253f
Vascular disease 326
Vascular sclerosis, signs of 225
Vasculitis 215
Vasospastic diseases 488
Venereal disease research laboratory
         73, 230
Ventral pontine syndrome 381
Verapamil 417
Vernal keratoconjunctivitis 19, 93,
         151, 152
Verteporfin 290
Vertical gaze pathways 419
Vessels, attenuation of 257
Videokeratography 114, 148
Viral keratitis 93, 96
   management of 104
   treatment protocol for 105t
VISA
   inflammatory index 41t
   scoring 40
Viscoelastics 159
Vision 40, 340
   acute loss of 236
   blurring of 121, 122, 147, 158, 164
   central 257
   diminution of 63, 77, 86, 174, 428
   gradual loss of 236
   loss 1, 141, 236, 323
         progressive 442
   sudden diminution of 309
Visual acuity 3, 16, 31, 45, 51, 63, 72,
         77, 86, 92, 110, 123, 133,
         141, 147, 164, 171, 174,
         193, 216, 223, 231, 237,
         244, 251, 259, 264, 269,
         300, 328, 335, 352, 361,
         368, 376, 382, 388, 395,
         418, 420, 422, 426, 429,
         435, 453, 458
   poor 368

Visual axis opacification 432
Visual evoked
  potential 389
  response 165, 218, 363, 430
Visual field 38, 191, 255, 348, 389, 423, 492
  analysis 187
  defects 264
  testing 21, 358
Visual loss 128, 269
  causes of 241
Visual potential assessment 460
Visual rehabilitation 358
  postoperative 431
Vitamin
  A palmitate 256
  C 290
  D
    excessive 159
    toxicity 159
  E 290
Vitelliform 360
Vitrectomy 219, 240
  anterior 431
  cutter 481, 482*f*
  indications of 219
  principles of 279
  with scleral buckle, role of 338
Vitreolysis, enzymatic 326
Vitreomacular adhesion 327
Vitreomacular interface, diseases of 266*t*
Vitreomacular traction 325, 326*f*
  syndrome 261
Vitreoretinal disorders, familial 270
Vitreoretinal scissors 484, 485*f*
Vitreoretinal surgery 344, 481
Vitreoretinal traction 275
Vitreoretinopathy, proliferative 268, 272, 277, 278*t*, 279*t*, 337

Vitreous 7, 45, 206, 245, 252, 270, 295, 300, 324, 370, 383, 430, 444, 446, 450, 454, 459
  anterior 216, 281, 336, 352
  base 273
  body 318
  cavity 342
  degeneration 217, 296
  haze 295*t*
  hemorrhage 214
    causes of 220, 221, 221*t*
    different forms of 216
    natural course of 217
  membranes 296
  strong adhesions of 273
  substitute 277*t*
    role of 265
  syneresis 336
Vitritis 217
Vogt's striae 111, 111*f*
Vogt's triad 184
Vogt–Koyanagi–Harada disease 201, 300
Vogt–Spielmeyer syndrome 311
Volkmann's ischemic contracture 31
Voltage-gated calcium channel antibodies 416
Volume deficient socket 29
von Graefe's knife 467
von Graefe's retractor 465, 465*f*
von Graefe's sign 5, 37
von Noorden modification 385*t*
Voriconazole 103, 104
Vossius ring 458
V-Y operation 58

W

Warburg syndrome 332
Warthin tumor 46, 47
Watzke–Allen test 260

Waxy disc pallor 253*f*
Wegener granulomatosis 2
Weill–Marchesani syndrome 434, 435, 450
Wells enucleation spoon 480, 480*f*
Westcott's scissors 469, 469*f*
Wet age-related macular degeneration
  management of 291
  neovascular 282
Wet socket 25
White-eye blowout fracture 30, 32, 34
Wide-angle viewing lenses 484
Wilder's sign 5, 37
Wildervanck syndrome 411, 413
Wilson disease 433
Wire vectis 469, 470*f*
Worth four-dot test 370, 398
Worth's Ivory ball test 429
Wound closure 431
Wrist sign 435

X

Xanthogranuloma, juvenile 175

Y

Y-V plasty, bilateral 66*f*

Z

Zeaxanthin 290
Zeiss gland 67
Ziehl–Neelsen stain 107
Zimmerman's hypothesis 308
Zinc 290
Zinn zonules 449
Zonular fibers 434
Zonular opacity 459
Zonular weakness, causes of 212
Zonules 436
Z-plasty 58

EU GSPR Authorised Reprsentative
Logos Europe, 9 rue Nicolas Poussin
1700, La Rochelle, France
Phone: +33 (0) 6 67 93 73 78
E-mail: contact@logoseurope.eu

www.ingramcontent.com/pod-product-compliance
Ingram Content Group UK Ltd.
Pitfield, Milton Keynes, MK11 3LW, UK
UKHW050251040725

460398UK00003B/22